T0210737

The Springer Series in Applied Machine Learning

Series Editor

Oge Marques, Florida Atlantic University, Boca Raton, FL, USA

The Springer Series in Applied Machine Learning focuses on monographs, textbooks, edited volumes, and reference books that provide suitable content and educate the reader on how the theoretical approaches, algorithms, and techniques of machine learning can be applied to address real-world problems in a principled way.

The goal is a series of state-of-the-art books for the libraries of both machine learning scientists interested in applying the latest techniques to novel problems as well as practitioners, technologists, and researchers in various fields interested in leveraging the latest advances in machine learning for developing solutions that work for practical problems. The scope spans the breadth of machine learning and AI as it pertains to all application areas — both through books that address techniques specific to one application domain — and books that show the applicability of different types of machine learning methods to a wide array of domains.

Ivo D. Dinov

Data Science and Predictive Analytics

Biomedical and Health Applications using R

Second Edition

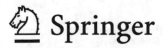 Springer

Ivo D. Dinov 🔘
University of Michigan–Ann Arbor
Ann Arbor, MI, USA

ISSN 2520-1298 ISSN 2520-1301 (electronic)
The Springer Series in Applied Machine Learning
ISBN 978-3-031-17485-8 ISBN 978-3-031-17483-4 (eBook)
https://doi.org/10.1007/978-3-031-17483-4

This Springer imprint is published by the registered company Springer Nature Switzerland AG
The registered company address is: Gewerbestrasse 11, 6330 Cham, Switzerland

Dedicated to my lovely and encouraging wife, Magdalena; our witty and persuasive kids, Anna-Sophia and Radina; my very insightful brother, Konstantin; and my nurturing parents, Yordanka and Dimitar.

Preface

Since the turn of the twenty-first century, the evidence overwhelming reveals that the rate of increase of the amount of data we collect doubles each 12–14 months (Kryder's law). The growth momentum of the volume and complexity of digital information we gather far outpaces the corresponding increase of computational power, which doubles each 18 months (Moore's law).[1] There is a substantial imbalance between the increase of data inflow and the corresponding computational infrastructure intended to process that data. This calls into question our ability to extract valuable information and actionable knowledge from the mountains of digital information we collect. Nowadays, it's very common for researchers to work with petabytes (PB) of data, 1 PB $= 10^{15}$ bytes, which may include non-homologous records that demand unconventional analytics. For comparison, the Milky Way galaxy has approximately 2×10^{11} stars. If each star represents a byte, then one petabyte of data corresponds to approximately 5000 Milky Way galaxies.

This data storage-computing asymmetry leads to an explosion of innovative data science methods and disruptive computational technologies that show promise to provide effective (semi-intelligent) decision support systems. Designing, understanding, and validating such new techniques require deep within-discipline basic science knowledge, trans-disciplinary team-based scientific collaboration, open-scientific endeavors, and a blend of exploratory and confirmatory scientific discovery. There is a pressing demand to bridge the widening gaps between the industry needs and skills of practicing data scientists, advanced techniques introduced by theoreticians, algorithms invented by computational scientists, models constructed by biosocial investigators, and network products and Internet of Things (IoT) services engineered by software architects.

The purpose of this book is to provide a sufficient methodological foundation for a number of modern data science techniques along with hands-on demonstration of implementation protocols, pragmatic mechanics of protocol execution, and

---

[1] https://doi.org/10.1186/s40537-015-0016-1

interpretation of the results of these methods applied on concrete case studies. Successfully completing the Data Science and Predictive Analytics (DSPA) training materials[2] will equip readers to (1) understand the computational foundations of big data science; (2) build critical inferential thinking; (3) lend a tool chest of *R* libraries for managing and interrogating raw, derived, observed, experimental, and simulated big healthcare datasets; and (4) furnish practical skills for handling complex datasets.

Prior to diving into DSPA, all readers are strongly encouraged to review the prerequisites[3] and complete the self-assessment pretest.[4] Sufficient remediation materials are provided or referenced throughout. The DSPA materials may be used for variety of graduate-level courses with durations of 10–30 weeks, with 3–4 instructional credit hours per week. Instructors can refactor and present the materials in alternative orders. The DSPA chapters in the book are organized sequentially. However, the content can be tailored to fit the audience's needs. Learning data science and predictive analytics is not a linear process—many alternative pathways can be completed to gain complementary competencies. We developed an interactive and dynamic flowchart[5] that highlights several tracks illustrating reasonable pathways starting with an introduction and ending with different specific competency topics (Fig. 1). The content of the book may also be used for self-paced learning or as a refresher for working professionals, as well as for formal and informal data science training, including massive open online courses (MOOCs). The DSPA materials are designed to build specific data science skills and predictive analytic competencies,[6] as described by the Michigan Institute for Data Science (MIDAS).

Throughout this book we use a constructive definition of "big data" derived by examining the common characteristics of many dozens of biomedical and healthcare case studies, involving complex datasets that required special handling, advanced processing, contemporary analytics, interactive visualization tools, and translational interpretation. These seven characteristics of "big data" are defined in the introductory chapter as size, heterogeneity and complexity, representation incongruency, incompleteness, multi-scale format, time-variability, and multi-source origins. All supporting electronic materials, including datasets, assessment problems, code, software tools, videos, and appendices, are available online at https://DSPA2.predictive.space.

This textbook presents a balanced view of the mathematical foundations, algorithmic implementations, computational statistics, and health applications of modern techniques for managing, processing, and interrogating big data. The intentional focus on human health applications is demonstrated by a diverse range of biomedical and healthcare case studies. However, the same techniques could be applied in other

---

[2] https://predictive.space

[3] https://www.socr.umich.edu/DSPA2/DSPA_Prereqs.html

[4] https://www.socr.umich.edu/DSPA2/DSPA_Pretest.html

[5] https://www.socr.umich.edu/DSPA2/DSPA_FlowChart.html

[6] https://www.socr.umich.edu/DSPA2/DSPA_Competencies.html

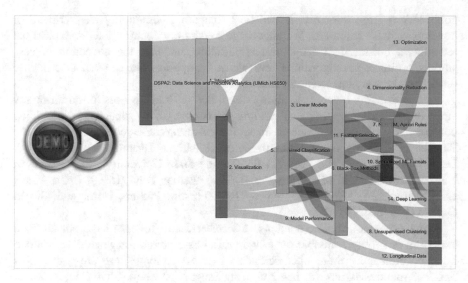

Fig. 1 DSPA2 topics flowchart; each node in this Sankey diagram dynamically links to the corresponding book chapter. https://www.socr.umich.edu/DSPA2/DSPA_FlowChart.html

domains that deal with complex data, for example, climate and environmental sciences, biosocial sciences, high-energy physics, and astronomy. Another specific feature of this book is that it solely utilizes the statistical computing language *R*, rather than any other scripting, user-interface based, or software programming alternatives. The choice for *R* is justified in the introductory chapter.

All techniques presented here aim to obtain data-driven and evidence-based scientific inference. This process starts with collecting or retrieving an appropriate dataset and identifying sources of data that need to be harmonized and aggregated into a joint computable data object. Next, the data is typically split into training and testing components. Model-based or model-free methods are fit, estimated, or learned on the training component and then validated on the complementary testing data. Different types of expected outcomes and results from this process include prediction, prognostication, or forecasting of specific clinical traits (computable phenotypes), clustering, or classification that labels units, subjects, or cases in the data. The final steps include algorithm fine-tuning, assessment, comparison, and statistical validation.

The work presented in this textbook relies on deep basic science, as well as holistic inter-disciplinary connections developed by scholars, teams of scientists, and transdisciplinary collaborations. Ideas, datasets, software, algorithms, and methods introduced by the wider scientific community were utilized throughout the DSPA resources. Specifically, methodological and algorithmic contributions from the fields of computer vision, statistical learning, mathematical optimization, scientific inference, biomedical computing, and informatics drove the concept presentations, data-driven demonstrations, and case study reports. The enormous contributions from the entire R statistical computing community were critical for developing these resources. We encourage community contributions to expand the techniques, bolster their scope and applications, enhance the collection of case studies, optimize the algorithms, and widen the applications to other data-intense disciplines or complex scientific challenges.

I am profoundly indebted to all my direct mentors and advisors for nurturing my curiosity, inspiring my studies, guiding the course of my career, and providing constructive and critical feedback throughout. Among these scholars are Guentcho Skordev (Sofia University), Kenneth Kuttler (Michigan Technological University), De Witt L. Sumners and Fred Huffer (Florida State University), Jan de Leeuw, Nicolas Christou, and Michael Mega (UCLA), Arthur Toga (USC), Brian Athey, Eric Michielssen, Kathleen Potempa, Janet Larson, Patricia Hurn, and Gilbert Omenn (University of Michigan).

Many other colleagues, students, researchers, and fellows have shared their expertise, creativity, valuable time, and critical assessment for generating, validating, and enhancing these open-science resources. Among these are Christopher Aakre, Simeone Marino, Jiachen Xu, Ming Tang, Nina Zhou, Chao Gao, Alexandr Kalinin, Syed Husain, Brady Zhu, Farshid Sepehrband, Lu Zhao, Sam Hobel, Hanbo Sun, Tuo Wang, Yueyang Shen, and many others. Many colleagues from the Statistics Online Computational Resource (SOCR) and the Michigan Institute for Data Science (MIDAS) provided encouragement and valuable suggestions.

The development of the DSPA materials was partially supported by the US National Science Foundation (grants 1916425, 1734853, 1636840, 1416953, 0716055 and 1023115) and the US National Institutes of Health (grants UL1 TR002240, R01 CA233487, R01 MH121079, R01 MH126137, T32 GM141746).

Ann Arbor, MI, USA   Ivo D. Dinov

Second Edition Preface

The original first edition of the Data Science and Predictive Analytics (DSPA) textbook was published in electronic and hardcover versions in fall 2018. Since then, the textbook has received significant coverage[7,8,9] has had over six million official downloads from Springer's website.[10] The book has been cited dozens of times in the scientific literature,[11] and the supporting website (containing supplementary materials) has served millions of readers and learners from across the globe.[12] As of 2022, the textbook is available at many academic, local, and governmental libraries across the world.[13]

Over the past several years, the textbook has been heavily used in a number of college classes, utilized in professional societies training events,[14] and used for massive open online courses (MOOCs). The techniques presented in the book have supported many research projects, collaborations, and partnerships. These activities identified possible improvements and necessary corrections. Aside from fixing typographical errors and rudimentary content polishing, the second edition also includes new material, which reflects recent scientific and technological progress and includes a substantial content reorganization to streamline the covered topics.[15] The first edition material is refactored from the original 23 chapters into 14 chapters in the revised second edition. These revisions are intended to (1) improve

---

[7] https://doi.org/10.1111/insr.12317

[8] https://doi.org/10.5195/jmla.2020.901

[9] https://en.wikipedia.org/wiki/Data_Science_and_Predictive_Analytics

[10] https://www.springer.com/us/book/9783319723464

[11] https://scholar.google.com/scholar?cites=774513957312424579&as_sdt=80000005&sciodt=0,23&hl=en

[12] https://DSPA2.predictive.space

[13] https://www.socr.umich.edu/people/dinov/courses/DSPA_Topics.html#DSPA_Availability

[14] https://wiki.socr.umich.edu/index.php/SOCR_News & https://myumi.ch/e6zyw

[15] https://www.socr.umich.edu/DSPA2/DSPA2_DSPA1_Chapter_Mapping.html

the experiences of readers, students, and learners; (2) provide course instructors with updated content and a more systematic pedagogical coverage; and (3) enhance the translational research of scholars, engineers, and STEM scientists using the techniques in the book to work on various data science projects.

Some of the specific second edition revisions include:

1. Content reorganization, restructuring the (original first edition) 23 chapters into 14 chapters.
2. Corrections of grammatical, stylistic, and typographical errors.
3. Translation of plots, graphics, and rasterized images into high-resolution interactive scale vector graphics (SVG) displays.
4. Improvements in the flow of text, mathematical notations, computational algorithms, code snippets, figures, and results.
5. Data science updates reflecting recent scientific developments (since 2017).
6. Some chapters include new material. For instance, Chap. 12 (Big Longitudinal Data Analysis) includes new material on recurrent (RNN) and long short-term memory (LSTM) networks; Chap. 13 (Function Optimization) includes new parallels between the mathematical formulation, computational implementation, and ML/AI utilization of optimization techniques; and Chap. 14 (Deep Learning, Neural Networks) contains new developments in transfer learning, general adversarial networks, and their broad applications.

DSPA Application and Use Disclaimer

The Data Science and Predictive Analytics (DSPA) resources are designed to help scientists, trainees, students, and professionals learn the foundations of data science and its practical applications, as well as actively learn with concrete datasets and experiment with specific case studies in dynamic sandbox environment. Neither the author nor the publisher have control over, or make any representation or warranties, expressed or implied, regarding the use of these resources by researchers, users, patients, or their healthcare provider(s), or the use or interpretation of any information stored on, derived from, computed with, suggested by, or received through any of the DSPA materials, code, scripts, or applications. All readers and users are solely responsible for obtaining, interpreting, and communicating any information to (and receiving feedback from) the user's representatives or healthcare providers.

Users, their proxies, or representatives (e.g., clinicians) are solely responsible for reviewing and evaluating the accuracy, relevance, and meaning of any information stored on, derived by, generated by, or received through the application of any of the DSPA software, protocols, or techniques. The author and the publisher cannot and do not guarantee said accuracy. The DSPA resources, their applications, and any information stored on, generated by, or received through them are not intended to be a substitute for professional or expert advice, diagnosis, or treatment. Always seek the advice of a physician or other qualified professional with any questions regarding any real case study (e.g., medical diagnosis, conditions, prediction, and prognostication). Never disregard professional advice or delay seeking it because of something read or learned through the use of the DSPA materials or any information stored on, generated by, or received through the SOCR resources.

All readers and users acknowledge that the DSPA copyright owners or licensors, in their sole discretion, may from time to time make modifications to the DSPA resources. Such modifications may require corresponding changes to be made in the code, protocols, learning modules, activities, case studies, and other DSPA materials. Neither the author, publisher, nor licensors shall have any obligation to furnish any maintenance or support services with respect to the DSPA resources.

The DSPA resources are intended for educational purposes only. They are not intended to offer or replace any professional advice nor provide expert opinion. Please speak to qualified professional service providers if you have any specific concerns, case studies, or questions.

Biomedical, Biosocial, Environmental, and Health Disclaimer

All DSPA information, materials, software, and examples are provided for general education purposes only. Persons using the DSPA data, models, tools, or services for any medical, social, healthcare, or environmental purposes should not rely on accuracy, precision, or significance of the DSPA reported results. While the DSPA resources may be updated periodically, users should independently check against other sources, latest advances, and most accurate peer-reviewed information.

Please consult appropriate professional providers prior to making any lifestyle changes or any actions that may impact those around you, your community, or various real, social, and virtual environments. Qualified and appropriate professionals represent the single best source of information regarding any Biomedical, Biosocial, Environmental and Health decisions. None of these resources have either explicit or implicit indication of FDA approval!

Any and all liability arising directly or indirectly from the use of the DSPA resources is hereby disclaimed. The DSPA resources are provided "as is" and without any warranty expressed or implied. All direct, indirect, special, incidental, consequential, or punitive damages arising from any use of the DSPA resources or materials contained herein are disclaimed and excluded.

Book Content

Instructors, formal and informal learners, working professionals, research scholars, engineers, and readers looking to refresh, update, or enhance their interactive data skills and expand their methodological knowledge may selectively go over specific sections, chapters, and examples they want to cover in more depth. Everyone who expects to gain new knowledge or acquire complementary computational abilities should review the overall textbook organization before they decide what to cover, how deeply, and in what order.

The revised second edition of the Data Science and Predictive Analytics (DSPA) textbook includes a substantial reorganization of the material, revisions based on community recommendations, error corrections, stylistic enhancements, content update to reflect recent scientific and technological advances, and significant expansions of several chapters. Many sections include improved graphics and some new material. The expanded Chap. 12 (Big Longitudinal Data Analysis) covers recurrent (RNN) and long short-term memory (LSTM) networks, and Chap. 13 (Function Optimization) includes additional details contrasting the mathematical formulation, computational implementation, and ML/AI utilization of objective function optimization. The redesigned Chap. 14 (Deep Learning, Neural Networks) contains some new developments in deep neural networks and transfer learning and illustrates their applications in neuroimaging and text mining. Finally, an expanded electronic appendix is provided online at the second edition supporting website (https://DSPA2.predictive.space). The organization of the chapters in the new edition of the book reflects an order that may appeal to many, albeit not all, readers.

Chapter 1 (*Introduction*) presents (1) the DSPA Mission and Objectives; (2) discusses several driving biomedical challenges including Alzheimer's disease, Parkinson's disease, drug and substance use, and amyotrophic lateral sclerosis; (3) provides demonstrations of brain visualization, neurodegeneration, and genomics computing; (4) identifies the six defining characteristics of big (biomedical and healthcare) data; (5) explains the concepts of *data science* and *predictive analytics*; (6) sets the DSPA expectations; (7) provides foundations of *R*; (8) presents fundamental R programming principles; (9) includes basic examples of data transformation, generation, ingestion, and export; (10) introduces main mathematical operators; and (11) provides data summaries, probability distributions, and simple synthetic data simulation.

In Chap. 2 (*Basic Visualization and Exploratory Data Analytics*), we present additional *R* programming details about (1) loading, manipulating, visualizing, and saving *R* data objects; (2) sample-based statistics measuring central tendency and dispersion; (3) understanding different types of variables; (4) scraping data from public websites; (5) missing observations and cohort-rebalancing; (6) graphical techniques for exposing composition, comparison, and relationships in multivariate data; and (7) visualizing and computing of 1D, 2D, 3D, and 4D distributions.

The foundations of *Linear Algebra, Matrix Computing, and Regression Modeling* are presented in Chap. 3. It covers (1) creation, interpretation, processing, and manipulation of second-order tensors (matrices); (2) illustrations of variety of matrix operations and their applications; (3) demonstrations of linear modeling and solutions of matrix equations; (4) discussion of the eigen-spectra of matrices; (5) the fundamentals of multivariate linear modeling and prediction; and (6) contrast regression trees and model trees. This chapter also includes several complete end-to-end predictive analytics examples.

Chapter 4 (*Linear and Nonlinear Dimensionality Reduction*) starts with a driving motivational example reducing a 2D dataset to a 1D signal. It covers (1) matrix rotations; (2) linear dimensionality techniques such as principal component analysis (PCA), singular value decomposition (SVD), independent component analysis (ICA), and factor analysis (FA); and (3) non-linear dimensionality reduction methods such as t-distributed stochastic neighbor embedding (t-SNE) and uniform manifold approximation and projection (UMAP).

The discussion of machine learning model-based and model-free techniques commences in Chap. 5 (*Supervised Classification*). This chapter covers (1) lazy learning classification using k-nearest neighbors (kNN) algorithm; (2) general divide-and-conquer approaches for splitting data into training and validation sets; (3) some basic strategies for evaluation of model performance; (4) probabilistic learning using Naïve Bayes classifier, linear and quadratic discriminant analysis classification; (5) decision tree divide and conquer classification; and (6) various classification metrics (e.g., entropy, misclassification error, Gini index) and strategies for pruning decision trees.

Chapter 6 (*Black Box Machine-Learning Methods*) lays out the foundation of neural networks as silicon analogues to biological neurons. This chapter covers (1) a discussion of the effects of network layers and topology on the resulting neural network classification; (2) support vector machines (SVM); and (3) ensemble methods based on bagging, boosting, random forest, and adaptive boosting. The chapter includes demonstrations of classification for optical character recognition (OCR), iris flowers clustering, Google trends and the stock market prediction, and quantifying quality of life in chronic disease.

Qualitative Learning Methods – Text Mining, Natural Language Processing, Apriori Association Rule Learning are presented in Chap. 7. In this chapter, we cover (1) the foundation of association rules and the Apriori algorithm; (2) discuss support and confidence measures for tracking association rules and demonstrate several examples based on grocery shopping and head and neck cancer treatment; and (3) utilize the term-frequency and inverse document frequency techniques for unstructured data using natural language processing (NLP) and text mining (TM) approaches.

Chapter 8 (*Unsupervised Clustering*) presents (1) the basics of machine learning clustering and classification tasks; (2) silhouette plots to quantify algorithmic performance; (3) k-means clustering, spectral clustering, hierarchical clustering, and Gaussian mixture modeling; and (4) strategies for tuning and improving of clustering techniques.

General protocols for measuring the performance of different types of classification and regression methods are presented in Chap. 9 (*Model Performance Assessment, Validation, and Improvement*). We discuss (1) evaluation strategies for binary, categorical, and continuous outcomes; (2) confusion matrices quantifying classification and prediction accuracy; (3) visualization of algorithm performance and ROC curves; (4) the foundations of internal statistical validation; (5) strategies for manual and automated model tuning; (6) improving model performance with meta-learning; (7) general prediction and forecasting methods; (8) internal statistical n-fold cross-validation; and (9) comparison strategies for multiple prediction models.

Chapter 10 (*Specialized Machine Learning Topics*) presents some technical details that may be useful to many data science practitioners, computational scientists, and engineers. Here, we discuss (1) data format conversion; (2) SQL data queries; (3) reading and writing XML, JSON, XLSX, and other data formats; (4) visualization of network bioinformatics data; (5) data streaming and on-the-fly stream classification and clustering; (6) optimization and improvement of computational performance; (7) parallel computing; and (8) integration of R, Python, C/C++, and other programming languages within a single *R* markdown electronic notebook.

The classical approaches for feature selection are presented in Chap. 11 (*Variable Importance and Feature Selection*). This chapter covers (1) filtering, wrapper, and embedded techniques for salient feature selection; (2) complete protocols, from data collection and preparation to model training, testing, evaluation, and comparison using recursive feature elimination; (3) regularized linear modeling (LASSO) and controlled variable selection (knockoff); (4) defining *fidelity* and *regularization* terms in the objective function used for model-based inference; (5) computational protocols for handling complex high-dimensional data; (6) model estimation by controlling the false-positive rate of selection of critical features; and (7) derivations of effective forecasting models.

Chapter 12 (*Big Longitudinal Data Analysis*) is focused on using classical and machine learning–based techniques for interrogating time-varying observations. We illustrate (1) time series analysis, for example, ARIMA modeling; (2) structural equation modeling (SEM) with latent variables; (3) longitudinal data analysis using linear mixed models; (4) the generalized estimating equations (GEE) modeling; and (5) recurrent (RNN) and long short-term memory (LSTM) networks.

Chapter 13 (*Function Optimization*) presents technical details about minimizing objective functions, which are present virtually in any data science–oriented inference or evidence-based translational study. In this chapter, we explain (1) constrained and unconstrained cost function optimization; (2) introduce Lagrange multipliers; (3) describe linear and quadratic programming; (4) formulate general non-linear optimization; (5) present a data denoising application; and (6) show examples illustrating the agreement between intuitive, manual, mathematical analysis, and computational algorithmic solutions of optimization problems.

The last chapter of the textbook is Chap. 14 (*Deep Learning, Neural Networks*). It covers (1) perceptron activation functions; (2) relations between artificial and biological neurons and networks; (3) neural nets for computing exclusive OR (XOR) and negative AND (NAND) operators; (4) classification of handwritten digits and network bases estimation of the square root function; (5) classification of natural images; (6) variational autoencoders (VAEs); (7) transfer learning; and (8) applications in text mining, image generation, pathological brain classification, and automated tumor mask segmentation.

We compiled several dozen biomedical and healthcare case studies[16] that are used to demonstrate the presented DSPA concepts, apply the methods, and validate the analytical protocols. For example, the *introductory chapter* includes high-level driving biomedical challenges including dementia and other neurodegenerative diseases, substance use, neuroimaging, and traumatic brain injury (TBI) case studies. Chapter 5 describes a heart attack case study, and Chap. 3 uses quality of life in chronic disease data and optical character recognition that can be applied to automatic reading of handwritten physician notes. Chapter 7 illustrates the applications of natural language processing to extract quantitative biomarkers from unstructured text, which can be used to study hospital admissions, medical claims, patient satisfaction, etc. Chapter 11 presents a predictive analytics Parkinson's disease study using neuroimaging-genetics data. Chapter 14 shows examples of predicting clinical outcomes for schizophrenia, amyotrophic lateral sclerosis, and irritable bowel syndrome cohorts, as well as quantitative and qualitative classification of biological images and volumes. Indeed, these represent just a few examples, and readers are encouraged to try the same methods, protocols, and analytics on their own datasets or on other research-derived, clinically acquired, aggregated, secondary-use, or simulated data.

The second edition of the textbook also includes an extended online appendix,[17] which is continuously updated with complementary materials, additional content, and DSPA recipes for a broader domain of applications. The topics in the electronic appendix include commonly used techniques for Bayesian simulation, statistical modeling and inference techniques, information-theoretic foundation of statistical learning, surface, shape, and manifold representation and visualization, statistical power analysis in experimental design, database SQL/noSQL queries and Google BigQuery, image convolution, filtering, Fourier transform, causality and transfer entropy, and agent-based reinforcement learning.

---

[16] https://umich.instructure.com/courses/38100/files/folder/Case_Studies

[17] https://DSPA2.predictive.space

Throughout the textbook, there are cross-references to appropriate chapters, sections, publications, datasets, Web services, and live demonstrations (Live Demos). The sequential arrangement of the chapters offers a suggested reading order; however, alternative sorting and pathways covering some parts of the materials may be appropriate in certain circumstances. Readers, instructors, formal and informal learners, and researchers may choose their own coverage paths based on specific intellectual interests and project needs. Community feedback, revision requests, and contributions are always welcome and appreciated.

Notations

The following common notations are used throughout the textbook (Fig. 2).

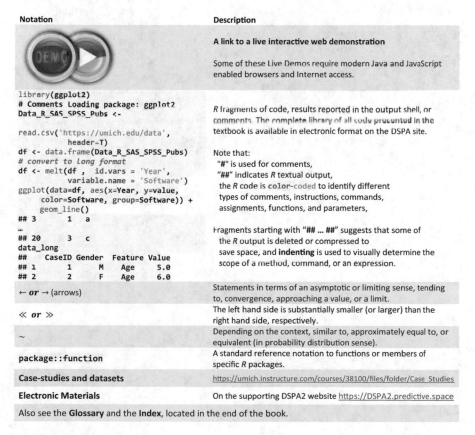

Notation	Description
	A link to a live interactive web demonstration
	Some of these Live Demos require modern Java and JavaScript enabled browsers and Internet access.
```library(ggplot2)``` ``# Comments Loading package: ggplot2`` ``Data_R_SAS_SPSS_Pubs <-`` ``read.csv('https://umich.edu/data',`` ``header=T)`` ``df <- data.frame(Data_R_SAS_SPSS_Pubs)`` ``# convert to Long format`` ``df <- melt(df , id.vars = 'Year',`` ``variable.name = 'Software')`` ``ggplot(data=df, aes(x=Year, y=value,`` ``color=Software, group=Software)) +`` ``geom_line()`` ``## 3      1    a`` ``...`` ``## 20     3    c`` ``data_long`` ``##   CaseID Gender  Feature Value`` ``## 1    1      M     Age    5.0`` ``## 2    2      F     Age    6.0``	R fragments of code, results reported in the output shell, or comments. The complete library of all code presented in the textbook is available in electronic format on the DSPA site. Note that: "#" is used for comments, "##" indicates R textual output, the R code is color-coded to identify different types of comments, instructions, commands, assignments, functions, and parameters, Fragments starting with "## … ##" suggests that some of the R output is deleted or compressed to save space, and **indenting** is used to visually determine the scope of a method, command, or an expression.
$\leftarrow$ *or* $\rightarrow$ (arrows)	Statements in terms of an asymptotic or limiting sense, tending to, convergence, approaching a value, or a limit.
$\ll$ *or* $\gg$	The left hand side is substantially smaller (or larger) than the right hand side, respectively.
~	Depending on the context, similar to, approximately equal to, or equivalent (in probability distribution sense).
``package::function``	A standard reference notation to functions or members of specific R packages.
Case-studies and datasets	https://umich.instructure.com/courses/38100/files/folder/Case_Studies
Electronic Materials	On the supporting DSPA2 website https://DSPA2.predictive.space
Also see the **Glossary** and the **Index**, located in the end of the book.	

Fig. 2 Common DSPA notations.

Contents

Chapter 1
Introduction

1.1 Motivation

Let's start with a quick overview illustrating some common data science challenges, qualitative descriptions of the fundamental principles, and awareness about the power and potential pitfalls of modern data-driven scientific inquiry.

1.1.1 DSPA Mission and Objectives

The second edition of this textbook (DSPA2) is based on the HS650 Data Science and Predictive Analytics (DSPA) course[1] the author teaches at the University of Michigan and the first DSPA edition.[2] These materials collectively aim to provide learners with a deep understanding of the challenges, appreciation of the enormous opportunities, and a solid methodological foundation for designing, collecting, managing, processing, interrogating, analyzing, and interpreting complex health and biomedical data. Readers that finish this course of training and successfully complete the examples and assignments included in the book will gain unique skills and acquire a tool-chest of methods, software tools, and protocols that can be applied to a broad spectrum of big data problems.

- *Vision*: Enable active-learning by integrating driving motivational challenges with mathematical foundations, computational statistics, and modern scientific inference.
- *Values*: Effective, reliable, reproducible, and transformative data-driven discovery supporting open-science.

---

[1] https://predictive.space/
[2] https://doi.org/10.1007/978-3-319-72347-1

- *Strategic priorities*: Trainees will develop scientific intuition, computational skills, and data-wrangling abilities to tackle big biomedical and health data problems. Instructors will provide well-documented R-scripts and software recipes implementing atomic data-filters as well as complex end-to-end predictive big data analytics solutions.

Before diving into the mathematical algorithms, statistical computing methods, software tools, and health analytics covered in the remaining chapters, we will discuss several *driving motivational problems*. These will ground all the subsequent scientific discussions, data modeling, and computational approaches.

1.1.2 Examples of Driving Motivational Problems and Challenges

For each of the studies below, we illustrate several clinically relevant scientific questions, identify appropriate data sources, describe the types of data elements, and pinpoint various complexity challenges.

1.1.2.1 Alzheimer's Disease

- Identify the relation between observed clinical phenotypes and expected behavior.
- Prognosticate future cognitive decline (3–12 months prospectively) as a function of imaging data and clinical assessment (both model-based and model-free machine learning prediction methods will be used).
- Derive and interpret the classifications of subjects into clusters using the harmonized and aggregated data from multiple sources (Table 1.1).

1.1.2.2 Parkinson's Disease

- Predict the clinical diagnosis of patients using all available data (with and without the UPDRS clinical assessment, which is the basis of the clinical diagnosis by a physician).
- Compute derived neuroimaging and genetics biomarkers that can be used to model the disease progression and provide automated clinical decisions support.
- Generate decision trees for numeric and categorical responses (representing clinically relevant outcome variables) that can be used to suggest an appropriate course of treatment for specific clinical phenotypes (Table 1.2).

Table 1.1   Alzheimer's disease neuroimaging initiative (ADNI) data archive

Data source	Sample size/data type	Summary
ADNI Archive[a]	Clinical data: demographics, clinical assessments, cognitive assessments; Imaging data: sMRI, fMRI, DTI, PiB/ FDG PET; Genetics data: Ilumina SNP genotyping; Chemical biomarker: lab tests, proteomics. Each data modality comes with a different number of cohorts. Generally, $200 \leq N \leq 1200$. For instance, previously conducted ADNI studies with $N > 500$ (https://doi.org/10.3233/ JAD-150335, https://doi.org/10.1111/jon. 12252, https://doi.org/10.3389/fninf. 2014.00041).	ADNI provides interesting data modalities, multiple cohorts (e.g., early-onset, mild, and severe dementia, controls) that allow effective model training and validation NACC Archive.

[a]https://www.adni-info.org/

Table 1.2   Parkinson's Progression Markers Initiative (PPMI) data archive

Data source	Sample size/data type	Summary
PPMI Archive[a]	Demographics: age, medical history, sex; Clinical data: physical, verbal learning and language, neurological and olfactory (University of Pennsylvania Smell Identification Test, UPSIT) tests), vital signs, MDS-UPDRS scores (Movement Disorder; Society-Unified Parkinson's Disease Rating Scale), ADL (activities of daily living), Montreal Cognitive Assessment (MoCA), Geriatric Depression Scale (GDS-15); Imaging data: structural MRI; Genetics data: Ilumina ImmunoChip (196,524 variants) and NeuroX (covering 240,000 exonic variants) with 100% sample success rate, and 98.7% genotype success rate genotyped for APOE e2/e3/ e4. Three cohorts of subjects; Group 1 = {de novo PD Subjects with a diagnosis of PD for 2 years or less who are not taking PD medications}, N1 = 263; Group 2 = {PD Subjects with Scans without Evidence of a Dopaminergic Deficit (SWEDD)}, N2 = 40; Group 3 = {Control Subjects without PD who are 30 years or older and who do not have a first-degree blood relative with PD}, N3 = 127	The longitudinal PPMI dataset including clinical, biological and imaging data (screening, baseline, 12-, 24-, and 48-month follow-ups) may be used to conduct model-based predictions as well as model-free classification and forecasting analyses.

[a]https://www.ppmi-info.org/

Table 1.3 Swiss cancer genetics database

Data source	Sample size/data type	Summary
Geneva University Hospital cancer genetics database	The dataset contained common reasons for genetic consultation, demographic, personal and family history, genetic sequences, family pedigree tracking, and detailed medical records. Regional Research Ethics Committee at the University Hospitals of Geneva has approved the data collection and management processes. Additional information collected for all participants included pathology reports, archived tumor tissue samples, and cancer treatments. The study contrasted the cancer risk estimations obtained via a model-based Breast and Ovarian Analysis of Disease Incidence and Carrier Estimation Algorithm (BOADICEA) against model-free AI/ML methods, adaptive boosting and random forest ensemble prediction.	The study demonstrated the significant power of ML/AI methods to correctly predict the lifelong risk of developing breast cancer in women. For instance, using testing data, in each of the low, moderate, and elevated risk categories, model-free methods outperformed model-based techniques, e.g., adaptive boosting and random forest methods improved the predictive accuracy by 20 – 25% compared to the BOADICEA model. These findings provide a basis for reexamining the recommendations for mammography surveillance used in the Swiss Surveillance Protocol. The main data science challenges in this study revolved around handling the intrinsic data heterogeneity, handling the significant levels of missing observations, accounting for the hierarchical structure of the familial observations, and computing the risk estimates using the large size of multivariate observations.

1.1.2.3   Swiss Cancer Study

This 2020 Swiss oncological study[3] examined the hereditary aggregation of breast, colorectal, and ovarian cancer in 2481 families including over 112, 000 family members. The Regional Research Ethics Committee at the University Hospitals of Geneva has approved the data collection and analysis processes, Table 1.3. The study goals included:

- Estimating the lifetime breast cancer risk for women of ages 20–80.
- Comparing classical statistical model-based strategies against advanced machine learning and artificial intelligence model-free approaches.
- Quantifying variability and precision of breast cancer risk estimation.

---

[3] https://doi.org/10.1038/s41416-020-0937-0

Table 1.4 Pooled Resource Open-Access ALS Clinical Trials (PRO-ACT) database

Data source	Sample size/data type	Summary
ProAct Archive[a]	Over 100 clinical variables are recorded for all subjects including: Demographics: age, race, medical history, sex; Clinical data: Amyotrophic Lateral Sclerosis Functional Rating Scale (ALSFRS), adverse events, onset_delta, onset_site, drugs use (riluzole). The PRO-ACT training dataset contains clinical and lab test information of 8635 patients. Information of 2424 study subjects with valid gold standard ALSFRS slopes will be used in out processing, modeling, and analysis.	The time points for all longitudinally varying data elements will be aggregated into signature vectors. This will facilitate the modeling and prediction of ALSFRS slope changes over the first 3 months (baseline to month 3).

[a] https://doi.org/10.1212/WNL.0000000000000951

1.1.2.4 Amyotrophic Lateral Sclerosis

- Identify the most highly significant variables that have power to jointly predict the progression of ALS (in terms of clinical outcomes like ALSFRS and muscle function).
- Provide a decision tree prediction of adverse events based on subject phenotype and 0 3 month clinical assessment changes (Table 1.4).

1.1.2.5 Normal Brain Visualization

The SOCR Brain Visualization App has preloaded sMRI, ROI labels, and fiber track models for a normal brain. It also allows users to drag-and-drop their data into the browser to visualize and navigate through the stereotactic data (including imaging, parcellations, and tractography) (Fig. 1.1).

1.1.2.6 Neurodegeneration

A study of Structural Neuroimaging in Alzheimer's disease[4] illustrates the big data challenges in modeling complex neuroscientific data. Specifically, 808 ADNI subjects were divided into 3 groups: 200 subjects with Alzheimer's disease (AD), 383 subjects with mild cognitive impairment (MCI), and 225 asymptomatic normal controls (NC). Their sMRI data were parcellated using BrainParser,[5] and the 80 most important neuroimaging biomarkers were extracted using the global shape analysis

---

[4] https://doi.org/10.3233/jad-150335
[5] https://dx.doi.org/10.1109%2FTMI.2007.908121

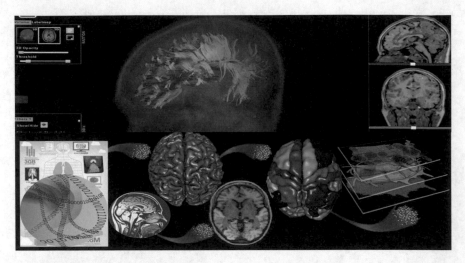

Fig. 1.1   Interactive SOCR Brain Viewer. (https://socr.umich.edu/HTML5/BrainViewer)

Pipeline workflow. Using a pipeline implementation of Plink, the authors obtained 80 SNPs highly associated with the imaging biomarkers. The authors observed significant correlations between genetic and neuroimaging phenotypes in the 808 ADNI subjects. These results suggest that differences between AD, MCI, and NC cohorts may be examined by using powerful joint models of morphometric, imaging, and genotypic data (Fig. 1.2).

1.1.2.7   Genomics Computing

1.1.2.7.1   Genetic Forensics—2013–2016 Ebola Outbreak

This HHMI disease detective activity[6] illustrates genetic analysis of sequences of Ebola viruses isolated from patients in Sierra Leone during the Ebola outbreak of 2013–2016. Scientists track the spread of the virus using the fact that most of the genome is identical among individuals of the same species, most similar for genetically related individuals, and more different as the hereditary distance increases. DNA profiling capitalizes on these genetic differences, specifically in regions of noncoding DNA, i.e., DNA that is not transcribed and translated into a protein. Variations in noncoding regions impact fewer individual traits. Such changes in noncoding regions may be immune to natural selection. DNA variations called *short tandem repeats (STRs)* are short bases, typically 2–5 bases long, which repeat multiple times. The repeat units are found at different locations, or loci, throughout the genome. Every STR has multiple alleles. These allele variants are defined by the

---

[6]https://www.hhmi.org/biointeractive/ebola-disease-detectives

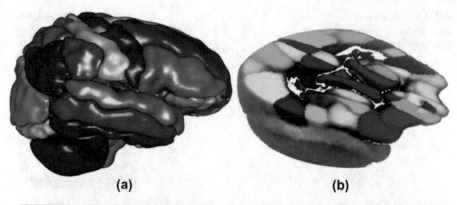

Fig. 1.2 Indices, labels, and names of the 56 regions of interest (ROIs) extracted using the LPBA40 brain atlas (https://dx.doi.org/10.1016%2Fj.neuroimage.2007.09.031). (a) Individual brain parcellation, (b) LPBA40 atlas

number of repeat units present or by the *length of the repeat sequence*. STRs are surrounded by nonvariable segments of DNA known as flanking regions. The STR allele in the Figure below could be denoted by "6," as the repeat unit (GATA) repeats six times, or as 70 base pairs (bps) because its length is 70 bases in length, including

Fig. 1.3 Fragment of the
short tandem repeats (STRs)
genotype data

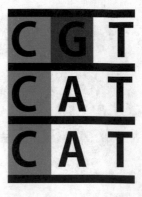

the starting/ending flanking regions. Different alleles of the same STR may correspond to different numbers of GATA repeats, with the same flanking regions
(Fig. 1.3).

1.1.2.7.2 Next-Generation Sequence (NGS) Analysis

Whole-genome and exome sequencing include essential clues for identifying genes
responsible for simple Mendelian inherited disorders. This paper proposed methods
that can be applied to study complex disorders using population genetics data.[7]
Next-generation sequencing (NGS) technologies include bioinformatics resources to
analyze the dense and complex sequence data. The Graphical Pipeline for Computational Genomics (GPCG) performs the computational steps required to analyze
NGS data. The GPCG implements flexible workflows for basic sequence alignment,
sequence data quality control, single nucleotide polymorphism analysis, copy number variant identification, annotation, and visualization of results. Applications of
NGS analysis provide clinical utility for identifying miRNA signatures in diseases.
Enabling hypotheses testing about the functional role of variants in the human
genome will help to pinpoint the genetic risk factors of many diseases (e.g.,
neuropsychiatric disorders) (Fig. 1.4).

1.1.2.7.3 Neuroimaging-Genetics

A computational infrastructure for high-throughput neuroimaging-genetics[8]
facilitates the data aggregation, harmonization, processing, and interpretation of
multisource imaging, genetics, clinical, and cognitive data. A unique feature of
this architecture is the graphical user interface to the Pipeline environment. Through

---

[7] https://doi.org/10.3390/genes3030545
[8] https://doi.org/10.3389/fninf.2014.00041

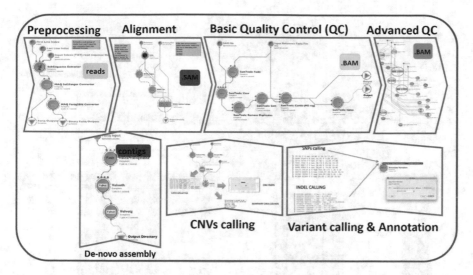

Fig. 1.4 Graphical pipelines for computational genomics (GPCG) used for analyzing NGS data

its client–server architecture, the Pipeline environment provides a graphical user interface for designing, executing, monitoring, validating, and disseminating complex protocols that utilize diverse suites of software tools and web-services. These pipeline workflows are represented as portable XML objects, which transfer the execution instructions and user specifications from the client user machine to remote pipeline servers for distributed computing. Using Alzheimer's and Parkinson's data, this study provides examples of translational applications using this infrastructure (Fig. 1.5).

1.1.3   *Common Characteristics of* Big (Biomedical and Health) Data

Software developments, student training, utilization of Cloud or IoT service platforms, and methodological advances associated with big data Discovery Science all present existing opportunities for learners, educators, researchers, practitioners, and policy makers alike. A review of many biomedical, health informatics and clinical studies suggests that there are indeed common characteristics of complex big data challenges. For instance, imagine analyzing observational data of thousands of Parkinson's disease patients based on tens-of-thousands of signature biomarkers derived from multisource imaging, genetics, clinical, physiologic, phenomics, and demographic data elements. IBM had defined the qualitative characteristics of big data as 4 V's: *Volume*, *Variety*, *Velocity*, and *Veracity* (there are additional V-qualifiers that can be added).

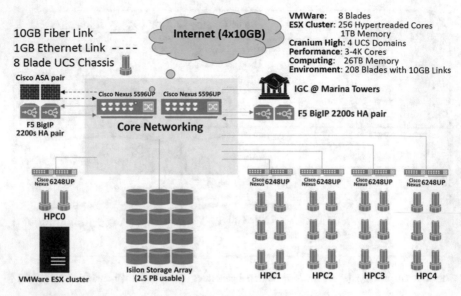

Fig. 1.5 Typical computational infrastructures supporting high-throughput neuroimaging-genetics studies require software, hardware, network, storage, and computing nodes to enable data aggregation, harmonization, processing and interpretation of multisource imaging, genetics, clinical, and cognitive data

Table 1.5 Characterization of the multifactorial properties of big data

BD dimensions	Existing gaps and necessary tools
Size	Harvesting and management of vast amounts of data
Complexity	Wranglers for dealing with heterogeneous data
Incongruency	Tools for data harmonization and aggregation
Multisource	Transfer, joint representation, and holistic modeling of disparate elements
Multiscale	Macro to meso to micro scale observations
Time	Techniques accounting for longitudinal patterns in the data
Incomplete	Reliable management of missing data, data imputation, and statistical obfuscation

An alternative constructive definition of big data (PMID:26998309)[9] explicitly identifies data characteristics with corresponding methodological gaps and tools needed to address specific data science challenges (Table 1.5).

---

[9]https://www.ncbi.nlm.nih.gov/pubmed/26998309

1.1.4 Data Science

Data science is an emerging new field that (1) is extremely transdisciplinary—bridging between the theoretical, computational, experimental, and applied sciences; (2) deals with enormous amounts of complex, incongruent, and dynamic data from multiple sources; and (3) aims to develop algorithms, methods, tools, and services capable of ingesting such datasets and generating semi-automated decision support systems. The latter can mine the data for patterns or motifs, predict expected outcomes, provide derived phenotypes, clusters or labels for both retrospective or prospective observations, compute data signatures or fingerprints, extract valuable information, and offer evidence-based actionable knowledge. Data science techniques often involve data manipulation (wrangling), data harmonization and aggregation, exploratory or confirmatory data analyses, predictive analytics, performance assessment, and model fine-tuning for transfer learning.

1.1.5 Predictive Analytics

Predictive analytics is the process of utilizing advanced mathematical formulations, powerful statistical computing algorithms, efficient software tools and services to represent, interrogate, and interpret complex data. As its name suggests, a core aim of predictive analytics is to forecast trends, predict patterns in the data, or prognosticate the process behavior either within the range or outside the range of the observed data (e.g., in the future, or at locations where data may not be available). In this context, *process* refers to a natural phenomenon that is being investigated by proxy measures and observational data. Presumably, by collecting and exploring the intrinsic data characteristics, we can track the behavior and unravel the underlying mechanisms governing the behavior of the system.

The fundamental goal of predictive analytics is to identify relationships, model associations, and explicate arrangements or motifs in the dataset in terms of space, time, and features. Such deep understanding of the variable relations and process mechanisms may reduce the complexity, or dimensionality, of the data and provide interpretability. Using these process characteristics, predictive analytics may predict unknown outcomes, produce estimations of likelihoods or parameters, generate classification labels, or contribute other aggregate or individualized forecasts. We will discuss how the outcomes of these predictive analytics can be refined, assessed, and compared, e.g., between alternative methods. The underlying assumptions of the specific predictive analytics technique determine its usability, affect the expected accuracy, and guide the (human) actions resulting from the (machine) forecasts. In this textbook, we will discuss supervised and unsupervised, model-based and model-free, classification and regression, as well as deterministic, stochastic, classical, and machine learning-based techniques for predictive analytics. The type of the expected outcome (e.g., binary, polytomous, probability, scalar, vector, tensor, etc.)

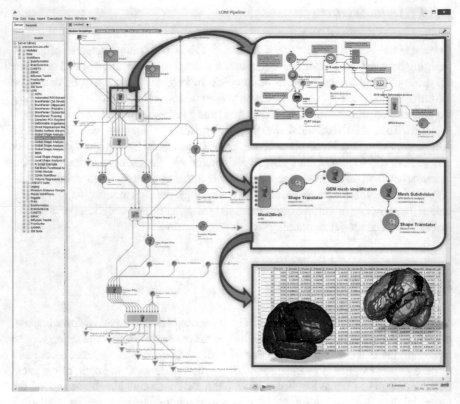

Fig. 1.6 The graphical pipeline environment supports the design, distributed execution, asynchronous tracking, and open-science collaborations involving complex data and computing protocols

determines if the predictive analytics strategy provides prediction, forecasting, labeling, likelihoods, groupings, or motifs.

1.1.6 High-Throughput Big Data Analytics

The Pipeline Environment provides a large tool chest of software and services that can be integrated, merged, and processed.[10] The Pipeline workflow library and the workflow miner illustrate much of the functionality that is available.[11] A Java-based and an HTML5 webapp-based graphical user interfaces provide access to a powerful 4000 core grid compute server (Fig. 1.6).

---

[10] https://doi.org/10.1371/journal.pone.0013070

[11] https://pipeline.loni.usc.edu

1.1.7 Examples of Data Repositories, Archives, and Services

There are many sources of data available on the Internet. A number of them provide open-access to the data via FAIR (Findable, Accessible, Interoperable, Reusable) principles. Below are examples of open-access data sources that can be used to test the techniques presented in the textbook. We demonstrate the tasks of retrieval, manipulation, processing, analytics, and visualization using example datasets from these archives:

- SOCR Wiki Data
- SOCR Canvas datasets
- SOCR Case-Studies
- IDA (https://ida.loni.usc.edu)
- NIH dbGaP (https://dbgap.ncbi.nlm.nih.gov/)
- Data.gov
- UCI Machine Learning Repository (https://archive.ics.uci.edu/ml/)
- Cancer Imaging Archive (https://www.cancerimagingarchive.net/access-data/)
- NASA EarthData (https://earthdata.nasa.gov/esds/ai-ml).

1.1.8 Responsible Data Science and Ethical Predictive Analytics

In addition to being data-literate and skilled artisans, all data scientists, quantitative analysts, and informaticians need to be aware of certain global societal norms and exhibit professional work ethics that ensure the appropriate use, result reproducibility, unbiased reporting, as well as expected and unanticipated interpretations of data, analytical methods, and novel technologies. Examples of this basic etiquette include (1) promoting FAIR (findable, accessible, interoperable, reusable, and reproducible resource) sharing principles; (2) ethical conduct of research; (3) balancing and explicating potential benefits and probable detriments of findings; (4) awareness of relevant legislation, codes of practice, and respect for privacy, security and confidentiality of sensitive data; and (5) document provenance, attributions, and longevity of resources.

1.1.8.1 Promoting FAIR Resource Sharing

The FAIR (findable, accessible, interoperable, reusable, and reproducible) resource sharing principles provide guiding essentials for appropriate development, deployment, use, management, and stewardship of data, techniques, tools, services, and information dissemination.

1.1.8.2   Research Ethics

Ethical data science and predictive analytics research demands responsible scientific conduct and integrity in all aspects of practical scientific investigation and discovery. All analysts should be aware of, and practice, established professional norms and ethical principles in planning, designing, implementing, executing, and assessing activities related to data-driven scientific research.

1.1.8.3   Understanding the Benefits and Detriments of Analytical Findings

Evidence and data-driven discovery is often bound to generate both questions and answers, some of which may be unexpected, undesired, or detrimental. Quantitative analysts are responsible for validating all their results, as well as for balancing and explicating all potential benefits and enumerating all probable detriments of positive and negative findings.

1.1.8.4   Regulatory and Practical Issues in Handling Sensitive Data

Decisions on security, privacy, and confidentiality of sensitive data collected and managed by data governors, manipulated by quantitative analysts, and interpreted by policy and decision makers is not trivial. The large number of people, devices, algorithms, and services that are within arms-length of the raw data suggests a multitier approach for sensible protection and security of sensitive information like personal health, biometric, genetic, and proprietary data. Data security, privacy, and confidentiality of sensitive information should always be protected throughout the data life cycle. This may require preemptive, on-going, and post-hoc analyses to identify and patch potential vulnerabilities. Often, there may be tradeoffs between data value benefits and potential risks of blind automated information interpretation. Neither of the extremes is practical, sustainable, or effective.

1.1.8.5   Protection of Sensitive Information Versus Data Utility

There are many organizational guidelines (e.g., IRB approvals), local requirements, state laws and regulations, and international agreements that require compliance with protection of personal, sensitive, and protected information. Examples of these include the US Health Insurance Portability and Accountability Act (HIPAA),[12]

---

[12] https://www.hhs.gov/hipaa

US Family Educational Rights and Privacy Act (FERPA),[13] and the EU General Data Protection Regulation (GDRP)[14] regulatory frameworks.

To complement the strong need for secure and appropriate use of observational data, there are recently developed strategies to measure and increase the *utility of the data* and provide mechanisms to *desensitize sensitive information*. Examples of such modern techniques include the data value metric (DVM),[15] which quantifies the information content (energy) contained in a given dataset, and the DataSifter method,[16] which statistically obfuscates data balancing the need for high level of protection (privacy) and the desire to preserve high data utility (value).

1.1.8.6 Resource Provenance and Longevity

The digitalization of human experiences, the growth of data science, and the promise of artificial intelligence have led to enormous societal investments, excitements, and anxieties. There is a strong sentiment and anticipation that the vast amounts of available information will ubiquitously translate into quick insights, useful predictions, optimal risk-estimations, and cost-effective decisions. Proper recording of the data, algorithmic, scientific, computational, and human factors involved in these forecasts represents a critical component of data science and its essential contributions to knowledge.

1.1.8.7 Examples of Inappropriate, Fake, or Malicious Use of Resources

Each of the complementary spaces of *appropriate* and *inappropriate* use of data science and predictive analytics resources are vast. The sections above outlined some of the guiding principles for ethical, respectful, appropriate, and responsible data-driven analytics and factual reporting. Below are some examples illustrating inappropriate use of data, resources, information, or knowledge to intentionally or unintentionally gain unfair advantage, spread fake news, misrepresent findings, or detrimental socioeconomic effects.

- Attempts to re-identify sensitive information or circumvent regulatory policies, common sense norms, or agreements. For instance, big data and advanced analytics were employed to re-identify the Massachusetts Governor William Weld's medical record using openly released insurance dataset stripped of direct personal identifiers.[17]

---

[13] https://www2.ed.gov/ferpa

[14] https://gdpr.eu

[15] https://doi.org/10.1186/s40537-021-00446-6

[16] https://doi.org/10.1177/17483026211065379

[17] https://doi.org/10.2139/ssrn.2076397

- Calibrated analytics that report findings relative to status-quo alternatives and level setting expected and computed inference in the context of the application domain. For example, ignoring placebo effects, methodological assumptions, potential conflicts and biases, randomization of unknown effects, and other strategies may significantly impact the efficacy of data-driven studies.
- Unintended misuse of resource access may be common practice. In 2014, an Uber employee ignored the company's policies and used his access to track the location of a journalist who was delayed for an Uber interview.[18] Obviously, tracking people without their explicit consent is unethical, albeit it represents an innovative use of the available technology to answer a good question.
- Between 2019 and 2021, personal data of 533 million Facebook users in 106 countries was hacked and repeatedly leaked on various hacking forums.[19] In response, the company indicated it expects more scraping incidents and suggested that this is a broader industry issue.
- There are plenty of examples of misuse of analytical strategies to fake the results or strengthen a point beyond the observed evidence,[20] and inappropriate use of information and advanced technology is covered by legislature such as the UK Computer Misuse Act.[21]
- Big data is naturally prone to *innocent errors*, e.g., selection bias, methodological development and applications, computational processing, empirical estimation instability, misunderstanding of data formats and metadata understanding, as well as *malicious manipulations*.
- Collecting, managing, and processing irrelevant big data may yield unnecessary details, skew the understanding of the phenomenon, or distract from the main discoveries. In these situations, there may be substantial socioeconomic costs, as well as negative returns associated with lost opportunities.

1.1.9 DSPA Expectations

The heterogeneity of data science makes it difficult to identify a complete and exact list of prerequisites necessary to succeed in learning all the appropriate methods. However, the reader is strongly encouraged to glance over the preliminary prerequisites,[22] the self-assessment pretest and remediation materials,[23] and the

---

[18] https://nypost.com/2017/08/15/uber-settles-federal-probe-over-god-view-spy-software/

[19] https://www.bbc.com/news/technology-56815478

[20] https://www.routledge.com/Misused-Statistics/Spirer-Spirer/p/book/9780367400392

[21] https://www.legislation.gov.uk/ukpga/1990/18/contents

[22] https://www.socr.umich.edu/DSPA2/DSPA_Prereqs.html

[23] https://www.socr.umich.edu/DSPA2/DSPA_Pretest.html

outcome competencies.[24] Throughout this journey, it is useful to *remember the following points*:

- You *don't have to* satisfy all prerequisites, be versed in all mathematical foundations, have substantial statistical analysis expertise, or be an experienced programmer.
- You *don't have to complete all chapters and sections* in the order they appear in the DSPA Topics Flowchart.[25] Completing one, or several of the suggested pathways may be sufficient for many readers.
- The *DSPA textbook aims* to expand the trainees' horizons, improve the understanding, enhance the skills, and provide a set of advanced, validated, and practice-oriented code, scripts, and protocols.
- To varying degrees, readers will develop abilities to skillfully utilize the *tool chest* of resources provided in the DSPA textbook. These resources can be revised, improved, customized, and applied to other biomedicine and biosocial studies, as well as to big data predictive analytics challenges in other disciplines.
- The DSPA *materials will challenge most readers*. When the going gets tough, seek help, engage with fellow trainees, search for help on the web, communicate via DSPA discussion forum/chat, review references and supplementary materials. Be proactive! Remember you will gain, but it will require commitment, prolonged immersion, hard work, and perseverance. If it were easy, its value would be compromised.
- When covering some chapters, few readers may be *underwhelmed or bored*. If you are familiar with certain topics, you can skim over the corresponding chapters/sections and move forward to the next topic. Still, it's worth reviewing some of the examples and trying the assignment problems to ensure you have a firm grasp of the material and your technical abilities are sound.
- Although the *return on investment* (e.g., time, effort) may vary between readers, those that complete the DSPA textbook will discover something new, acquire some advanced skills, learn novel data analytic protocols, or conceive of a cutting-edge idea.
- The complete R code (R markdown) for all examples and demonstrations presented in the textbook are available as electronic supplement.[26]
- The instructor acknowledges that these *materials may be improved*. If you discover problems, typos, errors, inconsistencies, or other problems, please contact us (DSPA.info@umich.edu) to correct, expand, or polish the resources, accordingly. If you have alternative ideas, suggestions for improvements, optimized code, interesting data and case-studies, or any other refinements, please send these along, as well. All suggestions and critiques will be carefully reviewed and potentially incorporated in revisions and new editions.

---

[24] https://www.socr.umich.edu/DSPA2/DSPA_Competencies.html

[25] https://www.socr.umich.edu/DSPA2/DSPA_FlowChart.html

[26] https://dspa2.predictive.space

1.2 Foundations of *R*

In this section, we will start with the foundations of R programming for visualization, statistical computing, and scientific inference. Specifically, we will (1) discuss the rationale for selecting R as a computational platform for all DSPA demonstrations; (2) present the basics of installing shell-based R and RStudio user-interface; (3) show some simple R commands and scripts (e.g., translate long-to-wide data format, data simulation, data stratification and subsetting); (4) introduce variable types and their manipulation; (5) demonstrate simple mathematical functions, statistics, and matrix operators; (6) explore simple data visualization; and (7) introduce optimization and model fitting. The chapter appendix includes references to R introductory and advanced resources, as well as a primer on debugging.

1.2.1 Why Use R?

There are many different classes of software that can be used for data interrogation, modeling, inference, and statistical computing. Among these are R, Python, Java, C/ C++, Perl, and many others. Table 1.6 compares R to various other statistical analysis software packages and more detailed comparison is available on the supporting website[27].

There exist substantial differences between distinct types of computational environments for data wrangling, preprocessing, analytics, visualization, and interpretation. Table 1.7 provides some rough comparisons between several of the most popular data computational platforms. With the exception of *ComputeTime*, higher scores represent better performance within the specific category. Note that these are just estimates and the scales are not normalized between categories.

Let's first look at some real peer-review publication data (1995–2015), specifically comparing all published scientific reports utilizing R, SAS, and SPSS as popular tools for data manipulation and statistical modeling. These data are retrieved using Google Scholar literature searches (Fig. 1.7).

---

[27] https://dspa2.predictive.space/

Table 1.6 Pros and cons of using R, SAS, Stata, and SPSS

Statistical Software	Advantages	Disadvantages
R	R is actively maintained ($\geq$100, 000 developers, $\geq$15, 000 packages). Excellent connectivity to various types of data and other systems. Versatile for solving problems in many domains. It's free, open-source code. Anybody can access/review/extend the source code. R is very stable and reliable. If you change or redistribute the R source code, you have to make those changes available for anybody else to use. R runs anywhere (platform agnostic). Extensibility: R supports extensions, e.g., for data manipulation, statistical modeling, and graphics. Active and engaged community supports R. Unparalleled question-and-answer (Q&A) websites. R connects with other languages (Java/C/JavaScript/Python/Fortran) & database systems, and other programs, SAS, SPSS, etc. Other packages have add-ons to connect with R. SPSS has incorporated a link to R, and SAS has protocols to move data and graphics between SAS and R	Mostly scripting language. Steeper learning curve
SAS	Large datasets. Commonly used in business & Government	Expensive. Somewhat dated programming language. Expensive/proprietary
Stata	Easy statistical analyses	Mostly classical stats
SPSS	Appropriate for beginners. Simple interfaces	Weak in more cutting-edge statistical procedures lacking in robust methods and survey methods

Table 1.7 Multifactor comparison between different data science computational platforms

Language	Open source	Speed	Compute time	Library extent	Ease of entry	Costs	Interoperability
Python	Yes	16	62	80	85	10	90
Julia	Yes	2941	0.34	100	30	10	90
R	Yes	1	745	100	80	15	90
IDL	No	67	14.77	50	88	100	20
Matlab	No	147	6.8	75	95	100	20
Scala	Yes	1428	0.7	50	30	20	40
C	Yes	1818	0.55	100	30	10	99
Fortran	Yes	1315	0.76	95	25	15	95

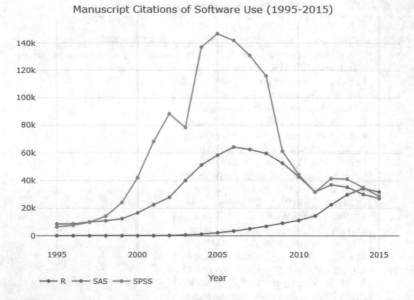

Fig. 1.7 Scientific publications citing use of different programming platforms (R, SAS, SPSS)

```
library(ggplot2)
library(reshape2)
library(plotly)
Data_R_SAS_SPSS_Pubs <-
  read.csv('https://umich.instructure.com/files/2361245/download?download_frd=1',
           header=T)
df <- data.frame(Data_R_SAS_SPSS_Pubs)
plot_ly(df, x = ~Year)  %>%
  add_trace(y = ~R, name = 'R', mode = 'lines+markers') %>%
  add_trace(y = ~SAS, name = 'SAS', mode = 'lines+markers') %>%
  add_trace(y = ~SPSS, name = 'SPSS', mode = 'lines+markers') %>%
  layout(title="Manuscript Citations of Software Use (1995-2015)", legend =
list(orientation = 'h'))
```

We can also look at a dynamic Google Trends map, which provides longitudinal tracking of the number of web-searches for each of these three statistical computing platforms (R, SAS, SPSS). The figure below shows one example of the evolving software interest over the past 15 years. You can expand this plot by modifying the trend terms, expanding the search phrases, and changing the time period.[28] Another static 2004–2018 monthly dataset tracking the popularity of SAS, SPSS, and R programming Google searches is available online.

The example below shows a dynamic pull of 18 years of Google queries about R, SAS, SPSS, and Python, traced between 2004-01-01 and 2022-03-16 (Fig. 1.8).

---

[28] https://trends.google.com/trends/explore?date=all&q=%2Fm%2F0212jm,%2Fm%2F018fh1,%2Fm%2F02l0yf8

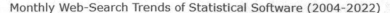

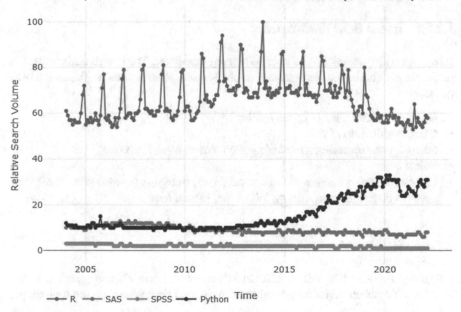

Fig. 1.8 Dynamic GoogleTrends data pull—monthly web-search queries for, SAS, SPSS, and Python (2004–2022)

```
# require(ggplot2)
# require(reshape2)
#   GoogleTrends_Data_R_SAS_SPSS_Worldwide_2004_2018.csv
library(gtrendsR)
library(ggplot2)
library(prophet)
df_GT1 <- gtrends(c("R", "SAS", "SPSS", "Python"),
                  gprop = "web", time = "2004-01-01 2022-03-16")[[1]]
head(df_GT1)
library(tidyr)
df_GT1_wide <- spread(df_GT1, key = keyword, value = hits)
# dim(df_GT1_wide ) # [1] 212    9

plot_ly(df_GT1_wide, x = ~date)  %>%
  add_trace(x = ~date, y = ~R, name = 'R', type = 'scatter',
            mode = 'lines+markers') %>%
  add_trace(x = ~date, y = ~SAS, name = 'SAS', type = 'scatter',
            mode = 'lines+markers') %>%
  add_trace(x = ~date, y = ~SPSS, name = 'SPSS', type = 'scatter',
            mode = 'lines+markers') %>%
  add_trace(x = ~date, y = ~Python, name = 'Python', type = 'scatter',
            mode = 'lines+markers') %>%
  layout(title="Monthly Web-Search Trends of Statistical Software (2004-2022)",
         legend = list(orientation = 'h'), xaxis = list(title = 'Time'),
         yaxis = list (title = 'Relative Search Volume'))
```

1.2.2　Getting Started with R

1.2.2.1　Install Basic Shell-Based R

R is a free software that can be installed on any computer. The R website is https://R-project.org. There you can install a shell-based R-environment following this protocol:

- Click download CRAN in the left bar
- Choose a download site
- Choose your operating system (e.g., Windows, Mac, Linux)
- Select *base*
- Choose the latest version to Download R (4.1, or higher (newer) version for your specific operating system, e.g., Windows, Linux, MacOS).

1.2.2.2　GUI-Based R Invocation (RStudio)

For many readers, it's best to also install and run R via *RStudio* graphical user interface. To install RStudio, go to https://www.rstudio.org/ and do the following.

- Click Download RStudio.
- Click Download RStudio Desktop.
- Click Recommended For Your System.
- Download the appropriate executable file (e.g., .exe) and run it (choose default answers for all questions).

1.2.2.3　RStudio GUI Layout

The RStudio interface consists of several windows.

- *Bottom left*: console window (also called command window). Here you can type simple commands after the ">" prompt and R will then execute your command. This is the most important window, because this is where R actually does stuff.
- *Top left*: editor window (also called script window). Collections of commands (scripts) can be edited and saved. When you don't get this window, you can open it with File > New > R script. Just typing a command in the editor window is not enough; it has to get into the command window before R executes the command. If you want to run a line from the script window (or the whole script), you can click Run or press CTRL+ENTER to send it to the command window.
- *Top right*: workspace / history window. In the workspace window, you can see which data and values R has in its memory. You can view and edit the values by clicking on them. The history window shows what has been typed before.

- *Bottom right*: files / plots / packages / help window. Here you can open files, view plots (also previous plots), install and load packages, or use the help function. You can change the size of the windows by dragging the gray bars between the windows.

1.2.2.4   Software Updates

Updating and upgrading the R environment involves a three-step process:

- *Updating the R-core*: This can be accomplished either by manually downloading and installing the latest version of R from CRAN or by auto-upgrading to the latest version of R using the R installr package. Type this in the R console: install.packages("installr");   library(installr); updateR(),
- *Updating RStudio*: This installs new versions of RStudio using RStudio itself. Go to the Help menu and click *Check for Updates*, and
- *Updating R libraries*: Go to the Tools menu and click *Check for Package Updates*. . ..

Just like any other software, services, or applications, these R updates should be done regularly; preferably monthly or at least semi-annually.

1.2.2.5   Some Notes

- The basic R environment installation comes with limited core functionality. Everyone eventually will have to install more packages, e.g., reshape2, ggplot2, and we will show how to expand your RStudio library throughout these materials.
- The core R environment also has to be upgraded occasionally, e.g., every 3– 6 months to get R patches, to fix known problems, and to add new functionality.
- The assignment operator in R is $<-$ (although $=$ may also be used), so to assign a value of 2 to a variable x, we can use $x < - 2$ or equivalently $x = 2$.

1.2.2.6   Help

R provides documentation for different R functions using the method help(). Typing help(topic) in the R console will provide detailed explanations for each R topic or function. Another way of doing it is to call ?topic, which is even easier. For example, if I want to check the function for linear models (i.e., function lm()), I will use the following function.

```
help(lm)
?lm
```

1.2.2.7   Simple Wide-to-Long Data Format Translation

Below is a simple R script for melting a small dataset that illustrates the R syntax for variable definition, instantiation, function calls, and parameter setting.

```
rawdata_wide <- read.table(header=TRUE, text='
 CaseID Gender Age  Condition1  Condition2
      1    M    5   13           10.5
      2    F    6   16           11.2
      3    F    8   10           18.3
      4    M    9        9.5     18.1
      5    M   10       12.1        19
')
# Make the CaseID column a factor
rawdata_wide$subject <- factor(rawdata_wide$CaseID)
rawdata_wide
##    CaseID Gender Age Condition1 Condition2 subject
## 1       1      M   5       13.0       10.5       1
## 2       2      F   6       16.0       11.2       2
## 3       3      F   8       10.0       18.3       3
## 4       4      M   9        9.5       18.1       4
## 5       5      M  10       12.1       19.0       5
library(reshape2)
# Specify id.vars: the variables to keep (don't split apart on!)
melt(rawdata_wide, id.vars=c("CaseID", "Gender"))
##    CaseID Gender   variable value
## 1       1      M        Age     5
## 2       2      F        Age     6
...
## 19      4      M    subject     4
## 20      5      M    subject     5
```

There are specific options for the `reshape2::melt()` function, from the `reshape2` R package, that control the transformation of the original (wide-format) dataset `rawdata_wide` into the modified (long-format) object `data_long`.

```
data_long <- melt(rawdata_wide,
        # ID variables - all the variables to keep but not split apart on
    id.vars=c("CaseID", "Gender"),
        # The source columns
    measure.vars=c("Age", "Condition1", "Condition2" ),
        # Name of the destination column that will identify the original
        # column that the measurement came from
    variable.name="Feature",
    value.name="Measurement"
)
data_long
```

For an elaborate justification, detailed description, and multiple examples of handling long-and-wide data, messy and tidy data, and data cleaning strategies, see the JSS Tidy Data article by Hadley Wickham.[29]

---

[29] https://www.jstatsoft.org/article/view/v059i10

1.2.2.8   Data Generation

Popular data generation functions include c (), seq (), rep (), and data.frame
(). Sometimes we use list () and array () to create data too.

c(): creates a (column) vector. With option recursive=T, it descends through
lists combining all elements into one vector.

```
a<-c(1, 2, 3, 5, 6, 7, 10, 1, 4)
a
## [1]  1  2  3  5  6  7 10  1  4
c(list(A = c(Z = 1, Y = 2), B = c(X = 7), C = c(W = 7, V=3, U=-1.9)), recursive =
TRUE)
##  A.Z  A.Y  B.X  C.W  C.V  C.U
##  1.0  2.0  7.0  7.0  3.0 -1.9
```

When combined with list (), c () successfully created a vector with all the
information in a list with three members A, B, and C.

seq(from, to): generates a sequence. Adding the option by= can help us specify
the increment, and option length= specifies the desired length. Also, seq
(along=x) generates a sequence 1, 2, ..., length(x). This is commonly
used in loops to create unique identifiers for each element in x.

```
seq(1, 20, by=0.5)
##  [1]  1.0  1.5  2.0  2.5  3.0  3.5  4.0  4.5  5.0  5.5  6.0  6.5  7.0  7.5  8.0
## [16]  8.5  9.0  9.5 10.0 10.5 11.0 11.5 12.0 12.5 13.0 13.5 14.0 14.5 15.0 15.5
## [31] 16.0 16.5 17.0 17.5 18.0 18.5 19.0 19.5 20.0
seq(1, 20, length=9)
## [1]  1.000  3.375  5.750  8.125 10.500 12.875 15.250 17.625 20.000
seq(along=c(5, 4, 5, 6))
## [1] 1 2 3 4
```

rep(x, times): creates a sequence that repeats x a specified number of times. The
option each= also allows us to repeat first over each element of x a certain number
of times.

```
rep(c(1, 2, 3), 4)
##  [1] 1 2 3 1 2 3 1 2 3 1 2 3
rep(c(1, 2, 3), each=4)
##  [1] 1 1 1 1 2 2 2 2 3 3 3 3
```

Compare this to replicating using replicate ().

```
X <- seq(along=c(1, 2, 3)); replicate(4, X+1)
##      [,1] [,2] [,3] [,4]
## [1,]    2    2    2    2
## [2,]    3    3    3    3
## [3,]    4    4    4    4
```

data.frame(): The function data.frame () creates a data frame object of
named or unnamed arguments. We can combine multiple vectors of different types
into data frames with each vector stored as a column. Shorter vectors are

automatically wrapped around to match the length of the longest vectors. With data.frame() you can mix numeric and characteristic vectors.

```
data.frame(v=1:4, ch=c("a", "B", "C", "d"), n=c(10, 11))
##   v ch  n
## 1 1  a 10
## 2 2  B 11
## 3 3  C 10
## 4 4  d 11
```

Note that the operator : generates a sequence and the expression 1:4 yields a vector of integers, from 1 to 4.

list(): Much like the column function c(), the function list() creates a *list* of the named or unnamed arguments—indexing rule: from 1 to n, including 1 and n. Remember that in R indexing of vectors, lists, arrays, and tensors starts at 1, not 0, as in some other programming languages.

```
l <- list(a=c(1, 2), b="hi", c=-3+3i); l
## $a
## [1] 1 2
## $b
## [1] "hi"
## $c
## [1] -3+3i
# Note Complex Numbers a <- -1+3i; b <- -2-2i; a+b
```

As R uses general *objects* to represent different constructs, object elements are accessible via $, @, ., and other delimiters, depending on the object type. For instance, we can refer to a member a and index i in the list of objects l containing an element a by l$a[[i]].

```
l$a[[2]]
## [1] 2
l$b
## [1] "hi"
```

array(x, dim=): creates an array with specific dimensions. For example, dim=c (3, 4, 2) means two 3×4 matrices. We use [] to extract specific elements in the array. [2, 3, 1] means the element at the second row third column on the first page. Leaving one number in the dimensions empty would help us to get a specific row, column, or page. [2, , 1] means the second row on the first page; see Fig. 1.9:

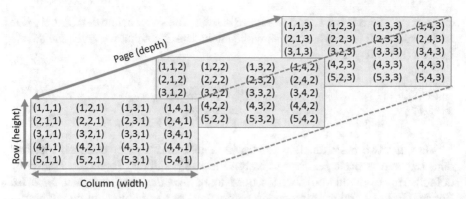

Fig. 1.9 Indexing of 3D arrays (volumes) as stacks of 2D matrices (images)

```
ar<-array(1:24, dim=c(3, 4, 2)); ar
## , , 1
##      [,1] [,2] [,3] [,4]
## [1,]    1    4    7   10
## [2,]    2    5    8   11
## [3,]    3    6    9   12
## , , 2
##      [,1] [,2] [,3] [,4]
## [1,]   13   16   19   22
## [2,]   14   17   20   23
## [3,]   15   18   21   24
ar[2, 3, 1]
## [1] 8
ar[2, ,1]
## [1]  2  5  8 11
```

In general, multidimensional arrays are called "tensors" (of order = number of dimensions). Other useful functions include the following:

- `matrix(x, nrow=, ncol=)`: creates matrix elements of `nrow` rows and `ncol` columns.
- `factor(x, levels=)`: encodes a vector `x` as a factor.
- `gl(n, k, length=n*k, labels=1:n)`: generates levels (factors) by specifying the pattern of their levels. *k* is the number of levels, and *n* is the number of replications.
- `expand.grid()`: a data frame from all combinations of the supplied vectors or factors.
- `rbind()` combine arguments by rows for matrices, data frames, and others.
- `cbind()` combine arguments by columns for matrices, data frames, and others.

1.2.2.9 Input/Output (I/O)

The first pair of functions we will talk about are `save()` and `load()`, which write and import objects between the current *R* environment RAM memory and long term storage, e.g., hard drive, Cloud storage, SSD, etc. The script below demonstrates the basic export and import operations with simple data. Note that we saved the data in `Rdata` (`Rda`) format.

```
x <- seq(1, 10, by=0.5)
y <- list(a = 1, b = TRUE, c = "oops")
save(x, y, file="xy.RData")
load("xy.RData")
```

There are two basic functions `data(x)` and `library(x)` that load specified data sets and R packages, respectively. The R *base* library is always loaded by default. However, add-on libraries need to be *installed* first and then *imported* (loaded) in the working environment before functions and objects in these libraries are accessible.

```
data("iris")
summary(iris)
##   Sepal.Length   Sepal.Width    Petal.Length   Petal.Width
##   Min.   :4.300  Min.   :2.000  Min.   :1.000  Min.   :0.100
##   1st Qu.:5.100  1st Qu.:2.800  1st Qu.:1.600  1st Qu.:0.300
##   Median :5.800  Median :3.000  Median :4.350  Median :1.300
##   Mean   :5.843  Mean   :3.057  Mean   :3.758  Mean   :1.199
##   3rd Qu.:6.400  3rd Qu.:3.300  3rd Qu.:5.100  3rd Qu.:1.800
##   Max.   :7.900  Max.   :4.400  Max.   :6.900  Max.   :2.500
##          Species
##   setosa    :50
##   versicolor:50
##   virginica :50
library(base)
```

read.table(file): reads a file in table format and creates a data frame from it. The default separator `sep=" "` is any whitespace. Use `header=TRUE` to read the first line as a header of column names. Use `as.is=TRUE` to prevent character vectors from being converted to factors. Use `comment.char=""` to prevent `"#"` from being interpreted as a comment. Use `skip=n` to skip n lines before reading data. See the help for options on row naming, NA treatment, and others. The example below uses `read.table()` to parse and load an ASCII text file containing a simple dataset, which is available on the supporting canvas data archive.

```
data.txt<-
     read.table("https://umich.instructure.com/files/1628628/download?download_frd=1",
        header=T, as.is = T) # 01a_data.txt
summary(data.txt)
##      Name              Team              Position            Height
##   Length:1034       Length:1034       Length:1034        Min.   :67.0
##   Class :character  Class :character  Class :character   1st Qu.:72.0
##   Mode  :character  Mode  :character  Mode  :character   Median :74.0
##                                                          Mean   :73.7
##                                                          3rd Qu.:75.0
##                                                          Max.   :83.0
##
##      Weight             Age
##   Min.   :150.0    Min.   :20.90
##   1st Qu.:187.0    1st Qu.:25.44
##   Median :200.0    Median :27.93
##   Mean   :201.7    Mean   :28.74
##   3rd Qu.:215.0    3rd Qu.:31.23
##   Max.   :290.0    Max.   :48.52
```

When using R to access (read/write) data on a Cloud web service, like Instructure (Canvas) or Google Drive (GDrive), mind that the direct URL reference to the raw file will be different from the URL of the pointer to the file that can be rendered in the browser window. For instance,

- This GDrive TXT file, *1Zpw3HSe-8HTDsOnR-n64KoMRWYpeBBek* (01a_data. txt)[30] can be downloaded and ingested in R via this separate URL.[31]
- While the file reference is unchanged (*1Zpw3HSe-8HTDsOnR-n64KoMRWYpeBBek*), note the change of syntax from viewing the file in the browser, **open?id**–, to auto downloading the file for R processing, **uc? export=download&id**=.

```
dataGDrive.txt <- read.table(
     "https://drive.google.com/uc?export=download&id=1Zpw3HSe-8HTDsOnR-n64KoMRWYpeBBek",
        header=T, as.is = T) # 01a_data.txt
summary(dataGDrive.txt)
```

read.csv("filename", header=TRUE) is identical to `read.table()` but with defaults set for reading comma-delimited files.

```
data.csv<-
     read.csv("https://umich.instructure.com/files/1628650/download?download_frd=1",
             header = T)  # 01_hdp.csv
summary(data.csv)
```

read.delim("filename", header=TRUE) is very similar to the first two. However, it has defaults set for reading tab-delimited files.

Also we have `read.fwf(file, widths, header=FALSE, sep="\t", as.is=FALSE)` to read a table of fixed width formatted data into a data frame.

---

[30] https://drive.google.com/open?id=1Zpw3HSe-8HTDsOnR-n64KoMRWYpeBBek

[31] https://drive.google.com/uc?export=download&id=1Zpw3HSe-8HTDsOnR-n64KoMRWYpeBBek

match(x, y) returns a vector of the positions of (first) matches of its first argument in its second. For a specific element in x if no element matches it in y, then the output would be NA.

```
match(c(1, 2, 4, 5), c(1, 4, 4, 5, 6, 7))
## [1]  1 NA  2  4
```

save.image(file) saves all objects in the current workspace.

write.table(x, file="", row.names=TRUE, col.names=TRUE, sep="") prints x after converting to a data frame and stores it into a specified file. If `quote` is TRUE, character or factor columns are surrounded by quotes ("). `sep` is the field separator. `eol` is the end-of-line separator. `na` is the string for missing values. Use `col.names=NA` to add a blank column header to get the column headers aligned correctly for spreadsheet input.

Most of the I/O functions have a file argument. This can often be a character string naming a file or a connection. The option `file=""` refers to the standard input or output. Connections can include files, pipes, zipped files, and R variables.

On windows, the file connection can also be used with `description = "clipboard"`. To read a table copied from Excel, use `x <- read.delim ("clipboard")`.

To write a table to the clipboard for Excel, use `write.table(x, "clipboard", sep="\t", col.names=NA)`.

For database interaction, see packages RODBC, DBI, RMySQL, RPgSQL, and ROracle, as well as packages XML, hdf5, and netCDF for reading other file formats. We will talk about some of them in later chapters. *Note*, an alternative library called `rio` handles import/export of multiple data types with simple syntax.

1.2.2.10   Slicing and Extracting Data

Table 1.8 summarizes the basic vector indexing operations.

Table 1.8 Vector indexing syntax

Expression	Explanation
x[n]	nth element
x[-n]	all but the nth element
x[1:n]	first n elements
x[-(1:n)]	elements from n + 1 to the end
x[c(1, 4, 2)]	specific elements
x["name"]	element named "name"
x[x > 3]	all elements greater than 3
x[x > 3 & x < 5]	all elements between 3 and 5
x[x %in% c("a", "and", "the")]	elements in the given set

Table 1.9 List object indexing syntax

Expression	Explanation
x[n]	list with n elements
x[[n]]	nth element of the list
x[["name"]]	element of the list named "name"

Table 1.10 Arrays and tensor object indexing syntax

Expression	Explanation
x[i, j]	element at row i, column j
x[i,]	row i
x[, j]	column j
x[, c(1, 3)]	columns 1 and 3
x["name",]	row named "name"

Indexing lists are similar but not identical to indexing vectors (Table 1.9).

Indexing for *matrices* and higher dimensional *arrays* (*tensors*) derive from vector indexing (Table 1.10).

1.2.2.11 Variable Conversion and Meta-Data

The following functions represent simple examples of converting between different data types.

```
as.array(x), as.data.frame(x), as.numeric(x), as.logical(x), as.
complex(x), as.character(x), ...
```

Typing methods(as) in the console will generate a complete list for variable conversion functions.

The following functions verify if the input is of a specific data type:

```
is.na(x), is.null(x), is.array(x), is.data.frame(x), is.numeric(x), is.
complex(x), is.character(x), ...
```

For a complete list, type methods(is) in the R console. The outputs for these functions are objects, either single values (TRUE or FALSE), or objects of the same dimensions as the inputs containing a Boolean TRUE or FALSE element for each entry in the dataset.

length(x) gives us the number of elements in x.

```
x<-c(1, 3, 10, 23, 1, 3)
length(x)
## [1] 6
is.na(x)
## [1] FALSE FALSE FALSE FALSE FALSE FALSE
is.vector(x)
## [1] TRUE
```

dim(x) retrieves or sets the dimension of an array and **length(y)** reports the length of a list or a vector.

```
x<-1:12
length(x)
## [1] 12
dim(x)<-c(3, 4)
x
##      [,1] [,2] [,3] [,4]
## [1,]    1    4    7   10
## [2,]    2    5    8   11
## [3,]    3    6    9   12
```

dimnames(x) retrieves or sets the dimension names of an object. For higher dimensional objects like matrices or arrays we can combine dimnames() with a list.

```
dimnames(x)<-list(c("R1", "R2", "R3"), c("C1", "C2", "C3", "C4"))
x
##    C1 C2 C3 C4
## R1  1  4  7 10
## R2  2  5  8 11
## R3  3  6  9 12
```

nrow(x) and **ncol(x)** report the number of rows and number of columns or a matrix.

```
nrow(x)
## [1] 3
ncol(x)
## [1] 4
```

class(x) gets or sets the class of x. Note that we can use unclass(x) to remove the class attribute of x.

```
class(x)
## [1] "matrix" "array"
class(x)<-"myclass"
x<-unclass(x)
x
##    C1 C2 C3 C4
## R1  1  4  7 10
## R2  2  5  8 11
## R3  3  6  9 12
```

attr(x, which) gets or sets the attribute `which` of *x*.

```
attr(x, "class")
## NULL
attr(x, "dim")<-c(2, 6)
x
##      [,1] [,2] [,3] [,4] [,5] [,6]
## [1,]    1    3    5    7    9   11
## [2,]    2    4    6    8   10   12
```

The above script shows that applying `unclass` to *x* sets its class to `NULL`.
attributes(obj) gets or sets the list of *attributes* of an object.

```
attributes(x) <- list(mycomment = "really special", dim = 3:4,
               dimnames = list(LETTERS[1:3], letters[1:4]), names = paste(1:12))
x
##   a b c  d
## A 1 4 7 10
## B 2 5 8 11
## C 3 6 9 12
## attr(,"mycomment")
## [1] "really special"
## attr(,"names")
##  [1] "1"  "2"  "3"  "4"  "5"  "6"  "7"  "8"  "9"  "10" "11" "12"
```

1.2.2.12   Data Selection and Manipulation

In this section, we will introduce some data manipulation functions. In addition,
tools from `dplyr` provide easy dataset manipulation routines.

which.max(x) returns the index of the greatest element (max) of *x*, **which.min(x)**
returns the index of the smallest element (min) of *x*, and **rev(x)** reverses the elements
of *x*.

```
x<-c(1, 5, 2, 1, 10, 40, 3)
which.max(x)
## [1] 6
which.min(x)
## [1] 1
rev(x)
## [1]  3 40 10  1  2  5  1
```

sort(x) sorts the elements of *x* in increasing order. To sort in decreasing order, we
can use `rev(sort(x))`.

```
sort(x)
## [1]  1  1  2  3  5 10 40
rev(sort(x))
## [1] 40 10  5  3  2  1  1
```

cut(x, breaks) divides *x* into intervals with the same length (sometimes factors).
The optional parameter `breaks` specifies the number of cut intervals or a vector of

cut points. cut divides the range of x into intervals coding the values in x according to the intervals they fall into.

```
x
## [1]  1  5  2  1 10 40  3
cut(x, 3)
## [1] (0.961,14] (0.961,14] (0.961,14] (0.961,14] (0.961,14] (27,40]
(0.961,14]
## Levels: (0.961,14] (14,27] (27,40]
cut(x, c(0, 5, 20, 30))
## [1] (0,5]  (0,5]  (0,5]  (0,5]  (5,20] <NA>    (0,5]
## Levels: (0,5] (5,20] (20,30]
```

which($x == a$) returns a vector of the indices of x if the comparison operation is true. For example, it returns the value i, if $x[i] == a$ is TRUE. Thus, the argument of this function (like x==a) must be a Boolean variable.

```
x
## [1]  1  5  2  1 10 40  3
which(x==2)
## [1] 3
```

na.omit(x) suppresses the observations with missing data (NA). It suppresses the corresponding line if x is a matrix or a data frame. **na.fail(x)** returns an error message if x contains at least one NA.

```
df<-data.frame(a=1:5, b=c(1, 3, NA, 9, 8))
df
##   a  b
## 1 1  1
## 2 2  3
## 3 3 NA
## 4 4  9
## 5 5  8
na.omit(df)
##   a b
## 1 1 1
## 2 2 3
## 4 4 9
## 5 5 8
```

unique(x) If x is a vector or a data frame, it returns a similar object suppressing the duplicate elements.

```
df1<-data.frame(a=c(1, 1, 7, 6, 8), b=c(1, 1, NA, 9, 8))
df1
unique(df1)
```

table(x) returns a table with the different values of x and their frequencies (typically used for integer or factor variables). The corresponding **prop.table()** function transforms these raw frequencies to relative frequencies (proportions, marginal mass).

```
v<-c(1, 2, 4, 2, 2, 5, 6, 4, 7, 8, 8)
table(v)
## v
## 1 2 4 5 6 7 8
## 1 3 2 1 1 1 2
prop.table(v)
## [1] 0.02040816 0.04081633 0.08163265 0.04081633 0.04081633 0.10204082
## [7] 0.12244898 0.08163265 0.14285714 0.16326531 0.16326531
```

subset(x, ...) returns a selection of *x* with respect to the specified criteria .... Typically ... are comparisons like x$V1 < 10. If *x* is a data frame, the option select= allows using a negative sign − to indicate values to keep or drop from the object.

```
sub <- subset(df1, df1$a>5)
sub
##   a  b
## 3 7 NA
## 4 6  9
## 5 8  8
sub <- subset(df1, select=-a)
sub
## Subsampling
x <- matrix(rnorm(100), ncol = 5)
y <- c(1, seq(19))
z <- cbind(x, y)
z.df <- data.frame(z)
z.df
##           V1         V2          V3          V4          V5 y
## 1  1.35106166  1.4150427  0.66723107  0.19623218  1.63026137 1
## 2  1.08529821  0.4494775 -1.28212047 -0.02539904  3.40851527 1
...
## 20 0.63302396 -1.3387503  0.03912024  0.96022419  0.47658683 19
names(z.df)
## [1] "V1" "V2" "V3" "V4" "V5" "y"
# subsetting rows
z.sub <- subset(z.df, y > 2 & (y<10 | V1>0))
z.sub
##           V1         V2          V3          V4          V5 y
## 4  0.39618603  1.5438144 -0.02360086 -0.7352154 -1.0428234  3
## 5  0.05386697  0.1473649 -1.20745077  1.1199621  0.4332058  4
...
## 17 0.39205807 -0.6750502  1.50978800 -0.1987926  2.3250238 16
## 20 0.63302396 -1.3387503  0.03912024  0.9602242  0.4765868 19
z.sub1 <- z.df[z.df$y == 1, ]
z.sub1
##         V1        V2         V3          V4         V5 y
## 1 1.351062 1.4150427  0.6672319  0.19623218 1.630261 1
## 2 1.085298 0.4494775 -1.2821205 -0.02539904 3.408515 1
z.sub2 <- z.df[z.df$y %in% c(1, 4), ]
z.sub2
##           V1        V2         V3          V4        V5 y
## 1 1.35106166 1.4150427  0.6672319  0.19623218 1.6302614 1
## 2 1.08529821 0.4494775 -1.2821205 -0.02539904 3.4085153 1
## 5 0.05386697 0.1473649 -1.2074508  1.11996205 0.4332058 4
# subsetting columns
z.sub6 <- z.df[, 1:2]
z.sub6
##           V1         V2
## 1  1.35106166  1.4150427
## 2  1.08529821  0.4494775
...
## 20 0.63302396 -1.3387503
```

sample(x, size) resamples randomly, without replacement, *size* elements in the vector *x*. The option `replace = TRUE` allows resampling with replacement.

```
df1 <- data.frame(a=c(1, 1, 7, 6, 8), b=c(1, 1, NA, 9, 8))
sample(df1$a, 20, replace = T)
## [1] 1 1 6 1 8 1 1 8 1 6 7 8 6 6 1 7 6 1 1 7
```

1.2.3 Mathematics, Statistics, and Optimization

Many mathematical functions, statistical summaries, and function optimizers will be discussed throughout the book. Below are the very basic functions to keep in mind.

1.2.3.1 Math Functions

Basic math functions like `sin`, `cos`, `tan`, `asin`, `acos`, `atan`, `atan2`, `log`, `log10`, `exp` and "set" functions `union(x, y)`, `intersect(x, y)`, `setdiff (x, y)`, `setequal(x, y)`, `is.element(el, set)` are available in R.

`lsf.str("package:base")` displays all base functions built in a specific R package (like `base`) (Table 1.11).

Note: many math functions have a logical parameter `na.rm=TRUE` to specify missing data (`NA`) removal.

1.2.3.2 Matrix Operations

Table 1.12 summarizes basic operation functions. We will discuss this topic in detail in Chap. 3.

```
mat1 <- cbind(c(1, -1/5), c(-1/3, 1))
mat1.inv <- solve(mat1)
mat1.identity <- mat1.inv %*% mat1
mat1.identity
##      [,1] [,2]
## [1,]    1    0
## [2,]    0    1
b <- c(1, 2)
x <- solve (mat1, b)
x
## [1] 1.785714 2.357143
```

Table 1.11 Core functions for most basic R calculations

Expression	Explanation
choose(n, k)	computes the combinations of k events among n repetitions. Mathematically it equals to $\frac{n!}{[(n-k)!k!]}$
max(x)	maximum of the elements of x
min(x)	minimum of the elements of x
range(x)	minimum and maximum of the elements of x
sum(x)	sum of the elements of x
diff(x)	lagged and iterated differences of vector x
prod(x)	product of the elements of x
mean(x)	mean of the elements of x
median(x)	median of the elements of x
quantile(x, probs=)	sample quantiles corresponding to the given probabilities (defaults to 0, 0.25, 0.5, 0.75, 1.0)
weighted.mean (x, w)	mean of x with weights w
rank(x)	ranks of the elements of x
var(x) or cov(x)	variance of the elements of x (calculated on n>1). If x is a matrix or a data frame, the variance-covariance matrix is calculated
sd(x)	standard deviation of x
cor(x)	correlation matrix of x if it is a matrix or a data frame (1 if x is a vector)
var(x, y) or cov (x, y)	covariance between x and y, or between the columns of x and those of y if they are matrices or data frames
cor(x, y)	linear correlation between x and y, or correlation matrix if they are matrices or data frames
round(x, n)	rounds the elements of x to n decimals
log(x, base)	computes the logarithm of x with base `base`
scale(x)	if x is a matrix, centers and reduces the data. Without centering use the option center=FALSE. Without scaling use scale=FALSE (by default center=TRUE, scale=TRUE)
pmin(x, y, ...)	a vector whose i-th element is the minimum of x[i], y[i], ...
pmax(x, y, ...)	a vector whose i-th element is the maximum of x[i], y[i], ...
cumsum(x)	a vector which i-th element is the sum from x[1] to x[i]
cumprod(x)	similar for the product
cummin(x)	similar for the minimum
cummax(x)	similar for the maximum
Re(x)	real part of a complex number
Im(x)	imaginary part of a complex number
Mod(x)	Modulus, abs(x) is the same
Arg(x)	angle in radians of the complex number
Conj(x)	complex conjugate
convolve(x, y)	compute the several kinds of convolutions of two sequences
fft(x)	Fast Fourier Transform of an array
mvfft(x)	FFT of each column of a matrix
filter(x, filter)	applies linear filtering to a univariate time series or to each series separately of a multivariate time series

Table 1.12 Basic matrix operations

Expression	Explanation
`t(x)`	transpose
`diag(x)`	diagonal
`%*%`	matrix multiplication
`solve(a, b)`	solves a `%*%` x = b for x
`solve(a)`	matrix inverse of a
`rowsum(x)`	sum of rows for a matrix-like object. `rowSums(x)` is a faster version
`colsum(x)`, `colSums(x)`	similar for columns
`rowMeans(x)`	fast version of row means
`colMeans(x)`	similar for columns

1.2.3.3   Optimization and Model Fitting

Chapter 13 will cover in detail the notion of (loss and objective) function optimization. Below are just some examples of standard R optimization functions.

- **optim(par, fn, method = c("Nelder-Mead", "BFGS", "CG", "L-BFGS-B", "SANN"))** general-purpose optimization; `par` is initial values, `fn` is a function to optimize (normally minimize).
- **nlm(f, p)** minimize function fusing a Newton-type algorithm with starting values p.
- **lm(formula)** fit linear models; `formula` is typically of the form `response ~ termA + termB + ...`; use `I(x*y) + I(x^2)` for terms made of nonlinear components.
- **glm(formula, family=)** fit generalized linear models, specified by giving a symbolic description of the linear predictor and a description of the error distribution; `family` is a description of the error distribution and link function to be used in the model; see `?family`.
- **nls(formula)** nonlinear least-squares estimates of the nonlinear model parameters.
- **approx(x, y=)** linearly interpolate given data points; *x* can be an *xy* plotting structure.
- **spline(x, y=)** cubic spline interpolation.
- **loess(formula)** (locally weighted scatterplot smoothing) fit a polynomial surface using local fitting.

Many of the formula-based modeling functions have several common arguments: `data=` the data frame for the formula variables, `subset=` a subset of variables used in the fit, `na.action=` action for missing values: `"na.fail"`, `"na.omit"`, or a function.

The following generics often apply to model fitting functions:

- `predict(fit, ...)` predictions from fit based on input data.
- `df.residual(fit)` returns the number of residual degrees of freedom.
- `coef(fit)` returns the estimated coefficients (sometimes with their standard-errors).
- `residuals(fit)` returns the residuals.
- `deviance(fit)` returns the deviance.
- `fitted(fit)` returns the fitted values.
- `logLik(fit)` computes the logarithm of the likelihood and the number of parameters.
- `AIC(fit)` computes the Akaike information criterion (AIC).

1.2.3.4 Statistics

Throughout the DSPA materials, we will see a number of statistical methods, functions, and techniques. Some of the basic statistical modeling functions include:

- **lm(formula)** linear modeling.
- **aov(formula)** analysis of variance model.
- **anova(fit, ...)** analysis of variance (or deviance) tables for one or more fitted model objects.
- **density(x)** kernel density estimates of x.

Other functions include: `binom.test()`, `pairwise.t.test()`, `power.t.test()`, `prop.test()`, `t.test()`, ... use `help.search("test")` to see details.

1.2.3.5 Distributions

The Probability Distributome Project[32] provides many details about univariate probability distributions. The SOCR R Shiny Distribution Calculators and the SOCR Bivariate and Trivariate Interactive Graphical Calculators provide additional demonstrations of multivariate probability distribution.[33]

In R, there are four complementary functions supporting each probability distribution. For *Normal distribution*, these four functions are `dnorm()` – density, `pnorm()` – distribution function, `qnorm()` – quantile function, and `rnorm()` – random generating function. For *Poisson distribution*, the corresponding functions are `dpois()`, `ppois()`, `qpois()`, and `rpois()` (Table 1.13).

---

[32] http://distributome.org

[33] https://doi.org/10.1007/s42979-022-01206-w

Table 1.13 Invocation syntax for generating random samples from different probability distributions

Expression	Distribution
rnorm(n, mean=0, sd=1)	Gaussian (normal)
rexp(n, rate=1)	exponential
rgamma(n, shape, scale=1)	gamma
rpois(n, lambda)	Poisson
rweibull(n, shape, scale=1)	Weibull
rcauchy(n, location=0, scale=1)	Cauchy
rbeta(n, shape1, shape2)	beta
rt(n, df)	Student's (t)
rf(n, df1, df2)	Fisher's (F) (df1, df2)
rchisq(n, df)	Pearson rbinom (n, size, prob) binomial
rgeom(n, prob)	geometric
rhyper(nn, m, n, k)	hypergeometric
rlogis(n, location=0, scale=1)	logistic
rlnorm(n, meanlog=0, sdlog=1)	lognormal
rnbinom(n, size, prob)	negative binomial
runif(n, min=0, max=1)	uniform
rwilcox(nn, m, n), rsignrank(nn, n)	Wilcoxon's statistics

Obviously, replacing the first letter r with d, p or q would reference the corresponding probability density (dfunc(x, ...)), the cumulative probability density (pfunc(x, ...)), and the value of quantile (qfunc(p, ...), with $0 < p < 1$).

1.2.4   Advanced Data Processing

In this section, we will introduce some functions that are useful in many data analytic protocols. The family of *apply() functions act on lists, arrays, vectors, data frames, and other objects.

apply(X, INDEX, FUN=) returns a vector or array or list of values obtained by applying a function FUN to margins (INDEX=1 means row, INDEX=2 means column) of *X*. Additional options may be specified after the FUN argument.

```
df1
##   a  b
## 1 1  1
## 2 1  1
## 3 7 NA
## 4 6  9
## 5 8  8
apply(df1, 2, mean, na.rm=T)
##    a    b
## 4.60 4.75
```

lapply(X, FUN) applies FUN to each member of the list *X*. If *X* is a data frame, then it will apply the FUN to each column and return a list.

```
lapply(df1, mean, na.rm=T)
## $a
## [1] 4.6
##
## $b
## [1] 4.75
lapply(list(a=c(1, 23, 5, 6, 1), b=c(9, 90, 999)), median)
## $a
## [1] 5
##
## $b
## [1] 90
```

tapply(X, INDEX, FUN=) applies FUN to each cell of a ragged array given by *X* with indexes equals to INDEX. Note that *X* is an atomic object, typically a vector.

```
# v<-c(1, 2, 4, 2, 2, 5, 6, 4, 7, 8, 8)
v
## [1] 1 2 4 2 2 5 6 4 7 8 8
fac <- factor(rep(1:3, length = 11), levels = 1:3)
table(fac)
## fac
## 1 2 3
## 4 4 3
tapply(v, fac, sum)
## 1  2  3
## 17 16 16
```

by(data, INDEX, FUN) applies FUN to data frame data subsetted by INDEX. In this example, we apply the sum function using column 1 (a) as an index.

```
by(df1, df1[, 1], sum)
```

merge(a, b) merges two data frames by common columns or row names. We can use option by= to specify the index column.

```
df2 <- data.frame(a=c(1, 1, 7, 6, 8), c=1:5)
df2
df3<-merge(df1, df2, by="a")
df3
```

xtabs(a ~ b, data=x) reports specific factorized contingency tables. The example below uses the 1973 UC Berkeley admissions dataset[34] to report gender-by-status breakdown.

---

[34] https://www.jstor.org/stable/1739581

```
DF <- as.data.frame(UCBAdmissions)
## 'DF' is a data frame with a grid of the factors and the counts
## in variable 'Freq'.
DF
##        Admit Gender Dept Freq
## 1  Admitted   Male    A  512
## 2  Rejected   Male    A  313
...
## 24 Rejected Female    F  317
## report marginal ...
xtabs(Freq ~ Gender + Admit, DF)
##          Admit
## Gender    Admitted Rejected
##   Male        1198     1493
##   Female       557     1278
## and for testing independence ...
summary(xtabs(Freq ~ ., DF))
## Call: xtabs(formula = Freq ~ ., data = DF)
## Number of cases in table: 4526
## Number of factors: 3
## Test for independence of all factors:
##   Chisq = 2000.3, df = 16, p-value = 0
```

aggregate(x, by, FUN) splits the data frame x into subsets, computes summary statistics for each part, and reports the results. by is a list of grouping elements, each of which has the same length as the variables in x. For example, we can apply the function sum to the data frame df3 subject to the index created by list(rep(1: 3, length=7)).

```
list(rep(1:3, length=7))
## [[1]]
## [1] 1 2 3 1 2 3 1
aggregate(df3, by=list(rep(1:3, length=7)), sum)
##   Group.1  a  b c
## 1       1 10 10 8
## 2       2  7 10 6
## 3       3  8 NA 4
```

stack(x, ...) transforms data stored as separate columns in a data frame, or list, into a single column vector; **unstack(x, ...)** is the inverse of stack().

```
stack(df3)
unstack(stack(df3))
```

reshape(x, ...) reshapes a data frame between *wide* format, with repeated measurements in separate columns of the same record, and *long* format, with the repeated measurements in separate records. We can specify the transformation direction, direction="wide" or direction="long".

```
df4 <- data.frame(school = rep(1:3, each = 4), class = rep(9:10, 6),
                  time = rep(c(1, 1, 2, 2), 3), score = rnorm(12))
wide <- reshape(df4, idvar = c("school", "class"), direction = "wide")
wide
##    school class    score.1     score.2
## 1       1     9 -1.01992631 -0.08005225
## 2       1    10 -2.02736163 -1.11179440
## 5       2     9 -0.57513435  0.17042075
## 6       2    10  0.07785447  1.71045196
## 9       3     9 -0.64234038 -0.56292494
## 10      3    10  0.30553690 -1.02195904
long <- reshape(wide, idvar = c("school", "class"), direction = "long")
long
##         school class time    score.1
## 1.9.1        1     9    1 -1.01992631
## 1.10.1       1    10    1 -2.02736163
## 2.9.1        2     9    1 -0.57513435
## 2.10.1       2    10    1  0.07785447
## 3.9.1        3     9    1 -0.64234038
## 3.10.1       3    10    1  0.30553690
## 1.9.2        1     9    2 -0.08005225
## 1.10.2       1    10    2 -1.11179440
## 2.9.2        2     9    2  0.17042075
## 2.10.2       2    10    2  1.71045196
## 3.9.2        3     9    2 -0.56292494
## 3.10.2       3    10    2 -1.02195904
```

Notes
- The *x* in this function has to be longitudinal data.
- The call to rnorm used in reshape might generate different results for each call, unless set.seed(1234) is used to ensure reproducibility of random-number generation.

1.2.4.1 Strings

The following functions are useful for handling strings in R.

paste(...) and **paste0**(...) concatenate vectors after converting the arguments to a vector of characters. There are several options, sep= to use a string to separate terms (a single space is the default), collapse= to separate "collapsed" results.

```
a<-"today"
b<-"is a good day"
paste(a, b)
## [1] "today is a good day"
paste(a, b, sep=", ")
## [1] "today, is a good day"
```

substr(x, start, stop) substrings in a character vector. Using substr(x, start, stop) <- value, it can also assign values (with the same length) to part of a string.

```
a<-"When the going gets tough, the tough get going!"
substr(a, 10, 40)
## [1] "going gets tough, the tough get"
## [1] "going gets tough, the tough get"
substr(a, 1, 9)<-"........."
a
## [1] ".........going gets tough, the tough get going!"
```

Note that characters at start and stop indexes are inclusive in the output.

strsplit(x, split) splits *x* according to the substring split. Use fixed=TRUE for nonregular expressions.

```
strsplit("a.b.c", ".", fixed = TRUE)
## [[1]]
## [1] "a" "b" "c"
```

grep(pattern, x) searches for pattern matches within *x* and returns a vector of the indices of the elements of *x* that had a match. Use regular expressions for pattern(unless fixed=TRUE), see ?regex for details.

```
letters
##  [1] "a" "b" "c" "d" "e" "f" "g" "h" "i" "j" "k" "l" "m" "n" "o" "p" "q" "r" "s"
## [20] "t" "u" "v" "w" "x" "y" "z"
grep("[a-z]", letters)
##  [1]  1  2  3  4  5  6  7  8  9 10 11 12 13 14 15 16 17 18 19 20 21 22 23 24 25
## [26] 26
```

gsub(pattern, replacement, x) replaces matching patterns in *x*, allowing for use of regular expression matching; **sub()** is the same but it only replaces the first occurrence of the matched pattern.

```
a<-c("e", 0, "kj", 10, ";")
gsub("[a-z]", "letters", a)
## [1] "letters"          "0"               "lettersletters" "10"
## [5] ";"
sub("[a-z]", "letters", a)
## [1] "letters" "0"          "lettersj" "10"          ";"
```

tolower(x) converts strings to lowercase and **toupper(x)** converts to uppercase.

match(x, table) yields a vector of the positions of first matches for the elements of *x* among table, x %in% table returns a logical vector.

```
x<-c(1, 2, 10, 19, 29)
match(x, c(1, 10))
## [1]  1 NA  2 NA NA
x %in% c(1, 10)
## [1]  TRUE FALSE  TRUE FALSE FALSE
```

pmatch(x, table) reports partial matches for the elements of *x*.

Table 1.14 Common data and time format specifications

Formats	Explanations
%a, %A	Abbreviated and full weekday name
%b, %B	Abbreviated and full month name
%d	Day of the month (01 ... 31)
%H	Hours (00 ... 23)
%I	Hours (01 ... 12)
%j	Day of year (001 ... 366)
%m	Month (01 ... 12)
%M	Minute (00 ... 59)
%p	AM/PM indicator
%S	Second as a decimal number (00 ... 61)
%U	Week (00 ... 53); the first Sunday as day 1 of week 1
%w	Weekday (0 ... 6, Sunday is 0)
%W	Week (00 ... 53); the first Monday as day 1 of week 1
%y	Year without century (00 ... 99). Don't use it
%Y	Year with century
%z (output only.)	Offset from Greenwich; −0800 is 8 hours west of
%Z (output only.)	Time zone as a character string (empty if not available)

Dates and Times

The class Date stores calendar dates, without times. POSIXct() has dates and times, including time zones. Comparisons (e.g., >), seq(), and difftime() are useful to compare dates. ?DateTimeClasses gives more information, see also package chron.

The functions as.Date(s) and as.POSIXct(s) convert to the respective class; format(dt) converts to a string representation. The default string format is 2001-02-21. These accept a second argument to specify a format for conversion (Table 1.14).

Where leading zeros are shown they will be used on output but are optional on input; see ?strftime for details.

1.2.5 Basic Plotting

The following functions represent the basic plotting functions in R (Table 1.15). In Chap. 2, we will discuss more elaborate visualization approaches and exploratory data analytic strategies.

- **plot(x)** plot of the values of x (on the y-axis) ordered on the x-axis.
- **plot(x, y)** bivariate plot of x (on the x-axis) and y (on the y-axis).
- **hist(x)** histogram of the frequencies of x.

- **barplot(x)** histogram of the values of x. Use `horiz=FALSE` for horizontal bars.
- **dotchart(x)** if x is a data frame, plots a Cleveland dot plot (stacked plots line-by-line and column-by-column).
- **pie(x)** circular pie-chart.
- **boxplot(x)** 'box-and-whiskers' plot.
- **sunflowerplot(x, y)** sunflowers plot with multiple leaves ('petals') such that overplotting is visualized instead of accidental and invisible.
- **stripplot(x)** plot of the values of x on a line (an alternative to `boxplot()` for small sample sizes).
- **coplot(x~y | z)** bivariate plot of x and y for each value or interval of values of z.
- **interaction.plot (f1, f2, y)** if f1 and f2 are factors, plots the means of y (on the y-axis) with respect to the values of f1 (on the x-axis) and of f2 (different curves). The option `fun` allows you to choose the summary statistic of y (by default `fun=mean`).
- **matplot(x, y)** bivariate plot of the first column of x vs. the first one of y, the second one of x vs. the second one of y, etc.
- **fourfoldplot(x)** visualizes, with quarters of circles, the association between two dichotomous variables for different populations (x must be an array with dim=c (2, 2, k), or a matrix with dim=c(2, 2) if k = 1).
- **assocplot(x)** Cohen's Friendly graph shows the deviations from independence of rows and columns in a two dimensional contingency table.
- **mosaicplot(x)** "mosaic"" graph of the residuals from a log-linear regression of a contingency table.
- **pairs(x)** if x is a matrix or a data frame, draws all possible bivariate plots between the columns of x.
- **plot.ts(x)** if x is an object of class "ts," plot of x with respect to time, x may be multivariate but the series must have the same frequency and dates. Detailed examples are in **Chapter 12: Big Longitudinal Data Analysis**.
- **ts.plot(x)** id. but if x is multivariate the series may have different dates and must have the same frequency.
- **qqnorm(x)** quantiles of x with respect to the values expected under a normal law.
- **qqplot(x, y)** quantiles of y with respect to the quantiles of x.
- **contour(x, y, z)** contour plot (data are interpolated to draw the curves), x and y must be vectors and z must be a matrix so that `dim(z)=c(length(x), length(y))` (x and y may be omitted).
- **filled.contour(x, y, z)** areas between the contours are colored, and a legend of the colors is drawn as well.
- **image(x, y, z)** plotting actual data with colors.
- **persp(x, y, z)** plotting actual data in perspective view.
- **stars(x)** if x is a matrix or a data frame, it draws a graph with segments or a star where each row of x is represented by a star and the columns are the lengths of the segments.
- **symbols(x, y, ...)** draws, at the coordinates given by x and y, symbols (circles, squares, rectangles, stars, thermometers or "boxplots") whose sizes, colors... are specified by supplementary arguments.
- **termplot(mod.obj)** plot of the (partial) effects of a regression model (`mod.obj`).

Table 1.15 Common parameters for many R basic plotting functions

Parameters	Explanations
add=FALSE	if TRUE superposes the plot on the previous one (if it exists)
axes=TRUE	if FALSE does not draw the axes and the box
type="p"	specifies the type of plot, "p": points, "l": lines, "b": points connected by lines, "o": id. But the lines are over the points, "h": vertical lines, "s": steps, the data are represented by the top of the vertical lines, "S": id. However, the data are represented at the bottom of the vertical lines
xlim=, ylim=	specifies the lower and upper limits of the axes, for example with xlim=c (1, 10) or xlim=range(x)
xlab=, ylab=	annotates the axes, must be variables of mode character
main=	main title, must be a variable of mode character
sub=	subtitle (written in a smaller font)

1.2.5.1 QQ Normal Probability Plot

Let's look at one simple visualization example—quantile–quantile probability plot. Assume $X \sim N(0, 1)$ and $Y \sim Cauchy$ represent the observed/raw and simulated/ generated data for one feature (variable) in the data (Fig. 1.10). The substantial differences between the QQ normal plots of the two variables suggest that their corresponding distributions are distinct.

```
# Sample different number of observations from all the 3 processes
X_norm1 <- rnorm(500)
X_norm2 <- rnorm(1000, m=-75, sd=3.7)
X_Cauchy <- rcauchy(1500)
# estimate the quantiles (scale the values to ensure measuring-unit invariance of
both processes)
qX_norm1 <- quantile(scale(X_norm1), probs = seq(from=0.01, to=0.99, by=0.01))
qX_norm2 <- quantile(scale(X_norm2), probs = seq(from=0.01, to=0.99, by=0.01))
qq.df.norm_norm <- data.frame(qX_norm1, qX_norm2)
# Normal(0,1) vs. Normal(-75, 3.7)
qq.df.norm_norm %>%
  plot_ly(x = ~qX_norm1) %>%
    add_markers(y = ~qX_norm2, name="Normal(0,1) vs. Normal(-75, 3.7) Data") %>%
    add_lines(x = ~qX_norm1, y = ~qX_norm1,
              mode="line", name="Theoretical Normal", line = list(width = 2)) %>%
    layout(title = "Q-Q Normal Plot", legend = list(orientation = 'h'))
# Normal(0,1) vs. Cauchy
qX_norm1 <- quantile(X_norm1, probs = seq(from=0.01, to=0.99, by=0.01))
qX_Cauchy <- quantile(X_Cauchy, probs = seq(from=0.01, to=0.99, by=0.01))
qq.df.norm_cauchy <- data.frame(qX_norm1, qX_Cauchy)
qq.df.norm_cauchy %>%
  plot_ly(x = ~qX_norm1) %>%
    add_markers(y = ~qX_Cauchy, name="Normal(0,1) vs. Cauchy Data") %>%
    add_lines(x = ~qX_norm1, y = ~qX_norm1,
              mode = "line", name = "Theoretical Normal", line=list(width=2)) %>%
    layout(title="Normal vs. Cauchy Q-Q Plot", legend = list(orientation = 'h'))
```

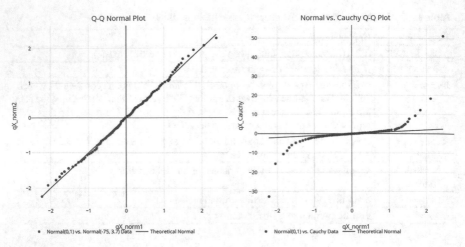

Fig. 1.10 Quantile-quantile (QQ) plots

1.2.5.2   Low-Level Plotting Commands

- **points(x, y)** adds points (the option type= can be used)
- **lines(x, y)** id. but with lines
- **text(x, y, labels, . . .)** adds text given by labels at coordinates (x, y). Typical use:
  plot(x, y, type="n"); text(x, y, names)
- **mtext(text, side=3, line=0, . . .)** adds text given by text in the margin specified
  by side (see axis() below); line specifies the line from the plotting area.
- **segments(x0, y0, x1, y1)** draws lines from points (x0, y0) to points (x1, y1)
- **arrows(x0, y0, x1, y1, angle= 30, code=2)** id. With arrows at points (x0, y0),
  if code=2. The arrow is at point (x1, y1), if code=1. Arrows are at both if
  code=3. Angle controls the angle from the shaft of the arrow to the edge of the
  arrow head.
- **abline(a, b)** draws a line of slope b and intercept a.
- **abline(h=y)** draws a horizontal line at ordinate y.
- **abline(v=x)** draws a vertical line at abscissa x.
- **abline(lm.obj)** draws the regression line given by lm.obj. abline(h=0, col=2)
  #color (col) is often used
- **rect(x1, y1, x2, y2)** draws a rectangle whose left, right, bottom, and top limits are
  x1, x2, y1, and y2, respectively.
- **polygon(x, y)** draws a polygon linking the points with coordinates given by x
  and y.
- **legend(x, y, legend)** adds the legend at the point (x, y) with the symbols given
  by legend.
- **title()** adds a title and optionally a subtitle.
- **axis(side, vect)** adds an axis at the bottom (side=1), on the left (side=2), at
  the top (side=3), or on the right (side=4); vect (optional) gives the abscissa
  (or ordinates) where tick-marks are drawn.

- **rug(x)** draws the data x on the x-axis as small vertical lines.
- **locator(n, type="n", ...)** returns the coordinates (x, y) after the user has clicked n times on the plot with the mouse; also draws symbols (type="p") or lines (type="l") with respect to optional graphic parameters (...); by default nothing is drawn (type="n").

1.2.5.3 General Graphics Parameters

These can be set globally with **par(...)**. Many can be passed as parameters to plotting commands (Table 1.16).

- **adj** controls text justification (adj=0 left-justified, adj=0.5 centered, adj=1 right-justified).
- **bg** specifies the color of the background (ex.: bg="red", bg="blue",...the list of the 657 available colors is displayed with colors()).
- **bty** controls the type of box drawn around the plot. Allowed values are: "o", "l", "7", "c", "u" ou "]" (the box looks like the corresponding character). If bty="n" the box is not drawn.
- **cex** a value controlling the size of texts and symbols with respect to the default. The following parameters have the same control for numbers on the axes-cex.axis, the axis labels-cex.lab, the title-cex.main, and the subtitle-cex.sub.
- **col** controls the color of symbols and lines. Use color names: "red", "blue" see colors() or as "#RRGGBB"; see rgb(), hsv(), gray(), and rainbow(); as for cex there are: col.axis, col.lab, col.main, col.sub.
- **font** an integer which controls the style of text (1: normal, 2: italics, 3: bold, 4: bold italics); as for cex there are: font.axis, font.lab, font.main, font.sub.
- **las** an integer which controls the orientation of the axis labels (0: parallel to the axes, 1: horizontal, 2: perpendicular to the axes, 3: vertical).
- **lty** controls the type of lines, can be an integer or string (1: "solid," 2: "dashed," 3: "dotted," 4: "dotdash," 5: "longdash," 6: "twodash," or a string of up to eight characters (between "0" and "9") which specifies alternatively the length, in points or pixels, of the drawn elements and the blanks, for example lty="44" will have the same effect as lty=2.
- **lwd** a numeric which controls the width of lines, default=1.
- **mar** a vector of 4 numeric values which control the space between the axes and the border of the graph of the form c(bottom, left, top, right), the default values are c(5.1, 4.1, 4.1, 2.1).
- **mfcol** a vector of the form c(nr, nc) which partitions the graphic window as a matrix of nr lines and nc columns, the plots are then drawn in columns.
- **mfrow** plots are drawn row-by-row.
- **pch** controls the type of symbol, either an integer between 1 and 25, or any single character within "".

Table 1.16 Examples of core R multivariate plots

Expression	Explanation
xyplot(y~x)	bivariate plots (with many functionalities)
barchart(y~x)	histogram of the values of y with respect to those of x
dotplot(y~x)	Cleveland dot plot (stacked plots line-by-line and column-by-column)
densityplot(~x)	density functions plot
histogram(~x)	histogram of the frequencies of x
bwplot(y~x)	"box-and-whiskers" plot
qqmath(~x)	quantiles of x with respect to the values expected under a theoretical distribution
stripplot(y~x)	single dimension plot, x must be numeric, y may be a factor
qq(y~x)	quantiles to compare two distributions, x must be numeric, y may be numeric, character, or factor but must have two "levels"
splom(~x)	matrix of bivariate plots
parallel(~x)	parallel coordinates plot
levelplot $(z \sim x * y \parallel g1 * g2)$	colored plot of the values of z at the coordinates given by x and y (x, y, and z are all of the same length)
wireframe $(z \sim x * y \parallel g1 * g2)$	3d surface plot
cloud $(z \sim x * y \parallel g1 * g2)$	3d scatter plot

- **ts.plot(x)** id. but if x is multivariate the series may have different dates by x and y.
- **ps** an integer which controls the size in points of texts and symbols.
- **pty** a character, which specifies the type of the plotting region, "s": square, "m": maximal.
- **tck** a value which specifies the length of tick-marks on the axes as a fraction of the smallest of the width or height of the plot; if `tck=1` a grid is drawn.
- **tcl** a value which specifies the length of tick-marks on the axes as a fraction of the height of a line of text (by default `tcl=-0.5`).
- **xaxt** if `xaxt="n"` the x-axis is set but not drawn (useful in conjunction with `axis(side=1, ...)`).
- **yaxt** if `yaxt="n"` the y-axis is set but not drawn (useful in conjunction with `axis(side=2, ...)`).

In the normal Lattice formula, `y~x|g1*g2`, combinations of optional conditioning variables `g1` and `g2` plotted on separate panels. Lattice functions take many of the same arguments as base graphics plus also `data=` the data frame for the formula variables and `subset=` for subsetting. Use `panel=` to define a custom panel function (see `apropos("panel")` and `?lines`). Lattice functions return an object of class trellis and have to be printed to produce the graph. Use `print (xyplot(...))` inside functions where automatic printing doesn't work. Use `lattice.theme` and `lset` to change Lattice defaults.

1.2.6 Basic *R* Programming

The standard setting for our **own function** is:

function.name <- function(x) { expr (an expression) return (value) }

Where *x* is the parameter in the expression.

```
adding <- function(x=0, y=0) {  z<-x+y; return(z) }
adding(x=5, y=10)
## [1] 15
```

Conditions setting: if (cond) {expr} or if (cond) cons.expr else alt.expr.

```
x<-10
if(x>10) z="T" else z="F"
z
## [1] "F"
```

Alternatively, ifelse represents a vectorized and extremely efficient conditional mechanism that provides one of the main advantages of R.

For loop: for (var in seq) expr.

```
x<-c()
for(i in 1:10) x[i]<-i
x
## [1]  1  2  3  4  5  6  7  8  9 10
```

Other loops: While loop: while (cond) expr, repeat: repeat expr. Applied to the innermost of nested loops: break, next. Use braces {} around statements.

ifelse(test, yes, no) returns a value with the same shape as test, filled with yes or no Boolean values.

do.call(funname, args) executes a function call from the name of the function and a list of arguments to be passed to it.

1.2.7 Data Simulation Primer

Before we demonstrate how to synthetically simulate data that resembles closely the characteristics of real observations from the same process, let's import some observed data for initial exploratory analytics.

Using the SOCR Parkinson's Disease Case-study available in the Canvas Data Archive, we can import some data and extract some descriptions of the sample data (05_PPMI_top_UPDRS_Integrated_LongFormat1.csv) (Fig. 1.11).

Fig. 1.11 Simulated age distribution of Parkinson's disease patients

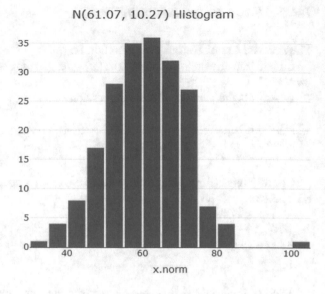

```
PPMI <- read.csv("https://umich.instructure.com/files/330397/download?download_frd=1")
# summary(PPMI)
Hmisc::describe(PPMI)
## PPMI
## 31  Variables      1764  Observations
##---------------------------------------------------------------------------
## FID_IID
##        n  missing distinct      Info      Mean       Gmd      .05      .10
##     1764        0      441         1      3534     390.9     3054     3089
##      .25      .50      .75       .90       .95
##     3272     3476     3817      4072      4102
## lowest : 3001 3002 3003 3004 3006, highest: 4122 4123 4126 4136 4139
## ---------------------------------------------------------------------------
…
## time_visit
##        n  missing distinct      Info      Mean       Gmd      .05      .10
##     1764        0       12     0.993      23.5     20.09     0.00     3.00
##      .25      .50      .75       .90       .95
##     8.25    21.00    37.50     48.00     54.00
##
## lowest :  0  3  6  9 12, highest: 30 36 42 48 54
##
## Value            0       3       6       9      12      18      24      30      36      42      48
## Frequency      147     147     147     147     147     147     147     147     147     147     147
## Proportion   0.083   0.083   0.083   0.083   0.083   0.083   0.083   0.083   0.083   0.083   0.083
# data driven age estimates
m  = round (mean(PPMI$Age), 2)
sd = round(sd(PPMI$Age), 2)
x.norm <- rnorm(n=200, m=m, sd=sd)
# hist(x.norm, main='N(10, 20) Histogram')
plot_ly(x = ~x.norm, type = "histogram") %>%
  layout(bargap=0.1, title=paste0('N(', m, ', ', sd, ') Histogram'))
```

```
mean(PPMI$Age)
## [1] 61.07281
sd(PPMI$Age)
## [1] 10.26669
```

Next, we will simulate new synthetic data to match the properties/characteristics of the observed PPMI data (using `Uniform`, `Normal`, and `Poisson` distributions) (Fig. 1.12).

```
# age m=62, sd=10
# Demographics variables; Define number of subjects
NumSubj <- 282
NumTime <- 4
# Define data elements; # Cases
Cases <- c(1:282)
# Imaging Biomarkers
L_caudate_ComputeArea <- rpois(NumSubj, 600)
L_caudate_Volume <- rpois(NumSubj, 800)
R_caudate_ComputeArea <- rpois(NumSubj, 893)
R_caudate_Volume <- rpois(NumSubj, 1000)
L_putamen_ComputeArea <- rpois(NumSubj, 900)
L_putamen_Volume <- rpois(NumSubj, 1400)
R_putamen ComputeArea <- rpois(NumSubj, 1300)
R_putamen_Volume <- rpois(NumSubj, 3000)
L_hippocampus_ComputeArea <- rpois(NumSubj, 1300)
L_hippocampus_Volume <- rpois(NumSubj, 3200)
R_hippocampus_ComputeArea <- rpois(NumSubj, 1500)
R_hippocampus_Volume <- rpois(NumSubj, 3800)
cerebellum_ComputeArea <- rpois(NumSubj, 16700)
cerebellum_Volume <- rpois(NumSubj, 14000)
L_lingual_gyrus_ComputeArea <- rpois(NumSubj, 3300)
L_lingual_gyrus_Volume <- rpois(NumSubj, 11000)
R_lingual_gyrus_ComputeArea <- rpois(NumSubj, 3300)
R_lingual_gyrus_Volume <- rpois(NumSubj, 12000)
L_fusiform_gyrus ComputeArea <- rpois(NumSubj, 3600)
L_fusiform_gyrus_Volume <- rpois(NumSubj, 11000)
R_fusiform_gyrus_ComputeArea <- rpois(NumSubj, 3300)
R_fusiform_gyrus_Volume <- rpois(NumSubj, 10000)
Sex <- 1felse(runif(NumSubj)<.5, 0, 1)
Weight <- as.integer(rnorm(NumSubj, 80, 10))
Age <- as.integer(rnorm(NumSubj, 62, 10))
# Diagnosis
Dx <- c(rep("PD", 100), rep("HC", 100), rep("SWEDD", 82))
# Genetics
chr12_rs34637584_GT <- c(ifelse(runif(100)<.3, 0, 1), ifelse(runif(100)<.6, 0,1),
                    ifelse(runif(82)<.4, 0, 1))     # NumSubj Bernoulli trials
chr17_rs11868035_GT <- c(ifelse(runif(100)<.7, 0, 1), ifelse(runif(100)<.4, 0,1),
                    ifelse(runif(82)<.5, 0, 1))     # NumSubj Bernoulli trials
# Clinical          # rpois(NumSubj, 15) + rpois(NumSubj, 6)
UPDRS_part_I <- c( ifelse(runif(100)<.7, 0, 1) + ifelse(runif(100) < .7, 0, 1),
ifelse(runif(100)<.6, 0, 1)+ ifelse(runif(100)<.6, 0, 1),
ifelse(runif(82)<.4, 0, 1)+ ifelse(runif(82)<.4, 0, 1) )
UPDRS_part_II <- c(sample.int(20, 100, replace=T), sample.int(14,100, replace=T),
sample.int(18, 82, replace=T) )
UPDRS_part_III <- c(sample.int(30, 100, replace=T),
     sample.int(20, 100, replace=T), sample.int(25, 82, replace=T) )
```

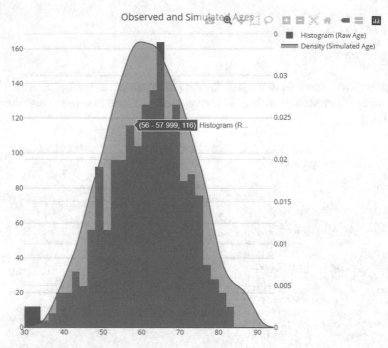

Fig. 1.12 Comparing observed Parkinson's disease patients ages vs. an age probability density model

```
# Time: VisitTime - done automatically below in aggregator
# Data (putting all components together)
sim_PD_Data <- cbind(
        rep(Cases, each= NumTime),                    # Cases
        rep(L_caudate_ComputeArea, each= NumTime),    # Imaging
        rep(Sex, each= NumTime),                      # Demographics
        rep(Weight, each= NumTime),
        rep(Age, each= NumTime),
        rep(Dx, each= NumTime),                       # Dx
        rep(chr12_rs34637584_GT, each= NumTime),      # Genetics
        rep(chr17_rs11868035_GT, each= NumTime),
        rep(UPDRS_part_I, each= NumTime),             # Clinical
        rep(UPDRS_part_II, each= NumTime),
        rep(UPDRS_part_III, each= NumTime),
        rep(c(0, 6, 12, 18), NumSubj)                 # Time
)
# Assign the column names
colnames(sim_PD_Data) <- c("Cases", "L_caudate_ComputeArea", "Sex", "Weight",
    "Age", "Dx", "chr12_rs34637584_GT", "chr17_rs11868035_GT", "UPDRS_part_I",
    "UPDRS_part_II", "UPDRS_part_III", "Time"
)
# some quality control (QC)
summary(sim_PD_Data)
dim(sim_PD_Data) ## [1] 1128    12
head(sim_PD_Data)
x <- PPMI$Age
fit <- density(as.numeric(as.data.frame(sim_PD_Data)$Age))
plot_ly(x = x, type = "histogram", name = "Histogram (Raw Age)") %>%
    add_trace(x = fit$x, y = fit$y, type = "scatter", mode = "lines",
            fill="tozeroy", yaxis = "y2", name = "Density (Simulated Age)") %>%
    layout(title='Observed and Simulated Ages', yaxis2 = list(overlaying = "y",
            side = "right"))
```

```
# Save Results; # Write out (save) the result to a file that can be shared
write.table(sim_PD_Data, "output_data.csv", sep=", ", row.names=FALSE, col.names=TRUE)
```

1.3 Practice Problems

1.3.1 Long-to-Wide Data Format Translation

Load in the long-format SOCR Parkinson's Disease data and export it as *wide format*. You can only select any five variables (not all), but note that there are several time observations for each subject. You can try using the reshape() method or Tidyverse techniques.

1.3.2 Data Frames

Create a Data Frame storing the SOCR Parkinson's Disease data and call summary() and Hmsc::describe() to summarize some of the feature characteristics.

1.3.3 Data Stratification

Complete the following protocol using the SOCR Parkinson's disease dataset.

- Extract the first 10 subjects.
- Find the cases for which L_caudate_ComputeArea<600.
- Sort the subjects based on L_caudate_Volume.
- Generate frequency and probability tables for Gender and Age.
- Compute the mean Age and the correlation between Age and Weight.
- Plot Histogram and density of R_fusiform_gyrus_Volume and scatterplot L_fusiform_gyrus_Volume and R_fusiform_gyrus_Volume.

Note: You don't have to apply these data filters sequentially, but this can also be done for deeper stratification.

1.3.4 Simulation

Generate 1000 standard normal variables and 1200 Cauchy distributed random variables and generate a *quantile–quantile* (Q–Q) probability plot of the pair of samples.

1.3.5   Programming

Generate an R function that given an object (e.g., vector, matrix, array, tensor, list), it computes the *arithmetic average* and compare it against the mean() function. Take special care to handle missing, non-numeric, and mixed-type objects.

1.4   Appendix

1.4.1   Tidyverse

The Tidyverse suite[35] integrates R packages that provide support for data science and big data analytics. It includes functionality for data import (readr), data manipulation (dplyr), data visualization (ggplot2), expanded data frames (tibble), data tidying (tidyr), and functional programming (purrr).

1.4.2   Additional R Documentation and Resources

- A very gentle stats intro using R Book (by Verzani).[36]
- R project Introduction.[37]
- UCLA ITS/IDRE R Resources.[38]

1.4.3   HTML SOCR Data Import

SOCR datasets can automatically be downloaded into the R environment using the following protocol, which uses the Parkinson's disease dataset as an example.

---

[35] https://www.tidyverse.org

[36] http://cran.r-project.org/doc/contrib/Verzani-SimpleR.pdf

[37] https://cran.r-project.org/manuals.html

[38] https://stats.idre.ucla.edu/r/

```
library(rvest)
# Loading required package: xml2; # UCLA SOCR Data
wiki_url <-
     read_html("http://wiki.stat.ucla.edu/socr/index.php/SOCR_Data_PD_BiomedBigMetadata")
html_nodes(wiki_url, "#content")
pd_data <- html_table(html_nodes(wiki_url, "table")[[2]])
head(pd_data); summary(pd_data)
## # A tibble: 6 x 33
...
## Max.    :18.0
```

1.4.4 R Debugging

Most programs that give incorrect results are impacted by logical errors. When errors (bugs, exceptions) occur, we need to explore deeper—this procedure to identify and fix bugs is "debugging".

R tools for debugging: traceback(), debug() browser() trace() recover().

traceback(): Failing R functions report to the screen immediately the run-time errors. Calling traceback() shows the place where the error occurred. The traceback() function prints the list of functions that were called before the error occurred. The stacked function calls are printed in reverse order.

```
f1 <- function(x) { r<- x-g1(x); `R` }
g1 <- function(y) { r<-y*h1(y); `R` }
h1 <- function(z) { r<-log(z); if(r<10) r^2 else   r^3}
f1(-1)
## Warning in log(z): NaNs produced
## Error in if (r < 10) r^2 else r^3: missing value where TRUE/FALSE needed
traceback()
3: h(y)
## Error in h(y): could not find function "h"
2: g(x)
## Error in g(x): could not find function "g"
1: f(-1)
## Error in f(-1): could not find function "f"
```

debug() – traceback() does not tell you where the error is. To find out which line causes the error, we may step through the function using debug().

debug(foo) flags the function foo() for debugging. undebug(foo) unflags the function. When a function is flagged for debugging, each statement in the function is executed one at a time. After a statement is executed, the function suspends and the user can interact with the R shell. This allows us to inspect a function line-by-line. Here is an example computing the sum squared error, SS.

```
## compute sum of squares
SS <- function(mu, x) {
  d<-x-mu;
  d2<-d^2;
  ss<-sum(d2);
  ss
}
set.seed(100);
x<-rnorm(100);
SS(1, x)
## to debug
debug(SS); SS(1, x)
## debugging in: SS(1, x)
## debug at <text>#2: {
##     d <- x - mu
##     d2 <- d^2
##     ss <- sum(d2)
##     ss
## }
## debug at <text>#3: d <- x - mu
## debug at <text>#4: d2 <- d^2
## debug at <text>#5: ss <- sum(d2)
## debug at <text>#6: ss
## exiting from: SS(1, x)
## [1] 202.5615
```

In the debugging shell ("Browse[1]>"), users can:

- Enter **n** (next) executes the current line and prints the next one.
- Typing **c** (continue) executes the rest of the function without stopping;
- Enter **Q** quits the debugging.
- Enter **ls()** list all objects in the local environment.
- Enter an object name or print() tells the current value of an object.

```
debug(SS)
SS(1, x)
## debugging in: SS(1, x)
## debug at <text>#2: {
##     d <- x - mu
##     d2 <- d^2
##     ss <- sum(d2)
##     ss
## }
## debug at <text>#3: d <- x - mu
## debug at <text>#4: d2 <- d^2
## debug at <text>#5: ss <- sum(d2)
## debug at <text>#6: ss
## exiting from: SS(1, x)
## [1] 202.5615
```

Browse[1]> n
debug: d <- x - mu ## the next command
Browse[1]> ls() ## current environment [1] "mu" "x" ## there is no d
Browse[1]> n ## go one step debug: d2 <- d^2 ## the next command

Browse[1]> ls() ## current environment [1] "d" "mu" "x" ## d has been created
Browse[1]> d[1:3] ## first three elements of d [1] -1.5021924 -0.8684688
    -1.0789171
Browse[1]> hist(d) ## histogram of d
Browse[1]> where ## current position in call stack where 1: SS(1, x)
Browse[1]> n
debug: ss <- sum(d2)
Browse[1]> Q ## quit

```
undebug(SS)        ## remove debug label, stop debugging process
SS(1, x)           ## now call SS again will without debugging
```

You can label a function for debugging while debugging another function.

```
f <- function(x) {
  r<-x-g(x);
  `R`
}
g <- function(y) {
  r<-y*h(y);
  `R`
}
h <- function(z) {
  r<-log(z);
  if(r<10) r^2
  else r^3
}

debug(f)           # ## If you only debug f, you will not go into g
f(-1)
## Warning in log(z): NaNs produced
## Error in if (r < 10) r^2 else r^3: missing value where TRUE/FALSE needed
```

Browse[1]> n
Browse[1]> n
But, we can also label g and h for debugging when we debug f
f(-1)
Browse[1]> n
Browse[1]> debug(g)
Browse[1]> debug(h)
Browse[1]> n

Inserting a call to **browser()** in a function will pause the execution of a function at the point where browser() is called. Similar to using **debug()**, except that you can control where execution gets paused. Here is another example.

```
h <- function(z) {
  browser()      ## a breakpoint inserted here
  r<-log(z)
  if(r<10)   r^2
  else r^3
}

f(-1)
## Error in if (r < 10) r^2 else r^3: missing value where TRUE/FALSE needed
```

Browse[1]> ls() Browse[1]> z
Browse[1]> n
Browse[1]> n
Browse[1]> ls()
Browse[1]> c

Calling **trace()** on a function allows inserting new code into a function.

```
as.list(body(h))
trace("h", quote(
if(is.nan(r))
{browser()}), at=3, print=FALSE)
f(1)
f(-1)
trace("h", quote(if(z<0) {z<-1}), at=2, print=FALSE)
f(-1)
untrace()
```

During the debugging process, **recover()** allows checking the status of variables in upper level functions. recover() can be used as an error handler using **options()** (e.g., `options (error = recover)`). When functions throw exceptions, execution stops at the point of failure. Browsing the function calls and examining the environment may indicate the source of the problem.

Chapter 2
Basic Visualization and Exploratory Data Analytics

2.1 Data Handling

A number of method for data wrangling, harmonization, manipulation, aggregation, visualization, and graphical exploration depend on the critical step of data `import` and `export (input/output)`. We will start with some basic approaches for processing different types of data. Specifically, we will illustrate common R data structures and strategies for loading (ingesting) and saving (regurgitating) data. In addition, we will (1) present some basic statistics, e.g., for measuring central tendency (mean, median, mode) or dispersion (variance, quartiles, range); (2) explore simple plots; (3) demonstrate the uniform and normal distributions; (4) contrast numerical and categorical types of variables; (5) present strategies for handling incomplete (missing) data; and (6) show the need for cohort-rebalancing when comparing imbalanced groups of subjects, cases, or units.

2.1.1 Saving and Loading R Data Structures

Let's start by extracting Edgar Anderson's Iris Data included in the R base. The iris dataset quantifies morphologic shape variations of 50 Iris flowers of three related genera—*Iris setosa*, *Iris virginica,* and *Iris versicolor*. Four shape features were measured from each sample—length and width of the sepals and petals (in centimeters), Fig. 2.1. These data were used by Ronald Fisher in his 1936 linear discriminant analysis paper[1].

---

[1] https://doi.org/10.1111/2Fj.1469-1809.1936.tb02137.x

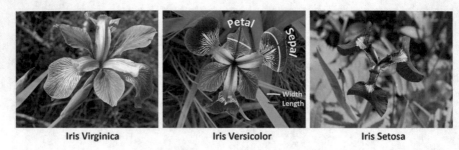

Iris Virginica   Iris Versicolor   Iris Setosa

Fig. 2.1 Three taxa of the iris flowers dataset

```
data()
data(iris)
class(iris) ## [1] "data.frame"
```

As an I/O (input/output) demonstration, after we load the `iris` data and examine its class type, we can save it into a file named "myData.RData" and then reload it back into R.

```
save(iris, file="myData.RData")
load("myData.RData")
```

2.1.2 Importing and Saving Data from CSV Files

Next we can show the process of importing outside data, e.g., `"CaseStudy07_WorldDrinkingWater_Data.csv"` from the case-studies available on the supporting website, and saving it into the R dataset named "water." The variables in the dataset are as follows:

- *Time*: Years (1990, 1995, 2000, 2005, 2010, 2012).
- *Demographic*: Country (across the world).
- *Residence Area Type*: Urban, rural, or total.
- *WHO Region*.
- *Population using improved drinking-water sources*: The percentage of the population using an improved drinking water source.
- *Population using improved sanitation facilities*: The percentage of the population using an improved sanitation facility.

By default, CSV files use comma as the element separator; however, the option `sep=","` in the command `read.csv()` provides more flexibility, if needed. Also, we can use `colnames()` to rename the column variables. This example shows the import of external CSV files that already include a header line containing the names of the variables. If we don't have a header in the dataset, we can use the `header=FALSE` option to read the first row in the file as data, rather than variable names. In such cases, R will assign default names to the column variables of the dataset.

```
water <-
    read.csv('https://umich.instructure.com/files/399172/download?download_frd=1',
        header=TRUE, fileEncoding = "UTF-8")
water[1:3, ]
##    Year..string. WHO.region..string. Country..string.
…
##                                                           0
colnames(water)<-c("year", "region", "country", "residence_area",
"improved_water", "sanitation_facilities")
water[1:3, ]
which.max(water$year);
## [1] 913
# row mean
mean(water[,6], trim=0.08, na.rm=T)
## [1] 71.63629
```

To save a data frame to CSV files, we could use the `write.csv()` function. The option `file = "/a/local/file/path/file"` allows us to specify the output file name and location.

```
write.csv(iris, file = "C:/Users/iris.csv")
```

2.1.3 Importing Data from ZIP and SAV Files

Just like the default RData file type uses compression to save disk storage space, many other information compressions (gz, zip, 7z, etc.) can be used to reduce the memory footprint of large and complex datasets. This example demonstrates data import from a compressed (zip) SPSS (sav) file. In this case, we utilize the DSPA case-study 25: National Ambulatory Medical Care Survey (NAMCS).

```
# install.packages("foreign")
library("foreign")
pathToZip <- tempfile()
download.file("https://umich.instructure.com/files/8111611/download?download_frd=1",
        pathToZip, mode = "wb")
dataset <- read.spss(unzip(pathToZip, files = "namcs2015-spss.sav",
            list = F, overwrite = TRUE), to.data.frame=TRUE)
dim(dataset) ## [1] 28332  1096
unlink(pathToZip)
```

2.1.4   Exploring the Structure of Data

We can use the command `str()` and to explore the structure of a dataset (in this case CaseStudy07_WorldDrinkingWater_Data).

```
str(water)
## 'data.frame': 3331 obs. of 6 variables:
## ...
```

We can see that this `World Drinking Water` dataset has 3331 observations and 6 variables. The output also includes the class of each variable and first few elements in the variable. Similarly, we see that the size of the first dataset (Case-Study 25: National Ambulatory Medical Care Survey) is much larger, 28, 332 × 1096.

2.1.5   Exploring Numeric Variables

Summary statistics for numeric variables in the dataset could be accessed by using the command `summary()`. The six summary statistics and `NA`'s (missing data) are reported in the output. Figure 2.2 shows a reconstructed probability density curve of the improved water quality.

```
library(plotly)
summary(water$year)
summary(water[c("improved_water", "sanitation_facilities")])
##  improved_water  sanitation_facilities
##  Min.   :  3.0   Min.   :  0.00
##  1st Qu.: 77.0   1st Qu.: 42.00
##  Median : 93.0   Median : 81.00
##  Mean   : 84.9   Mean   : 68.87
##  3rd Qu.: 99.0   3rd Qu.: 97.00
##  Max.   :100.0   Max.   :100.00
##  NA's   :32      NA's   :135
fit <- density(as.numeric(water$improved_water),na.rm = T)
plot_ly(x = fit$x, y = fit$y, type = "scatter", mode = "lines",
             fill = "tozeroy", name = "Density") %>%
    layout(title='Density of (%) Improved Water Quality',
            xaxis = list (title = 'Percent'), yaxis = list (title = 'Density'))
```

2.1.6   Measuring Central Tendency—Mean, Median, and Mode

The *mean* and *median* are two frequently used measurements of central tendency. The mean, or arithmetic average, is "the sum of all values divided by the number of elements." The median is the value in the middle of the ordered list of the sample

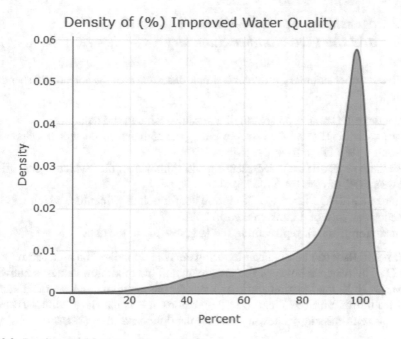

Fig. 2.2 Density model for improved water quality

data. In R, the functions mean() and median() can quickly access these two centrality measurements.

```
vec1<-c(40, 56, 99)
mean(vec1) ## [1] 65
mean(c(40, 56, 99)) ## [1] 65
median(vec1) ## [1] 56
median(c(40, 56, 99)) ## [1] 56
# install.packages("psych");
library("psych")
geometric.mean(vec1, na.rm=TRUE) ## [1] 60.52866
```

Another measure of centrality is the *mode*; the value that occurs most often in the dataset. The mode is often used for categorical data, where the mean and median may not be useful. We can have one or more modes. In the water dataset, we have "Europe" and "Urban" as the modes for region and residence area, respectively. These two variables are unimodal, indicating each has a single mode. For the year variable, we have two modes: 2000 and 2005, each having 570 observations. The *year* represents an example of a multimodal variable that has two, or more, modes.

As a measure for the central tendency, the mode may be used to contrast other data values and helps us determine whether one or several categories may be dominant. In numeric datasets, different modes correspond to local extremes in the histogram bins.

2.1.7   Measuring Spread—Variance, Quartiles, and the Five-Number Summary

The five-number summary provides a simple description of the spread and shape of a dataset:

- Minimum (Min.), representing the smallest value in the data.
- First quartile/Q1 (1st Qu.), representing the 25th percentile, which splits off the lowest 25% of data from the highest 75%.
- Median/Q2 (Median), representing the 50th percentile, which splits off the lowest 50% of data from the top 50%.
- Third quartile/Q3 (3rd Qu.), representing the 75th percentile, which splits off the lowest 75% of data from the top 25%.
- Maximum (Max.), representing the largest value in the data.

Min and Max can be obtained by using the corresponding functions min() and max(). The distance between the maximum and the minimum values is known as the range. In R, the function range() reports the minimum and the maximum. A combination of range() and diff() reports the actual range value. To avoid problems with missing values, we can use the option na.rm=TRUE.

```
range(water$improved_water, na.rm=TRUE)        ## [1]    3 100
diff(range(water$improved_water, na.rm=TRUE)) ## [1] 97
```

The first and third quartiles, Q1 and Q3, represent the 25th and 75th percentiles of the data. The second quartile, i.e., the median (Q2), is always located between Q1 and Q3 and represents the value splitting the top and bottom 50% of the data. The difference between Q3 and Q1 is called the interquartile range (IQR). The central half of the data lies within the IQR. In R, we use the IQR() to calculate the interquartile range. In the presence of missing values, these NA's may be ignored by using the option na.rm=TRUE.

```
IQR(water$improved_water, na.rm=TRUE) ## [1] 22
summary(water$improved_water)
##    Min. 1st Qu.  Median    Mean 3rd Qu.    Max.    NA's
##     3.0    77.0    93.0    84.9    99.0   100.0      32
```

In addition to using the command summary(), we can call the function quantile() to report the five-number summary of a numerical sample.

```
quantile(water$improved_water, na.rm = TRUE)
##   0%  25%  50%  75% 100%
##    3   77   93   99  100
```

We can also calculate specific percentiles in the data. For example, here is how we can compute the 20th and 60th percentiles for the improved water quality variable in the water dataset.

```
quantile(water$improved_water, probs = c(0.2, 0.6), na.rm = TRUE)
## 20% 60%
##  71  97
```

More generally, we can use the seq() function to generate evenly-spaced percentiles which can subsequently be used as inputs to the quartile() function.

```
quantile(water$improved_water, seq(from=0, to=1, by=0.2), na.rm = TRUE)
##   0%  20%  40%  60%  80% 100%
##    3   71   89   97  100  100
```

Let's re-examine the five-number summary for the improved_water variable. When we ignore the NA's, the difference between minimum and Q1 is 74 while the difference between Q3 and maximum is only 1. The interquartile range is 22%. Combining these facts, the data in the first quartile is more spread out than the middle 50% of values. The last quartile is the most condensed. Also, we can notice that the mean is smaller than the median. The mean is more sensitive to the extreme values than the median. Having very small values may spread out the first quartile, skew the distribution to the left, and make the mean smaller than the median (as measures of centrality).

Distribution models offer a way to characterize data using only a few parameters. For example, the normal distribution can be defined by only two parameters—center and spread, or statistically speaking, mean and standard deviation. The (sample) mean value is computed as the arithmetic average of all data points

$$\text{Mean}(X) = \mu = \frac{1}{n} \sum_{i=1}^{n} x_i.$$

The (sample) standard deviation is the square root of the variance. And the (sample) variance is the average sum of square deviation from the mean

$$\text{Var}(X) = \sigma^2 = \frac{1}{n-1} \sum_{i=1}^{n} (x_i - \mu)^2,$$

$$\text{StdDev}(X) = \sigma = \sqrt{\text{Var}(X)}.$$

Later on, we will demonstrate the power of fitting distribution models to observed datasets, Fig. 2.3. For now, we will include a simple illustration of fitting a normal distribution density model to a univariate dataset. Since the water dataset is not close

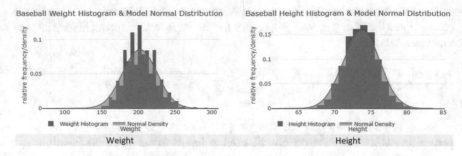

Fig. 2.3 Fitting Normal density models to the histogram of the baseball players weights (left) and heights (right)

to normal, we will use the MLB baseball players dataset to illustrate a normal distribution fit. The MLB dataset (01a_data.txt), available on the supporting Canvas website, has the following variables—*Name*, *Team*, *Position*, *Height*, *Weight*, and *Age*. We can use histograms to visually assess approximate normality of baseball players' *Height* and *Weight*.

```
baseball<-
    read.table("https://umich.instructure.com/files/330381/download?download_frd=1",
       header=T)
x <- rnorm(10000, mean=mean(baseball$Weight, na.rm=T), sd=sd(baseball$Weight,
na.rm=T))
fit <- density(x, bw=10)
plot_ly(x=~baseball$Weight, type = "histogram", name = "Weight Histogram",
            histnorm = "probability") %>%
    add_trace(x =~fit$x, y =~5*fit$y, type = "scatter", mode = "lines",
            opacity=0.1, fill = "tozeroy", name = "Normal Density") %>%
    layout(title='Baseball Weight Histogram & Model Normal Distribution',
            xaxis = list(title = "Weight"), legend = list(orientation='h'),
            yaxis = list(title = "relative frequency/density"))
x <- rnorm(10000, mean=mean(baseball$Height, na.rm=T),
            sd=sd(baseball$Height, na.rm=T))
fit <- density(x, bw=1)
plot_ly(x=~baseball$Height, type = "histogram", name = "Height Histogram",
            histnorm = "probability") %>%
    add_trace(x=~fit$x, y=~fit$y, type = "scatter", mode = "lines",
            opacity=0.1, fill = "tozeroy", name = "Normal Density") %>%
    layout(title='Baseball Height Histogram & Model Normal Distribution',
            xaxis = list(title = "Height"), legend = list(orientation='h'),
            yaxis = list(title = "relative frequency/density"))
```

We could also report the mean and standard deviation of the weight and height variables.

```
mean(baseball$Weight)  ## [1] 201.7166
mean(baseball$Height)  ## [1] 73.69729
var(baseball$Weight)   ## [1] 440.9913
sd(baseball$Weight)    ## [1] 20.99979
var(baseball$Height)   ## [1] 5.316798
sd(baseball$Height)    ## [1] 2.305818
```

Larger standard deviation, or variance, suggests the data is more spread out from the mean. Therefore, for MLB players, weights appear to be more spread than heights. Given the first two moments (mean and standard deviation), we can easily estimate how extreme a specific value is. Assuming we have a normal distribution, the values follow the $68 - 95 - 99.7$ rule. This means that 68% of the data is expected to be within the interval $[\mu - \sigma, \mu + \sigma]$; 95% of the data lies within the interval $[\mu - 2\sigma, \mu + 2\sigma]$; and 99.7% of the data lies within the interval $[\mu - 3\sigma, \mu + 3\sigma]$. The following graph plotted using $\texttt{plot\_ly()}$ illustrates visually this $68 - 95 - 99.7$ rule (Fig. 2.4).

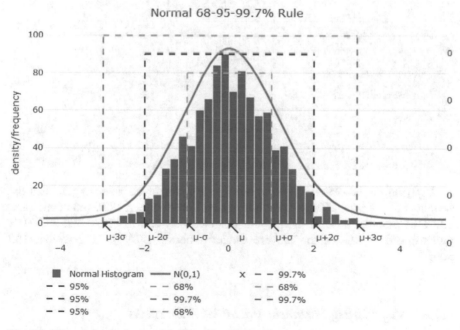

Fig. 2.4 Normal distribution model; $68 - 95 - 99.7$ rule

```
N <- 1000
norm <- rnorm(N, 0, 1)
normDensity <- density(norm, bw=0.5)
dens <- data.frame(x = normDensity$x, y = normDensity$y)
miny <- 0; maxy <- max(dens$y)
xLabels <- c("&mu;-3&#963;","&mu;-2&#963;", "&mu;-&#963;", "&mu;",
             "&mu;+&#963;", "&mu;+2&#963;", "&mu;+3&#963;")
labelColors <- c("green", "red", "orange", "black", "orange", "red", "green")
xLocation <- c(-3, -2, -1, 0, 1, 2, 3)
yLocation <- 0.2
data <- data.frame(xLabels, xLocation, yLocation)
plot_ly(dens) %>%
    add_histogram(x = norm, name="Normal Histogram") %>%
    add_lines(data = dens, x = ~x, y = ~y+0.05, yaxis = "y2",
              line = list(width = 3), name="N(0,1)") %>%
    add_annotations(x = ~xLocation, y = ~yLocation, type = 'scatter',
             ax = 20, ay = 20, mode = 'text', text = ~xLabels,
             textposition = 'middle right',
             textfont = list(color = labelColors, size = 16)) %>%
    add_segments(x=-3, xend=-3, y=0, yend=100, name="99.7%",
          line=list(dash="dash", color="green")) %>%
    add_segments(x=-2, xend=-2, y=0, yend=90, name="95%",
          line=list(dash="dash", color="red")) %>%
    add_segments(x=-1, xend=-1, y=0, yend=80, name="68%",
          line=list(dash="dash", color="orange")) %>%
    add_segments(x=1, xend=1, y=0, yend=80, name="68%",
          line = list(dash = "dash", color="orange")) %>%
    add_segments(x=2, xend=2, y=0, yend=90, name="95%",
          line=list(dash="dash", color="red")) %>%
    add_segments(x=3, xend=3, y=0, yend=100, name="99.7%",
          line=list(dash="dash", color="green")) %>%
    add_segments(x=-3, xend=3, y=100, yend=100, name="99.7%",
          line=list(dash="dash", color="green")) %>%
    add_segments(x=-2, xend=2, y=90, yend=90, name="95%",
          line=list(dash="dash", color="red")) %>%
    add_segments(x=-1, xend=1, y=80, yend=80, name="68%",
          line=list(dash="dash", color="orange")) %>%
    layout(bargap=0.1, xaxis=list(name=""),
      yaxis=list(title="density/frequency"),
      yaxis2 = list(overlaying = "y", side = "right",
               range = c(miny, maxy+0.1), showgrid = F, zeroline = F),
      legend = list(orientation = 'h'), title="Normal 68-95-99.7% Rule")
```

Applying the 68–95–99.7 rule to our baseball weight variable suggests that the weight of 68% of the MBL players is expected to be between 180.7168 pounds and 222.7164 pounds; 95% of the players weighted between 159.7170 and 243.7162 pounds; and 99.7% of the players weighted between 138.7172 and 264.7160 pounds.

2.1.8   Visualizing Numeric Variables—Boxplots

We can visualize the five-number summary using a boxplot (box-and-whiskers plot) (Fig. 2.5).

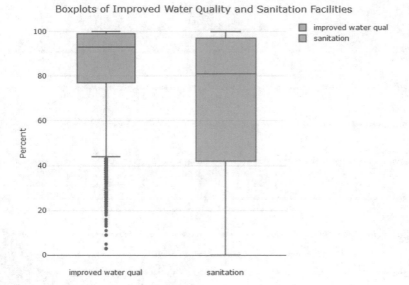

Fig. 2.5 Box plots of improvements in world water quality and sanitation

```
plot_ly(y=~water$improved_water, type="box", name="improved water qual") %>%
  add_trace(y = ~water$sanitation_facilities, name ="sanitation") %>%
    layout(yaxis = list (title = 'Percent'),
        title='Boxplots of Improved Water Quality and Sanitation Facilities')
```

All boxplots have five horizontal lines, each representing the corresponding value
in the five-number summary. The rectangular box in the middle represents the range of
the central 50% of the data. The bold line in the box center is the median (Q2). The
mean value is not illustrated on the graph. Boxplots only allow the two ends to extend
to a minimum or maximum of 1.5 times the IQR. Therefore, any value that falls
outside of the $3 \times IQR$ range will be considered atypical, represented as circles or dots,
and are considered as potential outliers. We can see that there are a number of potential
water quality outliers with small values on the low end of the graph on the left.

2.1.9 Visualizing Numeric Variables—Histograms

For numeric variables, histograms offer another way to show the (sample) distribution spread and shape. Histogram plots require specifications of a number of bins and
value containers to divide and stratify the original data. The heights of the bins
indicate the observed frequencies within each bin (Fig. 2.6).

```
plot_ly(x=~water$improved_water, type="histogram", name="improved_water") %>%
  add_trace(x = ~water$sanitation_facilities, type = "histogram",
      name="sanitation_facilities") %>%
  layout(bargap=0.1, title='Histograms', legend = list(orientation = 'h'),
      xaxis = list(title = 'Percent'), yaxis = list (title = 'Frequency'))
```

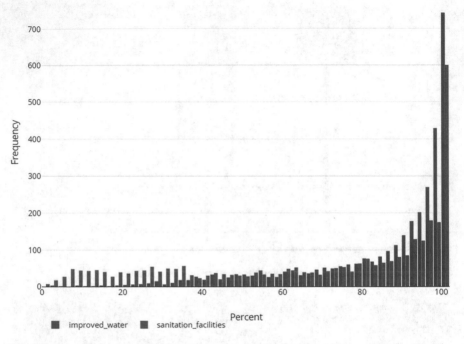

Fig. 2.6 Comparing water quality improvement and sanitation using histogram plots

We could see that the histogram shapes of the water quality (blue color) and sanitation facilities (orange color) are somewhat similar. They both appear to have left skewed patterns (*mean < median*). Other common skew patterns using simulated normal and negative binomial distributions are shown in the following graph (Fig. 2.7).

```
# Symmetric Normal process
N <- 10000
x <- rnorm(N, 15, 3.7)
fit <- density(x)
plot_ly(x = x, type = "histogram", name = "Data Histogram") %>%
    add_trace(x = fit$x, y = fit$y, type = "scatter", mode = "lines",
        opacity=0.3, fill = "tozeroy", yaxis = "y2",
        name = "Density (rnorm(N, 15, 3.7))") %>%
    layout(title='Symmetric Process', yaxis2 = list(overlaying = "y",
        side = "right"), legend = list(orientation = 'h'))
# Skewed Negative-binomial process
N <- 10000
x <- rnbinom(N, 5, 0.1)
fit <- density(x)
plot_ly(x = x, type = "histogram", name = "Data Histogram") %>%
    add_trace(x = fit$x, y = fit$y, type = "scatter", mode = "lines",
        opacity=0.3, fill = "tozeroy", yaxis = "y2",
        name = "Density (rnbinom(N, 5, 0.1))") %>%
    layout(title='Right Skewed Process', yaxis2 = list(overlaying = "y",
        side = "right"), legend = list(orientation = 'h'))
```

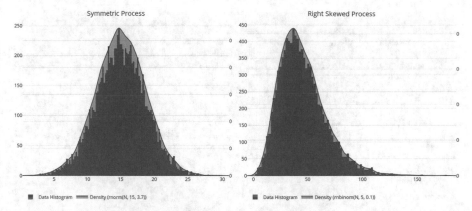

Fig. 2.7 Symmetric normal distribution (left) and skewed (right) negative-binomial distribution; sample histograms superimposed with corresponding density models

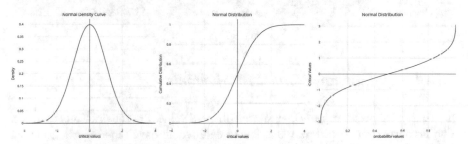

Fig. 2.8 Normal distribution density (left), cumulative distribution function (middle), and inverse CDF (quantile function) (right)

You can learn more about probability distributions in the SOCR Probability and Statistics EBook[2] and see density and cumulative distribution plots of over 80 different probability distributions using the Distributome HTML5 Distribution Calculators.[3]

For each probability distribution defined in R, there are four functions that provide the density (e.g., dnorm), the cumulative probability (e.g., pnorm), the inverse cumulative distribution (quantile) function (e.g., qnorm), and the random sampling (simulation) function (e.g., rnorm). The plots below show the *standard normal* density, cumulative probability, and the quantile functions. Even though the support of the normal distribution is infinite, the normal density is very small outside of the interval $[-4, 4]$ and the plots are restricted to this compact domain (Fig. 2.8).

---

[2] https://wiki.socr.umich.edu/index.php/EBook
[3] http://www.distributome.org/V3/calc/index.html

```
z<-seq(-4, 4, 0.1)  # points from -4 to 4 in 0.1 steps
q<-seq(0.001, 0.999, 0.001)  # quantile values from 0.1%-99.9% in 0.1% steps
dStandardNormal <- data.frame(Z=z, Density=dnorm(z, mean=0, sd=1),
                        Distribution=pnorm(z, mean=0, sd=1))
qStandardNormal <- data.frame(Q=q, Quantile=qnorm(q, mean=0, sd=1))
head(dStandardNormal)
# PDF
plot_ly(x = z, y= dStandardNormal$Density, name = "Normal Density Curve",
          mode = 'lines') %>%
   layout(title='Normal Density Curve', xaxis=list(title='critical values'),
          yaxis = list(title ="Density"),legend = list(orientation = 'h'))
# CDF
plot_ly(x = z, y= dStandardNormal$Distribution,
        name = "Normal Density Curve", mode = 'lines') %>%
   layout(title='Normal Distribution', xaxis=list(title='critical values'),
          yaxis = list(title ="Cumulative Distribution"),
          legend = list(orientation = 'h'))
# Quantile function (CDF^{-1})
plot_ly(x = q, y= qStandardNormal$Quantile,
        name = "Normal Quantile Function (Inverse CDF)", mode = 'lines') %>%
   layout(title='Normal Distribution',xaxis=list(title='probability values'),
        yaxis = list(title ="Critical Values"), legend=list(orientation='h'))
```

2.1.10   Uniform and Normal Distributions

If a dataset follows a *uniform distribution*, then all values are equally likely to occur. The histogram for a uniformly distributed data would have (approximately) equal heights for each bin like the following graph. The observed random frequency deviations are due to the small sample size (Fig. 2.9).

Often, but not always, real world processes may appear as normally distributed data. A *normal distribution* would have higher frequencies of observed values in the middle and lower frequencies of smaller or larger (extreme) values. Normal distribution characterization includes unimodal, symmetric, and bell-curved shape just as shown in the figure (right). Many parametric-based statistical approaches assume normality of the data. In cases where this parametric assumption is violated, variable transformations or distribution-free tests may be more appropriate.

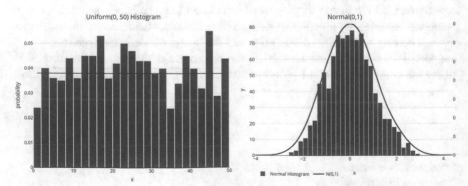

Fig. 2.9 Sample histograms and corresponding theoretical density models for uniform (left) and Normal (right) distributions

2.1.11 Exploring Categorical Variables

Let's go back to the water dataset and consider year as categorical rather than a numeric variable. Since year has only six distinctive values, it is rational to treat it as a categorical variable where each value is a category that could apply to multiple WHO regions. The region and residence area variables are also categorical.

Different from numeric variables, exploring categorical variables is more intuitive by constructing summary tables. A one-way table represents a single categorical variable. It contains the frequencies of counts of different categories. Let's use the `table()` function to create one-way tables for some categorical variables in the water dataset.

```
water <-
    read.csv('https://umich.instructure.com/files/399172/download?download_frd=1',
        header=T, fileEncoding = "UTF-8")
colnames(water) <- c("year", "region", "country", "residence_area",
                      "improved_water", "sanitation_facilities")
table(water$year)
## 1990 1995 2000 2005 2010 2012
##  520  561  570  570  556  554
table(water$region)
table(water$residence_area)
```

Given that we have a total of 3331 observations, the WHO region table tells us that about 27% (910/3331) of the areas examined in the study are in Europe. R can also directly report table proportions by using the `prop.table()` function. The proportion values can be transformed into percentage form and rounded, as needed.

```
year_table<-table(water$year)
prop.table(year_table)
##      1990      1995      2000      2005      2010      2012
## 0.1561093 0.1684179 0.1711198 0.1711198 0.1669168 0.1663164
year_pct <- prop.table(year_table)*100
round(year_pct, digits=1)
```

2.1.12 Exploring Relationships Between Variables

So far, we only considered univariate level methods and statistics. Sometimes, it is useful to examine bivariate or multivariate relationship between two or more variables. For example, does the percentage of the population that uses improved drinking-water sources increase over time? To address such multivariate problems, we need to look at bivariate or multivariate relationships.

2.1.12.1 Visualizing Relationships—Scatterplots

A scatterplot is a good way to visualize bivariate relationships. Each of the x and y axes represents one of the variables. Each (paired) observation is illustrated on the graph by a glyph, e.g., a solid point or a star. If the cumulative graph of scattered glyphs shows a clear pattern, rather than just a random scatter of points or a horizontal line, then the two variables may be correlated or associated with each other. In R, we can use the plot_ly() or plot() functions to create scatterplots. We have to explicitly map variables to the x-axis and the y-axis. Elaborate plots we will see later will demonstrate how to use additional data features to enhance scatter plots, e.g., include labels and use color, shape, and motion to communicate multivariate associations (Fig. 2.10).

```
plot_ly(x = ~water$sanitation_facilities, y = ~water$improved_water,
    type = "scatter", mode = "markers") %>%
layout(title='Scatterplot: Improved Water Quality vs. Sanitation Facilities',
        xaxis = list (title = 'Water Quality'),
        yaxis = list (title = 'Sanitation'))
```

This scatterplot shows an increasing pattern. In later years, there is a joint increase in the water quality and sanitation improvement.

2.1.12.2   Examining Relationships—Two-Way Cross-Tabulations

The scatterplot is a useful tool to examine the relationship between two variables where at least one of them is numeric. When both variables are nominal, two-way

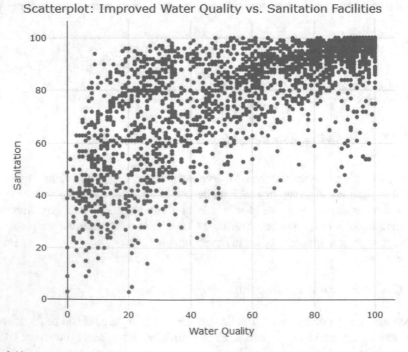

Fig. 2.10 An example of an interactive bivariate scatter plot—water quality vs. sanitation

cross-tabulation (also called crosstab or contingency table) represents a better choice of information compression. We can use the function gmodels::CrossTable (), in the package gmodels.

```
# install.packages("gmodels", repos = "http://cran.us.r-project.org")
library(gmodels)
```

Suppose we are interested in investigating the relationship between WHO region and residence area type in the water study. We might want to know if there is a difference in terms of residence area type between the African WHO region and all other WHO regions.

To address this problem, we need to create an indicator variable for the African WHO region first.

```
water$africa <- water$region == "Africa"
```

Then we can use the table() function to see how many WHO regions are in Africa.

```
table(water$africa)
## FALSE TRUE
## 2534 797
```

Now, let's create a two-way cross-tabulation using CrossTable().

```
CrossTable(x=water$residence_area, y=water$africa)
##      Cell Contents
## |-------------------------|
## |                       N |
## | Chi-square contribution |
## |           N / Row Total |
## |           N / Col Total |
## |         N / Table Total |
## |-------------------------|
## Total Observations in Table:  3331
##
##                      | water$africa
## water$residence_area |     FALSE |      TRUE | Row Total |
## --------------------|-----------|-----------|-----------|
##                Rural |       828 |       267 |      1095 |
##                      |     0.030 |     0.096 |           |
##                      |     0.756 |     0.244 |     0.329 |
##                      |     0.327 |     0.335 |           |
##                      |     0.249 |     0.080 |           |
## --------------------|-----------|-----------|-----------|
##                Total |       845 |       264 |      1109 |
##                      |     0.002 |     0.007 |           |
##                      |     0.762 |     0.238 |     0.333 |
##                      |     0.333 |     0.331 |           |
##                      |     0.254 |     0.079 |           |
## --------------------|-----------|-----------|-----------|
##                Urban |       861 |       266 |      1127 |
##                      |     0.016 |     0.050 |           |
##                      |     0.764 |     0.236 |     0.338 |
##                      |     0.340 |     0.334 |           |
##                      |     0.258 |     0.080 |           |
## --------------------|-----------|-----------|-----------|
##         Column Total |      2534 |       797 |      3331 |
##                      |     0.761 |     0.239 |           |
## --------------------|-----------|-----------|-----------|
```

Each cell in the table contains five numbers. The first one, N, gives us a count of all observations that fall into its corresponding category. The second value is the Chi-square contribution indicating the cell's contribution in the Pearson's Chi-squared test for independence between the two variables. This number measures the probability that the differences in cell counts are due to chance alone. The next two numbers, N/Row Total and N/Col Total, provide the relative counts over the row or column total, respectively. In this case, these numbers represent the distribution for residence area type among African regions and the regions in the rest of the world. We can see that for each type of residence area, these numbers are very close between African and non-African regions. Therefore, we can conclude that African WHO regions may not be dependent on the residence area types.

2.1.13   Missing Data

In the previous sections, we simply ignored the missing observations in our water dataset (na.rm = TRUE). Is this an appropriate strategy to handle incomplete data? Could the missingness pattern of those incomplete observations be important? It is possible that the arrangement of the missing observations may reflect an important factor that was not accounted for in our statistics or our models. The answer to all of these questions is—yes.

Missing Completely at Random (MCAR) is an assumption about the probability of missingness being equal for all cases; *Missing at Random (MAR)* assumes the probability of missingness has a known but random mechanism (e.g., different rates for different groups); *Missing not at Random (MNAR)* suggest a missingness mechanism linked to the values of predictors and/or response, e.g., some participants may drop out of a drug trial when they have side-effects.

There are a number of strategies to impute missing data. The expectation maximization (EM) algorithm provides one example for handling missing data.[4] The SOCR EM tutorial, activity, and documentations[5] provide the theory, applications, and practice for effective (multidimensional) EM parameter estimation. The simplest way to handle incomplete data is to substitute each missing value with its (feature or column) average. When the missingness proportion is small, the effect of substituting the means for the missing values will have little effect on the mean, variance, or other important statistics of the data. Also, this imputation process would facilitate the effective use of all observed data, even those included in rows or columns with missing entries. This figure shows a common tensor representation of data where cases (participants, records) and features (variables) are indexed in the rows and columns, respectively (Fig. 2.11).

---

[4]https://doi.org/10.1016/0167-9473(93)E0056-A

[5]https://wiki.socr.umich.edu/index.php/SOCR_EduMaterials_Activities_2D_PointSegmentation_
EM_Mixture

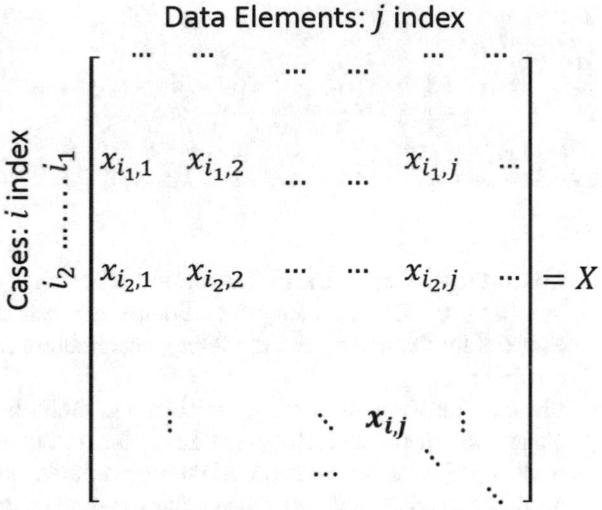

Fig. 2.11 Schematic of a common data frame representation of information

$$
\begin{array}{c}
\text{Data Elements: } j \text{ index} \\
\overset{\displaystyle \cdots \quad \cdots \qquad \cdots \quad \cdots \qquad \cdots \quad \cdots}{}
\end{array}
$$

$$
X =
\begin{bmatrix}
x_{i_1,1} & x_{i_1,2} & \cdots & \cdots & x_{i_1,j} & \cdots \\
x_{i_2,1} & x_{i_2,2} & \cdots & \cdots & x_{i_2,j} & \cdots \\
& & & & & \\
\vdots & & & \ddots & x_{i,j} & \vdots \\
& & \cdots & & & \ddots
\end{bmatrix}
= X
$$

Let's demonstrate the simplest approach of mean-value based data imputation.

```
m1<-mean(water$improved_water, na.rm = T)
m2<-mean(water$sanitation_facilities, na.rm = T)
water_imp<-water
for(i in 1:3331){
  if(is.na(water_imp$improved_water[i])){
    water_imp$improved_water[i]=m1
  }
  if(is.na(water_imp$sanitation_facilities[i])){
    water_imp$sanitation_facilities[i]=m2
  }
}
summary(water_imp) # all missing values are now imputed, the data is complete
```

A more sophisticated way of resolving missing data is to use a model (e.g., linear regression) to predict the missing feature and impute its missing values. This is called the `predictive mean matching approach`. This method is good for data with multivariate normality. However, a disadvantage of it is that it can only predict one value at a time, which is very time consuming. Also, the multivariate normality assumption might not be satisfied and there may be important multivariate relations that are not accounted for. We can use the `mi` package to demonstrate the predictive mean matching procedure.

```
# install.packages("mi")
library(mi)
```

First, we need to obtain the corresponding missing information matrix. To impute missing values in both variables (water and sanitation), we will use the imputation method pmm (predictive mean matching approach).

```
mdf <- missing_data.frame(water)
head(mdf)
show(mdf)
## Object of class missing_data.frame with 3331 observations on 7 variables
## There are 3 missing data patterns
…
mdf<-change(mdf, y="improved_water", what = "imputation_method", to="pmm")
mdf<-change(mdf,y="sanitation_facilities",what="imputation_method", to="pmm")
```

Notes

- Converting the input data.frame to a missing_data.frame allows us to include in the DF (data frame) additional metadata about each variable. This is essential for the subsequent modeling, interpretation, and imputation of the initial missing data.
- show() displays all missing variables and their class-labels (e.g., continuous), along with meta-data. The missing_data.frame constructor suggests the most appropriate classes for each missing variable, however, sometimes, we may need to correct, modify, or change these meta-data, using change().
- Use the change() function to change/correct any meta-data in the constructed missing_data.frame object.
- To get a sense of the raw data, use at the summary, image, or hist methods applied to the missing_data.frame.
- The mi (multiple imputation package) vignettes provide many useful examples of handling missing data.

Next, we will perform the initial imputation; here we imputed three times, which will create three different (complete) datasets, three *chains*, with slightly different imputed values.

```
imputations <- mi(mdf, n.iter=10, n.chains=3, verbose=T)
```

Let's extract several multiply imputed data.frames from imputations object and compare the summary statistics between the original dataset and the imputed datasets.

```
library(mi)
data.frames <- complete(imputations, 3)
summary(water)
mySummary <- lapply(data.frames, summary)
mySummary$`chain:1`    # report a summary just of the first (complete) chain
```

This is just a brief introduction for handling incomplete datasets. Later, we will discuss more about missing data with different imputation methods and show how to evaluate the complete imputed results.

2.1.13.1 Multivariate Data Simulation

Suppose we would like to generate a synthetic dataset.

$$\text{sim\_data} = \{y, x_1, x_2, x_3, x_4, x_5, x_6, x_7, x_8, x_9, x_{10}\}.$$

We can introduce a method that takes a dataset and a desired proportion of missingness and wipes out the same proportion of the data, i.e., introduces random patterns of missingness. Note that there are already R functions that automate the introduction of missingness, e.g., `missForest::prodNA()`, however writing such a method from scratch is helpful to illustrate R function definition and invocation.

```
set.seed(123)
# create MCAR missing-data generator
create.missing <- function (data, pct.mis = 10) {
    n <- nrow(data)
    J <- ncol(data)
    if (length(pct.mis) == 1) {
        if(pct.mis>=0 & pct.mis<=100) n.mis <- rep((n * (pct.mis/100)), J)
        else {
            warning("Percent missing values should be an integer between 0 and
                    100! Exiting"); break
        }
    } else {
        if (length(pct.mis) < J)
            stop("The length of the missing-vector is not equal to the
                number of columns in the data! Exiting!")
            n.mis <- n * (pct.mis/100)
    }
    for (i in 1:ncol(data)) {
        if (n.mis[i] == 0) { #if the column has no missing values, do nothing
            data[, i] <- data[, i]
        }
        else {
            data[sample(1:n, n.mis[i], replace = FALSE), i] <- NA
            # For each given column (i), sample the row indices (1:n),
            # a number of indices to replace as "missing", n.mis[i], "NA",
            # without replacement
        }
    }
    return(as.data.frame(data))
}
```

Next, let's synthetically generate (simulate) 1000 cases including all 11 features in the data ($\{y, x1, x2, x3, x4, x5, x6, x7, x8, x9, x10\}$) (Figs. 2.12, 2.13, and 2.14).

Show 10 ▼ entries   Search:

	y	x1	x2	x3	x4	x5	x6	x7	x8	x9	x10
1	1.14	0	0	0	5	d	6	1.3	4	0.51	6
2	10.43	4.01	5.24	0	2	d	8	-0.65	1	0.45	3
3	0.65	0	0	0	2	c	9	-1.04	4	0.51	5
4	11.49	5.75	6.22	0	4	b	2	0.17	5	0.13	3
5	6.53	3.49	0	0	3	f	9	2.23	1	0.45	5
6	5.77	0	4.38	1	2	b	4	-0.67	5	0.88	3
7	6.76	4.1	3.19	0	4	d	8	-1.49	5	0.5	4
8	2.24	2.93	0	1	3	i	2	-0.13	3	0.55	5
9	12.04	5.15	7.05	1	1	b	2	1.17	8	0.65	5
10	5.15	0	4.44	0	4	i	6	-0.28	9	0.75	4

Showing 1 to 10 of 1,000 entries   Previous | 1 | 2   3   4   5   ...   100   Next

Fig. 2.12 Paginated tabular form display of the raw simulated data

```
n <- 1000; u1 <- rbinom(n, 1, .5); v1 <- log(rnorm(n, 5, 1));
x1 <- u1*exp(v1)
u2 <- rbinom(n, 1, .5); v2 <- log(rnorm(n, 5, 1)); x2 <- u2*exp(v2)
x3 <- rbinom(n, 1, prob=0.45);
x4 <- ordered(rep(seq(1, 5), n)[sample(1:n, n)])
x5 <- rep(letters[1:10], n)[sample(1:n, n)]; x6 <- trunc(runif(n, 1, 10))
x7 <- rnorm(n); x8 <- factor(rep(seq(1, 10), n)[sample(1:n, n)])
x9 <- runif(n, 0.1, .99); x10 <- rpois(n, 4)
y <- x1 + x2 + x7 + x9 + rnorm(n)
# package the simulated data as a data frame object
sim_data <- cbind.data.frame(y, x1, x2, x3, x4, x5, x6, x7, x8, x9, x10)
# randomly create missing values
sim_data_30pct_missing <- create.missing(sim_data, pct.mis=30);
# head(sim_data_30pct_missing); summary(sim_data_30pct_missing)
# install.packages("DT")
library("DT")
library(dplyr)
df_raw <- sim_data %>% mutate_if(is.numeric, round, digits = 2)
datatable(df_raw)



df_miss <- sim_data_30pct_missing %>% mutate_if(is.numeric, round, digits=2)
# datatable(df_miss)
library("betareg"); library("mi")
# get show the missing information matrix
mdf <- missing_data.frame(sim_data_30pct_missing)
# show(mdf)
df_mdf <- as.data.frame(mdf) %>% mutate_if(is.numeric, round, digits = 2)
datatable(df_mdf)



# mdf@patterns   # to get the textual missing pattern
image(mdf)    # remember the visual pattern of this MCAR
```

In the missing data plot above, missing values are illustrated as black segments in the case-by-feature bivariate chart. The hot colormap represents the *normalized*

Show 10 ▼ entries   Search: [   ]

	y	x1	x2	x3	x4	x5	x6	x7	x8	x9	x10
1		0	0	0		d	6	1.3	4	0.51	6
2	10.43	4.01		2			8	-0.65			
3	0.65	0	0	0	2	c		-1.04	4		5
4	11.49	5.75		0	4		2	0.17		0.13	3
5		3.49		0		f		2.23	1	0.45	5
6	5.77		4.38	1	2	b	4	-0.67	5	0.88	3
7			3.19		4			-1.49			4
8	2.24	2.93	0	1	3	i	2	-0.13		0.55	
9	12.04	5.15			1	b	2	1.17	8		5
10		0	4.44	0	4	i	6	-0.28	9	0.75	

Showing 1 to 10 of 1,000 entries   Previous [1] 2   3   4   5   ...   100   Next

Fig. 2.13 Similarly, display in paginated tabular form all the simulated data with random missingness (30%)

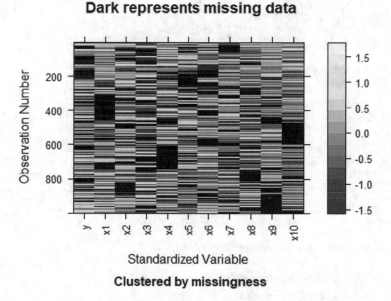

Fig. 2.14 Missing data frame plot illustrating the simulated (random) patters of missingness in the data

values of the corresponding feature-index pairs, see the mi::image() documentation. Also, test the order, cluster, and grayscale options, e.g., image(mdf, x.order = T, clustered = F, grayscale =T). In the next figure, the imputation-histogram plots display the distributions of the following:

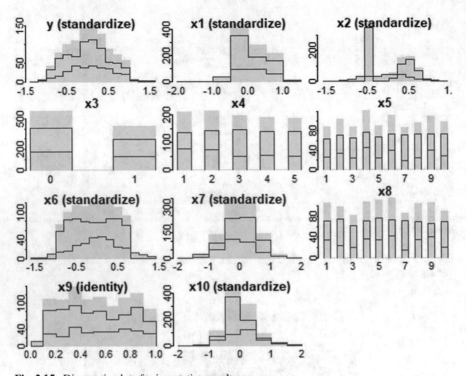

Fig. 2.15 Diagnostic plots for imputation results

Fig. 2.16 Completed data frame (imputation chain 1)

- The observed data (in *blue color*).
- The imputed data (in *red color*).
- The completed values (observed plus imputed, in *gray color*) (Figs. 2.15, 2.16, 2.17, and 2.18).

```
# Next try to impute the missing values.
par(mfcol=c(5, 5), oma=c(1,1,0,0), mar=c(1, 1, 1, 0), tcl=-0.1, mgp=c(0,0,0))
imputations <- mi(sim_data_30pct_missing, n.iter=5, n.chains=3, verbose=TRUE)
hist(imputations)
```

Show 10 ▾ entries   Search: [   ]

	V1	V2	V3	V4	V5	V6	V7
y	Min. :-3.886	1st Qu.: 2.579	Median : 5.540	Mean : 5.558	3rd Qu.: 8.278	Max. :16.526	
x1	Min. :0.000	1st Qu.:0.000	Median :0.000	Mean :2.472	3rd Qu.:4.996	Max. :8.390	
x2	Min. :0.000	1st Qu.:0.000	Median :2.687	Mean :2.516	3rd Qu.:5.007	Max. :8.421	
x3	Min. :0.000	1st Qu.:0.000	Median :0.000	Mean :0.431	3rd Qu.:1.000	Max. :1.000	
x4	1:200	2:200	3:200	4:200	5:200		
x5	Length:1000	Class :character	Mode :character				
x6	Min. :1.000	1st Qu.:3.000	Median :5.000	Mean :5.021	3rd Qu.:7.000	Max. :9.000	
x7	Min. :-3.289376	1st Qu.:-0.705687	Median : 0.020011	Mean : 0.002811	3rd Qu.: 0.761157	Max. : 3.715721	
x8	1 :100	2 :100	3 :100	4 :100	5 :100	6 :100	(Other):400
x9	Min. :0.1010	1st Qu.:0.3106	Median :0.5229	Mean :0.5350	3rd Qu.:0.7705	Max. :0.9881	

Table: summary(sim_data)

Showing 1 to 10 of 11 entries   Previous [1] 2 Next

Fig. 2.17 Summary for the original complete simulated data, all 11 variables—features (rows) by statistics (columns). Compare these with the results in the next figure

Show 10 ▾ entries   Search: [   ]

	V1	V2	V3	V4	V5	V6	V7
y	Min. :-4.404	1st Qu.: 2.670	Median : 5.545	Mean : 5.577	3rd Qu.: 8.301	Max. :16.526	
x1	Min. :-7.496	1st Qu.: 0.000	Median : 2.640	Mean : 2.603	3rd Qu.: 4.933	Max. :10.060	
x2	Min. :-5.242	1st Qu.: 0.000	Median : 2.099	Mean : 2.343	3rd Qu.: 4.751	Max. : 9.696	
x3	0:576	1:424					
x4	1:212	2:216	3:196	4:190	5:186		
x5	d :123	f :113	i :111	b :104	j :99	h : 97	(Other):353
x6	Min. :-2.707	1st Qu.: 3.000	Median : 5.000	Mean : 5.074	3rd Qu.: 7.000	Max. :12.057	
x7	Min. :-3.448821	1st Qu.:-0.671623	Median :-0.002201	Mean : 0.013433	3rd Qu.: 0.760535	Max. : 3.715721	
x8	6 :114	5 :111	4 :107	1 :106	9 :106	8 :103	(Other):353
x9	Min. :0.0001195	1st Qu.:0.3154341	Median :0.5177864	Mean :0.5328167	3rd Qu.:0.7672840	Max. :0.9940970	

Table: Imputed data: summary(chain:1)

Showing 1 to 10 of 22 entries   Previous [1] 2 3 Next

Fig. 2.18 Summary for the complete imputed (chain 1) data, all 11 variables—features (rows) by statistics (columns). Compare with the previous figure

```
# Extracts several multiply imputed data.frames from "imputations" object
data.frames <- complete(imputations, 3)
# compare the 3 objects, sim_data, sim_data_30pct_missing, and imputed chain1
df_miss <- sim_data_30pct_missing %>% mutate_if(is.numeric, round, digits=2)
datatable(df_miss, caption = htmltools::tags$caption(
    style = 'caption-side: bottom; text-align: center;',
    'Table: Initial sim_data'))
df_miss30pct <- sim_data_30pct_missing %>% mutate_if(is.numeric, round, digits=2)
datatable(df_miss30pct, caption = htmltools::tags$caption(
    style = 'caption-side: bottom; text-align: center;',
    'Table: sim_data 30% Missing'))
df_chain1 <- data.frames[[1]] %>% mutate_if(is.numeric, round, digits = 2)
datatable(df_chain1, caption = htmltools::tags$caption(
    style = 'caption-side: bottom; text-align: center;',
    'Table: Imputed data (chain 1)'))



# Compare the summary stats for the original data (prior to introducing
# missing values) with the corresponding missing data and
# completed data following imputation; # summary(sim_data)
datatable(data.frame(t(as.matrix(unclass(summary(sim_data))))), check.names =
    FALSE, stringsAsFactors = FALSE), caption = htmltools::tags$caption(
    style = 'caption-side: bottom; text-align: center;',
    'Table: summary(sim_data)'))



mySummary <- lapply(data.frames, summary)
datatable(data.frame(t(as.matrix(unclass(mySummary$`chain:1`)))), check.names=
    FALSE, stringsAsFactors = FALSE), caption = htmltools::tags$caption(
    style = 'caption-side: bottom; text-align: center;',
    'Table: Imputed data: summary(chain:1)'))
```

Let's check imputation convergence (details about convergence are provided below) (Fig. 2.19).

```
round(mipply(imputations, mean, to.matrix = TRUE), 3)
##              chain:1 chain:2 chain:3
## y             0.019   0.007   0.003
...
## missing_x10   0.300   0.300   0.300
Rhats(imputations, statistic="moments") #assess convergence of MI algorithm
##    mean_y    mean_x1    mean_x2    mean_x3    mean_x4    mean_x5    mean_x6    mean_x7
## 0.9661786 1.4349386 0.9083078 1.0909295 1.1222969 1.2982907 0.9806005 1.2013352
##    mean_x8    mean_x9   mean_x10       sd_y      sd_x1      sd_x2      sd_x3      sd_x4
## 0.9481337 1.5214104 1.1266608 0.9771095 1.9613922 1.0471710 1.0859335 0.9251055
##      sd_x5      sd_x6      sd_x7      sd_x8      sd_x9     sd_x10
## 1.3561015 0.9728600 1.2984525 1.1219111 1.1004689 1.1841799
plot(imputations); hist(imputations); image(imputations); summary(imputations)
```

Figure 2.20 shows the missingness pattern in the initial data (top) and the complete imputed.

After we first fit linear models to each chain, we can pool over and estimate an aggregate model over all completed chains ($m = 3$). As opposed to first pooling (averaging) the data across the chains and then computing a single linear model, the strategy of using the aggregate pooled model across the three chains is preferred as it generates more robust models and tighter parameter estimates (Fig. 2.21).

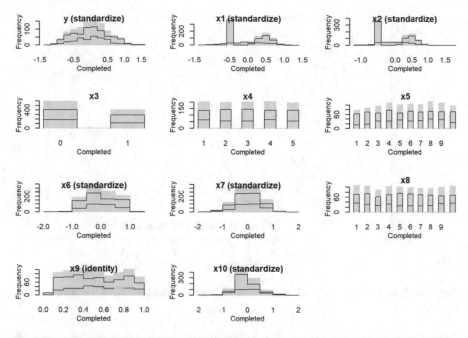

Fig. 2.19 For each imputation chain (there are three chains in this experiment) and all 11 variables plots of the distributions of the initial data (with missing values, blue), the synthetically imputed values alone (red), and the completed chain data (gray)

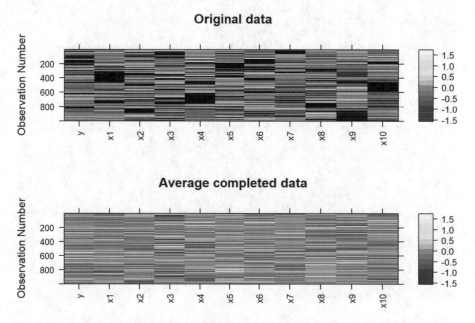

Fig. 2.20 Imputed chain-averaged complete data (bottom) compared to the initial data including 30% missingness (black areas on top). Color intensity saturation reflects the chance of missingness

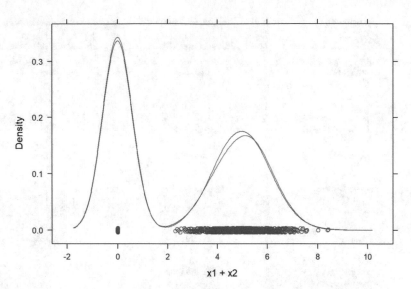

Fig. 2.21 Kernel densities of the first two covariate predictors estimated using the three chains of the imputed data

```
model_results <- pool(y~x1+x2+x3+x4+x5+x6+x7+x8+x9+x10, data=imputations,m=3)
## x1          0.950011   0.020957   45.332   < 2e-16 ***
## x2          0.926894   0.037807   24.516 4.54e-05 ***
...
## x10         0.081110   0.039087    2.075   0.0915 .
# Report the summaries of the imputations
data.frames <- complete(imputations, 3)    # extract the first 3 chains
mySummary <-lapply(data.frames, summary)
datatable(data.frame(t(as.matrix(unclass(mySummary$`chain:1`)))),
        check.names = FALSE, stringsAsFactors = FALSE),
        caption = htmltools::tags$caption(
            style = 'caption-side: bottom; text-align: center;',
            'Table: Imputed data: summary(chain:1)'))
datatable(data.frame(t(as.matrix(unclass(mySummary$`chain:2`)))),
        check.names = FALSE, stringsAsFactors = FALSE),
        caption = htmltools::tags$caption(
            style = 'caption-side: bottom; text-align: center;',
            'Table: Imputed data: summary(chain:2)'))
datatable(data.frame(t(as.matrix(unclass(mySummary$`chain:3`)))),
        check.names = FALSE, stringsAsFactors = FALSE),
        caption = htmltools::tags$caption(
            style = 'caption-side: bottom; text-align: center;',
            'Table: Imputed data: summary(chain:3)'))
coef(summary(model_results))[, 1:2] #report model coefficients & their SE's
##              Estimate Std. Error
## (Intercept) 0.093782649 0.36706499
## x1          0.950010616 0.02095653
...
## x10         0.081110499 0.03908680
library("lattice")
densityplot(y ~ x1 + x2, data=imputations)
```

Notes

- In general, it is recommended to generate multiple imputation chains and then analyze the data (e.g., estimate the model coefficients, obtain inference, compute likelihoods, etc.). *Pooling* the analytics across all chains accounts for between-chain as well as within-chain variability, cf. Rubin's rule.[6]
- When deciding on how many chains to compute, a general rule is to compute m chains if the rate of incomplete cases in the dataset is about $m\%$, i.e., 10-chains when 10% of cases are missing, see Royston and White.[7]
- For categorical features, e.g., binary predictors like x_3, the *display()* and *summary ()* functions will report coefficient estimates for each (category) level, relative to the base level.

2.1.13.2   TBI Data Example

Next, we will see a real example using the traumatic brain injury (TBI) dataset. More information about the clinical assessment scores (e.g., EGOS, GCS) is available in this publication[8] (Figs. 2.22, 2.23, 2.24, 2.25, 2.26, and 2.27).

```
# 1. Load the (raw) data "08_EpiBioSData_Incomplete.csv"
TBI_Data <-
    read.csv("https://umich.instructure.com/files/720782/download?download_frd=1",
        na.strings=c("", ".", "NA"))
summary(TBI_Data) # report a data summary matrix
# 2. create an object of class "missing_data.frame" from TBI_data data.frame
# Convert to a missing_data.frame # library("betareg"); library("mi")
mdf <- missing_data.frame(TBI_Data)
datatable(mdf)
```

image(mdf)

id	age	sex	mechanism	field.gcs	er.gcs	icu.gcs	worst.gcs	X6m.gose	X2013.gose	skull.fx	temp.injury	surgery	spikes.hr	min.hr	max.hr	acute.sz	late.sz	ever.sz
1	1	19	Male	Fall	10	10	10	10	5	5	0	1	1				1	1	1
2	2	55	Male	Blunt		3	3	3	5	7	1	1	1	168.74	14	757	0	1	1
3	3	24	Male	Fall	12	12	8	8	7	7	1	0	0	37.37	0	351	0	0	0
4	4	57	Female	Fall	4	4	6	4	3	3	1	1	1	4.35	0	59	0	0	0
5	5	54	Female	Peds_vs_Auto	14	11	8	8	5	7	0	1	1	54.59	0	284	0	0	0
6	6	16	Female	MVA	13	7	7	7	7	8	1	1	1	75.92	7	180	0	1	1
7	7	21	Male	Fall	3	3	6	3	3	3	1	0	1				0	0	0
8	8	25	Male	Fall	3	4	3	3	3	3	0	1	0	5.26	0	88	0	1	1
9	9	30	Male	GSW	3	9	3	3	3	5	1	1	1	43.88	0	367	0	1	1
10	10	38	Male	Fall	3	6	6	3	3	3	1	1	1	45.6	4	107	0	1	1

Show 10 entries   Search:

Showing 1 to 10 of 46 entries   Previous 1 2 3 4 5 Next

Fig. 2.22 Summary for the raw TBI data—participants/cases (rows) by features (columns)

---

[6] https://dx.doi.org/10.1186%2F1471-2288-9-57
[7] https://doi.org/10.18637/jss.v045.i04
[8] https://doi.org/10.1080/02699050701727460

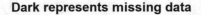

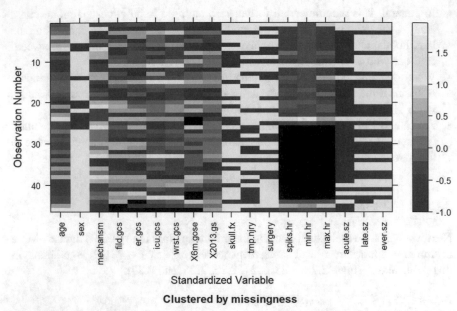

Fig. 2.23 The missing pattern in the TBI data suggests missingness is not at random

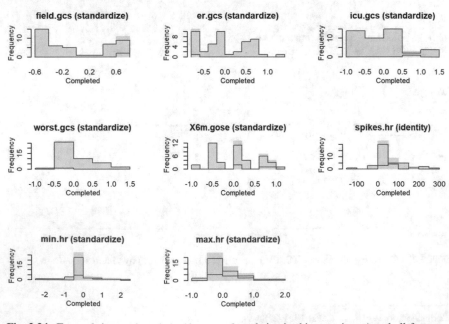

Fig. 2.24 For each imputation chain (there are five chains in this experiment) and all features, display the distributions of the initial data (with missing values, blue), the synthetically imputed values alone (red), and the completed chain data (gray)

Copy CSV PDF Print   Search:

	V1	V2	V3	V4	V5	V6	V7
id	Min. : 1.00	1st Qu.:12.25	Median :23.50	Mean :23.50	3rd Qu.:34.75	Max. :46.00	
age	Min. :16.00	1st Qu.:23.00	Median :33.00	Mean :36.89	3rd Qu.:47.25	Max. :83.00	
sex	Female: 9	Male :37					
mechanism	Bike_vs_Auto: 4	Blunt : 4	Fall :13	GSW : 2	MCA : 7	MVA :10	Peds_vs_Auto: 6
field.gcs	Min. :-4.217	1st Qu.: 3.000	Median : 7.000	Mean : 7.931	3rd Qu.:12.000	Max. :17.050	
er.gcs	Min. : 1.856	1st Qu.: 4.000	Median : 7.500	Mean : 8.403	3rd Qu.:12.750	Max. :24.700	
icu.gcs	Min. : 0.000	1st Qu.: 3.000	Median : 6.000	Mean : 6.363	3rd Qu.: 7.750	Max. :14.000	
worst.gcs	Min. : 0.000	1st Qu.: 3.000	Median : 3.000	Mean : 5.345	3rd Qu.: 7.000	Max. :14.000	
X6m.gose	Min. :0.4583	1st Qu.:3.0000	Median :5.0000	Mean :4.6999	3rd Qu.:6.0000	Max. :8.0000	
X2013.gose	Min. :2.000	1st Qu.:5.000	Median :7.000	Mean :5.804	3rd Qu.:7.000	Max. :8.000	

Table: Imputed data: summary(chain:1)

Showing 1 to 10 of 27 entries   Previous 1 2 3 Next

Fig. 2.25 Summary for the complete imputed (chain 1) data, all variables—features (rows) by statistics (columns)

Copy CSV PDF Print   Search:

	V1	V2	V3	V4	V5	V6	V7
id	Min. : 1.00	1st Qu.:12.25	Median :23.50	Mean :23.50	3rd Qu.:34.75	Max. :46.00	
age	Min. :16.00	1st Qu.:23.00	Median :33.00	Mean :36.89	3rd Qu.:47.25	Max. :83.00	
sex	Female: 9	Male :37					
mechanism	Bike_vs_Auto: 4	Blunt : 4	Fall :13	GSW : 2	MCA : 7	MVA :10	Peds_vs_Auto: 6
field.gcs	Min. : 3.000	1st Qu.: 3.250	Median : 7.000	Mean : 8.588	3rd Qu.:12.750	Max. :27.460	
er.gcs	Min. : 0.950	1st Qu.: 4.000	Median : 7.500	Mean : 8.064	3rd Qu.:12.000	Max. :15.000	
icu.gcs	Min. : 0.000	1st Qu.: 3.000	Median : 6.000	Mean : 6.535	3rd Qu.: 8.000	Max. :14.000	
worst.gcs	Min. : 0.000	1st Qu.: 3.000	Median : 3.000	Mean : 5.318	3rd Qu.: 7.000	Max. :14.000	
X6m.gose	Min. :-1.896	1st Qu.: 3.000	Median : 5.000	Mean : 4.578	3rd Qu.: 6.000	Max. : 8.000	
X2013.gose	Min. :2.000	1st Qu.:5.000	Median :7.000	Mean :5.804	3rd Qu.:7.000	Max. :8.000	

Table: Imputed data: summary(chain:5)

Showing 1 to 10 of 27 entries   Previous 1 2 3 Next

Fig. 2.26 Summary for the complete imputed (chain 5) data, all variables—features (rows) by statistics (columns). Compare to the statistics for chain 1 in the previous figure

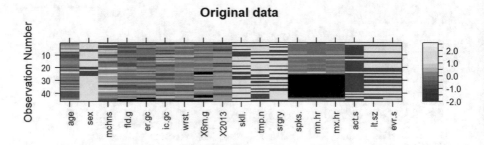

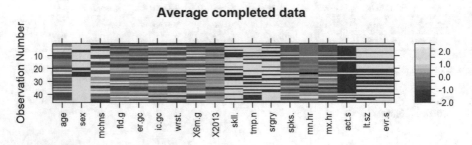

Fig. 2.27 Missing patterns in the raw and imputed TBI data

```
# 3. get description of the "family", "imputation_method", "size",
#    "transformation", "type", "link", or "model" of each incomplete variable
# show(mdf)
# 4. optional changes: mi::change() method changes the family, imputation
# method, size, type, and so forth of a missing variable. It's called
# before calling mi to affect how the conditional expectation of each
# missing variable is modeled.
mdf <- change(mdf, y = "spikes.hr", what = "transformation", to = "identity")
# The "to" choices include "identity" = no transformation, "standardize" =
standardization, "log" = natural logarithm transformation, "logshift" = log(y +
a) transformation, where a is a small constant, or "sqrt" = square-root variable
transformation. Changing the transformation will correspondingly change the
inverse transformation.
# 5. examine missingness patterns
summary(mdf); hist(mdf);
image(mdf)
# 6. Perform initial imputation
imputations1 <- mi(mdf, n.iter=10, n.chains=5, verbose=TRUE)
hist(imputations1)


# 7. Extract several multiply imputed data.frames from "imputations" object
data.frames1 <- complete(imputations1, 5)
# 8. Report a list of "summaries" for each element (imputation instance)
mySummary1 <- lapply(data.frames1, summary)
datatable(data.frame(t(as.matrix(unclass(mySummary1$`chain:1`)))),
    check.names = FALSE, stringsAsFactors = FALSE),
    caption = htmltools::tags$caption(
                style = 'caption-side: bottom; text-align: center;',
                'Table: Imputed data: summary(chain:1)'),
    extensions = 'Buttons', options = list(dom = 'Bfrtip',
    buttons = c('copy', 'csv', 'excel', 'pdf', 'print')))
```

```
datatable(data.frame(t(as.matrix(unclass(mySummary1$`chain:5`)))),
    check.names = FALSE, stringsAsFactors = FALSE),
    caption = htmltools::tags$caption(
    style = 'caption-side: bottom; text-align: center;',
    'Table: Imputed data: summary(chain:5)'),
    extensions = 'Buttons', options = list(dom = 'Bfrtip',
    buttons = c('copy', 'csv', 'excel', 'pdf', 'print')))
```

The *Rhat* convergence statistic $\left(\widehat{R}\right)$ compares the variance between chains to the variance within chains (similar to the ANOVA F-test). Classical Rhat interpretation suggests likely algorithmic convergence and stable complete chain results when $\widehat{R} \sim 1.0$, whereas $\widehat{R} \geq 1.2$ indicates that the chains should be run longer (use a large number of iterations) to reduce this statistic and improve the imputation results.

```
# 8.a. Cast imputed values as integers (not necessary, but may be useful)
indx <- sapply(data.frames1[[5]], is.numeric) #get indices of numeric columns
data.frames1[[5]][indx] <- lapply(data.frames1[[5]][indx], function(x)
as.numeric(as.integer(x)))           # cast each value as integer
# 9. Save results out
write.csv(data.frames1[[5]], "/path/TBI_MIData.csv")
# 10. Complete Data analytics, glmer.mi()
# 10.a Define LM Regression for multiply imputed dataset - also see Step (12)
## Linear regression for each imputed data set - 5 regression models are fit
fit_lm1 <- glm(ever.sz ~ surgery + worst.gcs + factor(sex) + age,
        data.frames1$`chain:1`, family = "binomial"); summary(fit_lm1);
display(fit_lm1)
# Fit the appropriate model and pool the results (estimates over MI chains)
model_results <- pool(ever.sz ~ surgery + worst.gcs + factor(sex) + age,
        family = "binomial", data=imputations1, m=5)
display (model_results); summary (model_results)
# Report the summaries of the imputations
data.frames <- complete(imputations1, 3)    # extract the first 3 chains
mySummary2 <- lapply(data.frames1, summary)
datatable(data.frame(t(as.matrix(unclass(mySummary2$`chain:1`)))),
        check.names = FALSE, stringsAsFactors = FALSE),
        caption = htmltools::tags$caption(
                style = 'caption-side: bottom; text-align: center;',
        'Table: Imputed data: summary(chain:1)'))
# 11. Validation: we now verify whether enough iterations were conducted.
# Validation criteria demands that the mean of each completed variable should
# be similar for each of the k chains (in this case k=5).
# mipply, a wrapper for sapply, for mi-class objects to compute the col means
round(mipply(imputations1, mean, to.matrix = TRUE), 3)
##                 chain:1 chain:2 chain:3 chain:4 chain:5
## age               0.000   0.000   0.000   0.000   0.000
## field.gcs        -0.008   0.029   0.069   0.007   0.065
...
## missing_max.hr    0.391   0.391   0.391   0.391   0.391
Rhats(imputations1, statistic="moments") # assess the convergence of MI algo
## mean_spikes.hr    mean_min.hr    mean_max.hr   sd_field.gcs    sd_er.gcs
##       1.920792       1.239771       1.984058       1.256564     1.276851
##     sd_icu.gcs   sd_worst.gcs   sd_X6m.gose    sd_spikes.hr     sd_min.hr
##       1.719536       2.938691       1.270407       2.030317     1.101942
# When convergence is unstable, we can continue the iterations for all chains
imputations1 <- mi(imputations1, n.iter=20) # add additional 20 iterations
# To plot the produced mi results, for all missing_variables we can generate
# a histogram of the observed, imputed, and completed data.
# We can compare of the completed data to the fitted model prediction values
```

```
# by plotting binned residuals. The hist() function works similarly as plot.
# image function gives a sense of the missingness patterns in the data
plot(imputations1); hist(imputations1); image(imputations1)
mySummary3 <-lapply(data.frames1, summary)
datatable(data.frame(t(as.matrix(unclass(mySummary3$`chain:1`)))),
    check.names = FALSE, stringsAsFactors = FALSE),
    caption = htmltools::tags$caption(
                    style = 'caption-side: bottom; text-align: center;',
                    'Table: Imputed data: summary(chain:1)'))
# 12. Finally, pool over the m=5 imputed datasets when we fit the "model"
# Pool from across the 5 chains, estimate a linear regression model, and
# quantify the impact of various predictors
model_results <- pool(ever.sz ~ surgery + worst.gcs + factor(sex) + age,
    data=imputations1, m=5); display(model_results); summary(model_results)
## Coefficients:
##                   Estimate Std. Error z value Pr(>|z|)
## (Intercept)       0.385385   1.265384   0.305   0.761
## surgery1          0.898961   0.649900   1.383   0.167
## worst.gcs        -0.080708   0.095915  -0.841   0.400
## factor(sex)Male  -0.309840   0.760390  -0.407   0.684
## age               0.002677   0.018080   0.148   0.882
```

2.1.13.3 Imputation via Expectation–Maximization

Below we present the theory and practice of one specific statistical computing
strategy for imputing incomplete datasets, which relies on estimation using expectation maximization.

2.1.13.3.1 Types of Missing Data

- *MCAR*: Data which is Missing Completely At Random has nothing systematic
  about which observations are missing. There is no relationship between
  missingness and either observed or unobserved covariates.
- *MAR*: Missing At Random is weaker than MCAR. The missingness is still
  random, but solely due to the observed variables. For example, those from a
  lower socioeconomic status (SES) may be less willing to provide salary information (but we know their SES). The key is that the missingness is not due to the
  values which are not observed. MCAR implies MAR, but not vice-versa.
- *MNAR*: If the data are Missing Not At Random, then the missingness depends on
  the values of the missing data. Examples include censored data, self-reported data
  for individuals who are heavier, who are less likely to report their weight, and
  response-measuring devices that can only measure values above 0.5, anything
  below that is missing.

2.1.13.3.2   General Idea of the EM Algorithm

Expectation–Maximization (EM)[9,10] is an iterative process involving two steps—
expectation and *maximization*, which are applied in tandem. EM can be employed to
find parameter estimates using maximum likelihood and is specifically useful when
the equations determining the relations of the data-parameters cannot be directly
solved. For example, a Gaussian mixture modeling assumes that each data point (X)
has a corresponding latent (unobserved) variable or a missing value (Y), which may
be specified as a mixture of coefficients determining the affinity of the data as a linear
combination of Gaussian kernels, determined by a set of parameters (θ), e.g., means
and variance-covariances. Thus, EM estimation relies on the following:

- An observed data set X.
- A set of missing (or latent) values Y.
- A parameter θ, which may be a vector of parameters.
- A likelihood function $L(\theta|X, Y) = p(X, Y|\theta)$.
- The maximum likelihood estimate (MLE) of the unknown parameter(s) θ that is
  computed using the marginal likelihood of the observed data:

$$L(\theta|X) = p(X|\theta) = \int p(X, Y|\theta)dY.$$

Most of the time, this equation may not be directly solved, e.g., when Y is
missing.

- *Expectation step (E step)*: computes the expected value of the *log likelihood
  function*, with respect to the conditional distribution of Y given X using the
  parameter estimates at the previous iteration (or at the position of initialization,
  for the first iteration), θ_t:

$$Q\left(\theta|\theta^{(t)}\right) = E_{Y|X,\theta^{(t)}}[\log(L(\theta|X, Y)]];$$

- *Maximization step (M step)*: Determine the parameter, θ, that maximizes the
  expectation above,

$$\theta^{(t+1)} = \arg\max_{\theta} Q\left(\theta|\theta^{(t)}\right).$$

---

[9] http://repositories.cdlib.org/socr/EM_MM
[10] https://doi.org/10.1109/79.543975

This SOCR EM Activity[11] shows the practical aspects of applying the EM algorithm. Also, in Chap. 3, we will illustrate the EM method for fitting single *distribution models* or (linear) *mixtures of distributions* to data that may represent a blend of heterogeneous observations from multiple different processes.

2.1.13.3.3   EM-Based Imputation

The EM algorithm is an alternative to Newton–Raphson (Chap. 13) or the method of scoring for computing MLE in cases where there are complications in calculating the MLE. It is applicable for imputing incomplete MAR data, where the missing data mechanism can be ignored and separate parameters may be estimated for each missing feature.

Complete Data:

$$Z = \begin{pmatrix} X \\ Y \end{pmatrix}, ZZ^T = \begin{pmatrix} XX^T & XY^T \\ YX^T & YY^T \end{pmatrix},$$

where X is the observed data and Y is the missing data.

- *E-step*: (Expectation) Get the expectations of Y and YY^T based on observed data, X.
- *M-step*: (Maximization) Maximize the conditional expectation in E-step to estimate the parameters.

Details If $o = $ obs and $m = $ mis stand for observed and missing, then the mean vector, $(\mu_{obs}, \mu_{mis})^T$, and the variance-covariance matrix, $\Sigma^{(t)} = \begin{pmatrix} \Sigma_{oo} & \Sigma_{om} \\ \Sigma_{mo} & \Sigma_{mm} \end{pmatrix}$, are represented by:

$$\mu^{(t)} = \begin{pmatrix} \mu_{obs} \\ \mu_{mis} \end{pmatrix}, \quad \Sigma^{(t)} = \begin{pmatrix} \Sigma_{oo} & \Sigma_{om} \\ \Sigma_{mo} & \Sigma_{mm.} \end{pmatrix}$$

---

[11] https://wiki.socr.umich.edu/index.php/SOCR_EduMaterials_Activities_2D_PointSegmentation_EM_Mixture

E-step:

$$E(Z|X) = \begin{pmatrix} X \\ E(Y|X) \end{pmatrix}, \quad E(ZZ^T|X) = \begin{pmatrix} XX^T & XE(Y|X)^T \\ E(Y|X)X^T & E(YY^T|X) \end{pmatrix}.$$

$$E(Y|X) = \mu_{\text{mis}} + \Sigma_{\text{mo}}\Sigma_{\text{oo}}^{-1}(X - \mu_{\text{obs}}).$$

$$E(YY^T|X) = \left(\Sigma_{\text{mm}} - \Sigma_{\text{mo}}\Sigma_{\text{oo}}^{-1}\Sigma_{\text{om}}\right) + E(Y|X)E(Y|X)^T.$$

M-step:

$$\mu^{(t+1)} = \frac{1}{n}\sum_{i=1}^{n} E(Z|X).$$

$$\Sigma^{(t+1)} = \frac{1}{n}\sum_{i=1}^{n} E(ZZ^T|X) - \mu^{(t+1)}\mu^{(t+1)^T}.$$

2.1.13.3.4 Manual Implementation of EM-Based Imputation

Below is a simple EM implementation demonstrating parameter estimation and missing data imputation using the above analytical representation, which will be tested using multivariate Normal distribution simulated data with 20 features and 200 cases (Figs. 2.28 and 2.29).

	Copy	CSV	PDF	Print														Search:		

	X1	X2	X3	X4	X5	X6	X7	X8	X9	X10	X11	X12	X13	X14	X15	X16	X17	X18	X19	X20
1		4.85	1.73	4.64	4.55	2.17	4.71	2.7	2.79	-0.93		5.56	6.15	2.21	0.11	1.09	8.43	2.1	3.63	-1.15
2	1.77	-1.7	0.42	6.26	-3.13	-1.8	1.29	0.99	1.08	1.16	6.29	-0.37	0.68	-1.69	4.5	3.48	-0.23	2.39	-0.02	
3	2.29	4.27	3.89	3.51	3	3.91	3.05	3.53		1.36	-1.18	6.02	1.1	4.32	-5.06	2.98		1.51	2.81	-3.57
4		6.93			-2.09	-0.88	5.65	1.33	0.65	4.71	6.37	-2.67	-5.04	4.56	11.13	3.31	-0.92	-4.43	3.92	
5	-0.03	2.31	0.73	1.25	-0.21	1.17	1.46	0.65	0.15	7.22		-0.7	5.95	3.71	6.11		8.22	-3.6	3.38	-1.13
6	1.94	3.66	6.3	0.35	1.09	1.31	0.03	-0.01		2.46	-1.88	10.45	-1.23	1.62	5.17	-1.07	6.67	6.28	1.03	9.85
7	0.52	4.22		4.37	5.71	0.47	4.58	0.25	-0.98	-2.62	1.24	0.02		-3.52	1.25	4.86	2.09	-2.01	0.66	3.4
8	3.31	0.12	0.98	4.78	4.98	-0.04	-0.32	4.36	2.75	3.77	2.37	0.37	1.19	-1.84	1.35		-7.08	-1.9	6.19	5.51
9	2.11			3.68	3.78	5.55	1.86	0.16	4.67		-2.8	1.65	2.27	-1.9	1.08	6.32	-0.22			-3.05
10	1.62	3.24	1.36	1.4	-1.35		3.17	-3.43	0.22	-2.29	7.02	5.12	-3.07	2.2	-4.67	-0.29	1.7	5.09	4.27	3.88

Table: Simulated Data (sim_data.df)

Showing 1 to 10 of 200 entries   Previous 1 2 3 4 5 ... 20 Next

Fig. 2.28 A snapshot of the initial (incomplete) data

Copy	CSV	PDF	Print												Search:				

	X1	X2	X3	X4	X5	X6	X7	X8	X9	X10	X11	X12	X13	X14	X15	X16	X17	X18	X19	X20
1	2.06	4.85	1.73	4.64	4.55	2.17	4.71	2.7	2.79	-0.93	10.04	5.56	6.15	2.21	0.11	1.09	8.43	2.1	3.63	-1.15
2	1.77	-1.7	0.42	6.26	-3.13	-1.8	1.29	0.99	1.08	1.16	6.29	-0.37	0.68	-1.69	4.5	3.48	-0.23	2.39	-0.02	5.03
3	2.29	4.27	3.89	3.51	3	3.91	3.05	3.53	1.09	1.36	-1.18	6.02	1.1	4.32	-5.06	2.98	-44.01	1.51	2.81	-3.57
4	2.17	6.93	-3.5	1.8	9.68	-2.09	-0.88	5.65	1.33	-0.65	4.71	6.37	-2.67	-5.04	4.56	11.13	3.31	-0.92	-4.43	3.92
5	-0.03	2.31	0.73	1.25	-0.21	1.17	1.46	0.65	0.15	7.22	0.75	-0.7	5.95	3.71	6.11	4.38	8.22	-3.6	3.38	-1.13
6	1.94	3.66	6.3	0.35	1.09	1.31	0.03	-0.01	4.32	2.46	-1.88	10.45	-1.23	1.62	5.17	-1.07	6.67	6.28	1.03	9.85
7	0.52	4.22	-10.03	4.37	5.71	0.47	4.58	0.25	-0.98	-2.62	1.24	0.02	2.35	-3.52	1.25	4.86	2.09	-2.01	0.66	3.4
8	3.31	0.12	0.98	4.78	4.98	-0.04	-0.32	4.36	2.75	3.77	2.37	0.37	1.19	-1.84	1.35	-1.81	-7.08	-1.9	6.19	5.51
9	2.11	5.84	-9.84	3.68	3.78	5.55	1.86	0.16	4.67	2.94	-2.8	1.65	2.27	-1.9	1.08	6.32	-0.22	0.33	0.97	-3.05
10	1.62	3.24	1.36	1.4	-1.35	4	3.17	-3.43	0.22	-2.29	7.02	5.12	-3.07	2.2	-4.67	-0.29	1.7	5.09	4.27	3.88

Table: EM-Imputed Simulated Data

Showing 1 to 10 of 200 entries　　　　　　　　　　Previous　1　2　3　4　5　...　20　Next

Fig. 2.29 A snapshot of the imputed (complete) data

```r
# install.packages(c("gridExtra", "MASS"))
library(ggplot2); library(gridExtra); library(MASS); library(knitr)
# You can choose multiple distribution for testing
# sim_data <- replicate(20, rpois(50, 10))
set.seed(202227)
mu <- as.matrix(rep(2,20))
sig <- diag(c(1:20) )
# Add noise \epsilon ~ MVN(as.matrix(rep(0,20)), diag(rep(1,20)))
sim_data <- mvrnorm(n = 200, mu, sig) +
                mvrnorm(n=200, as.matrix(rep(0,20)), diag( rep(1,20) ))
# save these in the "original" object
sim_data.orig <- sim_data
# install.packages("e1071")
# introduce 500 random missing indices (in the total of 4000=200*20)
# discrete distribution where the probability of the elements of values is
proportional to probs, which are normalized to add up to 1.
rand.miss <- e1071::rdiscrete(500, probs = rep(1,length(sim_data)),
                values = seq(1, length(sim_data)))
sim_data[rand.miss] <- NA
sum(is.na(sim_data))  # check now many missing (NA) are there < 500
# cast the data into a data.frame object and report 15*10 elements
sim_data.df <- data.frame(sim_data)
df_mdf <- sim_data.df %>% mutate_if(is.numeric, round, digits = 2)
datatable(df_mdf, caption = htmltools::tags$caption(
            style = 'caption-side: bottom; text-align: center;',
            'Table: Simulated Data (sim_data.df)'),
            extensions = 'Buttons', options = list(dom = 'Bfrtip',
            buttons = c('copy', 'csv', 'excel', 'pdf', 'print')))
```

```r
# Define the EM imputation method using the above analytical formulation
EM_algorithm <- function(x, tol = 0.001) {
  # identify the missing data entries (Boolean indices)
  missvals <- is.na(x)
  # instantiate the EM-iteration
  new.impute <- x
  old.impute <- x
  count.iter <- 1
  reach.tol  <- 0
  # compute \Sigma using complete data
  sigma <- as.matrix(var(na.exclude(x)))
  # compute the vector of feature (column) means
  mean.vec <- as.matrix(apply(na.exclude(x), 2, mean))
  # repeat until reaching convergence or meeting stopping criterion
  while (reach.tol != 1) {
    for (i in 1:nrow(x)) {
      pick.miss <- (c(missvals[i, ]))
      if (sum(pick.miss) != 0) {
        # compute inverse-Sigma_completeData, variance-covariance matrix
        inv.S <- solve(sigma[!pick.miss, !pick.miss], tol = 1e-40)
        # Expectation Step
        # $$E(Y/X)=\mu_{mis}+\Sigma_{mo}\Sigma_{oo}^{-1}(X-\mu_{obs})$$
        new.impute[i, pick.miss] <- mean.vec[pick.miss] +
          sigma[pick.miss,!pick.miss] %*% inv.S %*%
          (t(new.impute[i, !pick.miss]) - t(t(mean.vec[!pick.miss])))
      }
    }
    # Maximization Step
    # Recompute \Sigma and vector of feature (column) means
    # \Sigma^{(t+1)} = \frac{1}{n}\sum_{1=1}^nE(ZZ^T|X) -
    #         \mu^{(t+1)}{\mu^{(t+1)}}^T
    sigma <- var((new.impute))
       # \mu^{(t+1)} - \frac{1}{n}\sum_{i=1}^nE(Z|X)
    mean.vec <- as.matrix(apply(new.impute, 2, mean))
    # starting with the 2nd iteration, inspect for convergence (tolerance)
    if (count.iter > 1) {
      for (l in 1:nrow(new.impute)) {
        for (m in 1:ncol(new.impute)) {
          if (abs((old.impute[l, m]-new.impute[l, m]))>tol) { reach.tol<-0 }
          else {  reach.tol <- 1    }
        }
      }
    }
    count.iter <- count.iter + 1
    old.impute <- new.impute
  }
  # return the imputation output of current iteration that passed tolerance
  return(new.impute)
}
# call method EM_algorithm() and report complete data
sim_data.imputed <- EM_algorithm(sim_data.df, tol=0.0001)
df_mdf <- sim_data.imputed %>% mutate_if(is.numeric, round, digits = 2)
datatable(df_mdf, caption = htmltools::tags$caption(
                style = 'caption-side: bottom; text-align: center;',
                'Table: EM-Imputed Simulated Data'),
                extensions = 'Buttons', options = list(dom = 'Bfrtip',
                buttons = c('copy', 'csv', 'excel', 'pdf', 'print')))
```

2.1.13.3.5   Plotting the Complete and Imputed Data

Next, we will visually render the observed and the EM synthetically generated imputed values. Smaller *black* points represent the observed data, whereas circle-shapes colored in *magenta* denote the EM-imputed data (Fig. 2.30).

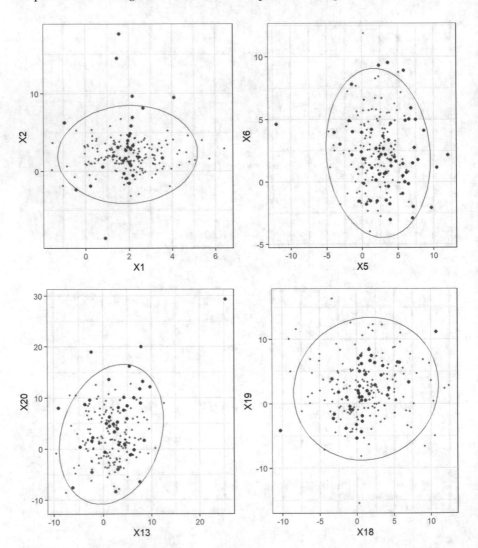

Fig. 2.30 Bivariate cross-sectional plots of four pairs of variables contrasting the EM synthetically imputed data (*magenta* color) against the observed (incomplete) data (*black*)

```
plot.me <- function(index1, index2){
  plot.imputed <- sim_data.imputed[row.names(
    subset(sim_data.df, is.na(sim_data.df[, index1]) |
        is.na(sim_data.df[, index2]))), ]
p=ggplot(sim_data.imputed,aes_string(paste0("X",index1),paste0("X",index2)))+
  geom_point(alpha = 0.5, size = 0.7) + theme_bw() +
  stat_ellipse(type = "norm", color = "#000099", alpha=0.5) +
  geom_point(data = plot.imputed, aes_string( paste0("X",index1) ,
paste0("X",(index2))),size = 1.5, color = "Magenta", alpha = 0.8)
}
gridExtra::grid.arrange( plot.me(1,2), plot.me(5,6), plot.me(13,20),
plot.me(18,19), nrow = 2)
```

2.1.13.3.6   Validation of EM-Imputation Using the R Package Amelia

The Amelia approach for data imputation is described in this manuscript[12] and the corresponding R package manual is available here.[13] Let's use the `amelia()` function to impute the original data *sim_data_df* and compare the results to our simpler manual `EM_algorithm()` imputation approach defined above.

```
# install.packages("Amelia")
library(Amelia)
dim(sim_data.df) ## [1] 200  20
amelia.out <- amelia(sim_data.df, m = 5)
```

In the figure below, circle-shapes colored in magenta denote the manual EM imputation via `EM_algorithm()`, whereas orange-colored squares denote the corresponding synthetic imputations using Amelia, and black dots represent the observed data (Fig. 2.31).

```
plot.ii2 <- function(index, index2){
  plot.imputed <- sim_data.imputed[row.names(
    subset(sim_data.df, is.na(sim_data.df[, index]) |
        is.na(sim_data.df[, index2]))), ]
  plot.imputed2 <- amelia.imputed.5[row.names(
    subset(sim_data.df, is.na(sim_data.df[, index]) |
        is.na(sim_data.df[, index2]))), ]
p =ggplot(sim_data.imputed,aes_string(paste0("X",index),paste0("X",index2)))+
  geom_point(alpha = 0.8, size = 0.7) + theme_bw() +
  stat_ellipse(type = "norm", color = "#000099", alpha=0.5) +
  geom_point(data = plot.imputed, aes_string( paste0("X",index),
    paste0("X",(index2))), size=2.5, color="Magenta", alpha=0.9, shape=16) +
    geom_point(data = plot.imputed2, aes( X1 , X2),size = 2.5,
        color = "#FF9933", alpha = 0.8, shape = 18)
  return(p)
}
plot.ii2(2, 4); plot.ii2(17, 18)
```

---

[12] https://doi.org/10.18637/jss.v045.i07

[13] https://cran.r-project.org/web/packages/Amelia/

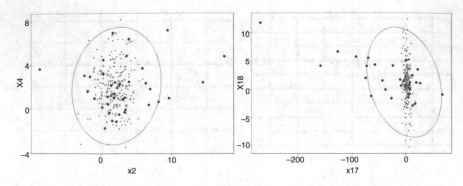

Fig. 2.31 Bivariate cross-sectional plots for two pairs of variables contrasting the EM synthetically imputed data (*magenta* color), the Amelia imputed data (*orange* color), and the observed data (*black* color)

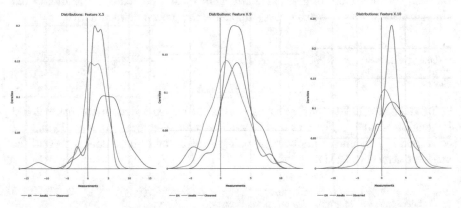

Fig. 2.32 Distributions of observed (green), EM-imputed values (blue), and Amelia-imputed values (orange) for three random features (left, middle, and right panels)

Finally, we can compare the densities of the original, manually EM-imputed, and Amelia-imputed datasets. Remember that in this simulation, we synthetically anni-hilated about 500 observations (missing data) out of the entire set of 4000 elements (Fig. 2.32).

```
library(tidyr)
myPlotly <- function(index){
  imputed <- sim_data.imputed[is.na(sim_data.df[, index]) , index]
  imputed.amelia <- amelia.imputed.5[is.na(sim_data.df[, index]) , index]
  observed <- sim_data.df[!is.na(sim_data.df[, index]) , index]
  imputed.df <- data.frame(x=c(observed,imputed,imputed.amelia),
        category=c(
          rep("obs",length(observed)),rep("simpleImplement",length(imputed)),
                        rep("amelia",length(imputed.amelia)) ) )
  df_long <- as.data.frame(cbind(index=c(1:length(imputed.df$x)),
                        category=imputed.df$category, x=imputed.df$x))
  df_wide <- spread(df_long, category, x)
  p = plot_ly() %>%
    add_lines(x = ~density(as.numeric(df_wide$simpleImplement), na.rm = T)$x,
        y= ~density(as.numeric(df_wide$simpleImplement), na.rm = T)$y,
            name = "EM", mode = 'lines') %>%
    add_lines(x = density(as.numeric(df_wide$amelia), na.rm = T)$x,
        y= density(as.numeric(df_wide$amelia), na.rm = T)$y,
            name = "Amelia", mode = 'lines') %>%
    add_lines(x = ~density(as.numeric(df_wide$obs), na.rm = T)$x,
        y= ~density(as.numeric(df_wide$obs), na.rm = T)$y,
            name = "Observed", mode = 'lines') %>%
    layout(title=sprintf("Distributions: Feature X.%d", index),
        xaxis =list(title = 'Measurements'), yaxis =list(title="Densities"),
        legend = list(title="Distributions", orientation = 'h'))
  return(p)
}
myPlotly(5); myPlotly(9); myPlotly(10)   # Plot a few features
```

2.1.14 Parsing Web Pages and Visualizing Tabular HTML Data

In this section, we will utilize the earthquakes dataset on SOCR website. It records information about earthquakes that happened between 1969 and 2007 with magnitudes larger than 5 on the Richter scale. Here is how we parse the data from the source webpage and ingest the information into R.

```
# install.packages("xml2")
library("XML"); library("xml2")
library("rvest")
wiki_url <-
read_html("https://wiki.socr.umich.edu/index.php/SOCR_Data_Dinov_021708_Earthquakes")
html_nodes(wiki_url, "#content")
earthquake<- html_table(html_nodes(wiki_url, "table")[[2]])
```

In this dataset, Magt (magnitude type) may be used as a grouping variable. We will display a "Longitude vs. Latitude" plot using plot_ly() with color and size reflecting earthquake magnitude type and underground depth (Fig. 2.33).

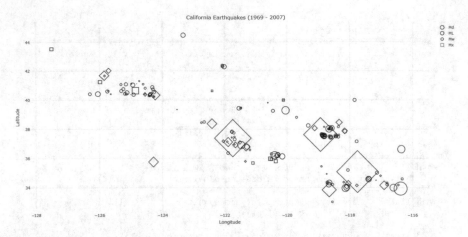

Fig. 2.33 Longitude, latitude, magnitude, and depth of powerful California earthquakes (1969–2007)

```
glyphication <- function (name) {
  glyph= vector()
  for (i in 1:length(name)) {
    glyph[i]="triangle-up"
    if (name[i]=="Md") { glyph[i]="diamond-open" }
    else if (name[i]=="ML") { glyph[i]="circle-open" }
    else if (name[i]=="Mw") { glyph[i]="square-open" }
    else if (name[i]=="Mx") { glyph[i]="x-open" }
  }
  return(glyph)
}
earthquake$glyph <- glyphication(earthquake$Magt)
plot_ly(earthquake) %>%
  add_markers(x = ~Longitude, y = ~Latitude, type="scatter",  color=~Magt,
       mode="markers", marker=list(size=~Depth, color=~Magt, symbol=~glyph,
                           line = list(color = "black",width = 2))) %>%
    layout(title="California Earthquakes (1969 - 2007)")
```

We can also compute and display a 2D kernel density and a 3D surface plots, which are often important and useful in multivariate exploratory data analytics. We will use the `plotly::plot_ly()` function, which takes data frame inputs. To create a surface plot, we use two vectors, x and y, of length m and n, respectively. We also need a matrix z of size $m \times n$ created using matrix operations (x and y outer product). The `kde2d()` function is needed for the 2D kernel density estimation.

```
kernal_density <- with(earthquake, MASS::kde2d(Longitude, Latitude, n=50))
```

The matrix z is an estimate of the kernel density function. Then we apply `plot_ly` to the list `kernal_density` via the `with()` function (Fig. 2.34).

```
library(plotly)
with(kernal_density, plot_ly(x=x, y=y, z=z, type="surface"))
```

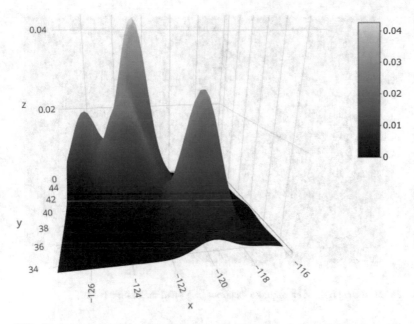

Fig. 2.34 Surface plot of spatial frequency distribution of the California earthquakes (longitude vs. latitude). The highest peaks show the seismically active areas in southern and northern California

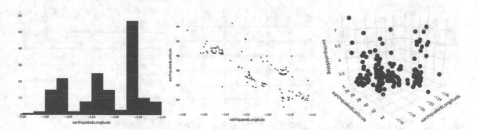

Fig. 2.35 Examples of 1D, 2D, and 3D plots of the California earthquakes

Note that we used the option "surface"; however, you can experiment with other type option. Alternatively, one can plot 1D, 2D, or 3D plots (Figs. 2.35 and 2.36).

```
plot_ly(x = ~ earthquake$Longitude)
plot_ly(x = ~ earthquake$Longitude, y = ~earthquake$Latitude)
plot_ly(x=~ earthquake$Longitude, y=~earthquake$Latitude, z=~earthquake$Mag)
```

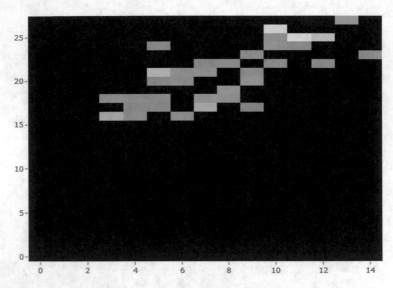

Fig. 2.36 Heat map plot of earthquake locations (x, y) and magnitude (color)

```
df3D <- data.frame(x=earthquake$Longitude,
            y=earthquake$Latitude, z=earthquake$Mag)
# Convert the Long (X, Y, Z) Earthquake format data into a Matrix Format
library("Matrix")
matrix_EarthQuakes <- with(df3D, sparseMatrix(i = as.numeric(180-x),
j=as.numeric(y), x=z, use.last.ij=T, dimnames=list(levels(x), levels(y))))
dim(matrix_EarthQuakes) ## [1] 307  44
library("ggplot2"); library("gplots")
plot_ly(z = ~as.matrix(matrix_EarthQuakes[280:307, 30:44]), type="heatmap")
    %>% hide_colorbar()
```

2.1.15   Cohort-Rebalancing (for Imbalanced Groups)

Comparing cohorts with imbalanced sample sizes (unbalanced designs) may present
hidden biases in the results. Frequently, a cohort-rebalancing protocol is necessary to
avoid such unexpected effects. Extremely unequal sample sizes can invalidate
various parametric assumptions (e.g., homogeneity of variances). Also, there may
be insufficient data representing the patterns belonging to the minority class
(es) leading to inadequate capturing of the feature distributions. Although the groups
do not have to have equal sizes, a general rule of thumb is that group sizes where one
group is more than an order of magnitude larger than the size of another group has
the *potential* for bias.

2.1.15.1   Example 1: Parkinson's Diseases Study

This Parkinson's diseases case-study involves neuroimaging, genetics, clinical, and phenotypic data for over 600 volunteers produced multivariate data for 3 cohorts— *HC=Healthy Controls (166), PD=Parkinson's (434), SWEDD= subjects without evidence for dopaminergic deficit (61)* (Fig. 2.37).

```
# load the data: 06_PPMI_ClassificationValidationData_Short.csv
ppmi_data <-
    read.csv("https://umich.instructure.com/files/330400/download?download_frd=1",
        header=TRUE)
table(ppmi_data$ResearchGroup)
# binarize the Dx classes
ppmi_data$ResearchGroup <- ifelse(ppmi_data$ResearchGroup == "Control",
            "Control", "Patient")
attach(ppmi_data)
head(ppmi_data)
# Model-free analysis, classification
# install.packages("crossval"); install.packages("ada")
library(crossval); library(ada)
#set up adaboosting prediction function
# Define a new classification result-reporting function
my.ada <- function (train.x, train.y, test.x, test.y, negative, formula){
  ada.fit <- ada(train.x, train.y)
  predict.y <- predict(ada.fit, test.x)
  #count TP, FP, TN, FN, Accuracy, etc.
  out <- confusionMatrix(test.y, predict.y, negative = negative)
  # negative  is the label of a negative "null" sample (default: "control")
  return (out)
}


# rebalance the groups
# SMOTE: Synthetic Minority Oversampling Technique to handle class imbalance in
binary classification.
set.seed(1000)
# install.packages("unbalanced") to deal with unbalanced group data
library(unbalanced)
ppmi_data$PD <- ifelse(ppmi_data$ResearchGroup=="Control", 1, 0)
uniqueID <- unique(ppmi_data$FID_IID)
ppmi_data <- ppmi_data[ppmi_data$VisitID==1, ]
ppmi_data$PD <- factor(ppmi_data$PD)
colnames(ppmi_data)
# ppmi_data.1<-ppmi_data[, c(3:281, 284, 287, 336:340, 341)]
n <- ncol(ppmi_data)
output.1 <- ppmi_data$PD
# remove Default Real Clinical subject classifications!
ppmi_data$PD <- ifelse(ppmi_data$ResearchGroup=="Control", 1, 0)
input <- ppmi_data[ , -which(names(ppmi_data) %in%
            c("ResearchGroup", "PD", "X", "FID_IID"))]
output <- as.factor(ppmi_data$PD)
```

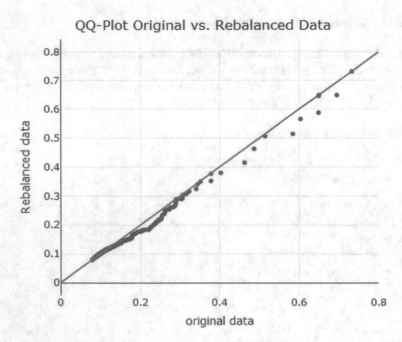

Fig. 2.37 A scatter plot illustrating the differences between the distributions of the raw (input) and rebalanced data (only for one variable)

```
c(dim(input), length(output))
# rebalance the dataset
data.1 <- ubBalance(X= input, Y=output, type="ubSMOTE", percOver=300,
            percUnder=150, verbose=TRUE)
# percOver = A number that drives the decision of how many extra cases from the
minority class are generated (known as over-sampling).
# k = A number indicating the number of nearest neighbors that are used to
generate the new examples of the minority class.
# percUnder = A number that drives the decision of how many extra cases from the
majority classes are selected for each case generated from the minority class
(known as under-sampling)
balancedData<-cbind(data.1$X, data.1$Y)
table(data.1$Y)
nrow(data.1$X); ncol(data.1$X)
nrow(balancedData); ncol(balancedData)
nrow(input); ncol(input)
colnames(balancedData) <- c(colnames(input), "PD")
# check visually for differences between the distributions of the raw (input) and
rebalanced data (for only one variable, in this case)
QQ <- qqplot(input[, 5], balancedData [, 5], plot.it=F)
plot_ly(x=~QQ$x, y = ~QQ$y, type="scatter", mode="markers", showlegend=F) %>%
  add_lines(x=c(0,0.8), y=c(0,0.8), showlegend=F) %>%
  layout(title="QQ-Plot Original vs. Rebalanced Data",
         xaxis=list(title="original data"),
         yaxis=list(title="Rebalanced data"))
```

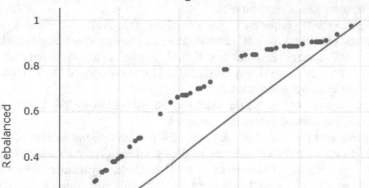

Fig. 2.38 FDR-adjusted p-values of the Wilcoxon tests comparing the distributions of the raw (input) and rebalanced data

The visual agreement between the quantiles of the raw and rebalanced datasets can also be confirmed quantitatively using the nonparametric Wilcoxon test (Fig. 2.38).

```
## Check cohort rebalancing using the Wilcoxon test
alpha.0.05 <- 0.05
test.results.bin <- NULL        # binarized/dichotomized p-values
test.results.raw <- NULL        # raw p-values
for (i in 1:(ncol(balancedData)-1)) {
    test.results.raw[i] <- wilcox.test(input[, i], balancedData[, i])$p.value
    test.results.bin [i] <- ifelse(test.results.raw [i] > alpha.0.05, 1, 0)
    print(c("i=", i, "Wilcoxon-test=", test.results.raw [i]))
}
print(c("Wilcoxon test results: ", test.results.bin))
test.results.corr <- stats::p.adjust(test.results.raw, method = "fdr",
                n = length(test.results.raw))
plot_ly(x=~test.results.raw, y = ~test.results.corr, type="scatter",
                mode="markers", showlegend=F) %>%
  add_lines(x=c(0,1), y=c(0,1), showlegend=F) %>%
  layout(title="Wilcoxon test results - Original vs. Rebalanced Data",
        xaxis=list(title="Original"),
        yaxis=list(title="Rebalanced"))
```

Notes

- SMOTE oversampling of the minority cohort is based on generation of synthetic minority samples within the neighborhoods of observed observations. Thus, new minority instances blend observations in the same class and create clusters around each observed minority element.

- The `percOver` parameter (perc.over/100) represents the number of new instances generated for each rare instance in the minority sample, when perc. over < 100, a single instance is generated. For example, `percOver=300` and `percOver=30` would triple (300/100) and leave unchanged (30/100) the size of the *minority sample*, respectively.
- The parameter *k* represents the number of neighbors to consider as the aggregate pool that the new examples are generated.
- The parameter `percUnder` (perc.under/100) represents the number of "normal" (majority class) instances that are randomly selected for each *smoted* (synthetically generated) observation. For instance, `percUnder=300` or `percUnder=30` would downsample the *majority sample* by choosing one-out-of-each-three or all of the majority sample points, respectively.

2.2 Exploratory Data Analytics (EDA)

In this section, we will see a broad range of simulations and hands-on activities to highlight some of the basic data visualization techniques using R. Starting with a brief discussion of alternative visualization methods, we will show plots of histograms, density, pie, jitter, bar, line, and scatter plots, as well as some strategies for displaying trees, graphs, and 3D surface plots. Many of such plots will be used throughout the textbook in the context of addressing the graphical needs of specific case-studies. It is practically impossible to cover all options of every different visualization routine. Readers are encouraged to experiment with each visualization type, change input data and parameters, explore the function documentation using R-help (e.g., `?plot_ly`), search for new R visualization packages, and test new functionality that are continuously released. Two common general questions that frequently arise in practice include the following:

- What exploratory graphical techniques are available to visually interrogate my specific data?
- How to examine paired associations and correlations in multivariate datasets?

2.2.1 Classification of Visualization Methods

Visualization methods are hard to classify; however, the following characteristics can be used for grouping different types of graphical representations of complex data:

- *Data Type*: structured/unstructured, small/large, complete/incomplete, time/ space, ASCII/binary, Euclidean/non-Euclidean, etc.
- *Task Type*: Task type is one of the aspects considered in classification of visualization techniques, which provides means of interaction between the researcher, the data, and the display software/platform.
- *Scalability*: Visualization techniques are subject to some limitations, such as the amount of data that a particular technique can meaningfully show.
- *Dimensionality*: Visualization techniques can also be classified according to the number of graph-specific attributes used to render the data.
- *Positioning and Attributes*: the distribution of attributes on the chart may affect the interpretation of the display representation, e.g., in correlation analysis, the relative distance among the plotted attributes represents a powerful clue relevant in the context of the study.
- *Investigative Need*: the specific scientific question or the exploratory need may also determine the type of visualization:

  - Examining the composition of the data.
  - Exploring the distribution of the data.
  - Contrasting or comparing several data elements, relations, or associations.
  - Unsupervised exploratory data mining, clustering, or classification.

The following figure shows examples of common data visualization methods according to task types (Fig. 2.39).

We can introduce common data visualization methods according to this classification schema, albeit this is not a unique or even broadly agreed upon ontological characterization of exploratory data visualization.

2.2.2 Composition

In this section, we will see composition plots for different types of variables and data structures.

2.2.2.1 Histograms and Density Plots

Histograms represent one of the first graphs we see in an introductory STEM class. In R, the functions hist() or plot_ly() represent two methods that can be applied to vectors or data frames to plot frequency histograms. The famous nineteenth-century statistician Karl Pearson introduced histograms as graphical

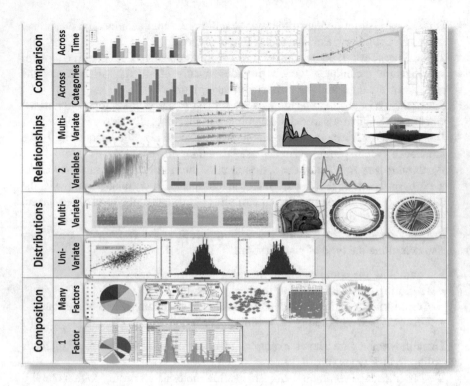

Fig. 2.39 Examples of different classes of exploratory and confirmatory data visualization plots

representations of the distribution of a sample of numeric data. Histogram plots display approximations to the corresponding probability distributions of the under- lying populations that the data are sampled from. Histograms are constructed by selecting a certain number of bins covering the range of values of the observed process. Typically, the number of bins for a data array of size N should be equal to $\sqrt{N}$. These bins form a partition (disjoint and covering sets) of the range. Finally, we compute the relative frequency, i.e., the proportion of observations that fall within each bin interval. Histogram plots represent piecewise step-functions defined over the union of the bin interfaces whose height values equal the observed relative frequencies within each bin (Fig. 2.40).

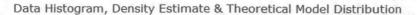

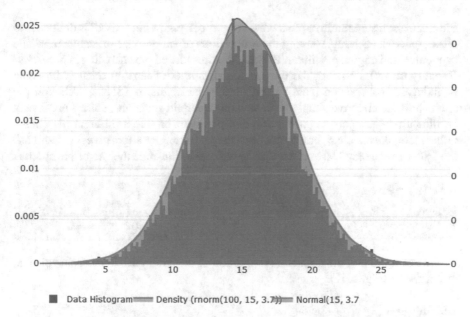

Fig. 2.40 Superposition of a data histogram, kernel density estimate, and a theoretical model distribution

```
library(plotly)
N <- 10000
mu <- 15; sd <- 3.7
set.seed(1234)
x <- rnorm(N, mean = mu, sd=sd)
fit <- density(x)
z<-seq(mu-4*sd, mu+4*sd, 0.1)  # points from -4 to 4 in 0.1 steps
q<-seq(0.001, 0.999, 0.001)  # probability quantiles 0.1%-99.9% in 0.1% steps
normDensity <- dnorm(z, mean=15, sd= 3.7)
plot_ly(x = x, type = "histogram", name = "Data Histogram",
        histnorm = "probability") %>%
    add_trace(x = fit$x, y = fit$y, type = "scatter", mode = "lines",
        opacity=0.1, fill = "tozeroy", yaxis = "y2",
        name = "Density (rnorm(100, 15, 3.7))") %>%
    add_trace(x = z, y = normDensity, type = "scatter", mode = "lines",
        opacity=0.1, fill = "tozeroy", yaxis = "y2",
        name = "Normal(15, 3.7)") %>%
    layout(title='Data Histogram, Density Estimate & Theoretical Model
Distribution',
            yaxis2 = list(overlaying = "y", side = "right"),
            legend = list(orientation = 'h'))
```

Not surprisingly, the shape of the histogram is very close to Normal distribution, because we sampled from $N(\mu = -15, \sigma^2 = 3.7^2)$ using rnorm(). Note the close alignment between the superimposed sample data histogram (blue color), the corresponding Normal density curve (green), and the kernel density estimate (orange).

2.2.2.2   Pie Chart

Pie charts represent intuitive plots where the whole, e.g., a big "cake," is divided into pieces (slices), each representing the proportions of various categorical factors. The economist and engineer William Playfair first introduced pie charts in his *Statistical Breviary* in 1801.[14] Later, the polymath and mother of nursing science, Florence Nightingale, generalized them to statistical polar charts in 1858.[15] Although pie charts provide effective simple visualization in certain situations, sometimes it may be difficult to compare segments within a pie chart or across different pie charts. Other plots like bar chart, box or dot plots may be attractive alternatives. We will use the Letter Frequency Data on the SOCR website to illustrate the use of pie charts.

```
library(rvest)
wiki_url <-
read_html("https://wiki.socr.umich.edu/index.php/SOCR_LetterFrequencyData")
html_nodes(wiki_url, "#content")
summary(letter)
```

We can try to plot the frequency proportion of the 26 English letters using pie and donut charts (Fig. 2.41).

```
plot_ly(letter, labels=~Letter, values=~English, type='pie', name="English",
        textposition='inside', textinfo='label+percent', showlegend=FALSE,
        domain = list(row = 0, column = 0)) %>%
  add_pie(labels = ~Letter, values = ~Spanish,  name = "Spanish",
          textposition='inside', textinfo='label+percent', showlegend=FALSE,
          domain = list(row = 0, column = 1)) %>%
  add_pie(labels = ~Letter, values = ~Swedish,  name = "Swedish",
          textposition='inside', textinfo='label+percent', showlegend=FALSE,
          domain = list(row = 1, column = 0)) %>%
  add_pie(labels = ~Letter, values = ~Polish,   name = "Polish",
          textposition='inside', textinfo='label+percent', showlegend=FALSE,
          domain = list(row = 1, column = 1)) %>%
  add_annotations(x=0.01, y=0.99,text="English",showarrow=F,ax=20,ay=-40) %>%
  add_annotations(x=0.58, y=0.99,text="Spanish",showarrow=F,ax=20,ay=-40) %>%
  add_annotations(x=0.01, y=0.01,text="Swedish",showarrow=F,ax=20,ay=-40) %>%
  add_annotations(x=0.58, y=0.01,text="Polish",showarrow=F, ax=20,ay=-40) %>%
  layout(title = 'Pie Charts of English, Spanish, Swedish & Polish Letters',
         grid=list(rows=2, columns=2),
         xaxis = list(showgrid=FALSE, zeroline=FALSE, showticklabels=FALSE),
         yaxis = list(showgrid=FALSE, zeroline=FALSE, showticklabels=FALSE))
```

2.2.2.3   Heat Map

Another common data visualization method is the heat map, or heatmap. Heat maps can help us visualize the individual values in a matrix intuitively. These plots

---

[14] https://doi.org/10.3102/2F10769986030004353

[15] https://www.jstor.org/stable/24969329

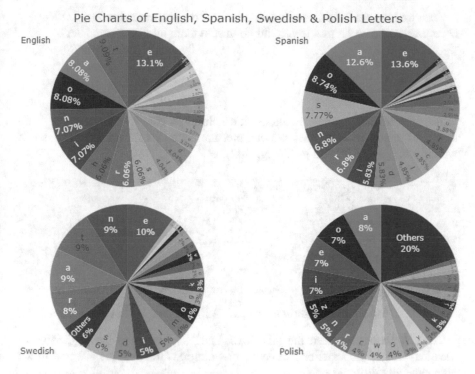

Fig. 2.41 Pie charts showing the frequencies of Latin letters in different languages: English, Spanish, Swedish, and Polish

are widely used in genetics research and financial applications. We will illustrate the use of heat maps to visualize data from a neuroimaging genetics case-study capturing the association (p-values) of different brain regions of interest (ROIs) and genetic traits (SNPs) for Alzheimer's disease (AD) patients, subjects with mild cognitive impairment (MCI), and normal healthy controls (NC/HC). First, let's import the data into R. The data are 2D arrays where the rows represent different genetic SNPs, columns represent brain ROIs, and the cell values represent the strength of the SNP-ROI association as probability values (smaller p-values indicate lower probability that the observed association is due to chance alone, i.e., stronger neuroimaging-genetic associations).

```
AD_Data <-
    read.table("https://umich.instructure.com/files/330387/download?download_frd=1",
        header=TRUE, row.names=1, sep=",", dec=".")
MCI_Data <-
    read.table("https://umich.instructure.com/files/330390/download?download_frd=1",
        header=TRUE, row.names=1, sep=",", dec=".")
NC_Data <-
    read.table("https://umich.instructure.com/files/330391/download?download_frd=1",
        header=TRUE, row.names=1, sep=",", dec=".")
```

Then we load the R packages we need for heat maps (use `install.packages` (`"package name"`) first if you did not install them into your computer).

```
library(graphics)
library(grDevices)
library(gplots)
```

Just like in many other situations, it's helpful to convert the input data into numerical matrix format. Then we can plot the heatmaps for all three cohorts of participants (AD, MCI, and HC) (Fig. 2.42).

```
AD_mat   <- as.matrix(AD_Data); class(AD_mat) <- "numeric"
MCI_mat  <- as.matrix(MCI_Data); class(MCI_mat) <- "numeric"
NC_mat   <- as.matrix(NC_Data); class(NC_mat) <- "numeric"
plot_ly(x=~colnames(AD_mat),y=~rownames(AD_mat),z=~AD_mat,type="heatmap") %>%
  layout(title="AD Neuroimaging-Genomic Associations (p-values)",
         xaxis=list(title="ROI Imaging Biomarkers"),yaxis=list(title="SNPs"))
plot_ly(x=~colnames(MCI_mat),y=~rownames(MCI_mat),z=~MCI_mat,type="heatmap") %>%
  layout(title="MCI Neuroimaging-Genomic Associations (p-values)",
         xaxis=list(title="ROI Imaging Biomarkers"),yaxis=list(title="SNPs"))
plot_ly(x=~colnames(NC_mat),y=~rownames(NC_mat),z=~NC_mat,type="heatmap") %>%
  layout(title="(Normal) HC Neuroimaging-Genomic Associations (p-values)",
         xaxis=list(title="ROI Imaging Biomarkers"),yaxis=list(title="SNPs"))
```

The differences between the AD, MCI, and NC heat maps are suggestive of variations of genetic traits or alternative brain regions that may be affected in the three clinically different cohorts.

2.2.3 Comparison

Plots used for comparing different individuals, groups of subjects, or multiple units represent another set of popular exploratory visualization tools.

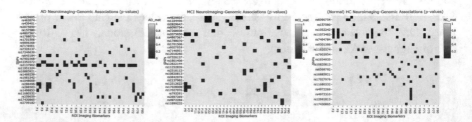

Fig. 2.42 Heat map plots of the neuroimaging genomic associations, region of interest (ROI) vs. genotype, for the Alzheimer's disease (AD) patients (left), the mild cognitive impairment (MCI) patients (middle), and the normal healthy control (HC) volunteers (right)

2.2.3.1 Paired Scatter Plots

Scatter plots use the 2D Cartesian plane to display a graph indexed by a pair of variables. 2D points in the graph represent values associated with the two variables corresponding to the two coordinate axes. The position of each 2D point is determined by the values of the first and second variables, tracked on the horizontal and vertical axes. If no clear dependent variable exists, either variable can be plotted on the X axis and the corresponding scatter plot will illustrate the degree of correlation (not necessarily causation) between two variables. Although we will mostly demonstrate the use of `plot_ly()`, which provides dynamic and interactive charts, many basic graphs, including scatter plots, can be rendered using the R function `plot(x, y)` (Fig. 2.43).

```
N <- 50; ind <- c(1:N)
x<-runif(N); y<-runif(N); z<-runif(N)
hoverText <- paste0("Point ", ind, ": (", round(x, 3), ",", round(y, 3), ")")
# plot(x, y, main="Scatter Plot")
plot_ly(x=~x[1:20], y=~y[1:20], type="scatter", size=2, name=ind[1:20],
        color=~z[1:20], mode="markers", text = hoverText[1:20]) %>%
   layout(title="Random Scatterplot", xaxis=list(title="X"),
          yaxis=list(title="Y")) %>% hide_colorbar()
```

Now let's illustrate paired scatter plots using a larger simulated dataset with five variables (Fig. 2.44).

Fig. 2.43 Bivariate scatter plot of random simulated data

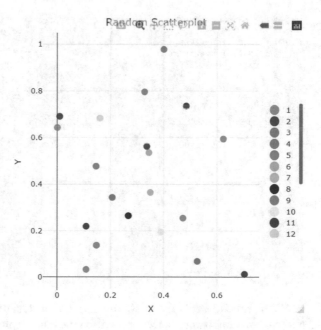

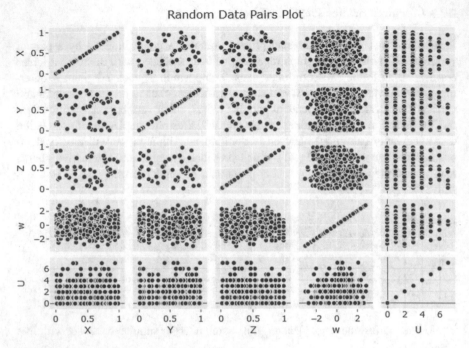

Fig. 2.44 Interactive pairs plot of random simulated data

```
N=1000; w <- rnorm(N); u <- rpois(N, lambda = 1.7)
# generate some random categorical labels for all N observations
class <- sample(LETTERS[1:3], N, replace=TRUE, prob=c(0.2, 0.5, 0.3))
df <- as.data.frame(cbind(x=x,y=y,z=z,w=w,u=u, class=class))
pl_colorscale = list(c(0.0, '#19d3f3'), c(0.333, '#19d3f3'),
                     c(0.333, '#e763fa'), c(0.666, '#e763fa'),
                     c(0.666, '#636efa'), c(1, '#636efa'))
axis = list(showline=FALSE, zeroline=FALSE, gridcolor='#ffff', ticklen=4)
plot_ly(df) %>%
    add_trace(type = 'splom', dimensions = list( list(label='X', values=~x),
              list(label='Y', values=~y),
              list(label='Z', values=~z), list(label='w', values=~w),
              list(label='U', values=~u)), text=~class,
              marker = list(color = as.integer(df$class),
                            colorscale = pl_colorscale, size = 7,
                            line=list(width=1, color='rgb(230,230,230)'))) %>%
    layout(title='Random Data Pairs Plot', hovermode='closest',
           dragmode='select', plot_bgcolor='rgba(240,240,240, 0.95)',
           xaxis=list(domain=NULL, showline=F, zeroline=F,
                      gridcolor='#ffff', ticklen=4),
           yaxis=list(domain=NULL, showline=F, zeroline=F,
                      gridcolor='#ffff', ticklen=4),
           xaxis2=axis, xaxis3=axis, xaxis4=axis,yaxis2=axis,
           yaxis3=axis, yaxis4=axis)
```

When run interactively in R, the result is a dynamic SVG pairs scatter plot allowing manipulation, selection, subsetting, and exploration of the associations between multiple variables across all pairs plots.

Let's see another example using the Mental Health Services Survey Data, which is available on the supporting website (Case_03_MentalHealthServicesSurvey). This survey data covers 10, 374 mental health facilities across the US, the District of Columbia, and US Territories with 237 variables representing various facility characteristics. We will use a subset of 10 variables for all 10,374 cases. Two of the characteristics are of particular interest (1) *supp*, representing the number of specialty and support services available at the mental health facility; and (2) *qual*, which is the number of quality indicators present at the mental health facility.

```
data1 <-
    read.table('https://umich.instructure.com/files/399128/download?download_frd=1',
        header=T)
head(data1)
attach(data1)
```

We can see from `head()` that there are some missing observations (*NA*'s) in the dataset and the pairs plot (`splom`) automatically ignores these (and posts a warning message). Below, we show examples of a bivariate scatter plot and a pairs ("splom") plot for the Mental Health Services Survey data (Figs. 2.45 and 2.46).

```
plot_ly(data1, x=~qual, y=~supp, type="scatter", size=2, name=STFIPS,
        color=~num, mode="markers", text = STFIPS) %>%
    layout(title="2010 National Mental Health Services Survey: Support Services
vs. Quality Indicators Scatterplot",
            xaxis=list(title="Support Services"),
            yaxis=list(title="Quality Indicators")) %>% hide_colorbar()
```

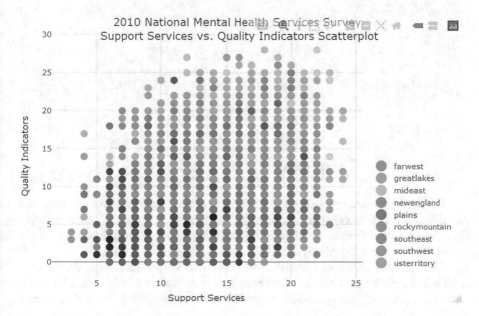

Fig. 2.45 Interactive bivariate scatter plot mental health services vs. quality indicators data

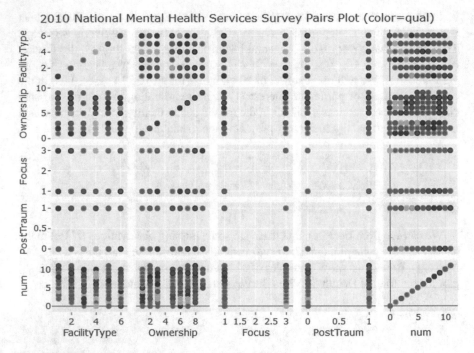

Fig. 2.46 Interactive pairs plot of the mental health data

```
plot_ly(data1) %>%
    add_trace(type = 'splom', dimensions = list(list(label='FacilityType',
                values=~FacilityType), list(label='Ownership',
                        values=~Ownership), list(label='Focus', values=~Focus),
                list(label='PostTraum', values=~PostTraum),
                list(label='num', values=~num)), text=~STFIPS,
                marker = list(color=as.integer(qual), colorscale=pl_colorscale,
                size = 7, line = list(width = 1, color = qual))) %>%
    layout(title= '2010 National Mental Health Services Survey Pairs Plot
(color=qual)', hovermode='closest', dragmode= 'select',
        plot_bgcolor='rgba(240,240,240, 0.95)',
        xaxis=list(domain=NULL, showline=F, zeroline=F, gridcolor='#ffff',
                ticklen=4),
        yaxis=list(domain=NULL, showline=F, zeroline=F, gridcolor='#ffff',
                ticklen=4),
        xaxis2=axis, xaxis3=axis, xaxis4=axis,yaxis2=axis, yaxis3=axis,
                yaxis4=axis)
```

The first (bivariate) plot shows the relation between *supp* (support services) and *qual* (quality indicators). The second more elaborate (pairs) plot illustrates multiple bivariate relations that can be interactively explored by selecting points in any of the plots, where points are color-coded by the *quality indicator* variable.

Later, in Chap. 3, we will demonstrate linear model-based prediction, forecasting, and inference. The next example illustrates how to model the trend, loess(supp ~ qual), of the support-services to quality relationship. This *locally estimated*

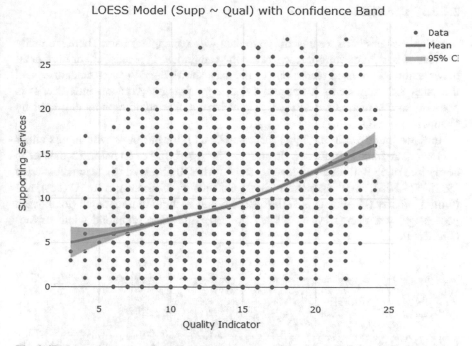

Fig. 2.47 Interactive scatter plot with model trajectory and confidence band for the mental health data (supporting services vs. quality indicators)

scatterplot smoothing (LOESS) model estimates a nonlinear smoothing regression between the two variables (Fig. 2.47).

```
# extract only the complete cases
library(dplyr)
df1 <- data1 %>% filter_at(vars(qual,supp), all_vars(!is.na(.)))
ll.smooth = loess(df1$supp ~ df1$qual, span=0.7)
ll.pred = predict(ll.smooth, se = TRUE)
ll.df = data.frame(x=ll.smooth$x, fit=ll.pred$fit,
      lb=ll.pred$fit-(1.96*ll.pred$se), ub=ll.pred$fit+(1.96*ll.pred$se))
ll.df = ll.df[order(ll.df$df1.qual),]
plot_ly(x=df1$qual,y=df1$supp,type="scatter",mode="markers", name="Data") %>%
  add_lines(x=df1$qual, y=ll.pred$fit, name="Mean",
      line=list(color="gray", width=4)) %>%
  add_ribbons(x=ll.df$df1.qual, ymin=ll.df$lb, ymax=ll.df$ub, name="95% CI",
          line=list(opacity=0.4, width=1, color="lightgray")) %>%
  layout(title = "LOESS Model (Supp ~ Qual) with Confidence Band",
        xaxis=list(title="Quality Indicator"),
        yaxis=list(title="Supporting Services"))
```

It may be useful to try some hands-on visualizations using the human height and weight dataset or the knee pain dataset to illustrate some interesting scatter plots.

2.2.3.2 Bar Plots

Bar plots, or bar charts, represent group data with rectangular bars. There are many variants of bar charts for comparison among categories. Typically, either horizontal or vertical bars are used where one of the axes shows the compared categories and the other axis represents a discrete value, e.g., frequency, count, intensity. It is possible, and sometimes desirable, to plot bar graphs including bars clustered by groups.

In R we can use `plot_ly()` or `barplot()` for bar plots with inputs either vectors, data frames, matrices, or arrays. The `ggplot2::diamonds` dataset is comprised of 53,940 diamond records (rows) with 10 observed characteristics: price ($326–$18,823); carat (diamond weight); cut (quality of the cut); color (D (best) to J (worst)); clarity (I1 (worst), ..., IF (best)); x, and z length in mm; depth (total depth percentage = z/mean(x, y) = 2 * z / (x + y)); and table (diamond width of top) (Fig. 2.48).

```
plot_ly(ggplot2::diamonds, x = ~cut, y = ~price, type = 'bar',
         color = ~clarity, text= ~clarity)
plot_ly(ggplot2::diamonds, y = ~log(price), color=~cut, type = "box") %>%
  layout(title = "Boxplot of Diamond (log) Price by Cut",
         xaxis=list(title="Diamond Cut"))
plot_ly(ggplot2::diamonds, x= ~clarity, y = ~log(price), color=~color,
         type = "box") %>%
  layout(boxmode = "group",
         title="Grouped Boxplot of Diamond (log) Price by Clarity and Color",
         legend=list(title=list(text='<b> Diamond Color </b>')),
         xaxis=list(title="Diamond Clarity"))
```

Let's look at a more complex example using a Child Trauma dataset (Case_04_ChildTrauma). This case study examines associations between post-traumatic psychopathology and service utilization by trauma-exposed children.

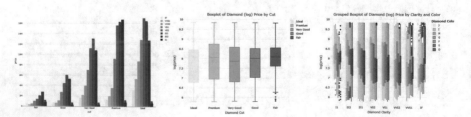

Fig. 2.48 Examples of simple, statistical, and grouped bar plots using the diamonds dataset

```
data2 <-
    read.table('https://umich.instructure.com/files/399129/download?download_frd=1',
        header=T)
attach(data2)
head(data2)
##   id sex age ses  race traumatype ptsd dissoc service
## 1  1   1   6   0 black   sexabuse    1      1      17
...
```

We have a pair of character-type variables and we can use bar plots to compare the means of `age` and `service` among different races in this study and perhaps add error bars to each bin. Note that bar plots require numerical inputs and typically a clear delineation of two, or more, character columns (labels).

```
data2.sub <- data2[, c(-5, -6)]
data2<-data2[, -6]
# separate groups and get group means
data2.df <- as.data.frame(data2)
Blacks <- data2[which(data2$race=="black"), ]
Other <- data2[which(data2$race=="other"), ]
Hispanic <- data2[which(data2$race=="hispanic"), ]
White <- data2[which(data2$race=="white"), ]
B <- c(mean(Blacks$age), mean(Blacks$service))
O <- c(mean(Other$age), mean(Other$service))
H <- c(mean(Hispanic$age), mean(Hispanic$service))
W <- c(mean(White$age), mean(White$service))
x <- cbind(B, O, H, W); x
##         B     O    H        W
## [1,] 9.165  9.12 8.67 8.950000
## [2,] 9.930 10.32 9.61 9.911667
```

Until now, we had a numerical matrix for the means available for plotting. Now, we can compute a second order statistic (standard deviation) and plot it along with the means to illustrate the amount of dispersion for each variable. Below we demonstrate bar plots using `plot_ly()` and `ggplot()`. These kinds of bar plots are quite different from the ones we previously saw. They plot the frequency counts of character variables, rather than the means of numerical variables. These plots help us compare the occurrences of different types of child-trauma among different races (Fig. 2.49).

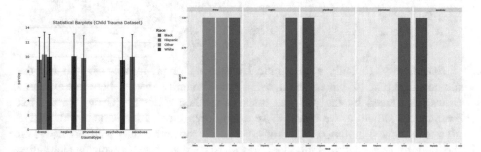

Fig. 2.49 Alternative bar plots using the Child Trauma dataset

```
library(plyr)
data_mean <- ddply(data2, c("traumatype", "race"), summarise,
            service = mean(service))
data_sd <- ddply(diamonds, c("traumatype", "race"), summarise,
            service = sd(service))
data2 <- data.frame(data_mean, sd=data_sd$service)
plot_ly(data = data2[which(data2$race == 'black'), ], x = ~traumatype,
    y = ~service, type = 'bar', name = 'Black',
    error_y = ~list(array = sd, color = '#000000')) %>%
  add_trace(data = data2[which(data2$race == 'hispanic'), ],
    name = 'Hispanic') %>%
  add_trace(data = data2[which(data2$race == 'other'), ], name = 'Other') %>%
  add_trace(data = data2[which(data2$race == 'white'), ], name = 'White') %>%
  layout(title="Statistical Barplots (Child Trauma Dataset)",
        legend=list(title=list(text='<b> Race </b>')))
library(ggplot2)
ggplot(data2, aes(race, fill=race)) + geom_bar() + facet_grid(. ~ traumatype)
```

2.2.3.3 Trees and Graphs

In general, a graph is an ordered pair $G = (V, E)$ of vertices (V), i.e., nodes or points, and a set of edges (E), arcs or lines connecting pairs of nodes V in the graph G. A tree is a special type of acyclic graph that does not include looping paths. Visualization of graphs is critical in many biosocial and health studies and we will see many examples throughout this textbook. In Chaps. 3 and 8, we will learn more about how to build hierarchical tree models and other clustering methods, and in Chap. 14, we will discuss deep learning and neural networks, which intrinsically represent AI decision graphs. In this section, will be focused on displaying tree graphs. Let's start with a simple demonstration using a flat data frame (02_Nof1_Data.csv) to generate a hierarchical graph structure (tree) using a clustering method. This process is a common in many data science applications and will be discuss in more detail in Chap. 8.

```
data3<-
    read.table("https://umich.instructure.com/files/330385/download?download_frd=1",
            sep=",", header = TRUE)
head(data3)
##    ID Day Tx SelfEff SelfEff25  WPSS SocSuppt PMss PMss3 PhyAct
## 1  1   1  1      33         8  0.97     5.00 4.03  1.03     53
## 2  1   2  1      33         8 -0.17     3.87 4.03  1.03     73
...
```

Specifically, to build a hierarchical clustering graph model, we will use the method `hclust()` whose input takes a dissimilarity matrix, between all cases (rows), produced by the pairwise distance method `dist()`. Using the derived hierarchical structure, we can display a top-down hierarchical structure depicting all tree branches, starting with a root node on the top and ending with leaf nodes on the bottom representing individual cases. Note that there are many alternative methods to generate the agglomeration. In this example, we used the `average`

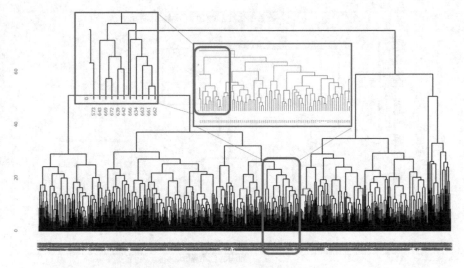

Fig. 2.50 Displaying a derived hierarchical structure (tree graph) with inserts showing magnified versions of the top-down clustering of all cases in the dataset.

method representing unweighted pair group method with arithmetic mean (UPGMA)[16] (Fig. 2.50).

```
hc <- hclust(dist(data3), method='average')
par (mfrow=c(1, 1))
library(plotly);  library(ggplot2); library(ggdendro)
pl <- ggdendrogram(hc, rotate = FALSE, size = 2); ggplotly(pl)
```

For large datasets and no limit on the maximum number of cluster groups, the above graph may be difficult to navigate and interpret. To limit the number of displayed clusters we can apply the method cutree(), to the output of the method hclust(), and obtain a vector of derived group indicators (labels) for all observations. Then, we can get the mean of each variable within groups using the following algorithm.

```
require(graphics)
mem <- cutree(hc, k = 10)
# mem; # to print the hierarchical tree labels for each case
# which(mem==5)  # to identify which cases belong to class/cluster 5
# To see the number of Subjects in which cluster: table(cutree(hc, k=5))
cent <- NULL
for(k in 1:10) cent <- rbind(cent, colMeans(data3[mem == k, , drop=FALSE]))
```

Now we can plot the new tree graph with only 10 groups representing computer-derived outcomes. Setting the option members=table(mem) indicates that the

---

[16]https://www.worldcat.org/oclc/11463855

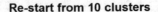

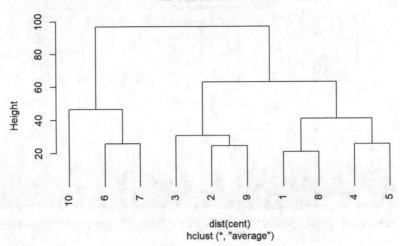

dist(cent)
hclust (*, "average")

Fig. 2.51 Limiting the number of clustered groups to 10 and displaying the graph tree structure of the derived hierarchy

matrix is taken to be a dissimilarity matrix between clusters instead of dissimilarities between singletons, and members specifies the number of observations per cluster (Fig. 2.51).

```
hc1 <- hclust(dist(cent), method = "average", members = table(mem))
plot(hc1, hang = -1, main = "Re-start from 10 clusters")
```

2.2.3.4   Correlation Plots

The corrplot package enables the graphical display of a correlation matrix, and confidence intervals, along with some tools for matrix reordering. There are seven visualization methods (parameter method) in the corrplot package, named "circle," "square," "ellipse," "number," "shade," "color," and "pie." Let's use 03_NC_SNP_ROI_Assoc_P_values.csv again to investigate the associations among SNPs using correlation plots. The corrplot() function we will be using takes correlation matrix only. So we need to get the correlation matrix of our data first via the cor() function.

```
# install.packages("corrplot")
library(corrplot)
NC_Associations_Data <-
    read.table("https://umich.instructure.com/files/330391/download?download_frd=1",
        header=TRUE, row.names=1, sep=",", dec=".")
M <- cor(NC_Associations_Data)
```

Let's explore the impact of different corrplot() parameter settings. In these examples, color shading is different and typically darker saturated colors represent

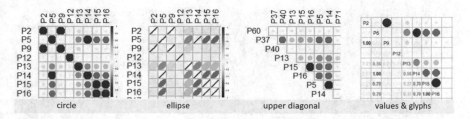

Fig. 2.52 Examples of (cropped) multivariate correlation plots with different parameter settings

high magnitude correlations between the corresponding pair of variables mapped on the x and y axes (Fig. 2.52).

```
# par specs c(bottom, left, top, right) set the margin size in inches
corrplot(M, method = "circle", title = "circle", tl.cex = 0.5,
         tl.col = 'black', mar=c(1, 1, 1, 1))
corrplot(M, method = "square", title = "square", tl.cex = 0.5,
         tl.col = 'black', mar=c(1, 1, 1, 1))
corrplot(M, method = "ellipse", title = "ellipse", tl.cex = 0.5,
         tl.col = 'black', mar=c(1, 1, 1, 1))
corrplot(M, method = "pie", title = "pie", tl.cex = 0.5,
         tl.col = 'black', mar=c(1, 1, 1, 1))
corrplot(M, type = "upper", tl.pos = "td", method = "circle", tl.cex = 0.5,
         tl.col = 'black', order = "hclust", diag=FALSE, mar=c(1, 1, 0, 1))
corrplot.mixed(M, number.cex = 0.4, tl.cex = 0.4)
```

2.2.4 Relationships

Line charts display a series of data points, e.g., observed intensities (Y) over time (X), by connecting them with straight-line segments. These can be used to either track temporal changes of a process or compare the trajectories of multiple cases, time series or subjects over time, space, or state.

We can visualize the distribution for different variables using density plots. The following segment of R code plots the distribution for latitude among different earthquake magnitude types. Also, it is using the ggplot() function combined with geom_density() (Fig. 2.53).

```
# library("ggplot2")
# table(earthquake$Magt) # to see the distribution of magnitude types
ggplot(earthquake, aes(Latitude, group=Magt, newsize=2))+
  geom_density(aes(color=Magt), size = 2) +
  theme(legend.position = 'right',
     legend.text = element_text(color= 'black', size = 12, face = 'bold'),
     legend.key = element_rect(size = 0.5, linetype='solid'),
     legend.key.size = unit(1.5, 'lines'))
```

Note how the green magt type (Local (ML) earthquakes) has a peak at latitude 37.5, which represents 37–38° North, corresponding to the Bay Area in California.

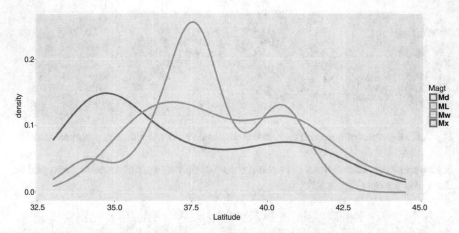

Fig. 2.53 Density line plots of earthquake magnitude types

Recall that there are dualities between *theoretical* and *empirical* mass, density, and distribution functions. Earlier, we saw the relations between these using the (continuous) Normal distribution, let's now look at the (discrete) Poisson distribution. The graph below plots (1) the histogram of a sample of 1000 Poisson (1) random observations (light blue color), (2) the theoretical density/mass function (magenta color), and (3) a smooth continuous (Gaussian) kernel density estimation based on the random sample (blue color). More interactive plots of univariate distributions and multivariate distributions are available at the Probability Distributome Project and SOCR (Fig. 2.54).

```
set.seed(1234)
poisson_sample <- rpois(1000, 1)
# slightly offset the histogram bins to align with mass function
hist_breakes <- c(-0.5, 0.5, 1.5, 2.5, 3.5, 6.5)
h <-hist(poisson_sample, breaks = hist_breakes, plot = F)
t <- seq(0, 6, by=0.01)
Pois <- density(poisson_sample, kernel = "gaussian")
plot_ly(x = h$mids, y = h$density, type = "bar", name="Sample Histogram") %>%
  add_lines(x=t, y=dpois(t,1), type="scatter", mode="lines",
            name="(Theoretical) Poisson Mass Function") %>%
  add_lines(x=Pois$x, y=Pois$y,
         type="scatter", mode="lines",
         name="Gaussian kernel density estimate (sample)") %>%
  layout(bargap=0.1, title="Histogram (Simulated Poisson Data)",
         legend = list(orientation = 'h'))
```

2.2.4.1 Data Modeler

A common task in data-driven inference involves the *fitting* of appropriate distribution models to specific observed data elements (features). In general, this is a difficult task as there are uncountably many possible distributions that can be used as models for various types of processes. The Probability Distributome Project (see

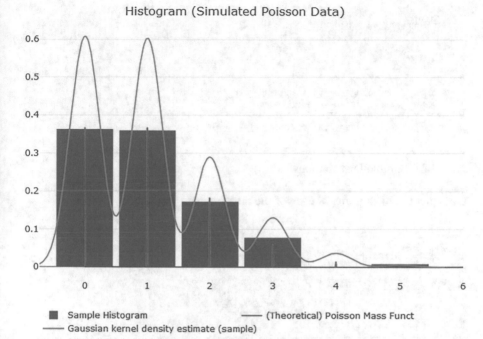

Fig. 2.54 Sampling histogram, probability mass function, and Gaussian kernel density estimate line plots of simulated Poisson data

Distributome Navigator) provides a deeper understanding of the notion of a probability distribution and the relations between various distributions.

We will demonstrate the concept of a *data modeler* by using *crystallographic data*[17] from the Ivanova Lab at the University of Michigan,[18] which includes the crystal spectra of nine length samples and nine width samples (all data are available on the supporting website). For both, the length and width spectra, the nine samples include "AC1338," "AC1432," "AC1593," "AC1679," "AC1860," "AC1874," "AC1881," "AC1903," and "Rec." Notice that the nine spectra are not congruent; different samples have different sampling rates. We will employ the fitdistrplus R-package to estimate the parameters of three complementary distributions; however, there are many alternative packages that can also be used.

2.2.4.1.1 Loading the Spectral Crystallography Data

The data include two separate signals capturing the spectral *length* and the *width* of the crystallographic sample.

---

[17] https://doi.org/10.1038/nature15368

[18] https://www.umich.edu/~mivanova

```
# You may choose which of the 2 CSV files (width or Length) to work with
crystallography_Length_data <-
 read.csv(file="https://umich.instructure.com/files/11653615/download?download_frd=1",
     header=TRUE)
crystallography_Width_data <-
 read.csv(file="https://umich.instructure.com/files/11653614/download?download_frd=1",
     header=TRUE)
crystallography_data <- crystallography_Length_data
# crystallography_data <- crystallography_Width_data
# Get the sample names (IDs)
colNames <- colnames(crystallography_data); colNames
```

2.2.4.1.2   Sample Distributions

Let's plot the histograms of each of the nine samples (Fig. 2.55).

```
# plot all histograms
library(tidyr)
crystalCompleteData <-
        crystallography_data[complete.cases(crystallography_data), ]
df_crystal <- apply(crystalCompleteData, 2, density, kernel="gaussian",bw=15)
df <- data.frame(x = unlist(lapply(df_crystal, "[[", "x")),
                 y = unlist(lapply(df_crystal, "[[", "y")),
                 sample = rep(names(df_crystal), each =
length(df_crystal[[1]]$x)))
plot_ly(df, x = ~x, y = ~y, color = ~sample, type = "scatter", mode = "lines")
%>%
    layout(title='Crystallography Sample Densities',
           legend=list(title=list(text='<b> Samples </b>')),
           xaxis=list(title='X'), yaxis=list(title='Density'))
```

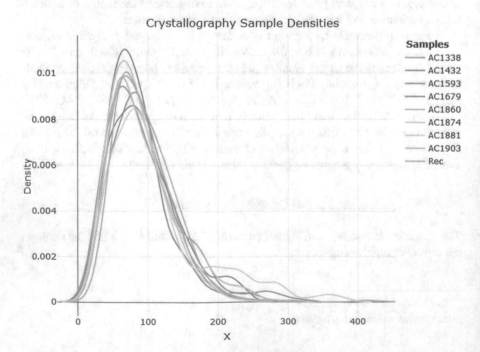

Fig. 2.55 Line plots of the kernel density estimates for different crystallography samples

2.2.4.1.3 Fitting Single-Sample Univariate Distribution Models

We will fit Weibull, Gamma, and Log-Normal distribution models to each sample in the data.

```r
# install.packages("fitdistrplus")
library(fitdistrplus)
col_num <- dim(crystallography_data)[2]; col_num
# Store the Weibull, Gamma, and Log-Normal Distribution models for 9 samples
fit_W <- vector(mode = "list", length = col_num)
fit_G <- vector(mode = "list", length = col_num)
fit_LN <- vector(mode = "list", length = col_num)
for(i in 1:col_num) {
data_no_NA<-crystallography_data[complete.cases(crystallography_data[,i]), i]
  length(data_no_NA)
  fit_W[[i]]  <- fitdist(data_no_NA, "weibull"); summary(fit_W[i])
  fit_G[[i]]  <- fitdist(data_no_NA, "gamma"); summary(fit_G[i])
  fit_LN[[i]] <- fitdist(data_no_NA, "lnorm"); summary(fit_LN[i])
}
# extract the model parameters for all 3 models
W_mod_p1_name = array(dim=c(col_num,2))  # param name
W_mod_p1_val = array(dim=c(col_num,2))   # parameter-estimate value
G_mod_p1_name = array(dim=c(col_num,2))  # param name
G_mod_p1_val = array(dim=c(col_num,2))   # parameter-estimate value
LN_mod_p1_name = array(dim=c(col_num,2)) # param name
LN_mod_p1_val = array(dim=c(col_num,2))  # parameter-estimate value
# Compute the mean (m) and standard deviation (sd) for each dist model
W_mod_mean = array(dim=c(col_num,1)) # Weibull mean or mode
W_mod_sd = array(dim=c(col_num,1))   # Weibull SD
G_mod_mean = array(dim=c(col_num,1)) # Gamma mean or mode
G_mod_sd = array(dim=c(col_num,1))   # Gamma SD
LN_mod_mean = array(dim=c(col_num,1))# Log-normal mean or mode
LN_mod_sd = array(dim=c(col_num,1))  # Log-normal SD
for(i in 1:col_num) {
  W_mod_p1_name[i, 1] <- names(fit_W[[i]]$estimate[1])  # Weibull "shape"
  W_mod_p1_val[i, 1] <- fit_W[[i]]$estimate[[1]]
  W_mod_p1_name[i, 2] <- names(fit_W[[i]]$estimate[2])  # Weibull "scale"
  W_mod_p1_val[i, 2] <- fit_W[[i]]$estimate[[2]]
  W_mod_mean[i] = W_mod_p1_val[i, 2] * gamma(1+1/W_mod_p1_val[i, 1]) # mean
  W_mod_mean[i] = W_mod_p1_val[i, 2] *
   ((W_mod_p1_val[i, 1]-1)/W_mod_p1_val[i, 1])^(1/W_mod_p1_val[i,1]) # mode
  W_mod_sd[i] = W_mod_p1_val[i, 2]*sqrt(gamma(1+2/W_mod_p1_val[i, 1])-
     (gamma(1+1/W_mod_p1_val[i, 1]))^2)  # Weibull SD
  G_mod_p1_name[i, 1] <- names(fit_G[[i]]$estimate[1])  # Gamma "shape"
  G_mod_p1_val[i, 1] <- fit_G[[i]]$estimate[[1]]
  G_mod_p1_name[i, 2] <- names(fit_G[[i]]$estimate[2])  # Gamma "scale"
  G_mod_p1_val[i, 2] <- fit_G[[i]]$estimate[[2]]
  G_mod_mean[i] = G_mod_p1_val[i, 1] / G_mod_p1_val[i, 2]   # Gamma mean
  G_mod_mean[i] = (G_mod_p1_val[i, 1]-1) / G_mod_p1_val[i, 2]  # Gamma mode
  G_mod_sd[i] = sqrt(G_mod_p1_val[i, 1]) / G_mod_p1_val[i, 2]  # Gamma SD
  LN_mod_p1_name[i, 1] <- names(fit_LN[[i]]$estimate[1]) # Log-normal "shape"
  LN_mod_p1_val[i, 1] <- fit_LN[[i]]$estimate[[1]]
  LN_mod_p1_name[i,2] <- names(fit_LN[[i]]$estimate[2]) # Log-normal "scale"
  LN_mod_p1_val[i, 2] <- fit_LN[[i]]$estimate[[2]]
  LN_mod_mean[i] = exp(LN_mod_p1_val[i, 1]+ (LN_mod_p1_val[i, 2])^2/2) # mean
  LN_mod_mean[i] = exp(LN_mod_p1_val[i, 1] - LN_mod_p1_val[i, 2]^2)    # mode
  LN_mod_sd[i] = sqrt((exp(LN_mod_p1_val[i, 2]^2)-1)*
     exp(2*LN_mod_p1_val[i, 1]+LN_mod_p1_val[i, 2]^2)) # Log-normal SD
}
# Check results, just for one model
str(fit_W[[1]])
```

2.2.4.1.4   Visual Inspection

Let's examine graphically the quality of the *fitted* distribution models. We'll plot the histograms of the samples, the fitted probability densities. Similarly, we can plot the corresponding cumulative distribution function (CDF) models and compare them to their sample counterparts (Fig. 2.56).

```
windows(width=20, height=8)
par(mfrow=c(3,3))
for(i in 1:col_num) {
  # get plot labels
  plot.legend <- c(sprintf("Weibull(%s=%s,%s=%s) (m=%s,sd=%s)",
                  W_mod_p1_name[i, 1], format(W_mod_p1_val[i, 1], digits=2),
                  W_mod_p1_name[i, 2], format(W_mod_p1_val[i, 2], digits=2),
                          format(W_mod_mean[i], digits=2),
                          format(W_mod_sd[i], digits=2)),
                  sprintf("Gamma(%s=%s,%s=%s) (m=%s,sd=%s)",
                    G_mod_p1_name[i,1], format(G_mod p1 val[i, 1], digits=2),
                    G_mod_p1_name[i,2], format(G_mod_p1_val[i, 2], digits=2),
                          format(G_mod_mean[i], digits=2),
                          format(G_mod_sd[i], digits=2)),
                  sprintf("Log-normal(%s=%s,%s=%s) (m=%s,sd=%s)",
                    LN_mod_p1_name[i,1], format(LN_mod_p1_val[i,1],digits=2),
                    LN_mod_p1_name[i,2], format(LN_mod_p1_val[i,2],digits=2),
                          format(LN_mod_mean[i], digits=2),
                          format(LN_mod_sd[i], digits=2)))
  denscomp(list(fit_W[[i]], fit_G[[i]], fit_LN[[i]]), legendtext=plot.legend,
          xlegend = "topright", ylegend ="right",
          main=sprintf("Width: Feature: %s: Histogram & Model Densities",
colnames(crystallography_data)[i]))
  abline(v = format(W_mod_mean[i], digits=2), col ="red", lty=1)
  abline(v = format(G_mod_mean[i], digits=2), col = "green", lty=2)
  abline(v = format(LN_mod_mean[i], digits=2), col = "blue", lty=3)
  # cdfcomp (list(fit_w, fit_g, fit_Ln), legendtext = plot.legend)
  # qqcomp  (list(fit_w, fit_g, fit_Ln), legendtext = plot.legend)
  # ppcomp  (list(fit_w, fit_g, fit_Ln), legendtext = plot.legend)
}
```

Fig. 2.56 Plots of crystallography sample histograms and their corresponding Weibull, Gamma, and Log-Normal kernel density models derived using MLE parameter estimates

An interactive `plot_ly()` line plots of these three distribution models are also available on the DSPA2 website.

2.2.4.1.5   Quantitative Summaries

Often, it's useful to export the numerical results of various models. This may include various distribution characteristics like distribution parameter estimates, measures of centrality (e.g., mean, median, mode), measures of dispersion (e.g., standard deviation), and metrics of the model performance (e.g., Kolmogorov–Smirnov test p-values). Below is one example of reporting such quantitative summaries using the crystallography models (Fig. 2.57).

```
# Save the summary outputs (mode & SD) across 9 samples, 3 models and 2 measures
into a dataframe
df_matrix = array(dim=c(col_num,3*2*2)); dim(df_matrix)
## [1]   9 12
for(i in 1:col_num) {
  data1 <- crystallography_data[complete.cases(crystallography_data[,i]), i]
  df_matrix[i, 1] = format(W_mod_mean[i], digits=2)   # Weibull mode
  df_matrix[i, 2] = format(W_mod_sd[i], digits=2)     # Weibull SD
  ks_W <- ks.test(data1, "pweibull", scale=W_mod_p1_val[i, 2],
            shape=W_mod_p1_val[i, 1])
  df_matrix[i,3]=format(ks_W$statistic[[1]],digits=4)  # KS-test-stat Weibull
  df_matrix[i,4]=format(ks_W$p.value, digits=5)       # KS-test-p-value Weibull
  df_matrix[i, 5] = format(G_mod_mean[i], digits=2)  # Gamma mode
  df_matrix[i, 6] = format(G_mod_sd[i], digits=2)     # Gamma SD
  ks_G <- ks.test(data1, "pgamma", rate=G_mod_p1_val[i, 2],
              shape=G_mod_p1_val[1, 1])
  df_matrix[i,7]=format(ks_G$statistic[[1]], digits=4)  # KS-test-stat Gamma
  df_matrix[i, 8] = format(ks_G$p.value, digits=5)     # KS-test-p-value Gamma
  df_matrix[i, 9] = format(LN_mod_mean[i], digits=2)  # Log-normal mode
  df_matrix[i, 10] = format(LN_mod_sd[i], digits=2)    # Log-normal SD
  ks_LN <- ks.test(data1, "plnorm", sdlog=LN_mod_p1_val[i, 2],
              meanlog=LN_mod_p1_val[i, 1])
df_matrix[i,11]=format(ks_LN$statistic[[1]],digits=4)#KS-test-stat Log-normal
  df_matrix[i,12]=format(ks_G$p.value,digits=5)  # KS-test-p-value Log-normal
}
df_summary <- as.data.frame(df_matrix, row.names=colNames)
colnames(df_summary) <- c("Weibull_mode", "Weibull_sd",
    "Weibull_KS.test.stat", "Weibull_KS.p.val", "Gamma_mode",
    "Gamma_sd","Gamma_KS.test.stat", "Gamma_KS.p.val", "Lognormal_mode",
    "Lognormal_sd","Lognormal_KS.test.stat", "Lognormal_KS.p.val")
df_summary
library("DT")
datatable(t(df_summary))
```

2.2.4.1.6   Mixture Distribution Data Modeling

Earlier, we discussed the *expectations–maximization* (EM) algorithm for parameter estimation. Now, we will illustrate the use of EM to estimate the mixture weights and the distribution parameters needed to obtain mixture-distribution data models. For

Show 10 ▾ entries   Search: [   ]

	AC1338	AC1432	AC1593	AC1679	AC1860	AC1874	AC1881	AC1903	Rec
Weibull_mode	71	75	81	81	78	75	72	80	76
Weibull_sd	42	40	54	49	45	42	58	48	41
Weibull_KS.test.stat	0.0411	0.07218	0.05572	0.0462	0.06798	0.06495	0.0821	0.07426	0.05729
Weibull_KS.p.val	0.4284	0.047982	0.10341	0.36208	0.088752	0.032324	0.00069318	0.059275	0.027524
Gamma_mode	64	69	75	73	73	68	70	73	68
Gamma_sd	42	38	52	49	42	41	55	47	40
Gamma_KS.test.stat	0.02878	0.03942	0.03823	0.03222	0.03691	0.03431	0.05289	0.06417	0.03865
Gamma_KS.p.val	0.84738	0.63424	0.4885	0.80172	0.74826	0.61239	0.073267	0.14456	0.28357
Lognormal_mode	57	63	67	64	67	61	63	66	62
Lognormal_sd	48	40	58	56	45	45	60	51	44

Showing 1 to 10 of 12 entries   Previous [1] 2 Next

Fig. 2.57 Reporting quantitative summaries of the estimated Weibull, Gamma, and Log-Normal density models for each of the crystallography samples

each sample, we fit mixtures of $k = 3$ distribution models. The specific types of mixtures for each of the nine samples are indicated below.

```
sampleColNames <- c("AC1338","AC1432","AC1593", "AC1679", "AC1860", "AC1874",
                    "AC1881", "AC1903", "Rec")
sampleMixtureParam <- c(3, 3, 3, 3, 3, 3, 3, 3, 3)
df_sampleMixtureParam <- data.frame(t(sampleMixtureParam))
colnames(df_sampleMixtureParam) <- sampleColNames; # df_sampleMixtureParam
```

2.2.4.1.7   Mixture-Distribution Model Fitting and Parameter Estimation

We will use the R package *mixtools* to obtain the EM estimates of the mixture distribution weights and the corresponding distribution parameters.

```
library(mixtools)  # install.packages("mixtools")
col_num <- dim(crystallography_data)[2]; col_num
# Fit mixture models
capture.output(
  for(i in 1:col_num) {    # remove all non-numeric elements (if any)
    data_no_NA <- crystallography_data[complete.cases(
              crystallography_data[, i]), i]
    # length(data_no_NA)
    fit_W[[i]]<-weibullRMM_SEM(data_no_NA,k=df_sampleMixtureParam[1,i],verb=F)
    # summary(fit_W[i])
    fit_G[[i]] <- gammamixEM(data_no_NA, k=df_sampleMixtureParam[1,i], verb=F)
    # summary(fit_G[i])
    fit_LN[[i]] <- normalmixEM(data_no_NA,k=df_sampleMixtureParam[1,i],verb=F)
    },
  file='NUL'
)
```

2.2.4.1.8   Plotting the Mixture Distribution Models

We will define custom plots for the mixtures of *Gamma*, *Weibull*, and *Normal* distributions. Alternatively, we can also use some of the `mixtools::plot()` function to display mixture distribution models.

```r
# Custom design of Gamma-Mixture Model plot
gammaMM.plot <- function(mix.object, k = 2, main = "") {
 data_no_NA<-crystallography_data[complete.cases(crystallography_data[,i]),i]
 d3 <- function(x) { # construct the mixture using the estimated parameters
    mix.object$lambda[1]*dgamma(x, shape=mix.object$gamma.pars[1,1],
        1/mix.object$gamma.pars[2,1]) +
      mix.object$lambda[2]*dgamma(x, shape=mix.object$gamma.pars[1,2],
        1/mix.object$gamma.pars[2,2]) +
      mix.object$lambda[3]*dgamma(x, shape=mix.object$gamma.pars[1,3],
        1/mix.object$gamma.pars[2,3])
 }
 x <- seq(min(data_no_NA), max(data_no_NA), 0.001)
 hist(data_no_NA,col="pink",freq=F,breaks=10, main=main, xlab="Intensities")
 lines(x, d3(x), lwd=3, col="black", xlim=c(4,23), ylim=c(0, 0.25))
 mixColors <- colorRampPalette(c("blue", "red"))(k)
 for (i in 1:k) {
   d = function(x) { # Build Gamma components using the estimated parameters
     mix.object$lambda[i]*dgamma(x, shape=mix.object$gamma.pars[1, i],
        1/mix.object$gamma.pars[2,i])
   }
   lines(x, d(x), lwd=3, col=mixColors[i])
 }
}
# Custom design of Weibull-Mixture Model plot
weibullMM.plot <- function(mix.object, k = 2, main = "") {
 data_no_NA<-crystallography_data[complete.cases(crystallography_data[,i]),i]
 d3 <- function(x) { # construct the mixture using the estimated parameters
    mix.object$lambda[1]*dweibull(x, shape=mix.object$shape[1],
        scale=mix.object$scale[1]) +
      mix.object$lambda[2]*dweibull(x, shape=mix.object$shape[2],
        scale=mix.object$scale[2]) +
      mix.object$lambda[3]*dweibull(x, shape=mix.object$shape[3],
        scale=mix.object$scale[3])
 }
 x <- seq(min(data_no_NA), max(data_no_NA), 0.001)
 hist(data_no_NA, col="pink", freq=F, breaks=15, main = main,
        xlab="Intensities")
 lines(x, d3(x), lwd=3, col="black", xlim=c(4,23), ylim=c(0, 0.25))
 mixColors <- colorRampPalette(c("blue", "red"))(k)
 for (i in 1:k) {
   d = function(x) { # Build Weibull components using estimated parameters
     mix.object$lambda[i]*dweibull(x, shape=mix.object$shape[i],
        scale=mix.object$scale[i])
   }
   lines(x, d(x), lwd=3, col=mixColors[i])
 }
}
```

```
# Custom design of Normal-Mixture Model plot
normalMM.plot <- function(mix.object, k = 2, main = "") {
 data_no_NA<-crystallography_data[complete.cases(crystallography_data[,i]),i]
  d3 <- function(x) { # construct the mixture using the estimated parameters
    mix.object$lambda[1]*dnorm(x, mean=mix.object$mu[1],
        sd=mix.object$sigma[1]) +
     mix.object$lambda[2]*dnorm(x, mean=mix.object$mu[2],
        sd=mix.object$sigma[2]) +
     mix.object$lambda[3]*dnorm(x, mean=mix.object$mu[3],
        sd=mix.object$sigma[3])
  }
  x <- seq(min(data_no_NA), max(data_no_NA), 0.001)
  hist(data_no_NA, col="pink", freq=F, breaks=20, main = main,
       xlab="Intensities", xlim = c(4,180), ylim = c(0.0, 0.2))
  lines(x, d3(x), lwd=3, col="black")
  mixColors <- colorRampPalette(c("blue", "red"))(k)
  for (i in 1:k) {
    d = function(x) {#Build the Weibull components using estimated parameters
      mix.object$lambda[i]*dnorm(x, mean=mix.object$mu[i],
           sd=mix.object$sigma[i])
    }
    lines(x, d(x), lwd=3, col=mixColors[i])
  }
}
```

Next, we will display the three alternative mixture distribution models juxtaposed on the sample histograms of each of the nine samples (Fig. 2.58).

```
for(i in 1:2) {       # this only plots the first 2 samples to save space
  weibullMM.plot(fit_W[[i]], df_sampleMixtureParam[1,i],
          paste0("Mixture of ", df_sampleMixtureParam[1, sampleColNames[i]],
                 " Weibull Models of ", sampleColNames[i]))
  gammaMM.plot(fit_G[[i]], df_sampleMixtureParam[1,i],
          paste0("Mixture of ", df_sampleMixtureParam[1, sampleColNames[i]],
                 " Gamma Models of ", sampleColNames[i]))
  normalMM.plot(fit_LN[[i]], df_sampleMixtureParam[1,i],
          paste0("Mixture of ", df_sampleMixtureParam[1, sampleColNames[i]],
                 " Normal Models of ", sampleColNames[i]))
}
```

2.2.4.1.9 Reporting Model Parameter Estimates

For each of the nine samples in this dataset and each of the three types of mixture distribution models (Weibull, Gamma, and Normal), we will summarize the parameter estimates:

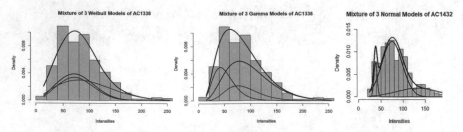

Fig. 2.58 Three-component mixture distribution models of the crystallographic data

- *lambda*: The weights (impacts) of each of the three mixture components to the overall mixture model
- *parameters*: of each mixture distribution component, *mean* and *sd*
- *loglik*: the overall mixture distribution log-likelihood value

```r
# Generate the summary DF
getSummaryTable <- function (crystalSampleIndex) {
  mat <- matrix(0, nrow = 3, ncol = 10)
  # Weibull estimates for all 3 model components
  mat[1,1] <- round(fit_W[[crystalSampleIndex]]$lambda[1],3) # Lambda
  mat[1,2] <- round(fit_W[[crystalSampleIndex]]$scale[1] *
           gamma(1+1/fit_W[[crystalSampleIndex]]$shape[1]),3)  # mean
  mat[1,3] <- round(fit_W[[crystalSampleIndex]]$scale[1] *
           sqrt(gamma(1+2/fit_W[[crystalSampleIndex]]$shape[1])-
           (gamma(1+1/fit_W[[crystalSampleIndex]]$shape[1]))^2),3)  # sd
  mat[1,4] <- round(fit_W[[crystalSampleIndex]]$lambda[2],3) # Lambda
  mat[1,5] <- round(fit_W[[crystalSampleIndex]]$scale[2] *
           gamma(1+1/fit_W[[crystalSampleIndex]]$shape[2]),3)  # mean
  mat[1,6] <- round(fit_W[[crystalSampleIndex]]$scale[2] *
           sqrt(gamma(1+2/fit_W[[crystalSampleIndex]]$shape[2])-
           (gamma(1+1/fit_W[[crystalSampleIndex]]$shape[2]))^2),3)  # sd
  mat[1,7]  <- round(fit_W[[crystalSampleIndex]]$lambda[3],3) # Lambda
  mat[1,8] <- round(fit_W[[crystalSampleIndex]]$scale[3] *
           gamma(1+1/fit_W[[crystalSampleIndex]]$shape[3]),3)  # mean
  mat[1,9] <- round(fit_W[[crystalSampleIndex]]$scale[3] *
           sqrt(gamma(1+2/fit_W[[crystalSampleIndex]]$shape[3])-
           (gamma(1+1/fit_W[[crystalSampleIndex]]$shape[3]))^2),3)  # sd
  mat[1,10] <- round(fit_W[[crystalSampleIndex]]$loglik,3)    # Log-lik
  # Gamma estimates for all 3 model components
  mat[2,1] <- round(fit_G[[crystalSampleIndex]]$lambda[1],3)        # Lambda
  mat[2,2] <- round(fit_G[[crystalSampleIndex]]$gamma.pars[1,1]*
               fit_G[[crystalSampleIndex]]$gamma.pars[2,1],3)  # mean
  mat[2,3] <- round(sqrt(fit_G[[crystalSampleIndex]]$gamma.pars[1,1])*
               fit_G[[crystalSampleIndex]]$gamma.pars[2,1],3)  # SD
  mat[2,4] <- round(fit_G[[crystalSampleIndex]]$lambda[2],3)     # Lambda
  mat[2,5] <- round(fit_G[[crystalSampleIndex]]$gamma.pars[1,2]*
               fit_G[[crystalSampleIndex]]$gamma.pars[2,2],3)  # mean
  mat[2,6] <- round(sqrt(fit_G[[crystalSampleIndex]]$gamma.pars[1,2])*
               fit_G[[crystalSampleIndex]]$gamma.pars[2,2],3)  # sd
  mat[2,7]  <- round(fit_G[[crystalSampleIndex]]$lambda[3],3)     # Lambda
  mat[2,8] <- round(fit_G[[crystalSampleIndex]]$gamma.pars[1,3]*
               fit_G[[crystalSampleIndex]]$gamma.pars[2,3],3)  # mean
  mat[2,9] <- round(sqrt(fit_G[[crystalSampleIndex]]$gamma.pars[1,3])*
               fit_G[[crystalSampleIndex]]$gamma.pars[2,3],3)  # sd
  mat[2,10] <- round(fit_G[[crystalSampleIndex]]$loglik,3)    # Log-lik
  # Normal estimates for all 3 model components
  mat[3,1] <- round(fit_LN[[crystalSampleIndex]]$lambda[1],3)       # Lambda
  mat[3,2] <- round(fit_LN[[crystalSampleIndex]]$mu[1],3)  # shape
  mat[3,3] <- round(fit_LN[[crystalSampleIndex]]$sigma[1],3)  # scale
  mat[3,4] <- round(fit_LN[[crystalSampleIndex]]$lambda[2],3)      # Lambda
  mat[3,5] <- round(fit_LN[[crystalSampleIndex]]$mu[2],3)  # shape
  mat[3,6] <- round(fit_LN[[crystalSampleIndex]]$sigma[2],3)  # scale
  mat[3,7]  <- round(fit_LN[[crystalSampleIndex]]$lambda[3],3)      # Lambda
  mat[3,8] <- round(fit_LN[[crystalSampleIndex]]$mu[3],3)  # shape
  mat[3,9] <- round(fit_LN[[crystalSampleIndex]]$sigma[3],3)  # scale
  mat[3,10] <- round(fit_LN[[crystalSampleIndex]]$loglik,3)    # Log-lik
  return(as.data.frame(mat))
}
# render the summary DT tables
library("DT")
```

Show 10 ▼ entries   Search:

	MC 1 Weight	MC 1 Mean	MC 1 SD	MC 2 Weight	MC 2 Mean	MC 2 SD	MC 3 Weight	MC 3 Mean	MC 3 SD	MixMod LogLik
Weibull	0.279	69.106	28.285	0.338	79.823	34.023	0.383	100.381	50.513	-2299.981
Gamma	0.506	62.115	26.317	0.318	107.296	50.359	0.176	110.455	26.041	-2294.6
Normal	0.404	53.77	18.279	0.578	102.23	34.889	0.018	235.415	13.654	-2295.334

Showing 1 to 3 of 3 entries   Previous 1 Next

Fig. 2.59 Parameter estimates for each of the three-component mixture distribution models

Below we summarize the mixture-distribution models just for the first crystallographic sample (Fig. 2.59).

```
df_summary <- getSummaryTable(1)
rownames(df_summary) <- c("Weibull", "Gamma", "Normal")
colnames(df_summary) <- c("MC 1 Weight", "MC 1 Mean","MC 1 SD","MC 2 Weight",
   "MC 2 Mean","MC 2 SD","MC 3 Weight","MC 3 Mean","MC 3 SD","MixMod LogLik")
datatable(df_summary, rownames = TRUE)
```

for the first crystallographic sample

2.2.4.2 2D Kernel Density and 3D Surface Plots

The univariate density estimation we saw above illustrates the process of using observed data to compute an estimate of an underlying process probability density function. There are several approaches to obtain density estimation, but the most basic technique is to use a rescaled histogram. Below we will show how this approach can be used for multivariate density estimation, in particular, for plotting 2D kernel density and 3D surface plots, which are important and useful in multivariate exploratory data analytics.

We will use the plot_ly() function in the plotly package, which works with data frame objects. To create a surface plot, we use two vectors x and y of length m and n, respectively. We also need a matrix z of size $m \times n$. This z matrix is created from matrix multiplication involving x and y. To demonstrate the 2D kernel density estimation plot, we will use the eruptions data from the "Old Faithful" geyser in Yellowstone National Park, Wyoming, stored in object geyser. Also, the kde2d () function is needed for 2D kernel density estimation.

```
kd <- with(MASS::geyser, MASS::kde2d(duration, waiting, n = 50))
kd$x[1:5]
```

We will make use of the matrix multiplication operator %*%, which is defined in Chap. 3, to compute z=t(x)%*%y. Then we apply plot_ly to the list kd using the with() function (Fig. 2.60).

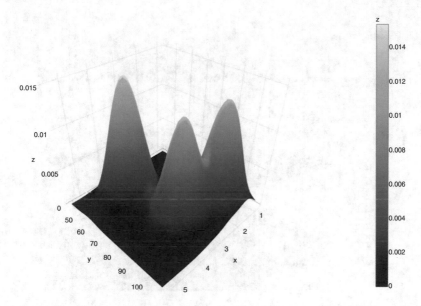

Fig. 2.60 2D (geyser duration and eruption waiting) kernel density estimation for the Old Faithful geyser

```
library(plotly)
with(kd, plot_ly(x=x, y=y, z=z, type="surface"))
```

Similarly, we can stack multiple surfaces in the same 3D scene, as in the stack of 2D image surface plots shown below (Fig. 2.61).

```
library(jpeg)
# Get an image file downloaded (default: MRI_ImageHematoma.jpg)
img_url  <- "https://umich.instructure.com/files/1627149/download?download_frd=1"
img_file <- tempfile(); download.file(img_url, img_file, mode="wb")
img <- readJPEG(img_file)
file.remove(img_file) # cleanup
img <- img[, , 1] # extract the first channel (from RGB spectrum) as 2D array
library(spatstat)
img_s <- as.matrix(blur(as.im(img), sigma=10)) # smooth the image
z2 <- img_s + 1   # abs(rnorm(1, 1, 1)) # Upper confidence surface
z3 <- img_s - 1   # abs(rnorm(1, 1, 1)) # Lower confidence limit
# Plot the image surfaces
p <- plot_ly(z=img, type="surface", showscale=FALSE) %>%
 add_trace(z=z2, type="surface", showscale=FALSE, opacity=0.98) %>%
 add_trace(z=z3, type="surface", showscale=FALSE, opacity=0.98)
p # Plot the mean-surface along with lower and upper confidence services.
```

2.2.4.3 3D and 4D Visualizations

Many datasets have intrinsic multi-dimensional characteristics. For instance, the human body is a 3D solid of matter (three spatial dimensions can be used to describe

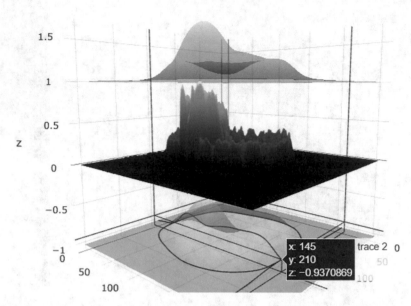

Fig. 2.61 Interactive 3D scene showing a stack of 2D surface representations of brain images

the position of every component, e.g., sMRI volume) that changes over time (the fourth longitudinal dimension, e.g., fMRI hyper-volume time-series). The SOCR BrainViewer[19] shows how to use a web-browser to visualize 2D cross-sections of 3D volumes, display volume-rendering, and show 1D (e.g., 1-manifold curves embedded in 3D) and 2D (e.g., surfaces, shapes) models jointly into the same 3D scene. We will now illustrate an example of 3D/4D visualization in R using the packages brainR and rgl.

```
# install.packages("brainR") ## if necessary
library(brainR)
brainURL <- "https://socr.umich.edu/HTML5/BrainViewer/data/TestBrain.nii.gz"
brainFile <- file.path(tempdir(), "TestBrain.nii.gz")
download.file(brainURL, dest=brainFile, quiet=TRUE)
brainVolume <- readNIfTI(brainFile, reorient=FALSE)
brainVolDims <- dim(brainVolume); brainVolDims ## [1] 181 217 181
# try different levels to construct contour surfaces (10 fast & smooth)
contour3d(brainVolume, level = 20, alpha = 0.1, draw = TRUE)
contour3d(brainVolume, level = c(10, 120), alpha = c(0.3, 0.5),
        add = TRUE, color=c("yellow", "red"))
# create text for orientation of right/left
text3d(x=brainVolDims[1]/2, y=brainVolDims[2]/2, z=brainVolDims[3]*0.98,
        text="Top")
text3d(x=brainVolDims[1]*0.98, y=brainVolDims[2]/2, z = brainVolDims[3]/2,
        text="Right")
```

---

[19] https://socr.umich.edu/HTML5/BrainViewer/

The supplementary website provides some additional 3D/4D PET, sMRI, and fMRI volumes in *.nii.gz format:

- sMRI (3D real-valued structural MRI volume)
- fMRI (4D real-valued functional MRI hyper-volume)
- PET (3D perfusion positron emission tomography volume).

For 4D fMRI time-series, we can load the hyper-volumes similarly and then display some lower dimensional projections (Fig. 2.62).

```
fMRIURL<-"https://socr.umich.edu/HTML5/BrainViewer/data/fMRI_FilteredData_4D.nii.gz"
fMRIFile <- file.path(tempdir(), "fMRI_FilteredData_4D.nii.gz")
download.file(fMRIURL, dest=fMRIFile, quiet=TRUE)
(fMRIVolume <- readNIfTI(fMRIFile, reorient=FALSE))
# dimensions: 64 x 64 x 21 x 180 ; 4mm x 4mm x 6mm x 3 sec
fMRIVolDims <- dim(fMRIVolume); fMRIVolDims
time_dim <- fMRIVolDims[4]; time_dim
# Plot the 4D array of imaging data in a 5x5 grid of images
image(fMRIVolume, zlim=range(fMRIVolume)*0.95)
```

Below is an orthographic display of the fMRI data using the axial plane containing the left-and-right thalamus to approximately center the crosshairs (Figs. 2.63 and 2.64).

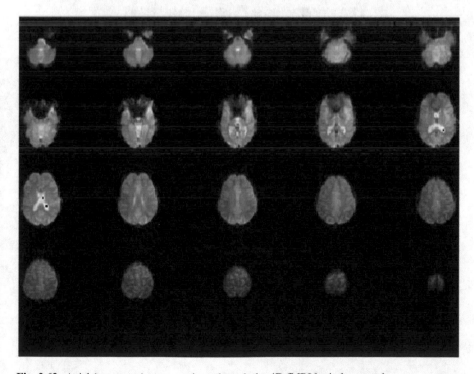

Fig. 2.62 Axial (transverse) cross-sections through the 4D fMRI brain hyper-volume

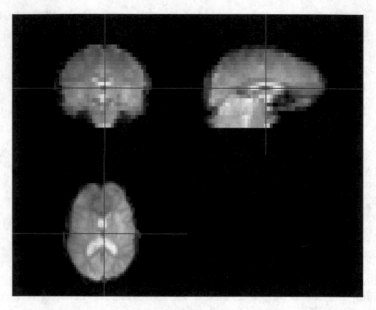

Fig. 2.63 An orthographic projection through the 4D fMRI brain hyper-volume

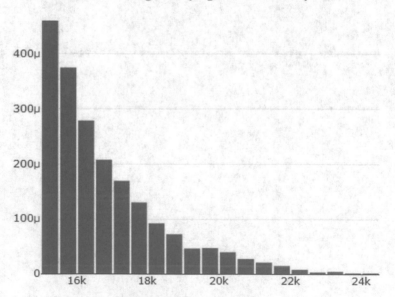

Fig. 2.64 Intensity histogram of the 4D fMRI brain hyper-volume

```
orthographic(fMRIVolume, xyz=c(34,29,10), zlim=range(fMRIVolume)*0.9)
```

```
stat_fmri_test <- ifelse(fMRIVolume > 15000, fMRIVolume, NA)
h <- hist(stat_fmri_test, plot = F)
plot_ly(x = h$mids, y = h$density, type = "bar") %>%
   layout(bargap=0.1, title="fMRI Histogram (high intensities)")
```

Next we will show the time dynamics of the longitudinal fMRI data at a fixed spatial voxel location (Fig. 2.65).

```
x1 <- c(1:180)
y1 <- loess(fMRIVolume[30, 30, 10,]~ x1, family = "gaussian")
plot_ly(x = x1, y = fMRIVolume[30, 30, 10,],
        name="Raw fMRI", type = 'scatter', mode = 'lines') %>%
   add_trace(y = smooth(fMRIVolume[30, 30, 10,]), name = 'loess fMRI')  %>%
   add_trace(y = ksmooth(x1, fMRIVolume[30, 30, 10,], kernel="normal",
        bandwidth = 5)$y, name='kSmooth fMRI')  %>%
   layout(title="Time Series of 3D Voxel (x=30, y=30, z=10)",
        legend = list(orientation = 'h'))
```

Chapter 12 provides more details about longitudinal and time-series data analysis. Finally, the online DSPA Appendix 3 includes examples of topological classification, representation, modeling, and visualization of parametric and implicit surfaces, as well as open and closed manifolds.

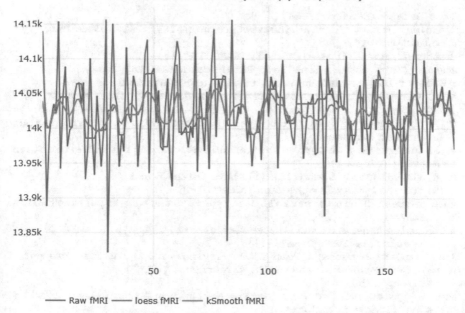

Fig. 2.65 Longitudinal dynamics of the raw and smoothed fMRI time-series at a fixed spatial location

2.3   Practice Problems

2.3.1   Data Manipulation

Practice simple data importing, plotting, summarizing, and exporting. Load the following two datasets, generate summary statistics for all variables, plot some of the features (e.g., using histograms, box plots, density plots, etc.), and save the data locally as CSV files:

- ALS case-study data
- SOCR Knee Pain Data

2.3.2   Bivariate Relations

Explore some data bivariate relations. Use ALS case-study data or SOCR Knee Pain Data to explicate some bivariate relations (e.g., use bivariate plots, correlations, table cross tables, etc.)

Use 07_UMich_AnnArbor_MI_TempPrecipitation_HistData_1900_2015 data to show the relations between *temperature* and *time*. [Hint: use geom_line(), geom_bar(), or plot_ly()]. Sample code for dealing with the temperatures data:

```
Temp_Data <- as.data.frame(
 read.csv("https://umich.instructure.com/files/706163/download?
download_frd=1",
 header=T, na.strings=c("",".","NA","NR")))
summary(Temp_Data) # View(Temp_Data); colnames(Temp_Data)
# Wide-to-Long transformation: reshape arguments include
# (1) list of variable names that define the different times or metrics
(varying),
# (2) the name we wish to give the variable containing these values in our
long dataset (v.names),
# (3) the name we wish to give the variable describing the different times
or metrics (timevar),
# (4) the values this variable will have (times), and
# (5) the end format for the data (direction)
# Before reshaping make sure all data types are the same as putting them in
1 column will
# otherwise generate inconsistencies/errors
colN <- colnames(Temp_Data[,-1])
longTempData <- reshape(Temp_Data, varying = colN, v.names = "Temps",
 timevar="Months", times = colN, direction = "long")
# View(longTempData)
bar2 <- ggplot(longTempData, aes(x = Months, y = Temps, fill = Months)) +
 geom_bar(stat = "identity")
print(bar2)
bar3 <- ggplot(longTempData, aes(x = Year, y = Temps, fill = Months)) +
```

```
geom_bar(stat = "identity") print(bar3)
p <- ggplot(longTempData, aes(x=Year, y=as.integer(Temps),
color=Months)) +
 geom_line()
p
```

2.3.3 Missing Data

Using one of the above datasets, introduce (artificially) some missing data, impute the missing values, and examine the differences between the original, incomplete, and imputed datasets.

2.3.4 Surface Plots

Generate a surface plot for the (RF=right knee, frontal view) Knee Pain data illustrating the 2D distribution of locations of the patient reported knee pain (use plot_ly() and kernel density estimation).

2.3.5 Unbalanced Groups

Rebalance the groups of ALS (training data) patients according to Age > 50 and Age ≤ 50 using synthetic minority oversampling (SMOTE) to ensure approximately equal cohort sizes.

2.3.6 Common Plots

Use the TBI dataset (CaseStudy11_TBI) to display some interactive (SVG) visualization plots—e.g., histograms, density plots, pie charts, heatmaps, bar plots, and paired correlation plots.

2.3.7 Trees and Graphs

Use the SOCR Resource Hierarchical Dataset (JSON) or the DSPA Dynamic Certificate Map (JSON) to generate tree/graph displays of the corresponding structural information contained in the JSON object.

Processing a JSON hierarchy

```
library(jsonlite); library(RCurl); library(data.tree)
url <- "https://socr.umich.edu/html/navigators/D3/xml/
SOCR_HyperTree.json"
raw_data <- getURL(url)
document <- fromJSON(raw_data)
tree <- Node$new(document$name)
for(i in seq_len(length(document))) {
tree$AddChild(document$children$name[[i]])
 for(j in seq_len(length(document$children$children[[i]]))) {
tree$children[[i]]$AddChild(document$children$children[[i]]$name
[[j]])
 for(k in seq_len(length(
document$children$children[[i]]$children[[j]]))){
 tree$children[[i]]$children[[j]]$AddChild((
document$children$children[[i]]$children[[j]]$name[[k]]))
 }
 }
}
suppressMessages(library(igraph))
plot(as.igraph(tree, directed = T, direction = "climb"))
suppressMessages(library(networkD3))
treenetwork <- ToDataFrameNetwork(tree, "name")
simpleNetwork(treenetwork, fontSize = 10)
```

2.3.8   Data EDA Examples

- Use the SOCR_OilGasData to generate three individual bar plots for Fossil Fuels, Nuclear Electric Power and Renewable Energy respectively (*Hint*: you may use plot_ly(), ggplot() and facet_grid()). Include two lines for *Productions* and *Consumption*. The x-axis should be *time* (you may use year as numeric type directly), draw *Consumption* slightly wider and noticeable (e.g., using magenta color).
- Use the SOCR_OzoneData to generate a correlation plot with the variables "MTH_1," "MTH_2," ..., "MTH_12." (*Hint*: you need to compute the correlation matrix first, then apply corrplot() or plot_ly(), try to use multiple chart types, "circle," "pie," "mixed," etc.)
- Use the SOCR_ CA_OzoneData to generate a 3D surface plot (using the variables *Longitude*, *Latitude*, and *O3*).
- Generate random numbers from the Cauchy distribution. Draw a histogram and compare it with the histogram of normal distribution. What do you find? You may try different seeds to re-generate the Cauchy random numbers.
- Use the SOCR_Data_PD_BiomedBigMetadata to generate a *heatplot*. Set RowSideColors and ColSideColors and use rainbow colors.

- Use SOCR_Data_2011_US_JobsRanking to draw a scatter plot *Overall_Score - Average_Income(USD)*. Specify title, legend, and axes labels. Then try `plot_ly()` or qplot()` to display *Overall_Score* vs. *Average_Income(USD)*, color the blobs according to the *Stress_Level* and size them, according to *Hiring_Potential*, blob labels should represent *Job_Title*.
- Use the SOCR_TurkiyeStudentEvalData to generate trees and graphs using `cutree()`. (use variables *Q1–Q28*).

2.3.9   Data Reports

Use the California Ozone Data to generate a summary report. Make sure to include summary for every variable, structure, and type of data elements; discuss the tendency of the ozone average concentration; explore the differences of the ozone concentration for separate regions (e.g., focus just on 2006); and explore the change of ozone concentration by season.

Chapter 3
Linear Algebra, Matrix Computing, and Regression Modeling

Before continuing on, readers may find it useful to first review some of the fundamental mathematical representations, analytical modeling techniques, and basic concepts.[1] These foundations play critical roles in all subsequent chapters and sections. Examples of core mathematical principles include calculus of differentiation and integration; representation of scalars, vectors, matrices, and tensors; displacement, velocity, and acceleration; polynomials, exponents, and logarithmic functions; Taylor's series; complex numbers; ordinary and partial differential equations; probability and statistics; statistical moments; and probability distributions. In this chapter, we will cover the basics of linear algebra, matrix computing, solving systems of linear equations, computing sample statistics as estimates of population parameters, least squares method, linear modeling, eigenvalues and eigenvectors, correlations, simple and multivariate linear regression.

3.1 Linear Algebra

Linear algebra is a branch of mathematics that studies linear associations using vectors, vector-spaces, linear equations, linear transformations, and matrices. Although it is generally challenging to visualize complex data, e.g., large vectors, tensors, and tables in n-dimensional Euclidean spaces ($n \geq 3$), linear algebra allows us to represent, model, synthesize, and summarize such complex data.

Virtually all natural processes permit first-order linear approximations, which are useful because linear equations are easy to write, interpret, and solve. These first-order approximations may be convenient to practically assess the process, determine general trends, identify potential patterns, and suggest associations in the data. Linear equations represent the simplest type of models for many processes.

---

[1] https://socr.umich.edu/BPAD/

© The Author(s), under exclusive license to Springer Nature Switzerland AG 2023
I. D. Dinov, *Data Science and Predictive Analytics*, The Springer Series in Applied Machine Learning, https://doi.org/10.1007/978-3-031-17483-4_3

Higher-order models may include additional nonlinear terms, e.g., Taylor-series expansion. Linear algebra provides the foundation for linear representation, analytics, solutions, inference, and visualization of first-order affine models. Linear algebra is a small part of the larger mathematics *functional analysis* field, which is actually the infinite-dimensional version of linear algebra. Specifically, *linear algebra* allows us to *computationally* manipulate, model, solve, and interpret complex systems of equations that represent large numbers of dimensions/variables. Arbitrarily large problems can be mathematically transformed into simple matrix equations in the form of $Ax = b$ or $Ax = \lambda x$.

In this chapter, we review the fundamentals of linear algebra, matrix manipulation, and their applications to representation, modeling, and analysis of real data. Specifically, we will cover: (1) construction of matrices and matrix operations; (2) general matrix algebra notations; (3) eigenvalues and eigenvectors of linear operators; (4) least squares estimation; (5) linear regression and variance-covariance matrices; and (6) regression decision tree prediction.

3.1.1   Building Matrices

The easiest way to create a matrix in R is by using the `matrix()` or `array()` functions, both allow splicing a long vector into a matrix or a tensor of a certain size.

```
seq1 <- seq(1:6)
m1 <- matrix(seq1, nrow=2, ncol=3); m1
##      [,1] [,2] [,3]
## [1,]    1    3    5
## [2,]    2    4    6
m2 <- diag(seq1); m2
m3 <- matrix(rnorm(20), nrow=5); m3
```

The function `diag()` is very useful. When the object is a vector, it creates a diagonal matrix with the vector in the principal diagonal.

```
diag(c(1, 2, 3))
```

When the object is a matrix, `diag()` returns its principal diagonal.

```
diag(m1) ## [1] 1 4
```

When the object is a scalar, `diag(k)` returns a $k \times k$ identity matrix.

```
diag(4)
```

The functions `cbind()` and `rbind()` are also useful for building matrices from vectors by column or row concatenation.

```
c1 <- 1:5
m4 <- cbind(m3, c1); m4
r1 <- 1:4
m5 <- rbind(m3, r1); m5
```

Note that the matrix m5 has a row named r1, which appears as the 4th row in the matrix. Sometimes, we may need to remove row and column names by naming them NULL.

```
dimnames(m5) <- list(NULL, NULL); m5
```

3.1.2 Matrix Subscripts

Each element in a matrix has a location indexed by the corresponding row and column. A[i, j] stores the element in the i-th row and j-th column in the matrix A. We can also access some specific rows or columns using matrix subscripts.

```
m6 <- matrix(1:12, nrow=3); m6
m6[1, 2] ## [1] 4
m6[1, ]  ## [1]  1  4  7 10
m6[, 2]  ## [1] 4 5 6
m6[, c(2, 3)]
```

The ordinal scalar operations, addition, subtraction, multiplication, and division, can be generalized as matrix operations.

3.1.3 Addition and Subtraction

Matrix addition and subtraction require matrices of the same dimensions. The sum or difference of two matrices is matrices containing elements representing the scalar sum or difference, respectively, of the values in corresponding positions in the two matrices.

```
m7 <- matrix(1:6, nrow=2);   m7
m8 <- matrix(2:7, nrow = 2); m8
m7 + m8
##      [,1] [,2] [,3]
## [1,]   3    7   11
## [2,]   5    9   13
m8 - m7
m8 - 1
```

3.1.4 Multiplication

Element-wise matrix multiplication is valid for matrices of the same sizes. However, *matrix multiplication* is different from component-wise scalar multiplication and requires a special match between the dimensions of the multiplied matrices, $P_{m \times k} = L_{m \times n} \cdot R_{n \times k}$. That is, the number of *columns* in the left matrix, L, must equal to the number of *rows* of the right matrix, R. Then, the *row × column* matrix multiplication rule yields a product matrix of dimensions corresponding to the number of rows (m) of L and the number of columns (k) of R, i.e., $P_{m \times k}$.

3.1.4.1   Element-Wise Multiplication

Element-wise matrix multiplication (∗) involves scalar products of the elements in the same positions.

```
m8 * m7
## [,1] [,2] [,3]
## [1,] 2 12 30
## [2,] 6 20 42
```

3.1.4.2   Matrix Multiplication (Product)

Matrix product (% ∗ %) generates an output matrix having the same number of rows as the left matrix and the same number of columns as the right matrix.

```
dim(m8)  ## [1] 2 3
m9 <- matrix(3:8, nrow=3); m9; dim(m9) ## [1] 3 2
M <- m8 %*% m9; M
##      [,1] [,2]
## [1,]   52   88
## [2,]   64  109
```

The product of multiplying two matrices $m^8_{2 \times 3} * m^9_{3 \times 2}$ is another matrix $M_{2 \times 2}$ of size 2×2. The process of multiplying two vectors is called the *outer product*. Assume we have two vectors u and v. Using matrix multiplication, their outer product is $u \%o\% v \equiv u \underbrace{\% * \%}_{product} \overbrace{t(v)}^{transpose}$, or mathematically uv^t. In R, the vector outer product operator is %o% generates outputs that are second-order tensors (matrices).

```
u <- c(1, 2, 3, 4, 5)
v <- c(4, 5, 6, 7, 8)
u %o% v
##      [,1] [,2] [,3] [,4] [,5]
## [1,]    4    5    6    7    8
## [2,]    8   10   12   14   16
## [3,]   12   15   18   21   24
## [4,]   16   20   24   28   32
## [5,]   20   25   30   35   40
u %*% t(v)
```

Try to explain the differences between $u \% * \% v$, $u \% * \% t(v)$, $u * t(v)$, and $u * v$.

3.1.4.3   Matrix Inversion (Division)

Element-wise matrix (or scalar) division is well defined for matrices of the same dimensions.

```
m8 / m7
##      [,1]     [,2]     [,3]
## [1,]  2.0 1.333333 1.200000
## [2,]  1.5 1.250000 1.166667
m8 / 2
```

However, matrix inversion is different. Recall that the *transpose* of a matrix is a matrix with swapped columns and rows. In R, matrix transposition is done by the function t().

```
m8; t(m8)
## [,1] [,2]
## [1,] 2 3
## [2,] 4 5
## [3,] 6 7
```

Notice that the $[1, 2]$ element in m8[1, 2] is the same as the $[2, 1]$ element in t (m8)[2, 1].

The *right inverse* of a matrix, $(A^{-1}_{m \times n})$, is a special matrix with the property that multiplying the original matrix $(A_{n \times m})$ on the *right* by this inverse $(A^{-1}_{m \times n})$ yields the identity matrix, which has 1's on the main diagonal and 0's off the diagonal, i.e.,

$$A_{n \times m} A^{-1}_{m \times n} = I_{n \times n}.$$

Similarly, a *left matrix inverse* is defined as a matrix, $(A^{-1}_{m \times n})$, with the property that multiplying the original matrix $(A_{n \times m})$ on the *left* by this inverse $(A^{-1}_{m \times n})$ yields the identity matrix, i.e.,

$$A^{-1}_{m \times n} A_{n \times m} = I_{m \times m}.$$

A *matrix* inverse is only defined for square matrices, $m = n$. For example, given four numbers satisfying $ad - bc \neq 0$, the following 2×2 matrix.

$$A_{2 \times 2} = \begin{pmatrix} a & b \\ c & d \end{pmatrix},$$

has an inverse matrix given by

$$A_{2\times 2}^{-1} = \frac{1}{ad-bc}\begin{pmatrix} d & -b \\ -c & a \end{pmatrix}.$$

It's easy to validate that $A_{2\times 2}A_{2\times 2}^{-1} = I_{2\times 2}$. In higher dimensions, the Cramer's rule may be used to compute the matrix inverse. Matrix inversion is available in R via the `solve()` function.

```
m10 <- matrix(1:4, nrow=2); m10
solve(m10)   # the inverse matrix
m10 %*% solve(m10)
##      [,1] [,2]
## [1,]   1    0
## [2,]   0    1
```

Note that only special matrices are invertible, not all. These matrices are *square* (have the same number of rows and columns) and nonsingular. Another function that can help us to get the inverse of a matrix is the `ginv()` function in the MASS package. This function gives us the Moore–Penrose Generalized Inverse of a matrix.

```
library(MASS)
ginv(m10)
```

In addition, the function `solve()` can be used to solve matrix equations. For instance, `solve(A, b)` returns a vector x satisfying the equation $b = Ax$, i.e., $x = A^{-1}b$.

```
s1 <- diag(c(2, 4, 6, 8))
s2 <- c(1, 2, 3, 4)
solve(s1, s2)
## [1] 0.5 0.5 0.5 0.5
```

The following table summarizes some of the basic matrix operation functions (Table 3.1).

```
mat1 <- cbind(c(1, -1/5), c(-1/3, 1))
mat1.inv <- solve(mat1)
mat1.identity <- mat1.inv %*% mat1; mat1.identity
##      [,1] [,2]
## [1,]   1    0
## [2,]   0    1
b <- c(1, 2)
x <- solve (mat1, b); x
## [1] 1.785714 2.357143
```

Table 3.1 Basic R matrix operators

Expression	Explanation
t(x)	transpose
diag(x)	diagonal
%*%	matrix multiplication
solve(a, b)	solves a %*% x = b for x
solve(a)	matrix inverse of a
rowsum(x)	sum of rows for a matrix-like object. rowSums(x) is a faster version
colSums(x), colSums(x)	id. for columns
rowMeans(x)	fast version of row means
colMeans(x)	id. for columns

3.2 Matrix Computing

Let's look at the basics of matrix notation and matrix algebra. The product AB between matrices A and B is defined only if the number of columns in A equals the number of rows in B. That is, we can multiply an $m \times n$ matrix A by an $n \times k$ matrix B and the result will be $(AB)_{m \times k}$ matrix. Each element of the product matrix, $(AB_{i, j})_{i, j}$, represents the product of the i-th row in A and the j-th column in B, which are of the same size n. Matrix multiplication is row-by-column. Linear algebra notation simplifies the mathematical descriptions and manipulations of linear models, as well as coding in R. The main point is to show how we can write *linear models* using matrix notation. Later, we'll explain how this is useful for solving the *least squares problems*.

3.2.1 Solving Systems of Equations

Linear algebra notation enables the mathematical analysis and derivation of solutions of systems of linear equations and provides a generic machinery for solving linear problems

$$\begin{matrix} a + b + 2c = 6 \\ 3a - 2b + c = 2 \\ 2a + b - c = 3 \end{matrix} \Longleftrightarrow \underbrace{\begin{pmatrix} 1 & 1 & 2 \\ 3 & -2 & 1 \\ 2 & 1 & -1 \end{pmatrix}}_{A} \underbrace{\begin{pmatrix} a \\ b \\ c \end{pmatrix}}_{x} = \underbrace{\begin{pmatrix} 6 \\ 2 \\ 3 \end{pmatrix}}_{b}.$$

That is, $Ax = b$, which implies that

$$\begin{pmatrix} a \\ b \\ c \end{pmatrix} = \begin{pmatrix} 1 & 1 & 2 \\ 3 & -2 & 1 \\ 2 & 1 & -1 \end{pmatrix}^{-1} \begin{pmatrix} 6 \\ 2 \\ 3 \end{pmatrix}.$$

In other words, $A^{-1}Ax \equiv x = A^{-1}b$. Notice that this approach parallels the strategy for solving of simple (univariate) linear equations like

$$\underbrace{2}_{\text{(design matrix) } A} \overbrace{x}^{\text{unknown}} \underbrace{-3}_{\text{simple constant term}} = \overbrace{5}^{b}.$$

The constant term, -3, can be moved and integrated into the right-hand-side, b, to form a new (bias) term $b' = 5 + 3 = 8$. Thus, the shifting factor is mostly ignored in linear models, or linear equations, which simplifies the linear matrix equation to:

$$\underbrace{2}_{\text{(design matrix) } A} \overbrace{x}^{\text{unknown}} = \underbrace{5 + 3}_{b'} = \overbrace{8}^{b'}.$$

This simple linear equation is solved by multiplying both hand sides by the inverse (reciprocal) of the x multiplier, 2,

$$\frac{1}{2}2x = \frac{1}{2}8.$$

Thus, the unique solution is $x = \frac{1}{2}8 = 4$.

So, let's utilize the same strategy to solve the corresponding *matrix equation* (linear equation, $Ax = b$) using R, where the *unknown* is x, and the *design matrix A* and the *constant* vector b are known.

$$\underbrace{\begin{pmatrix} 1 & 1 & 2 \\ 3 & -2 & 1 \\ 2 & 1 & -1 \end{pmatrix}}_{A} \underbrace{\begin{pmatrix} a \\ b \\ c \end{pmatrix}}_{x} = \underbrace{\begin{pmatrix} 6 \\ 2 \\ 3 \end{pmatrix}}_{b}.$$

```
A_matrix_values <- c(1, 1, 2, 3, -2, 1, 2, 1, -1)
# matrix elements are arranged by columns, so, we need to transpose them to
arrange them by rows.
A <- t(matrix(A_matrix_values, nrow=3, ncol=3))
b <- c(6, 2, 3)
x <- solve (A, b); x # to solve Ax = b, x=A^{-1}*b # Ax = b ==> x = A^{-1}*b
## [1] 1.35 1.75 1.45
# Check the Solution x=(1.35 1.75 1.45)
LHS <- A %*% x
round(LHS-b, 6)
##        (0, 0, 0)
```

How about if we want to triple-check the consistency of the `solve()` method to provide accurate solutions to matrix-based systems of linear equations? We can generate the solution (x) to the equation $Ax = b$ by using first principles,

$$x = A^{-1}b.$$

```
A.inverse <- solve(A) # the inverse matrix A^{-1}
x1 <- A.inverse %*% b
# check if X and x1 are the same
x; x1
round(x - x1, 6)
```

3.2.2 The Identity Matrix

The *identity matrix* is the matrix analog to the multiplicative numeric identity, the number 1. Multiplying the identity matrix by any other matrix (B) does not change the matrix B. This property requires that the *multiplicative identity matrix* must look like this

$$
I = \begin{pmatrix}
1 & 0 & 0 & \cdots & 0 & 0 \\
0 & 1 & 0 & \cdots & 0 & 0 \\
0 & 0 & 1 & \cdots & 0 & 0 \\
\vdots & \vdots & \vdots & \ddots & \vdots & \vdots \\
0 & 0 & 0 & \cdots & 1 & 0 \\
0 & 0 & 0 & \cdots & 0 & 1
\end{pmatrix}.
$$

The identity matrix is always a square matrix with diagonal elements 1 and 0 at the off-diagonal elements. Following the above matrix multiplication rules, we can see that

$$
X \times I = \begin{pmatrix}
x_{1,1} & \cdots & x_{1,p} \\
\vdots & \ddots & \vdots \\
x_{n,1} & \cdots & x_{n,p}
\end{pmatrix}
\begin{pmatrix}
1 & 0 & 0 & \cdots & 0 & 0 \\
0 & 1 & 0 & \cdots & 0 & 0 \\
0 & 0 & 1 & \cdots & 0 & 0 \\
\vdots & \vdots & \vdots & \ddots & \vdots & \vdots \\
0 & 0 & 0 & \cdots & 1 & 0 \\
0 & 0 & 0 & \cdots & 0 & 1
\end{pmatrix}
= \begin{pmatrix}
x_{1,1} & \cdots & x_{1,p} \\
\vdots & \ddots & \vdots \\
x_{n,1} & \cdots & x_{n,p}
\end{pmatrix} = X.
$$

In R, we can express the identity matrix as follows:

```
n <- 3 # pick number of dimensions
I <- diag(n); I
A %*% I; I %*% A
```

3.2.3   Vectors, Matrices, and Scalars

Let's look at this notation deeper using the baseball players dataset, which contains three quantitative variables, Height, Weight, and Age. Suppose the variable Weight is considered as a random response (outcome vector) denoted by Y_1, Y_2, $\cdots$, Y_n. We can express each player's Weight as a function of Age and Height.

```
# Data: https://umich.instructure.com/courses/38100/files/folder/data (01a_data.txt)
data <-
    read.table('https://umich.instructure.com/files/330381/download?download_frd=1',
        as.is=T, header=T)
attach(data); head(data)
##                     Name Team        Position Height Weight   Age
## 1    Adam_Donachie  BAL          Catcher     74    180 22.99
## 2       Paul_Bako  BAL          Catcher     74    215 34.69
## 3 Ramon_Hernandez  BAL          Catcher     72    210 30.78
## 4    Kevin_Millar  BAL  First_Baseman     72    210 35.43
## 5     Chris_Gomez  BAL  First_Baseman     73    188 35.71
## 6   Brian_Roberts  BAL Second_Baseman     69    176 29.39
```

In matrix form, we can express the outcome using one symbol, **Y**. Usually, but not always, we use **bold face** characters to distinguish scalars from vectors, matrices, and tensors

$$\mathbf{Y} = \begin{pmatrix} Y_1 \\ Y_2 \\ \vdots \\ Y_n \end{pmatrix}.$$

In R, the default representation of vector data is as *columns*, i.e., our outcome vector dimension is $n \times 1$, as opposed to $1 \times n$ used for row vectors (e.g., $\mathbf{Y}^t$). Similarly, we can use matrix notation to represent the covariates, or predictors, Age and Height. In a case with two predictors, we can represent them like this

$$\mathbf{X}_1 = \begin{pmatrix} x_{1,1} \\ \vdots \\ x_{n,1} \end{pmatrix} \text{ and } \mathbf{X}_2 = \begin{pmatrix} x_{1,2} \\ \vdots \\ x_{n,2} \end{pmatrix}.$$

In the baseball players study, $x_{1,1} = \text{Age}_1$ and $x_{i,1} = \text{Age}_i$, with Age_i representing the Age of the i-th player, and similarly, $x_{i,2} = \text{Height}_i$ is the height of the i-th player. These vectors can be thought of as $n \times 1$ matrices. For instance, it is convenient to represent the covariates as *design matrices*

$$X = [X_1 X_2] = \begin{pmatrix} x_{1,1} & x_{1,2} \\ \vdots & \vdots \\ x_{n,1} & x_{n,2} \end{pmatrix}.$$

The size of this design matrix is $n \times 2, n = 1,034$.

```
X <- cbind(Age, Height)
head(X) ##  Age Height
dim(X)  ##  [1] 1034    2
```

We can also use this notation to denote an arbitrary number (k) of covariates with the following $n \times k$ matrix

$$X = \begin{pmatrix} x_{1,1} & \cdots & x_{1,k} \\ x_{2,1} & \cdots & x_{2,k} \\ \vdots & \vdots & \vdots \\ x_{n,1} & \cdots & x_{n,k} \end{pmatrix}.$$

You can simulate such a design matrix in R using the method `matrix()`, instead of `cbind()`.

```
n <- 1034; k <- 5
X <- matrix(1:(n*k), n, k)
head(X); dim(X) ## [1] 1034    5
```

By default, matrices are filled *column-by-column order*, however using the `byrow=TRUE` argument allows us to change the order to *row-by-row*.

```
n <- 1034; k <- 5
X <- matrix(1:(n*k), n, k, byrow=TRUE)
head(X); dim(X) ## [1] 1034    5
```

Scalars are just one-dimensional values, typically numbers, that are different from their higher-dimensional counterparts, vectors, matrices, and tensors, which are usually denoted by bold characters.

3.2.4   Sample Statistics

To compute the sample *average* and *variance* of a dataset, we use the formulas:

$$\overline{Y} = \frac{1}{n} \sum_{i=1}^{n} Y_i$$

and

$$\underbrace{\mathrm{Var}(Y)}_{s} = \frac{1}{n-1} \sum_{i=1}^{n} \left(Y_i - \overline{Y}\right)^2,$$

which can be represented as matrix multiplications. Define an $n \times 1$ matrix made of 1's

$$A = \begin{pmatrix} 1 \\ 1 \\ \vdots \\ 1 \end{pmatrix}.$$

This implies that

$$\frac{1}{n} A^t Y = \frac{1}{n} (1 \quad 1 \quad \cdots \quad 1) \begin{pmatrix} Y_1 \\ Y_2 \\ \vdots \\ Y_n \end{pmatrix} = \frac{1}{n} \sum_{i=1}^{n} Y_i = \overline{Y}.$$

Recall that we multiply matrices and scalars, like $\frac{1}{n}$, by *, whereas we multiply matrices using the matrix product operator, %*%.

```
# Using the Baseball dataset
y <- data$Height
print(mean(y)) ## [1] 73.69729
n <- length(y)
Y <- matrix(y, n, 1)
A <- matrix(1, n, 1)
barY <- (t(A) %*% Y) / n
print(barY) ## [1,] 73.69729
# double-check the result
mean(data$Height) ## [1] 73.69729
```

Multiplying the transpose of a matrix with another matrix is very common in linear modeling and statistical computing, so there is an appropriate function in R, crossprod().

```
barY <- (crossprod(A, Y)) / n
print(barY) ## [1,] 73.69729
```

There is a similar matrix algebra for computing the variance

$$Y' \equiv \begin{pmatrix} Y_1 - \bar{Y} \\ \vdots \\ Y_n - \bar{Y} \end{pmatrix}, \quad \frac{1}{n-1} Y'^t Y' = \frac{1}{n-1} \sum_{i=1}^{n} (Y_i - \bar{Y})^2.$$

A crossprod with only one matrix computes $Y^t Y$.

```
Y1 <- y - mean(y)
crossprod(Y1)/(n-1)   # Y1.man <- (1/(n-1))* t(Y1) %*% Y1
##           [,1]
## [1,] 5.316798      # Check the result
var(y)
## [1] 5.316798
```

3.2.5 Applications of Matrix Algebra in Linear Modeling

Let's use the following matrices

$$\overset{\text{outcome}}{\overbrace{Y}} = \begin{pmatrix} Y_1 \\ Y_2 \\ \vdots \\ Y_n \end{pmatrix}, \quad \underset{\text{design}}{\underbrace{X}} = \begin{pmatrix} 1 & x_1 \\ 1 & x_2 \\ \vdots & \vdots \\ 1 & x_n \end{pmatrix}, \quad \overset{\text{effects}}{\overbrace{\beta}} = \begin{pmatrix} \beta_0 \\ \beta_1 \end{pmatrix} \quad \text{and} \quad \underset{\text{error}}{\underbrace{\varepsilon}} = \begin{pmatrix} \varepsilon_1 \\ \varepsilon_2 \\ \vdots \\ \varepsilon_n \end{pmatrix}.$$

Then, we can express the problem as a linear model

$$Y_i = \beta_0 + \beta_1 x_i + \varepsilon_i, \quad i = 1, \cdots, n.$$

We can also write the complete problem formulation into a corresponding succinct matrix notation formula

$$\begin{pmatrix} Y_1 \\ Y_2 \\ \vdots \\ Y_n \end{pmatrix} = \begin{pmatrix} 1 & x_1 \\ 1 & x_2 \\ \vdots & \vdots \\ 1 & x_n \end{pmatrix} \begin{pmatrix} \beta_0 \\ \beta_1 \end{pmatrix} + \begin{pmatrix} \varepsilon_1 \\ \varepsilon_2 \\ \vdots \\ \varepsilon_n \end{pmatrix}.$$

In matrix form

$$Y = X\beta + \varepsilon,$$

which represents a simpler way to write the same (linear) model equation.

One way to obtain an *optimal solution* is by minimizing all residuals (ε_i). This *high-fidelity* criterion indicates a good model fit. The *least squares (LS) solution* represents one way to solve this matrix equation ($Y = X\beta + \varepsilon$). The LS solution is obtained by minimizing the *residual sum square error*

$$\langle \varepsilon^t, \varepsilon \rangle = (Y - X\beta)^t \times (Y - X\beta).$$

Let's define the LS objective function using the cross-product notation.

$$f(\beta) = (Y - X\beta)^t (Y - X\beta).$$

We can determine the *effect size estimates*, $\widehat{\beta}$, by minimizing the function above. Of course, we can derive an analytic solution using calculus to find the minimum of the cost (objective) function, $f(\beta)$.

3.2.6   *Finding Function Extrema (Min/Max) Using Calculus*

There are several rules that help with solving partial derivative equations in matrix forms. Recall that the *critical points* of the objective functions are either at the domain border or at values where the derivative of the objective function is trivial, $f'(x) = 0$. Hence, solving for the unknown parameter β requires identifying the critical points, $\widehat{\beta}$, which will represent candidate solution(s). The derivative of the above equation is

$$2X^t\left(Y - X\widehat{\beta}\right) = 0,$$
$$X^t X\widehat{\beta} = X^t Y,$$
$$\widehat{\beta} = (X^t X)^{-1} X^t Y.$$

This estimate $\widehat{\beta}$ represents the desired LS solution to the linear modeling problem. The hat notation, $\widehat{}$, is used to denote *estimates*. For instance, the solution for the unknown β parameter vector is denoted by the data-driven (vector) estimate $\widehat{\beta}$. The least squares minimization works because minimizing a function corresponds to finding the roots of its first derivative. We will see more details about function optimization in Chap. 13. With ordinary least squares (OLS), the objective function is the sum of the squared residuals

$$f(\beta) = (Y - X\beta)^t (Y - X\beta).$$

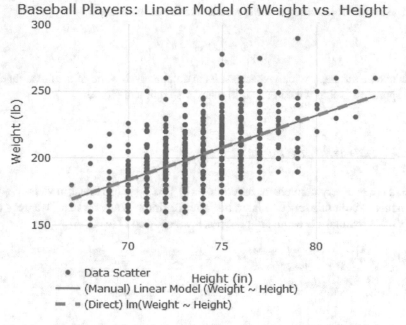

Fig. 3.1 Manual and automated simple linear modeling of weight vs. height of baseball players

Notice that the minimum of $f(x)$ and $f^2(x)$ are achieved at the same roots of $f'(x)$, as the derivative of $f^2(x)$ is $\frac{d}{dx}f^2(x) = 2f(x)f'(x)$. Here is how we obtain the Least Squares parameter vector estimation in R.

```
library(plotly)
x <- data$Height
y <- data$Weight
X <- cbind(1, x)
beta_hat <- solve( t(X) %*% X ) %*% t(X) %*% y  ### or alternatively
beta_hat <- solve( crossprod(X) ) %*% crossprod( X, y )
```

Now we can see the results of this by computing the estimated $\widehat{\beta}_0 + \widehat{\beta}_1 x$ (fitted model prediction) corresponding to any covariate input value of x (Fig. 3.1).

```
X <- cbind(1, x)
fitted <- X%*%beta_hat
plot_ly(x = ~x) %>%
  add_markers(y = ~y, name="Data Scatter") %>%
  add_lines(x = ~x, y = ~fitted[,1],
      name="(Manual) Linear Model (Weight ~ Height)") %>%
  add_lines(x = ~x, y = ~lm(y ~ x)$fitted,
      name="(Direct) lm(Weight ~ Height)",
      line = list(width = 4, dash = 'dash')) %>%
    layout(title='Baseball Players: Linear Model of Weight vs. Height',
      xaxis = list(title="Height (in)"), yaxis = list(title="Weight (lb)"),
      legend = list(orientation = 'h'))
```

The closed-form analytical expression for the LS estimate

$$\widehat{\beta} = (X^t X)^{-1} X^t Y$$

is one of the most widely used results in data analysis. One of the advantages of this approach is that we can use it in many different situations.

3.2.7   Linear Modeling in R

In R, there is a very convenient function `lm()` that fits these linear models. We will learn more about this function later, but here we simply show that `lm()` agrees with the simple manual LS estimation approach we showed above.

```
# X <- cbind(data$Height, data$Age) # more complicated model
X <- data$Height    # simple model
y <- data$Weight
fit <- lm(y ~ X)
```

3.3   Eigenspectra—Eigenvalues and Eigenvectors

Starting in the eighteenth century, the work of Euler on rotational motion and later Lagrange on the study of inertia matrices led to the notions of principal axes (*eigenvectors*) and characteristic roots (*eigenvalues*). However, it took close to 200 years until Hilbert and others working on integral operators settled on using the terminology *eigen*, "own," to denote eigenvalues (proper characteristic values) and eigenvectors (principal axes). The *eigenspectrum* (eigenspace) decomposition of linear operators (matrices) into *eigenvalues* and *eigenvectors* enables us to understand linear transformations and characterize their properties. The eigenvectors represent the "axes" (directions) along which a linear transformation acts by *stretching*, *compressing*, or *flipping*.

The eigenvalues represent the amounts of this linear transformation into the specified eigenvector direction. In higher dimensions, there are more directions along which we need to understand the behavior of the linear transformation. The eigenspectrum makes it easier to understand the linear transformation especially when many (all?) of the eigenvectors are linearly independent (orthogonal).

For a given matrix A, if we have $A\vec{v} = \lambda\vec{v}$, then we say that a nonzero vector $\vec{v}$ is a right eigenvector of the matrix A and the scale factor λ is the eigenvalue corresponding to that eigenvector. With some calculations we can show that $A\vec{v} = \lambda\vec{v}$ is the same as $(\lambda I_n - A)\vec{v} = \vec{0}$, where I_n is the $n \times n$ identity matrix. So, when we solve this equation, we get the corresponding eigenvalues and

Table 3.2 Examples of R functions corresponding to commonly used mathematical operators

Functions	Math expression or explanation
crossprod(A, B)	$A^T B$ Where A, B are matrices
y<-svd(A)	the output has the following components
-y$d	vector containing the singular values of A
-y$u	matrix with columns contain the left singular vectors of A
-y$v	matrix with columns contain the right singular vectors of A
k <- qr(A)	the output has the following components
-k$qr	has an upper triangle that contains the decomposition and a lower triangle that contains information on the Q decomposition
-k$rank	is the rank of A
-k$qraux	a vector which contains additional information on Q
-k$pivot	contains information on the pivoting strategy used
rowMeans(A)/ colMeans(A)	returns vector of row/column means
rowSums(A)/ colSums(A)	returns vector of row/column sums

eigenvectors. As this is a very common operation, we don't need to do that by hand - the method `eigen()` provides this functionality.

```
m11 <- diag(nrow = 2, ncol=2); m11
eigen(m11)
## eigen() decomposition ## $values ## $vectors
```

We can easily validate that $(\lambda I_n - A)\vec{v} = \vec{0}$.

```
(eigen(m11)$values*diag(2)-m11) %*% eigen(m11)$vectors
##       [,1] [,2]
## [1,]    0    0
## [2,]    0    0
```

As we mentioned earlier, `diag(n)` creates a $n \times n$ identity matrix. Thus, `diag(2)` is the I_2 matrix in the above equation. The output matrix of zeros proves that the equation $(\lambda I_n - A)\vec{v} = \vec{0}$ holds true.

Other important matrix operation functions are listed in the following Table 3.2.

3.4 Matrix Notation

Some flexible matrix operations can help us save time calculating row or column averages. For example, *column averages* can be calculated by the following matrix operation.

$$AX = \left(\frac{1}{N} \quad \frac{1}{N} \quad \cdots \quad \frac{1}{N}\right) \begin{pmatrix} X_{1,1} & \cdots & X_{1,p} \\ X_{2,1} & \cdots & X_{2,p} \\ \vdots & \vdots & \ddots & \vdots \\ X_{N,1} & \cdots & X_{N,p} \end{pmatrix} = \left(\overline{X}_1 \quad \overline{X}_2 \quad \cdots \quad \overline{X}_N\right).$$

The *row averages* can be calculated similarly.

$$XB = \begin{pmatrix} X_{1,1} & \cdots & & X_{1,p} \\ X_{2,1} & \cdots & & X_{2,p} \\ \vdots & \vdots & \ddots & \vdots \\ X_{N,1} & \cdots & & X_{N,p} \end{pmatrix} \begin{pmatrix} \frac{1}{p} \\ \frac{1}{p} \\ \vdots \\ \frac{1}{p} \end{pmatrix} = \begin{pmatrix} \overline{X}_1 \\ \overline{X}_2 \\ \vdots \\ \overline{X}_N \end{pmatrix}.$$

Expeditious matrix calculations can be done by multiplying a matrix on the left or at the right by another matrix. In general, multiplying by a vector on the left amounts to *weight averaging*.

$$AX = \left(a_1 \quad a_2 \quad \cdots \quad a_N\right) \begin{pmatrix} X_{1,1} & \cdots & & X_{1,p} \\ X_{2,1} & \cdots & & X_{2,p} \\ \vdots & \vdots & \ddots & \vdots \\ X_{N,1} & \cdots & & X_{N,p} \end{pmatrix} =$$

$$\left(\sum_{i=1}^{N} a_i \overline{X}_{i,1} \quad \sum_{i=1}^{N} a_i \overline{X}_{i,2} \quad \cdots \quad \sum_{i=1}^{N} a_i \overline{X}_{i,N}\right).$$

Now let's try this matrix notation to look at genetic expression data including 8793 different genes for 208 subjects. These gene expression data represent a microarray experiment—GSE5859—comparing Gene Expression Profiles from Lymphoblastoid cells.[2] Specifically, the data compare the expression level of genes in lymphoblasts from individuals in three HapMap populations {*CEU*, *CHB*, *JPT*}. The study found that the mean expression levels between the {CEU} and {CHB + JPT} samples were significantly different ($p < 0.05$) for more than a thousand genes. The gene expression profiles data have two components (CaseStudy16_GeneExpression_GSE5859)[3]:

---

[2] https://www.ncbi.nlm.nih.gov/geo/query/acc.cgi?acc=GSE5859
[3] https://umich.instructure.com/courses/38100/files/folder/Case_Studies/

- The gene expression intensities (*exprs_GSE5859.csv*): rows represent features on the microarray (e.g., genes), and columns represent different microarray samples, and
- Meta-data about each of the samples (*exprs_MetaData_GSE5859.csv*) rows represent samples and columns represent meta-data (e.g., sex, age, treatment status, the date of the sample processing).

```
gene <-
    read.csv("https://umich.instructure.com/files/2001417/download?download_frd=1",
        header = T) # exprs_GSE5859.csv
info <-
    read.csv("https://umich.instructure.com/files/2001418/download?download_frd=1",
        header=T)  # exprs_MetaData_GSE5859.csv
```

Recall that the `lapply()` function that we talked about in Chap. 2 and the `sapply()` function can be used to calculate column and row averages. Let's compare the outputs of `sapply` and the corresponding matrix algebra process.

```
colmeans <- sapply(gene[, -1], mean)
gene1 <- as.matrix(gene[, -1])
# can also use built in functions e.g., colMeans <- colMeans(gene1)
colmeans.matrix <- crossprod(rep(1/nrow(gene1), nrow(gene1)), gene1)
colmeans[1:15]
##   GSM25581.CEL.gz  GSM25681.CEL.gz GSM136524.CEL.gz GSM136707.CEL.gz
##         5.703998         5.721779         5.726300         5.743632
...

colmeans.matrix[1:15]
```

The same outputs are generated by both protocols. Note that we used `rep (1/nrow(gene1), nrow(gene1))` to create the vector

$$\left(\frac{1}{N} \quad \frac{1}{N} \quad \cdots \quad \frac{1}{N} \right)$$

needed to obtain manually the column averages by matrix algebra. Similarly, we can compute the column means (Fig. 3.2).

```
colmeans <- as.matrix(colmeans)
h <- hist(colmeans, plot=F)
plot_ly(x = h$mids, y = h$counts, type = "bar", name = "Column Averages") %>%
    layout(title='Average Gene Expression Histogram',
        xaxis = list(title = "Column Means"),
        yaxis = list(title = "Average Expression", side = "left"),
        legend = list(orientation = 'h'))
```

The histogram shows that the distribution is somewhat symmetric, unimodal, and bell-shaped, i.e., approximately normal. We can also solve harder problems using matrix algebra. For example, let's calculate the differences between genders for each gene. First, we need to get the gender information for each subject and reorder the columns to make them consistent with the feature matrix `gene1`.

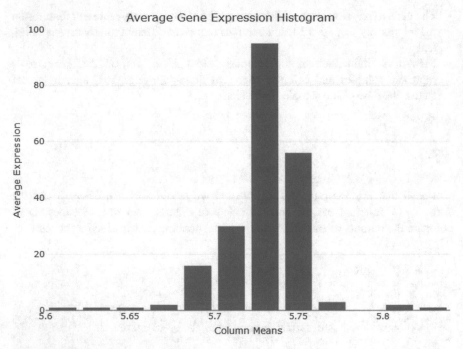

Fig. 3.2 Average gene expression histogram

```
gender <- info[, c(3, 4)]
rownames(gender) <- gender$filename
gender <- gender[colnames(gene1), ]
```

Next, we are going to design an appropriate weight matrix that can be multiplied by the feature matrix to obtain the desired gene-specific gender effects.

$$
\begin{pmatrix} X_{1,1} & \cdots & X_{1,p} \\ X_{2,1} & \cdots & X_{2,p} \\ \vdots & \ddots & \vdots \\ X_{N,1} & \cdots & X_{N,p} \end{pmatrix} \begin{pmatrix} \dfrac{1}{p} & a_1 \\ \dfrac{1}{p} & a_2 \\ \vdots & \vdots \\ \dfrac{1}{p} & a_p \end{pmatrix} = \begin{pmatrix} \overline{X}_1 & \text{gender.diff}_1 \\ \overline{X}_2 & \text{gender.diff}_2 \\ \vdots & \vdots \\ \overline{X}_N & \text{gender.diff}_N \end{pmatrix},
$$

where $a_i = -\frac{1}{N_F}$ if the subject is *female* and $a_i = \frac{1}{N_M}$ if the subject is *male*. Thus, we gave each female and male the same weight before the subtraction, i.e., for each gene, we compute the differences between gender averages. $\overline{X}_i$ is the average across both genders and gender. diff$_i$ represents the gender difference for the i-th gene.

```
table(gender$sex) ##    F   M  ## 86 122
gender$vector <- ifelse(gender$sex=="F", -1/86, 1/122)
vec1 <- as.matrix(data.frame(rowavg=rep(1/ncol(gene1), ncol(gene1)),
                 gender.diff=gender$vector))
gender.matrix <- gene1 %*% vec1
gender.matrix[1:15, ]
##         rowavg  gender.diff
...
```

3.5 Linear Regression

As we mentioned earlier, the formula for linear regression can be written as

$$Y_i = \beta_0 + X_{i,1}\beta_1 + \cdots + X_{i,p}\beta_p + \epsilon_i, \ i = 1, \cdots, N.$$

This formula can also be expressed in matrix form

$$\begin{pmatrix} Y_1 \\ Y_2 \\ \vdots \\ Y_N \end{pmatrix} = \begin{pmatrix} 1 \\ 1 \\ \vdots \\ 1 \end{pmatrix}\beta_0 + \begin{pmatrix} X_{1,1} \\ X_{2,1} \\ \vdots \\ X_{N,1} \end{pmatrix}\beta_1 + \cdots + \begin{pmatrix} X_{1,p} \\ X_{2,p} \\ \vdots \\ X_{N,p} \end{pmatrix}\beta_p + \begin{pmatrix} \epsilon_1 \\ \epsilon_2 \\ \vdots \\ \epsilon_N \end{pmatrix},$$

which can be compressed into a simple matrix equation $Y = X\beta + \epsilon$

$$\begin{pmatrix} Y_1 \\ Y_2 \\ \vdots \\ Y_N \end{pmatrix} = \begin{pmatrix} 1 & X_{1,1} & \cdots & X_{1,p} \\ 1 & X_{2,1} & \cdots & X_{2,p} \\ \vdots & \vdots & \ddots & \vdots \\ 1 & X_{N,1} & \cdots & X_{N,p} \end{pmatrix}\begin{pmatrix} \beta_o \\ \beta_1 \\ \vdots \\ \beta_p \end{pmatrix} + \begin{pmatrix} \epsilon_1 \\ \epsilon_2 \\ \vdots \\ \epsilon_N \end{pmatrix}.$$

As $Y = X\beta + \epsilon$ implies that $X^t Y \sim X^t(X\beta) = (X^t X)\beta$, and thus, the LS solution for β is obtained by multiplying both hand sides by the inverse of the square cross product matrix $(X^t X)^{-1}$:

$$\hat{\beta} = (X^t X)^{-1} X^t Y.$$

Matrix calculations are much faster, especially on specialized computer chips, than fitting multiple piecewise regression models. Let's apply this to the Lahman Baseball data representing yearly stats and standings. Let's download it and save it in the R working directory. We can use the load() function to import the local RData. For this example, we subset the dataset by evaluating the following Boolean expressions G==162 and yearID < 2002. Also, we create a new feature named Singles that is equal to H(Hits by batters) - X2B(Doubles) -

X3B(Tripples) - HR(Home Runs by batters). Finally, we only pick four features: *R* (Runs scored), *Singles*, *HR* (Home Runs by batters), and *BB* (Walks by batters).

```
#If you downloaded the .RData locally first, then you can easily load it into
the`R`workspace by load("Teams.RData")
# Alternatively you can also download the data in CSV format (teamsData.csv)
Teams <-
    read.csv('https://umich.instructure.com/files/2798317/download?download_frd=1',
       header=T)
dat <- Teams[Teams$G==162&Teams$yearID<2002, ]
dat$Singles <- dat$H-dat$X2B-dat$X3B-dat$HR
dat <- dat[, c("R", "Singles", "HR", "BB")]; head(dat)
##         R Singles  HR  BB
## 439  505     997   11 344
...
```

In this example, let's work with *R* as the response variable and *BB* as the independent variable. For a full (simple) linear model, we need to add another column of 1's to the design matrix *X*.

```
Y <- dat$R
X <- cbind(rep(1, n=nrow(dat)), dat$BB); X[1:10, ]
##        [,1] [,2]
## [1,]     1  344
## [2,]     1  580
...
```

We use the LS analytical formula to obtain the beta (effects) estimates

$$\widehat{\beta} = (X^t X)^{-1} X^t Y.$$

```
beta <- solve(t(X) %*% X) %*% t(X) %*% Y
beta ## [1,] 326.8241628  ## [2,]   0.7126402
```

To confirm this manual calculation, we can refit the linear equation using the lm() function, and compare the computational times. In this simple example, is there evidence of higher computational efficiency using matrix calculations?

```
fit <- lm(R~BB, data=dat)
fit    ## lm(formula = R ~ BB, data = dat)
## Coefficients:
## (Intercept)           BB
##    326.8242       0.7126
summary(fit)
## Call:
## lm(formula = R ~ BB, data = dat)
## Residuals:
##       Min       1Q   Median       3Q      Max
## -187.788  -53.977   -2.995   55.649  258.614
## Coefficients:
##              Estimate Std. Error t value Pr(>|t|)
## (Intercept) 326.82416   22.44340   14.56   <2e-16 ***
## BB            0.71264    0.04157   17.14   <2e-16 ***
## ---
## Signif. codes:  0 '***' 0.001 '**' 0.01 '*' 0.05 '.' 0.1 ' ' 1
## Residual standard error: 76.95 on 661 degrees of freedom
## Multiple R-squared:  0.3078, Adjusted R-squared:  0.3068
## F-statistic:   294 on 1 and 661 DF,  p-value: < 2.2e-16
system.time(fit <- lm(R~BB, data=dat))
##     user  system elapsed
##     0.02    0.00    0.02
system.time(beta1 <- solve(t(X) %*% X) %*% t(X) %*% Y)
##     user  system elapsed
##        0       0       0
```

For a better model, we can expand the covariates to include multiple predictors
and compare the resulting estimates.

```
X <- cbind(rep(1, n=nrow(dat)), dat$BB, dat$Singles, dat$HR)
system.time(fit <- lm(R ~ BB+ Singles + HR, data=dat))
system.time(beta2 <- solve(t(X) %*% X) %*% t(X) %*% Y)
fit$coefficients; t(beta2)
## (Intercept)           BB      Singles           HR
## -401.0057242    0.3666606    0.6705535    1.7175775
##            [,1]       [,2]       [,3]      [,4]
## [1,] -401.0057 0.3666606 0.6705535 1.717577
```

A 2D scatter plot can be used to show visually the relationship between the
outcome R and one of the predictors BB (Fig. 3.3).

```
plot_ly(x = ~dat$BB) %>%
  add_markers(y = ~dat$R, name="Data Scatter") %>%
  add_lines(x = ~dat$BB, y = ~lm(dat$R ~ dat$BB)$fitted,
     name="lm(Runs scored ~ Walks by batters)", line = list(width = 4)) %>%
    layout(title='Scatter plot/regression for baseball data',
     xaxis = list(title="(BB) Walks by batters"),
     yaxis = list(title="(R) Runs scored"), legend = list(orientation='h'))
```

Here, the orange model line represents our regression model estimated using
matrix algebra. The power of matrix algebra becomes more apparent when we use
multiple variables. In the following figure, we demonstrate using fundamental linear
algebra to estimate predictive (linear and planar) models of R using two covariates;
home runs and walks by batters (HR and BB). Of course, the same strategy can be
extended inductively to any number of predicting variables and higher-order hyper-
linear models (hyperplanes) (Fig. 3.4).

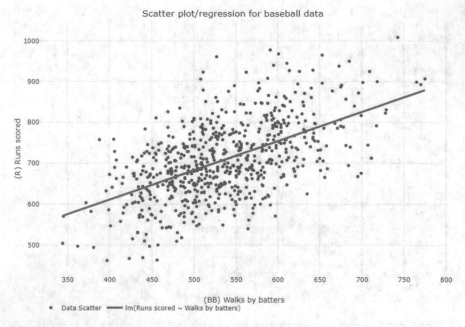

Fig. 3.3 Baseball data scatter plot with a linear model—runs (vertical axis) and walks by batters

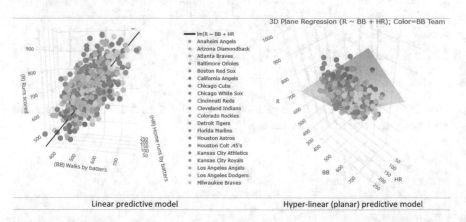

Fig. 3.4 Baseball data 3D scatter plots with a bivariate linear (left) and hyper-linear (right) models

```
library(reshape2)
X <- cbind(rep(1, n=nrow(dat)), dat$BB, dat$HR)
beta <- solve(t(X) %*% X) %*% t(X) %*% Y; beta
dat$name <- Teams[Teams$G==162&Teams$yearID<2002, "name"]
fit = lm(dat$R ~ dat$BB + dat$HR, data = dat)
# Plot the Linear model # get the BB & HR ranges summary(dat$BB); cf =
fit$coefficients
pltx = seq(344, 775,length.out = length(dat$BB))
plty = seq(11,264,length.out = length(dat$BB))
pltz = cf[1] + cf[2]*pltx + cf[3]*plty
plot_ly() %>%        # Plot Scatter and add the LM line to the plot
  add_trace(x = ~pltx, y = ~plty, z = ~pltz, type="scatter3d", mode="lines",
        line = list(color = "red", width = 4), name="lm(R ~ BB + HR") %>%
  add_markers(x = ~dat$BB, y = ~dat$HR, z = ~dat$R, color = ~dat$name,
        mode="markers") %>%
  layout(scene = list(xaxis = list(title = '(BB) Walks by batters'),
        yaxis = list(title = '(HR) Home runs by batters'),
        zaxis = list(title = '(R) Runs scored')))
# Plot Scatter and add the LM PLANE (hyper-linear model) to the plot
lm <- lm(R ~ 0 + HR + BB, data = dat)
axis_x <- seq(min(dat$HR), max(dat$HR), length.out=100) # Setup the Axes
axis_y <- seq(min(dat$BB), max(dat$BB), length.out=100)
# Sample points
lm_surface <- expand.grid(HR = axis_x, BB = axis_y, KEEP.OUT.ATTRS = F)
lm_surface$R <- predict.lm(lm, newdata = lm_surface)
lm_surface <- acast(lm_surface, HR ~ BB, value.var = "R") #`R`~ 0 + HR + BB
plot_ly(dat, x = ~HR, y = ~BB, z = ~R,
        text = ~name, type = "scatter3d", mode = "markers", color=~dat$name) %>%
  add_trace(x = ~axis_x, y = ~axis_y, z = ~lm_surface, type="surface",
        color="gray", opacity=0.3) %>%
  layout(title="3D Plane Regression (R ~ BB + HR); Color=BB Team",
        showlegend=F, xaxis = list(title = '(BB) Walks by batters'),
        yaxis = list(title = '(HR) Home runs by batters'),
        zaxis = list(title = '(R) Runs scored')) %>% hide_colorbar()
```

3.5.1 Sample Covariance Matrix

We can also express the covariance matrix for our features using matrix operation. Suppose

$$X_{N \times K} = \begin{pmatrix} X_{1,1} & \cdots & X_{1,K} \\ X_{2,1} & \cdots & X_{2,K} \\ \vdots & \ddots & \vdots \\ X_{N,1} & \cdots & X_{N,K} \end{pmatrix} = [X_1, X_2, \cdots, X_N]^t.$$

Then the covariance matrix is $\Sigma = (\Sigma_{i,j})$, where $\Sigma_{i,j} = \text{Cov}(X_i, X_j) = E((X_i - \mu_i)(X_j - \mu_j))$, $1 \leq i, j, \leq N$. For a given dataset, the sample covariance matrix is

$$\Sigma_{i,j} = \frac{1}{N-1} \sum_{m=1}^{N} (x_{m,i} - \bar{x}_i)(x_{m,j} - \bar{x}_j),$$

where

$$\bar{x}_i = \frac{1}{N} \sum_{m=1}^{N} x_{m,i}, \quad i = 1, \cdots, K.$$

In general,

$$\Sigma = \frac{1}{n-1}(X - \bar{X})'(X - \bar{X}).$$

Suppose that we want to get the sample covariance matrix of the following $5 * 3$ feature matrix x.

```
x <- matrix(c(4.0, 4.2, 3.9, 4.3, 4.1, 2.0, 2.1, 2.0, 2.1, 2.2, 0.60,
            0.59, 0.58, 0.62, 0.63), ncol=3); x
##      [,1] [,2] [,3]
## [1,]  4.0  2.0 0.60
## [2,]  4.2  2.1 0.59
## [3,]  3.9  2.0 0.58
## [4,]  4.3  2.1 0.62
## [5,]  4.1  2.2 0.63
```

Notice that this matrix represents the design matrix of 3 features and 5 observations. Let's compute the column means first.

```
vec2 <- matrix(c(1/5, 1/5, 1/5, 1/5, 1/5), ncol=5)
#column means
x.bar <- vec2 %*% x; x.bar
##      [,1] [,2]  [,3]
## [1,]  4.1 2.08 0.604
x.bar <- matrix(rep(x.bar, each=5), nrow=5)
S <- 1/4*t(x-x.bar) %*% (x-x.bar); S
##         [,1]     [,2]     [,3]
## [1,] 0.02500 0.00750 0.00175
## [2,] 0.00750 0.00700 0.00135
## [3,] 0.00175 0.00135 0.00043
```

In the covariance matrix, $S[i, i]$ is the variance of the i-th feature and $S[i, j]$ is the covariance of i-th and j-th features. Compare this to the automated calculation of the variance–covariance matrix.

```
autoCov <- cov(x) ; autoCov
##      [,1]    [,2]    [,3]
## [1,] 0.02500 0.00750 0.00175
## [2,] 0.00750 0.00700 0.00135
## [3,] 0.00175 0.00135 0.00043
```

3.6 Linear Multivariate Regression Modeling

Later, in Chap. 5, we will cover some classification methods that use this mathematical framework for model-based and model-free ML/AI prediction. However, let's start with linear model-based statistical methods providing forecasting and classification functionality. Specifically, in this section, we will (1) demonstrate the predictive power of multivariate linear regression, (2) show the foundation of regression trees and model trees, and (3) examine two complementary case-studies (Baseball Players and Heart Attack). Regression represents a model of a relationship between a *dependent variable* (value to be predicted) and a group of *independent variables* (predictors or features). We assume the relationships between the outcome dependent variable and the independent variables is linear.

3.6.1 Simple Linear Regression

Earlier, we discussed the straightforward case of regression as simple linear regression, which involves a single predictor

$$y = a + bx.$$

In this *slope-intercept* formula, *a* is the model *intercept* and *b* is the model *slope*. Thus, simple linear regression may be expressed as a bivariate equation. If we know *a* and *b*, for any given *x* we can estimate, or predict, *y* via the regression formula. When the two variables are exactly linearly related, plotting *x* against *y* in a 2D coordinate system will result in a straight line. However, this is an idealized case that is rarely observed in practice. Bivariate scatterplots using real world data may show patterns that are not necessarily precisely linear, see Chap. 2. Let's look at a bivariate scatterplot and try to fit a simple linear regression line using two variables, e.g., hospital charges, or CHARGES, as a dependent variable, and length of stay in the hospital, or LOS, as an independent predictor. The data are available in the DSPA data archive as CaseStudy12_AdultsHeartAttack_Data. For simplicity, we can first remove the pair of observations with missing values using the command (Fig. 3.5)

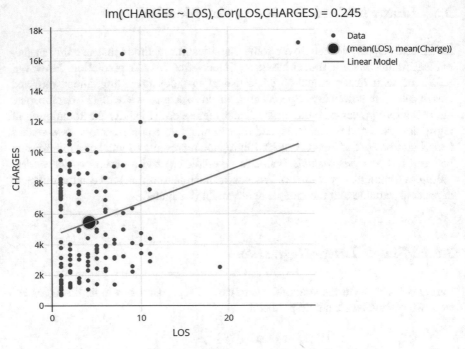

Fig. 3.5 Linear model of hospitalization charges and length of hospital stay. Note that the least square linear model (green line) goes through the point of gravitational balance $(\bar{x}, \bar{y})$, blue point

```
heart_attack <- heart_attack[complete.cases(heart_attack), ].
```

```r
library(plotly)
heart_attack <-
    read.csv("https://umich.instructure.com/files/1644953/download?download_frd=1",
        stringsAsFactors = F)
heart_attack$CHARGES <- as.numeric(heart_attack$CHARGES)
heart_attack <- heart_attack[complete.cases(heart_attack), ]
fit1 <- lm(CHARGES ~ LOS, data=heart_attack)
plot_ly(heart_attack, x = ~LOS, y = ~CHARGES, type = 'scatter', mode = "markers",
name="Data") %>%
    add_trace(x=~mean(LOS), y=~mean(CHARGES), type="scatter", mode="markers",
        name="(mean(LOS), mean(Charge))", marker=list(size=20, color='blue',
            line=list(color='yellow', width=2))) %>%
    add_lines(x = ~LOS, y = fit1$fitted.values, mode = "lines",
        name="Linear Model") %>%
    layout(title=paste0("lm(CHARGES ~ LOS), Cor(LOS,CHARGES) = ",
            round(cor(heart_attack$LOS, heart_attack$CHARGES),3)))
```

As expected, longer hospital stays are expected to be associated with higher medical costs, or hospital charges. The scatterplot shows dots for each pair of observed measurements (x = LOS and y = CHARGES), and an increasing linear trend. The estimated expression for this regression line is

$$\hat{y} = 4582.70 + 212.29 \times x$$

or equivalently

$$\text{CHARGES} = 4582.70 + 212.29 \times \text{LOS}.$$

Once the linear model is fit, i.e., its coefficients are estimated, we can make predictions using this `explicit` regression model. Assume we have a patient that spent 10 days in hospital, then we have `LOS` = 10. The corresponding predicted charge is likely to be around $4582.70 + $212.29 × 10 = $6705.6. Plugging x into the expression equation automatically gives us an estimated value of the outcome y.

3.6.2   Ordinary Least Squares Estimation

How did we get the estimated expression? The most common estimating method in statistics is *ordinary least squares* (OLS). OLS estimators are obtained by minimizing the sum of the squared errors—that is the sum of squared vertical distance from each dot on the scatter plot to the regression line (Fig. 3.6).

OLS is minimizing the following expression

$$\langle c, c \rangle^2 = \sum_{i=1}^{n} (y_i - \hat{y}_i)^2 = \sum_{i=1}^{n} \left(\underbrace{y_i}_{\text{observed outcome}} - \underbrace{(a + b x_i)}_{\text{predicted outcome}} \right)^2 = \sum_{i=1}^{n} \underbrace{e_i^2}_{\text{squared residual}} .$$

Simple calculus-based calculations suggest that the (slope parameter) value b minimizing the squared error is

$$b = \frac{\sum (x_i - \bar{x})(y_i - \bar{y})}{\sum (x_i - \bar{x})^2}.$$

Then, the corresponding constant term (y-intercept) is $a = \bar{y} - b\bar{x}$, where the x and y sample averages are denoted by $\bar{x}$ and $\bar{y}$.

These expressions would become apparent as we recall that the variance is obtained by averaging sums of squared deviations $\left(\sigma = \text{Var}(x) = \frac{1}{n} \sum_{i=1}^{n} (x_i - \mu)^2 \right)$, where μ is the population mean, $\bar{x}$ is the sample mean of the process x, and we have the following formula for the (sample) variance $s = \widehat{\text{Var}}(x) = \frac{1}{n-1} \sum_{i=1}^{n} (x_i - \bar{x})^2$, which is just a factor $\left(\frac{1}{n-1} \right)$ of the denominator of the slope parameter, b. Similar to the variance, the covariance of x and y measures the average sum of the deviance of x times the deviance of y

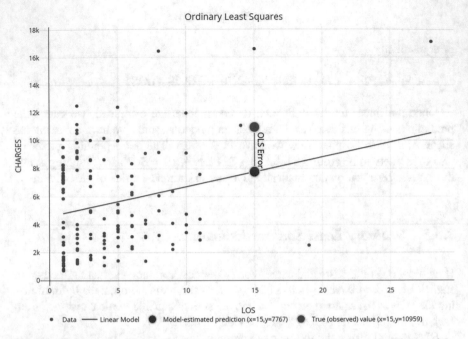

Fig. 3.6 Geometric motivation of ordinary least squares model estimation as an equilibrium of the aggregate spring forces pooling the model line toward all observed data points

$$\text{Cov}(x, y) = \frac{1}{n} \sum_{i=1}^{n} (x_i - \mu_x)(y_i - \mu_y).$$

If we utilize the sample average vector $(\bar{x}, \bar{y})$ as a vector of estimates of the corresponding population means, we have the sample covariance

$$\widehat{\text{Cov}}(x, y) = \frac{1}{n-1} \sum_{i=1}^{n} (x_i - \bar{x})(y_i - \bar{y}),$$

which is the same factor $\left(\frac{1}{n-1}\right)$ of the numerator of b. Thus, combining this pair of expressions we get an estimate of the slope coefficient (effect-size of LOS on Charge) expressed as

$$b = \frac{\widehat{\text{Cov}}(x, y)}{\widehat{\text{Var}}(x)}.$$

Let's use the heart attack data to demonstrate these calculations.

```
b <- cov(heart_attack$LOS, heart_attack$CHARGES)/var(heart_attack$LOS); b
## [1] 212.2869
a <- mean(heart_attack$CHARGES)-b*mean(heart_attack$LOS); a
## [1] 4582.7
# compare these estimates to the lm() estimate
fit1$coefficients[1] ## (Intercept)   ##        4582.7
# we can do the same for the slope parameter (b=fit1$coefficients[2]
```

We can see that this is exactly the same as the previously computed estimate of the constant intercept terms using `lm()`.

3.6.3   Regression Model Assumptions

Regression modeling has five key assumptions:

- Linear relationship between dependent outcome and the independent predictor(s),
- Multivariate normality,
- No or controlled (low level) multicollinearity,
- No autocorrelation, approximate independence of model covariates,
- Homoscedasticity, which is the homogeneity (approximate similarity) property of variances, a common assumption in many parametric statistical tests trying to quantify group dissimilarities.

If these assumptions are violated, the estimated linear models may provide invalid estimates and unreliable predictions.

3.6.4   Correlations

The readers are encouraged to develop an R protocol with dynamic interface demonstrating data-driven linear models, identification of trends, correlations, slopes, and residuals.

Based on the covariance, we can calculate the correlation, which indicates how closely the relationship between two variables follows a straight line,

$$\rho_{x,y} = \mathrm{Corr}(x, y) = \frac{\mathrm{Cov}(x, y)}{\sigma_x \sigma_y} = \frac{\mathrm{Cov}(x, y)}{\sqrt{\mathrm{Var}(x)\mathrm{Var}(y)}}.$$

In R, the correlation may be computed using the method `cor()` and the square root of the variance, i.e., the standard deviation computed by `sd()`.

```
r <- cov(heart_attack$LOS,
    heart_attack$CHARGES)/(sd(heart_attack$LOS)*sd(heart_attack$CHARGES)); r
## [1] 0.2449743
cor(heart_attack$LOS, heart_attack$CHARGES)
## [1] 0.2449743
```

Again, the manual and automated correlation estimates coincide. This correlation is a positive number that is relatively small indicating a weak positive linear association between these two variables. If we have a negative correlation estimate, then it is indicative of a negative linear association. We have a weak linear association when $0.1 \leq |\text{Cor}| < 0.3$, a moderate association for $0.3 \leq |\text{Cor}| < 0.5$, and a strong association for $0.5 \leq |\text{Cor}| \leq 1.0$. A correlation below 0.1 suggests little to no linear relation between the variables.

3.6.5 Multiple Linear Regression

In practice, we usually have more situations with multiple predictors and one dependent variable, which may follow a multiple linear model. That is,

$$y = \beta_0 + \beta_1 x_1 + \beta_2 x_2 + \cdots + \beta_k x_k + \epsilon.$$

This equation shows the linear relationship between k predictors $\{x_i\}_{i=1}^{k}$ and a dependent variable, y. In total, we have $k + 1$ coefficients to estimate, $\{\beta_i\}_{i=0}^{k}$, including the constant term β_o. The matrix notation for the above equation is

$$Y = X\beta + \epsilon,$$

where

$$\underbrace{Y}_{\text{outcome}} = \begin{pmatrix} y_1 \\ y_2 \\ \vdots \\ y_n \end{pmatrix}, \underbrace{X}_{\substack{\text{data} \\ \text{design}}} = \begin{pmatrix} 1 & x_{11} & x_{21} & \cdots & x_{k1} \\ 1 & x_{12} & x_{22} & \cdots & x_{k2} \\ \vdots & \vdots & \vdots & \ddots & \vdots \\ 1 & x_{1n} & x_{2n} & \cdots & x_{kn} \end{pmatrix}, \underbrace{\beta}_{\text{effects}} = \begin{pmatrix} \beta_0 \\ \beta_1 \\ \vdots \\ \beta_k \end{pmatrix}, \underbrace{\epsilon}_{\text{error}} = \begin{pmatrix} \epsilon_1 \\ \epsilon_2 \\ \vdots \\ \epsilon_n \end{pmatrix}.$$

Similar to simple linear regression, our goal is to minimize the sum of squared errors. Solving the matrix equation for β, we get the OLS solution for the parameter vector

$$\widehat{\beta} = (X^t X)^{-1} X^t Y.$$

The solution is presented in a matrix form, where X^t and $(X^t X)^{-1}$ are the *transpose* of the original design matrix X and the *inverse* of the square cross product matrix, respectively. The next example demonstrates making *de novo* a simple regression (least squares estimating) function `reg()`.

```
reg <- function(y, x){
  x <- as.matrix(x)
  x <- cbind(Intercept=1, x)
  solve(t(x)%*%x)%*%t(x)%*%y
}
```

We saw earlier that a clever use of matrix multiplication (`%*%`) and `solve()` can help with the explicit OLS solution. Next, we will apply our function `reg()` to the heart attack data and demonstrate that the simple linear regression (`lm()`) output coincides with the results of our manual regression estimator, `reg()`.

```
reg(y=heart_attack$CHARGES, x=heart_attack$LOS)
## Intercept 4582.6997
##           212.2869
fit1 # recall that fit1 <- lm(CHARGES ~ LOS, data=heart_attack)
## lm(formula = CHARGES ~ LOS, data = heart_attack)
## Coefficients:
## (Intercept)          LOS
##      4582.7        212.3
```

The results of the automated (`lm()`) and the manual (`reg()`) simple linear models agree and we can proceed with testing the multivariate functionality using additional variables as predictors, e.g., just adding `age` as a second variable into the model.

```
str(heart_attack)
## 'data.frame':    148 obs. of  8 variables:
##  $ Patient  : int  1 2 3 4 5 6 7 8 9 10 ...
##  $ DIAGNOSIS: int  41041 41041 41091 41081 41091 41091 41091 41091 ...
##  $ SEX      : chr  "F" "F" "F" "F" ...
##  $ DRG      : int  122 122 122 122 122 121 121 121 121 123 ...
##  $ DIED     : int  0 0 0 0 0 0 0 0 0 1 ...
##  $ CHARGES  : num  4752 3941 3657 1481 1681 ...
##  $ LOS      : int  10 6 5 2 1 9 15 15 2 1 ...
##  $ AGE      : int  79 34 76 80 55 84 84 70 76 65 ...
reg(y=heart_attack$CHARGES, x=heart_attack[, c(7, 8)]) # covariates LOS + AGE
## Intercept 7280.55493
## LOS         259.67361
## AGE         -43.67677
# and compare the result to lm()
fit2 <- lm(CHARGES ~ LOS + AGE, data=heart_attack); fit2
## lm(formula = CHARGES ~ LOS + AGE, data = heart_attack)
## Coefficients:
## (Intercept)          LOS          AGE
##      7280.55       259.67       -43.68
```

The following sections provide additional examples of simple and multivariate regression. To facilitate joint model fitting and feature selection, in Chap. 9, we will introduce regularized linear modeling by generalizing the OLS regression model estimation.

3.7   Case Study 1: Baseball Players

3.7.1   Step 1: Collecting Data

In this example, we will utilize the MLB data (01a_data.txt). The data contain 1034 records of heights and weights for some recent Major League Baseball (MLB) Players. These data were obtained from different resources (e.g., IBM Many Eyes).
Variables:

- *Name*: MLB Player Name
- *Team*: The Baseball team the player was a member of at the time the data was acquired
- *Position*: Player field position
- *Height*: Player height in inch
- *Weight*: Player weight in pounds
- *Age*: Player age at time of record

3.7.2   Step 2: Exploring and Preparing the Data

Let's first load this dataset using `as.is=T` to keep non-numerical vectors as characters. Also, we will delete the `Name` variable because we don't need the players' names in this case study.

```
mlb <-
    read.table('https://umich.instructure.com/files/330381/download?download_frd=1',
        as.is=T, header=T)
str(mlb)
## 'data.frame':    1034 obs. of  6 variables:
## $ Name    : chr  "Adam_Donachie" "Paul_Bako" "Ramon_Hernandez" ...
## $ Team    : chr  "BAL" "BAL" "BAL" "BAL" ...
## $ Position: chr  "Catcher" "Catcher" "Catcher" "First_Baseman" ...
## $ Height  : int  74 74 72 72 73 69 69 71 76 71 ...
## $ Weight  : int  180 215 210 210 188 176 209 200 231 180 ...
## $ Age     : num  23 34.7 30.8 35.4 35.7 ...
mlb <- mlb[, -1]
```

By looking at the `str()` output we notice that the variables TEAM and Position are misspecified as characters. To fix this, we can use the function `as.factor()` to convert numeric or character vectors to factors.

```
mlb$Team <- as.factor(mlb$Team)
mlb$Position <- as.factor(mlb$Position)
```

The data are now ready to compute some summary statistics and generate simple plots.

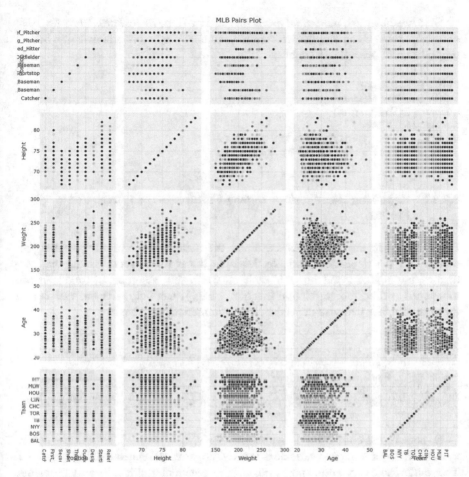

Fig. 3.7 Pairs plot or scatter plot matrix (splom) of the baseball dataset

As we saw in Chap. 1, distribution of `Weight` appears a little right-skewed. `Pairs plots` provide a convenient display of bivariate relations for multivariate processes (Fig. 3.7).

```
plot_ly(mlb) %>%
    add_trace(type = 'splom', dimensions = list( list(label='Position',
            values=~Position), list(label='Height', values=~Height),
    list(label='Weight', values=~Weight), list(label='Age', values=~Age),
    list(label='Team', values=~Team)), text=~Team,
    marker = list(color = as.integer(mlb$Team), size = 7,
        line = list(width = 1, color = 'rgb(230,230,230)'))) %>%
    layout(title= 'MLB Pairs Plot', hovermode='closest', dragmode= 'select',
        plot_bgcolor='rgba(240,240,240, 0.95)')
```

Here, we have two *numerical predictors* and two *categorical predictors* for 1034 observations. We can summarize certain candidate predictors and examine how R treats different classes of variables.

```
table(mlb$Team)
table(mlb$Position)
summary(mlb$Height)
summary(mlb$Age)
## Min. 1st Qu. Median Mean 3rd Qu. Max.
## 20.90 25.44 27.93 28.74 31.23 48.52
```

3.7.2.1 Exploring Relationships Among Features—The Correlation Matrix

Before fitting linear models, let's examine the independence of our potential predictors and the dependent variable. Multiple linear regressions assume that predictors are all independent with each other. Is this assumption valid? As we mentioned earlier, the correlation function, cor(), can help with this question in the case of linear pairwise dependencies for numerical variables.

```
cor(mlb[c("Weight", "Height", "Age")])
##              Weight       Height          Age
## Weight 1.0000000  0.53031802   0.15784706
## Height 0.5303180  1.00000000  -0.07367013
## Age    0.1578471 -0.07367013   1.00000000
```

Of course, the correlation is symmetric, $cor(y, x) = cor(x, y)$, and further $cov(x, x) = 1$. Also, our Height variable is weakly (negatively) related to the players' age. The results look very good and do not suggest potential multicollinearity problems. If two of our predictors are highly correlated, they both provide similar information. Such multicollinearity may cause undue bias in the model and one common practice is to remove one of the highly correlated predictors prior to fitting the model.

In general multivariate regression analysis, we can use the variance inflation factors (VIFs) to detect potential multicollinearity between all covariates. The variance inflation factor quantifies the amount of artificial inflation of the variance due to observed multicollinearity in the covariates. The VIF_l's represent the expected inflation of the corresponding estimated variances. In a simple linear regression model with a single predictor x_l, $y_i = \beta_o + \beta_1 x_{i,l} + \epsilon_i$, relative to the *baseline variance*, σ, the *lower bound (min) of the variance* of the estimated effect-size, β_l, is

$$\text{Var}(\beta_l)_{\min} = \frac{\sigma^2}{\sum_{i=1}^{n} (x_{i,l} - \bar{x}_l)^2}.$$

This allows us to track the inflation of the β_l variance ($\text{Var}(\beta_l)$) in the presence of correlated predictors in the regression model. Suppose the linear model includes k covariates with some of them being multicollinear or correlated

$$y_i = \beta_o + \beta_1 x_{i,1} + \beta_2 x_{i,2} + \cdots + \underbrace{\beta_l x_{i,l}}_{\text{effect} \times \text{feature}} + \cdots + \beta_k x_{i,k} + \epsilon_i.$$

Assume some of the predictors are correlated with the feature x_l, then the variance of its effect, $\text{Var}(\beta_l)$, will be inflated as follows

$$\text{Var}(\beta_l) - \frac{\sigma^2}{\sum_{i=1}^{n}(x_{i,l} - \bar{x}_l)^2} \times \frac{1}{1 - R_l^2},$$

where R_l^2 is the R^2-value computed by regressing the lth feature on the remaining $(k-1)$ predictors. The stronger the *linear dependence* between the lth feature and the remaining predictors, the larger the corresponding R_l^2 value will be, the smaller the denominator in the inflation factor (VIF_l), and the larger the variance estimate of β_l.

The *variance inflation factor* (VIF_l) is the ratio of the two variances – the variance of the effect (numerator) and the lower bound minimum variance of the effect (denominator).

$$\text{VIF}_l = \frac{\text{Var}(\beta_l)}{\text{Var}(\beta_l)_{\text{min}}} = \frac{\frac{\sigma^2}{\sum_{i=1}^{n}(x_{i,l} - \bar{x}_l)^2} \times \frac{1}{1 - R_l^2}}{\frac{\sigma^2}{\sum_{i=1}^{n}(x_{i,l} - \bar{x}_l)^2}} = \frac{1}{1 - R_l^2}.$$

The regression model's VIFs measure how much the variance of the estimated regression coefficients, β_l, may be "inflated" by unavoidable presence of multicollinearity among the model predictor features. $\text{VIF}_l \sim 1$ implies that there is no substantial multicollinearity involving the lth predictor and the remaining features, and hence, the variance estimate of β_l is not inflated. On the other hand, when $\text{VIF}_l > 4$, potential multicollinearity is likely, and when $\text{VIF}_l > 10$, there may be serious multicollinearity in the data, which may require some model correction to account for variance estimates that may be significantly biased.

We can use the function `car::vif()` to compute and report the VIF factors.

```
car::vif(lm(Weight ~ Height + Age, data=mlb))
##   Height      Age
## 1.005457 1.005457
```

3.7.2.2 Multicollinearity and Feature-Selection in High-Dimensional Data

In Chap. 11, we will discuss various methods and computational strategies to identify salient features in high-dimensional datasets. Let's briefly identify some practical approaches to address multicollinearity problems and tackle challenges related to large numbers of inter-dependencies in the data. Data that contain a large number of predictors are likely to include completely unrelated variables having high sample correlation. To see the nature of this problem, assume we are generating a random Gaussian $n \times k$ matrix, $X = (X_1, X_2, \cdots, X_k)$ of k feature vectors, X_i, $1 \leq i \leq k$, using IID standard normal random samples. Then, the expected maximum correlation between any pair of columns, $\rho(X_{i_1}, X_{i_2})$, can be as large as $k \ll n$.

Even in this IID sampling problem, we still expect a high rate of intrinsic and strong feature correlations. In general, this phenomenon is amplified for high-dimensional observational data, which would be expected to have a high degree of multicollinearity. This problem presents a number of computational, model-fitting, model-interpretation, and selection of salient predictors challenges, e.g., function singularities and indefinite Hessian matrices. There are some techniques that allow us to resolve such multicollinearity issues in high-dimensional data. Let's denote n to be the number of cases (samples, subjects, units, etc.) and k be the number of features. Using a divide-and-conquer strategy, we can split the problem into two special cases:

- When $n \geq k$, we can use the VIF to solve the problem parametrically.
- When $n \gg k$, VIF is not applicable and other creative approaches are necessary. In this case, examples of strategies that can be employed include

  - Use dimensionality-reduction (PCA, ICA, FA, SVD, PLSR, t-SNE, see Chap. 4) to simplify the problem to $n \geq k'$ (using only the top k' bases, functions, or directions).
  - Compute the (Spearman's rank-order based) pair correlation (matrix) and do some kind of feature selection, e.g., choosing only features with lower paired-correlations.

The Sure Independence Screening (SIS) technique[4] is based on correlation learning utilizing the sample correlation between a response and a given predictor. SIS reduces the feature-dimension (k) to a moderate dimension $O(n)$.

- The basic SIS method estimates marginal linear correlations between predictor and responses, which can be done by fitting a simple linear model. Nonparametric Independence Screening (NIS)[5] expands this model-based SIS strategy to use nonparametric models and allow more flexibility for the predictor ranking. Models' diagnostics for predictor-ranking may use the magnitude of the marginal

---

[4] https://doi.org/10.18637/jss.v083.i02

[5] https://doi.org/10.1198/jasa.2011.tm09779

estimators, nonparametric marginal-correlations, or marginal residual sum of squares.

- Generalized Correlation screening[6] employs an empirical sample-driven estimate of a generalized correlation to rank the individual predictors.
- *Forward Regression* using best subset regression is computationally very expensive because of the large combinatorial space, as the utility of each predictor depends on many other predictors. It generates a nested sequence of models, each having one additional predictor than the prior model. The model expansion adds new variables to the model based on their effect to improve the model quality, e.g., the largest decrease of the regression sum of squares, compared to the prior model.
- Model-Free Screening strategy[7] basically uses empirical estimates for conditional densities of the response given the predictors. Most methods have consistency in ranking (CIR) property,[8] which ensures that the objective utility function ranks unimportant predictors lower than important predictors with high probability (as $p \to 1$).

3.7.2.3   Visualizing Relationships Between Features

There are many alternative ways to visualize correlations, e.g., pairs(), ggpairs(), or plot_ly(). We already saw the pairs (splom) plot for the baseball data earlier. Some of these plots may give a sense of variable associations or show specific patterns in the data. The psych::pairs.panels() function provides another sophisticated display (splom = scatter plot matrix) that is often useful in exploring multivariate relations.

3.7.3   Step 3: Training a Model on the Data

The base R method we are going to use now is the linear modeling function, lm(). No extra package is needed when using the lm() function, which has the following invocation protocol

m <- lm(dv ~ iv, data=mydata)
- *dv*: dependent variable.
- *iv*: independent variables. Also see the function OneR() in Chap. 5. If we use . as iv, then all of the variables, except the dependent variable (*dv*), are included as model predictors.

---

[6]https://doi.org/10.1198/jcgs.2009.08041
[7]https://dx.doi.org/10.1198%2Fjasa.2011.tm10563
[8]https://dl.acm.org/doi/abs/10.5555/2999134.2999272

- *data*: specifies the data object containing both a dependent variable and independent variables.

```
fit <- lm(Weight ~ ., data=mlb); fit
## lm(formula = Weight ~ ., data = mlb)
## …
```

The output model report includes both numeric and factor predictors. For each factor variable, the model creates a set of several indicators (one-hot-encoding, dummy variables) with corresponding coefficients matching each factor level (except for all reference factor levels, as the effects of all factors are reported *relative* to the corresponding reference level). For each numerical variable, there is just one coefficient (the matching effect).

3.7.4   Step 4: Evaluating Model Performance

Let's examine the linear model performance (Fig. 3.8).

```
summary(fit)
## Call:
## lm(formula = Weight ~ ., data = mlb)
## Residuals:
##    Min     1Q  Median     3Q     Max
## -48.692 -10.909  -0.778   9.858  73.649
## Coefficients:
##                            Estimate Std. Error t value Pr(>|t|)
## (Intercept)              -164.9995    19.3828  -8.513  < 2e-16 ***
## TeamARZ                     7.1881     4.2590   1.688 0.091777 .
## TeamATL                    -1.5631     3.9757  -0.393 0.694278
...
## TeamWAS                    -1.7555     4.0038  -0.438 0.661142
## PositionDesignated_Hitter   8.9037     4.4533   1.999 0.045842 *
...
## PositionThird_Baseman      -4.6035     3.1689  -1.453 0.146613
## Height                      4.7175     0.2563  18.405  < 2e-16 ***
## Age                         0.8906     0.1259   7.075 2.82e-12 ***
## ---
## Signif. codes:  0 '***' 0.001 '**' 0.01 '*' 0.05 '.' 0.1 ' ' 1
## Residual standard error: 16.78 on 994 degrees of freedom
## Multiple R-squared:  0.3858,  Adjusted R-squared:  0.3617
## F-statistic: 16.01 on 39 and 994 DF,  p-value: < 2.2e-16
plot_ly(x=fit$fitted.values,y=fit$residuals,type="scatter",mode="markers") %>%
  layout(title="LM: Fitted-values vs. Model-Residuals",
         xaxis=list(title="Fitted"), yaxis = list(title="Residuals"))
```

The model *summary* shows how well the model fits the dataset:

- *Residuals*: This tells us about the residuals. If we have extremely large or extremely small residuals for some observations compared to the rest of residuals, either they are outliers due to reporting error or the model fits data poorly. We have 73.649 as our maximum and −48.692 as our minimum. Their extremeness could be examined by residual diagnostic plots.

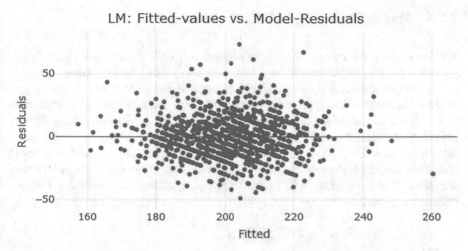

Fig. 3.8 Linear model diagnostic plot—residuals vs. fitted values

- *Coefficients*: In this section, strong effects are indicated by more stars (∗) in the right-most column. Stars, or dots, next to probability-value for each variable indicate whether the variable is a significant predictor of the outcome, and therefore should be included in the model. However, an empty field there suggests that (statistically speaking) this variable does not contribute significantly (in the specified model) to predicting the outcome, i.e., there is no strong evidence to suggest its estimated effect is nonzero. The column $Pr(>|t|)$ contains the estimated probability corresponding to the t-statistic for this covariate. Smaller values (close to 0$) indicate the variable is a significant covariate, and conversely, larger values indicate lack of significance and indication that the variable may be dropped from the model. In our examples, only some of the teams and positions are not significant, whereas Age and Height are significant predictors of the outcome, Weight.
- *R-squared*: Quantifies what percent in Y (outcome) is explained by included predictors (X). Here, we have $R^2 = 38.58\%$, which indicates the model is not bad but could be improved. Usually, a well-fitted linear regression would have over $R^2 > 50\%$.

In general, *diagnostic plots* may be helpful for understanding the model performance relative to the data:

- *Residual vs Fitted*: This is the residual diagnostic plot. We can see that the residuals of observations indexed 65, 160, and 237 are relatively far apart from the rest. They are potential influential points or outliers.
- *Normal Q-Q*: This plot examines the normality assumption of the model. If these dots follow the line on the graph, the normality assumption is valid. In our case, it is relatively close to the line. So, we can say that our model is valid in terms of normality.

3.7.5   Step 5: Improving Model Performance

We can employ the `step` function to perform *forward* or *backward* selection of important features/predictors. It works for both `lm()` and `glm()` models. In most cases, backward-selection is preferable because it tends to retain much larger models. On the other hand, there are various criteria to evaluate a model. Commonly used criteria include Akaike Information Criterion (*AIC*), Bayesian Information Criterion (*BIC*), *Adjusted R^2*, etc. Let's compare the backward and forward model selection approaches. The `step` function argument `direction` allows this control (default is `both`, which will select the better result from either backward or forward selection). Later, in Chap. 11, we will present details about alternative feature selection approaches.

```
step(fit,direction = "backward")
## Start:  AIC=5871.04
## Weight ~ Team + Position + Height + Age
##             Df Sum of Sq    RSS    AIC
## - Team      29      9468 289262 5847.4
## <none>                   279793 5871.0
## - Age        1     14090 293883 5919.8
## - Position   8     20301 300095 5927.5
## - Height     1     95356 375149 6172.3
##
## Step:  AIC=5847.45
## Weight ~ Position + Height + Age
##             Df Sum of Sq    RSS    AIC
## <none>                   289262 5847.4
## - Age        1     14616 303877 5896.4
## - Position   8     20406 309668 5901.9
## - Height     1    100435 389697 6153.6
## Call:
## lm(formula = Weight ~ Position + Height + Age, data = mlb)
## Coefficients:
##              (Intercept)  PositionDesignated_Hitter
##                -168.0474                     8.6968
##     PositionFirst_Baseman         PositionOutfielder
##                   2.7780                    -6.0457
##    PositionRelief_Pitcher     PositionSecond_Baseman
##                  -7.7782                   -13.0267
##          PositionShortstop    PositionStarting_Pitcher
##                 -16.4821                    -7.3961
##      PositionThird_Baseman                     Height
##                  -4.1361                     4.7639
##                      Age
##                   0.8771
```

```
step(fit,direction = "forward")
## Start:   AIC=5871.04
## Weight ~ Team + Position + Height + Age
## Call:
## lm(formula = Weight ~ Team + Position + Height + Age, data = mlb)
## Coefficients:
##                      (Intercept)                        TeamARZ
##                         -164.9995                         7.1881
##                          TeamATL                        TeamBAL
...
##                           4.7175                         0.8906
step(fit,direction = "both")
## Start:   AIC=5871.04
## Weight ~ Team + Position + Height + Age
##                Df Sum of Sq    RSS    AIC
## - Team       29      9468 289262 5847.4
## <none>                    279793 5871.0
## - Age         1     14090 293883 5919.8
## - Position    8     20301 300095 5927.5
## - Height      1     95356 375149 6172.3
## Step:  AIC=5847.45
## Weight ~ Position + Height + Age
##                Df Sum of Sq    RSS    AIC
## <none>                    289262 5847.4
## + Team       29      9468 279793 5871.0
## - Age         1     14616 303877 5896.4
## - Position    8     20400 309660 5901.9
## - Height      1    100435 389697 6153.6
```

We can observe that forward selection retains the whole model. The better feature selection model uses backward stepwise selection. Both backward and forward feature selection methods utilize greedy algorithms and do not guarantee an optimal model selection result. Identifying the best feature selection requires exploring every possible combination of the predictors, which is often not practically feasible due to computational complexity associated with model selection using $\binom{n}{k}$ combinations of features. Alternatively, we can choose models based on various *information criteria*.

```
step(fit, k=2)
## Start:  AIC=5871.04
## Weight ~ Team + Position + Height + Age
##
##           Df Sum of Sq    RSS    AIC
## - Team    29      9468 289262 5847.4
## <none>                 279793 5871.0
## - Age      1     14090 293883 5919.8
## - Position 8     20301 300095 5927.5
## - Height   1     95356 375149 6172.3
## Step:   AIC=5847.45
## Weight ~ Position + Height + Age
##           Df Sum of Sq    RSS    AIC
## <none>                 289262 5847.4
## - Age      1     14616 303877 5896.4
## - Position 8     20406 309668 5901.9
## - Height   1    100435 389697 6153.6
## Call:
## lm(formula = Weight ~ Position + Height + Age, data = mlb)
##
## Coefficients:
##              (Intercept)  PositionDesignated_Hitter
##                -168.0474                     8.6968
##      PositionFirst_Baseman        PositionOutfielder
##                   2.7780                    -6.0457
##   PositionRelief_Pitcher     PositionSecond_Baseman
##                  -7.7782                   -13.0267
##        PositionShortstop    PositionStarting_Pitcher
##                 -16.4821                    -7.3961
##    PositionThird_Baseman                     Height
##                  -4.1361                     4.7639
##                      Age
##                   0.8771
step(fit, k=log(nrow(mlb)))
## Start:  AIC=6068.69
## Step:   AIC=5901.8
```

Setting the parameter $k = 2$ yields the genuine AIC criterion, and $k = \log(n)$ refers to BIC. Let's try to evaluate the model performance again (Fig. 3.9).

```
fit2 = step(fit,k=2,direction = "backward")
## Start:  AIC=5871.04
## Step:   AIC=5847.45
plot_ly(x=fit2$fitted.values, y=fit2$residuals, type="scatter",
        mode="markers") %>%      # this plot is suppressed to save space
  layout(title="LM: Fitted-values vs. Model-Residuals",
         xaxis=list(title="Fitted"), yaxis = list(title="Residuals"))
# compute the quantiles
QQ <- qqplot(fit2$fitted.values, fit2$residuals, plot.it=FALSE)
# take a smaller sample size to expedite the viz
ind <- sample(1:length(QQ$x), 1000, replace = FALSE)
plot_ly() %>%
  add_markers(x=~QQ$x, y=~QQ$y, name="Quantiles Scatter", type="scatter",
              mode="markers") %>%
  add_trace(x = ~c(160,260), y = ~c(-50,80), type="scatter", mode="lines",
            line = list(color = "red", width = 4), name="Line", showlegend=F) %>%
  layout(title='Quantile plot', xaxis = list(title="Fitted"),
         yaxis = list(title="Residuals"), legend = list(orientation = 'h'))
```

Sometimes, simpler models are preferable, even when there is a little bit of loss of (fidelity) performance. In this case, we have a simpler model and $R^2 = 0.365$. The

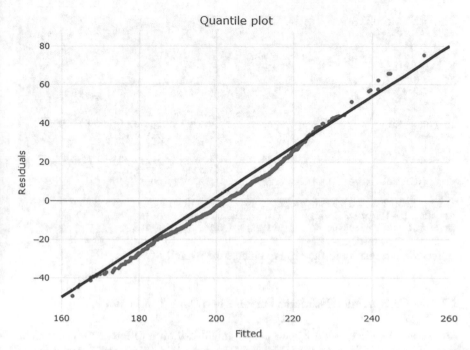

Fig. 3.9 Quantile–quantile model diagnostic plot—residuals vs. fitted values

whole model is still very significant. We can see that observations 65, 160, and 237 are relatively far from the bulk of other residuals. These cases represent potentially influential points, or outliers.

Also, we can observe the *leverage points*—those that are either outliers, influential points, or both. In a regression model setting, *observation leverage* is the relative distance of the observation (data point) from the mean of the explanatory variable. Observations near the mean of the explanatory variable have *low leverage* and those far from the mean have *high leverage*. Yet, not all points of high leverage are necessarily influential. A deeper discussion of variable selection, controlling the false discovery rate, is provided in Chap. 11.

3.7.5.1   Adding Nonlinear Relationships

In linear regression, the relationship between independent and dependent variables is assumed to be affine. However, in general, this might not be the case. The relationship between age and weight could be quadratic, logarithmic, exponential, etc. For instance, if middle-aged people are expected to gain weight dramatically and then lose it as they age. This is an example of adding a nonlinear (quadratic) term to the linear model. Note that the model is still referred to as *linear*, as it still has a linear matrix representation.

```
mlb$age2 <- (mlb$Age)^2
fit2      <- lm(Weight ~ ., data=mlb)
summary(fit2)
## lm(formula = Weight ~ ., data = mlb)
## Residuals:
##     Min     1Q  Median     3Q     Max
## -49.068 -10.775  -1.021  9.922  74.693
## Coefficients:
##                             Estimate Std. Error t value Pr(>|t|)
## (Intercept)                -209.07068   27.49529  -7.604 6.65e-14 ***
## TeamARZ                       7.41943    4.25154   1.745 0.081274 .
...
## Age                           3.82295    1.30621   2.927 0.003503 **
## age2                         -0.04791    0.02124  -2.255 0.024327 *
## Signif. codes:  0 '***' 0.001 '**' 0.01 '*' 0.05 '.' 0.1 ' ' 1
##
## Residual standard error: 16.74 on 993 degrees of freedom
## Multiple R-squared:  0.3889, Adjusted R-squared:  0.3643
## F-statistic:  15.8 on 40 and 993 DF,  p-value: < 2.2e-16
```

Including a quadratic factor may change the overall R^2.

3.7.5.2 Converting a Numeric Variable to a Binary Indicator

As discussed earlier, middle-aged people might exhibit a different weight pattern, compared to younger or older people. The overall pattern may not always be cumulative, i.e., weight may represent two separate trajectories for young and middle-aged people. For concreteness, let's use the age of 30 as a threshold segregating young and middle-aged people. People over 30 may have a steeper line for weight change than those under 30. Here we use an `ifelse()` conditioning statement to create a new indicator variable (age30) based on this threshold value.

```
mlb$age30 <- ifelse(mlb$Age>=30, 1, 0)
fit3      <- lm(Weight ~ Team+Position+Age+age30+Height, data=mlb)
summary(fit3)
## lm(formula = Weight ~ Team + Position + Age + age30 + Height,
##     data = mlb)
## Residuals:
##     Min     1Q  Median     3Q     Max
## -48.313 -11.166  -0.916  10.044  73.630
## Residual standard error: 16.77 on 993 degrees of freedom
## Multiple R-squared:  0.3866, Adjusted R-squared:  0.3619
## F-statistic: 15.65 on 40 and 993 DF,  p-value: < 2.2e-16
```

This model performs worse than the quadratic model in terms of R^2. Moreover, age30 does not appear as a significant predictor of weight. Therefore, such a pseudo factor does not contribute to explaining the observed variability in the dataset. However, if including such binary indicator (dummy variable, or one-hot-encoding feature) improved the model (e.g., increased R^2), then we can leave the binary feature in the model and interpret its coefficient estimate in terms of a difference of expectations

- $E(\text{Weight}_i| \text{age30}_i{=}0){=}\beta_o{+}\beta_{\text{Team}}\text{Team}{+}\beta_{\text{Position}}\text{Position}{+}\beta_{\text{Age}}\text{Age}{+}\beta_{\text{Height}}\text{Height}$, is the expected Weight where $\text{age30}_i = 0$, i.e., for younger people,

- $E(\text{Weight}_i | \text{age30}_i = 1)$

$$= \beta_o + \beta_{\text{Team}}\text{Team} + \beta_{\text{Position}}\text{Position} + \beta_{\text{Age}}\text{Age} + \underbrace{\beta_{\text{age30}}}_{\text{effect size}} \overbrace{Age30}^{\text{dummy var.}} + \beta_{\text{Height}}\text{Height}$$

is the expected Weight, where age30$_i = 1$, i.e., for older people. In other words, $\beta_{\text{age30}} \equiv E(\text{Weight}_i | \text{age30}_i = 1) - E(\text{Weight}_i | \text{age30}_i = 0)$. Therefore, β_{age30} is the difference in age-group specific expectations, i.e., the difference in expected Weight between older and younger people.

3.7.5.3   Adding Interaction Effects

So far, we only accounted for the individual and independent effects of each variable included in the linear model. It is also possible that pairs of features *jointly* affect the independent outcome variable. *Interactions* represent combined effects of two features on the outcome. If we are uncertain whether two variables interact, we could include them along with their interaction in the model, and then test the significance of the interaction term. If the interaction is significant, then it remains in the model; if not, this term can be dropped.

```
fit4 <- lm(Weight ~ Team + Height + Age*Position + age2, data=mlb)
summary(fit4)
## lm(formula = Weight ~ Team + Height + Age * Position + age2,
##     data = mlb)
## Residuals:
##     Min      1Q  Median      3Q     Max
## -48.761 -11.049  -0.761   9.911  75.533
## Coefficients:
##                               Estimate Std. Error t value Pr(>|t|)
## (Intercept)                 -199.15403   29.87269  -6.667 4.35e-11 ***
## TeamARZ                        8.10376    4.26339   1.901   0.0576 .
## TeamATL                       -0.81743    3.97899  -0.205   0.8373
...
## TeamWAS                       -1.43933    4.00274  -0.360   0.7192
## Height                         4.70632    0.25646  18.351  < 2e-16 ***
## Age                            3.32733    1.37088   2.427   0.0154 *
## PositionDesignated_Hitter    -44.82216   30.68202  -1.461   0.1444
...
## PositionThird_Baseman        -10.20102   23.26121  -0.439   0.6611
## age2                          -0.04201    0.02170  -1.936   0.0531 .
## Age:PositionDesignated_Hitter  1.77289    1.00506   1.764   0.0780 .
## Age:PositionFirst_Baseman     -0.71111    0.67848  -1.048   0.2949
## Age:PositionOutfielder         0.24147    0.53650   0.450   0.6527
## Age:PositionRelief_Pitcher     0.30374    0.50564   0.601   0.5482
## Age:PositionSecond_Baseman     0.46281    0.68281   0.678   0.4981
## Age:PositionShortstop          0.38257    0.70998   0.539   0.5901
## Age:PositionStarting_Pitcher  -0.17104    0.51976  -0.329   0.7422
## Age:PositionThird_Baseman      0.18968    0.79561   0.238   0.8116
## ---
## Signif. codes:  0 '***' 0.001 '**' 0.01 '*' 0.05 '.' 0.1 ' ' 1
## Residual standard error: 16.73 on 985 degrees of freedom
## Multiple R-squared:  0.3945, Adjusted R-squared:  0.365
## F-statistic: 13.37 on 48 and 985 DF,  p-value: < 2.2e-16
```

In this example, we see that the overall R^2 improved by including a Age × Position interaction and we can interpret its significance level.

3.8   Regression Trees and Model Trees

In Chap. 5, we will discuss decision trees built by multiple conditional logical decisions that lead to natural classifications of all observations. We could also add regression into decision tree modeling to make numerical predictions.

3.8.1   Adding Regression to Trees

Numeric prediction trees are built in the same way as classification trees. In Chap. 5, we will show how data are partitioned first by a *divide-and-conquer* strategy based on features. The homogeneity of the resulting classification trees is measured by various metrics, e.g., entropy. In regression-tree prediction, node homogeneity (which is used to determine if a node needs to be split) is measured by various statistics such as variance, standard deviation, or absolute deviation from the mean. A common splitting criterion for decision trees is the *standard deviation reduction (SDR)*.

$$\text{SDR} = \text{sd}(T) - \sum_{i=1}^{n} \left| \frac{T_i}{T} \right| \times \text{sd}(T_i),$$

where $\text{sd}(T)$ is the standard deviation for the original data. After the summation of all segments, $\left| \frac{T_i}{T} \right|$ is the proportion of observations in the ith segment compared to total number of observations, and $\text{sd}(T_i)$ is the standard deviation for the ith segment.

Let's look at a simple example

$$\text{Original data} : \{1, 2, 3, 3, 4, 5, 6, 6, 7, 8\},$$

$$\text{Split method 1} : \left\{ \underbrace{1, 2, 3}_{T_1} \mid \underbrace{3, 4, 5, 6, 6, 7, 8}_{T_2} \right\},$$

$$\text{Split method 2} : \left\{ \underbrace{1, 2, 3, 3, 4, 5}_{T_1'} \mid \underbrace{6, 6, 7, 8}_{T_2'} \right\}.$$

In split method 1, $T_1 = \{1, 2, 3\}$, $T_2 = \{3, 4, 5, 6, 6, 7, 8\}$, and in the alternative split method 2, $T'_1 = \{1, 2, 3, 3, 4, 5\}$, $T'_2 = \{6, 6, 7, 8\}$. Clearly the first splitting method appears inferior as it separates the pair of observations $(3, 3)$ into each of the two children nodes T_1 and T_2.

```
ori <- c(1, 2, 3, 3, 4, 5, 6, 6, 7, 8)
at1 <- c(1, 2, 3)
at2 <- c(3, 4, 5, 6, 6, 7, 8)
bt1 <- c(1, 2, 3, 3, 4, 5)
bt2 <- c(6, 6, 7, 8)
sdr_a <- sd(ori)-
          (length(at1)/length(ori)*sd(at1)+length(at2)/length(ori)*sd(at2))
sdr_b<-sd(ori)-
          (length(bt1)/length(ori)*sd(bt1)+length(bt2)/length(ori)*sd(bt2))
sdr_a    ## [1] 0.7702557
sdr_b    ## [1] 1.041531
```

The method `length()` is used above to get the number of elements in a specific vector.

Larger SDR indicates greater reduction in standard deviation after splitting. Here, we have split method 2 yielding greater SDR, so the tree splitting decision would prefer the *second method*, which is expected to produce more homogeneous subsets (children nodes), compared to *method 1*. Now, the tree will be split under bt1 and bt2 following the same rules (greater SDR wins). Assume we cannot split further (bt1 and bt2 are terminal nodes). The observations classified into bt1 will be predicted with mean(bt1) = 3 and those classified as bt2 with mean(bt2) = 6.75.

3.9 Bayesian Additive Regression Trees (BART)

Bayesian Additive Regression Trees (BART) represent sums of regression trees models that rely on boosting the constituent Bayesian regularized trees. The R packages `BayesTree` and `BART` provide computational implementation of fitting BART models to data. In supervised settings where x and y represent the predictors and the outcome, the BART model is mathematically represented as

$$y = f(x) + \epsilon = \sum_{j=1}^{m} f_j(x) + \epsilon.$$

More specifically,

$$y_i = f(x_i) + \epsilon = \sum_{j=1}^{m} f_j(x_i) + \epsilon, \forall 1 \leq i \leq n.$$

The residuals are typically assumed to be white noise, $\epsilon_i \sim N(o, \sigma^2)$, IID. The function f represents the boosted ensemble of weaker regression trees, $f_i = g(\cdot | T_j, M_j)$, where T_j and M_j represent the jth tree and the set of values, $\mu_{k,j}$, assigned to each terminal node k in T_j, respectively. The BART model may be estimated via Gibbs sampling, e.g., Bayesian backfitting Markov chain Monte Carlo (MCMC) algorithm. For instance, iteratively sampling (T_j, M_j) and σ, conditional on all other variables, (x, y), for each j until meeting a certain convergence criterion. Given σ, conditional sampling of (T_j, M_j) may be accomplished via the partial residual

$$\epsilon_{j_o} = \sum_{i=1}^{n} \left(y_i - \sum_{j \neq j_o}^{m} g(x_i | T_j, M_j) \right).$$

For prediction on *new data*, X, data-driven priors on σ and the parameters defining (T_j, M_j) may be used to allow sampling a model from the posterior distribution

$$p(\sigma, \{(T_1, M_1), (T_2, M_2), \cdots,$$

$$(T_2, M_2)\} | X, Y) = p(\sigma) \prod_{(\text{tree})j=1}^{m} \left(\left(\prod_{(\text{node})k} p(\mu_{k,j} | T_j) \right) p(T_j) \right).$$

In this posterior factorization, model regularization is achieved by four criteria:

- Enforcing reasonable marginal probabilities, $p(T_j)$, to ensure that the probability of a depth d node in the tree T_j has children decreases as d increases. That is, the probability a current bottom node, at depth l, is split into a left and right child nodes is $\frac{\alpha}{(1+l)^\beta}$, where the base ($\alpha$) and power ($\beta$) parameters are selected to optimize the fit (including regularization).
- For each interior (nonterminal) node, the distribution on the splitting variable assignments is uniform over the range of values taken by a variable.
- For each interior (nonterminal) node, the distribution on the splitting rule assignment, conditional on the splitting variable, is uniform over the discrete set of splitting values.

- All other priors are chosen as $p(\mu_{k_j}|T_j) = N(\mu_{k_j}|\mu, \sigma)$ and $p(\sigma)$ where σ^2 is inverse chi-square distributed. To facilitate the calculations, this introduces prior conjugate structure with the corresponding hyper-parameters estimated using the observed data.

Using the BART model to forecast a response corresponding to newly observed data x is achieved by using one individual (or ensembling/averaging multiple) prediction model(s) near the point of algorithmic convergence. The BART algorithm involves three steps

- Initialize a prior on the model parameters (f, σ), where $f = \{f_i = g(\cdot | T_j, M_j)\}_i$.
- Run a Markov chain with state (f, σ) where the stationary distribution is the posterior $p((f, \sigma)|\text{Data} = \{(x_i, y_i)\}_{i=1}^n)$.
- Examine the draws as a representation of the full posterior. Even though f is complex and changes its dimensional structure, for a given x, we can explore the marginals of σ and $f(x)$ by selecting a set of data $\{x_j\}_j$ and computing $f(x_j)$. If f_l represents the lth MCMC draw, then the homologous Bayesian tree structures at every draw will yield results of the same dimensions $(f_l(x_i), f_l(x_2), \cdots)$.

3.9.1   1D Simulation

This example illustrates a simple 1D BART simulation, based on an analytical process modeled by $h(x) = x^3 \sin(x)$, where we can nicely track the performance of the BART classifier (Fig. 3.10).

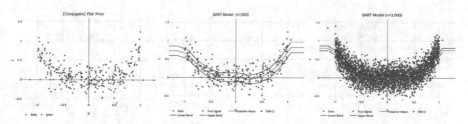

Fig. 3.10 Weighted BART model estimation using uninformative Jeffrey's flat prior (left) and smaller (middle) or larger (right) number of MCMC Gibbs samples

```r
# simulate training data
sig = 0.2  # sigma
func = function(x) {    return (sin(x) * (x^(3))) }
set.seed(1234)
n = 300
x = sort(2*runif(n)-1)          # define the input
y = func(x) + sig * rnorm(n)  # define the output
# xtest: values we want to estimate func(x) at; this is also our prior prediction
for y.
xtest = seq(-pi, pi, by=0.2)
plot_ly(x=x, y=y, type="scatter", mode="markers", name="data") %>%
  add_trace(x=xtest,y=rep(0,length(xtest)), mode="markers", name="prior") %>%
  layout(title='(Conjugate) Flat Prior',
     xaxis= list(title="X", range = c(-1.3, 1.3)),
     yaxis= list(title="Y", range=c(-0.6, 1.6)), legend=list(orientation='h'))
# run the weighted BART (BART::wbart) on the simulated data
# install.packages("BART")
library(BART)
set.seed(1234) # set seed for reproducibility of MCMC
# nskip=Number of burn-in MCMC iterations
# ndpost=number of posterior draws to return
model_bart <- wbart(x.train=as.data.frame(x), y.train=y,
         x.test=as.data.frame(xtest), nskip=300, ndpost=1000, printevery=1000)
## *****Into main of wbart
## *****Data:
## data:n,p,np: 300, 1, 32
# result is a list containing the BART run
# explore the BART model fit
names(model_bart)
##  [1] "sigma"         "yhat.train.mean" "yhat.train"     "yhat.test.mean"
##  [5] "yhat.test"     "varcount"        "varprob"        "treedraws"
##  [9] "proc.time"     "mu"              "varcount.mean"  "varprob.mean"
## [13] "rm.const"
dim(model_bart$yhat.test)
## [1] 1000   32
# The (l,j) element of the matrix `yhat.test` represents the l^{th} draw of
`func` evaluated at the j^{th} value of x.test
# A matrix with ndpost rows and nrow(x.train) columns where
# each row corresponds to a draw f* from the posterior of f
# and each column corresponds to a row of x.train. The (i,j) value is f*(x)
# for the i^th kept draw of f and the j^th row of x.train
quant_marg = apply(model_bart$yhat.test, 2, quantile, probs=c(0.025, 0.975)) #
plot the 2.5% and 97.5% quantiles
plot_ly(x=x, y=y, type="scatter", mode="markers", name="Data") %>%
  add_trace(x=xtest, y=func(xtest), mode="markers", name="True Signal") %>%
  add_trace(x=xtest, y=apply(model_bart$yhat.test, 2, mean), mode="lines",
        name="Posterior Mean") %>%
  add_trace(x=xtest, y=apply(model_bart$yhat.test, 2, quantile,
            probs=c(0.025,0.975)), mode="markers", name="95% CI") %>%
  add_trace(x=xtest, y=quant_marg[1,], mode="lines", name="Lower Band") %>%
  add_trace(x=xtest, y=quant_marg[2,], mode="lines", name="Upper Band") %>%
  layout(title='BART Model (n=300)', xaxis=list(title="X",range=c(-1.3,1.3)),
     yaxis=list(title="Y", range=c(-0.6, 1.6)), legend=list(orientation='h'))
names(model_bart)
```

```
dim(model_bart$yhat.train) ## [1] 1000  300
summary(model_bart$yhat.train.mean-apply(model_bart$yhat.train, 2, mean))
##      Min.    1st Qu.     Median       Mean    3rd Qu.       Max.
## -4.441e-16 -8.327e-17  6.939e-18 -8.130e-18  9.714e-17  5.551e-16
summary(model_bart$yhat.test.mean-apply(model_bart$yhat.test, 2, mean))
##      Min.    1st Qu.     Median       Mean    3rd Qu.       Max.
## -2.776e-16  1.535e-16  3.331e-16  2.661e-16  4.441e-16  4.441e-16
# yhat.train(test).mean: Average the draws to get the estimate of the posterior
mean of func(x)
# Let's increase the sample size, n, the BART model bounds should get tighter
n = 3000 # 300 --> 3,000
set.seed(1234)
x = sort(2*runif(n)-1)
y = func(x) + sig*rnorm(n)
model_bart_2 <- wbart(x.train=as.data.frame(x), y.train=y,
        x.test=as.data.frame(xtest), nskip=300, ndpost-1000, printevery=1000)
## data:n,p,np: 3000, 1, 32
quant_marg2 = apply(model_bart_2$yhat.test, 2, quantile, probs=c(0.025, 0.975)) #
plot the 2.5% and 97.5% CI
plot_ly(x=x, y=y, type="scatter", mode="markers", name="Data") %>%
  add_trace(x=xtest, y=func(xtest), mode="markers", name="True Signal") %>%
  add_trace(x=xtest, y=apply(model_bart_2$yhat.test, 2, mean), mode="lines",
        name="Posterior Mean") %>%
  add_trace(x=xtest, y=apply(model_bart_2$yhat.test, 2, quantile,
        probs=c(0.025, 0.975)), mode="markers", name="95% CI") %>%
  add_trace(x=xtest, y=quant_marg2[1,], mode="lines", name="Lower Band") %>%
  add_trace(x=xtest, y=quant_marg2[2,], mode="lines", name="Upper Band") %>%
  layout(title='BART Model (n=3,000)',
      xaxis=list(title="X", range=c(-1.3,1.3)),
      yaxis=list(title="Y", range=c(-0.6, 1.6)), legend=list(orientation='h'))
```

3.9.2 Higher-Dimensional Simulation

In this second BART example, we will simulate $n = 5,000$ cases with $p = 20$ features (Fig. 3.11).

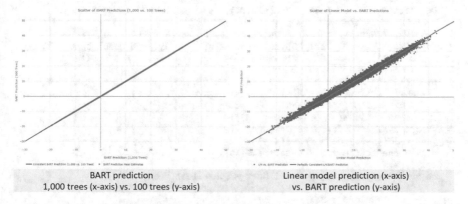

| BART prediction 1,000 trees (x-axis) vs. 100 trees (y-axis) | Linear model prediction (x-axis) vs. BART prediction (y-axis) |

Fig. 3.11 Effect of the number of trees for BART model prediction (left) and contrasting linear model and BART model predictions (right)

```
# simulate data
set.seed(1234)
n=5000; p=20
beta = 3*(1:p)/p
sig=1.0
X = matrix(rnorm(n*p), ncol=p) # design matrix)
y = as.double(10 + X %*% matrix(beta, ncol=1) + sig*rnorm(n)) # outcome
np=100000
Xp = matrix(rnorm(np*p), ncol=p)
set.seed(1234)
t1 <- system.time(model_bart_MD <-
        wbart(x.train=as.data.frame(X), y.train=y, x.test=as.data.frame(Xp),
        nkeeptrain=200, nkeeptest=100, nkeeptestmean=500, nkeeptreedraws=100,
        printevery=1000) )
## data:n,p,np: 5000, 20, 100000
## y1,yn: -6.790191, 5.425931
…
dim(model_bart_MD$yhat.train) ## [1]  200 5000
dim(model_bart_MD$yhat.test)  ## [1]  100 100000
names(model_bart_MD$treedraws)
# str(model_bart_MD$treedraws$trees)
# The trees are stored in a long character string and there are 100 draws each
consisting of 200 trees.
# To predict using the Multi-Dimensional BART model (MD)
t2 <- system.time({pred_model_bart_MD2 <-
                    predict(model_bart_MD, as.data.frame(Xp), mc.cores=6)})


dim(pred_model_bart_MD2) ## [1]     100 100000
t1
##    user  system elapsed
##  162.94    0.07  163.39
t2
##    user  system elapsed
##   47.66    0.05   47.81
# pred_model_bart_MD2 has row dimension equal to the number of kept tree draws
(100) and column dimension equal to the number of rows in Xp (100,000).
# Compare the BART predictions using 1K trees vs. 100 kept trees (very similar
results)
plot_ly() %>%
  add_trace(x = c(-30,50), y = c(-30,50), type="scatter", mode="lines",
      line = list(width = 4),
      name="Consistent BART Prediction (1,000 vs. 100 Trees)") %>%
  add_markers(x=model_bart_MD$yhat.test.mean, y=apply(pred_model_bart_MD2,
      2, mean), name="BART Prediction Mean Estimates", type="scatter",
      mode="markers") %>%
  layout(title='Scatter of BART Predictions (1,000 vs. 100 Trees)',
      xaxis = list(title="BART Prediction (1,000 Trees)"),
      yaxis = list(title="BART Prediction (100 Trees)"),
      legend = list(orientation = 'h'))
# Compare BART Prediction to a linear fit
lm_func = lm(y ~ ., data.frame(X,y))
pred_lm = predict(lm_func, data.frame(Xp))
plot_ly() %>%
  add_markers(x=pred_lm, y=model_bart_MD$yhat.test.mean,
      name="Consistent LM/BART Prediction", type="scatter",
      mode="markers") %>%
  add_trace(x = c(-30,50), y = c(-30,50), type="scatter", mode="lines",
      line = list(width = 4), name="LM vs. BART Prediction") %>%
  layout(title='Scatter of Linear Model vs. BART Predictions',
      xaxis = list(title="Linear Model Prediction"),
      yaxis = list(title="BART Prediction"),legend = list(orientation = 'h'))
```

3.9.3   Heart Attack Hospitalization Case-Study

Let's use BART to model the heart attack dataset (CaseStudy12_
AdultsHeartAttack_Data.csv). The data include about 150 observations and 8 features, including hospital charges (CHARGES), which will be used as a response variable.

```
heart_attack <-
    read.csv("https://umich.instructure.com/files/1644953/download?download_frd=1",
        stringsAsFactors = F)
str(heart_attack)
## 'data.frame':    150 obs. of  8 variables:
# convert the CHARGES (independent variable) to numerical form.
# NA's are created so let's remain only the complete cases
heart_attack$CHARGES <- as.numeric(heart_attack$CHARGES)
heart_attack <- heart_attack[complete.cases(heart_attack), ]
heart_attack$gender <- ifelse(heart_attack$SEX=="F", 1, 0)
heart_attack <- heart_attack[, -c(1,2,3)]
dim(heart_attack); colnames(heart_attack) ## [1] 148    6
x.train <- as.matrix(heart_attack[ , -3]) #x training, excl. charges (output)
y.train = heart_attack$CHARGES #y-output for modeling (BART, lm, lasso, etc.)
# Data should be standardized for all model-based predictions (e.g., lm,
lasso/glmnet), but this is not critical for BART
# We'll just do some random train/test splits and report the out of sample
performance of BART and lasso
RMSE <- function(y, yhat) { return(sqrt(mean((y-yhat)^2))) }
nd <- 10 # number of train/test splits (ala CV validation)
n <- length(y.train)
ntrain <- floor(0.8*n) # 80:20 train:test split each time
RMSE_BART <- rep(0, nd) # initialize BART and LASSO RMSE vectors
RMSE_LASSO <- rep(0, nd)
pred_BART <- matrix(0.0, n-ntrain,nd) # Initialize the BART and LASSO out-of-
sample predictions
pred_LASSO <- matrix(0.0, n-ntrain,nd)
```

In Chap. 11, we will learn more about *LASSO* regularized linear modeling. Now, let's use the glmnet::glmnet() method to fit a LASSO model and compare it to BART using the Heart Attack hospitalization case-study (Fig. 3.12).

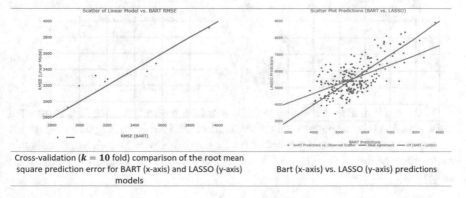

Cross-validation ($k = 10$ fold) comparison of the root mean square prediction error for BART (x-axis) and LASSO (y-axis) models

Bart (x-axis) vs. LASSO (y-axis) predictions

Fig. 3.12 LASSO vs. BART model prediction—RMSE (left) and prediction scatter (right)

```r
library(glmnet)
for(i in 1:nd) {
   set.seed(1234*i)
   # train/test split index
   train_ind <- sample(1:n, ntrain)
   # Outcome (CHARGES)
   yTrain <- y.train[train_ind]; yTest <- y.train[-train_ind]
   # Features for BART
   xBTrain <- x.train[train_ind, ]; xBTest <- x.train[-train_ind, ]


   # Features for LASSO (scale)
   xLTrain <- apply(x.train[train_ind, ], 2, scale)
   xLTest <- apply(x.train[-train_ind, ], 2, scale)
   # BART: parallel version of mc.wbart, same arguments as in wbart
   model_BART <- wbart(xBTrain, yTrain, xBTest, printevery=1000)
   # LASSO
   cv_LASSO <- cv.glmnet(xLTrain, yTrain, family="gaussian",standardize=TRUE)
   best_lambda <- cv_LASSO$lambda.min
   model_LASSO <- glmnet(xLTrain, yTrain, family="gaussian",
                         lambda=c(best_lambda), standardize=TRUE)
   #get predictions on testing data
   pred_BART1 <- model_BART$yhat.test.mean
   pred_LASSO1<-predict(model_LASSO,xLTest,s=best_lambda,type="response")[,1]
   #store results
   RMSE_BART[i] <- RMSE(yTest, pred_BART1); pred_BART[, i] <- pred_BART1
   RMSE_LASSO[i] <- RMSE(yTest, pred_LASSO1); pred_LASSO[, i] <- pred_LASSO1;
}
# Plot BART vs. LASSO predictions, compare the out of sample RMSE measures
plot_ly() %>%
  add_markers(x=RMSE_BART, y=RMSE_LASSO,
              name="", type="scatter", mode="markers") %>%
  add_trace(x = c(2800,4000), y = c(2800,4000), type="scatter", mode="lines",
            line = list(width = 4), name="") %>%
  layout(title='Scatter of Linear Model vs. BART RMSE',
            xaxis = list(title="RMSE (BART)"), legend = list(orientation='h')
            yaxis = list(title="RMSE (Linear Model)"))
# Next compare the out of sample predictions
model_lm <-lm(B~L,data.frame(B=as.double(pred_BART),L=as.double(pred_LASSO)))
x1 <- c(2800,9000)
y1 <- model_lm$coefficients[1] + model_lm$coefficients[2]*x1
plot_ly() %>%
  add_markers(x=as.double(pred_BART), y=as.double(pred_LASSO),
              name="BART Predictions vs. Observed Scatter", type="scatter",
              mode="markers") %>%
  add_trace(x = c(2800,9000), y = c(2800,9000), type="scatter", mode="lines",
            line = list(width = 4), name="Ideal Agreement") %>%
  add_trace(x = x1, y = y1, type="scatter", mode="lines",
            line = list(width = 4), name="LM (BART ~ LASSO)") %>%
  layout(title='Scatter Plot Predictions (BART vs. LASSO)',
            xaxis = list(title="BART Predictions"), legend=list(orientation='h')
            yaxis = list(title="LASSO Predictions"))
```

When the default prior estimate (`sigest` of the error variance (σ^2) is inverted chi-squared, i.e., computed using a standard conditionally conjugate prior) yields reasonable results, we can try longer BART runs (`ndpost=5000`). Mind the stable distribution of the $\widehat{\sigma}^2$ (y-axis) with respect to the number of posterior draws (x-axis) (Figs. 3.13 and 3.14).

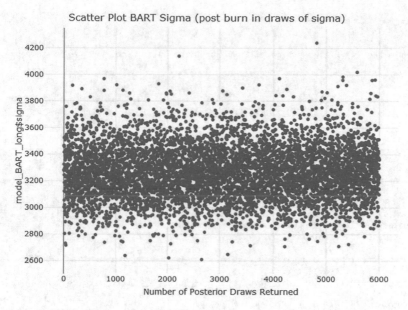

Fig. 3.13 Stable distribution of the BART model error variance against number of posterior distribution draws

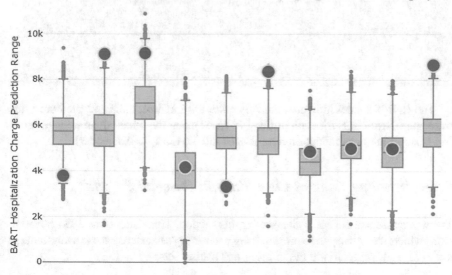

Fig. 3.14 Magnification showing BART prediction of hospitalization charges. The green dots indicate the actual charges and purple box-and-whisker plots indicate the distributions of the corresponding BART-derived (posterior distribution) hospitalization charge predictions for several patients

```
model_BART_long <- wbart(x.train, y.train, nskip=1000,
                         ndpost=5000, printevery=5000)
plot_ly() %>%
  add_markers(x=c(1:length(model_BART_long$sigma)), y=model_BART_long$sigma,
          name="BART vs. LASSO Scatter", type="scatter", mode="markers") %>%
  layout(title='Scatter Plot BART Sigma (post burn in draws of sigma)',
          xaxis = list(title="Number of Posterior Draws Returned"),
          yaxis = list(title="model_BART_long$sigma"),
          legend = list(orientation = 'h'))
```

```
ind <- order(model_BART_long$yhat.train.mean)
# boxplot(model_BART_Long$yhat.train[ , ind], ylim=range(y.train),
# xlab="case", ylab="BART Hospitalization Charge Prediction Range")
caseIDs <- paste0("Case",rownames(heart_attack))
rowIDs <- paste0("", c(1:dim(model_BART_long$yhat.train)[1]))
colnames(model_BART_long$yhat.train) <- caseIDs
rownames(model_BART_long$yhat.train) <- rowIDs
df1 <- as.data.frame(model_BART_long$yhat.train[ , ind])
df2_wide <-
      as.data.frame(cbind(index=c(1:dim(model_BART_long$yhat.train)[1]), df1))
# colnames(df2_wide); dim(df2_wide)
df_long <- tidyr::gather(df2_wide, case, measurement, Case138:Case8)
# str(df_long )
# 'data.frame': 74000 obs. of  3 variables:
# $ index      : int  1 2 3 4 5 6 7 8 9 10 ...
# $ case       : chr  "Case138" "Case138" "Case138" "Case138" ...
# $ measurement: num  5013 3958 4604 2602 2987 ...
actualCharges <- as.data.frame(cbind(cases=caseIDs, value=y.train))
plot_ly() %>%
  add_trace(data=df_long, y = ~measurement, color = ~case, type = "box") %>%
  add_trace(x=~actualCharges$cases, y=~actualCharges$value, type="scatter",
       mode="markers", name="Observed Charge", marker=list(size=20,
            color='green', line=list(color='yellow', width=2))) %>%
  layout(title="Box-and-whisker Plots across all 148 Cases
      (Highlighted True Charges)", xaxis = list(title="Cases"),
      yaxis = list(title="BART Hospitalization Charge Prediction Range"),
      showlegend=F)
```

The BART model indicates there is quite a bit of uncertainty in predicting the outcome (CHARGES) for each of the 148 cases using the other covariate features in the heart attack hospitalization data (DRG, DIED, LOS, AGE, gender).

3.9.4 Another Look at Case Study 2: Baseball Players

We will again use the MLB dataset for this section. This dataset has 1034 observations which we will separate into *training* and *testing* sets. Here we use a randomized split (75 − 25%) to divide the training and testing sets.

```
set.seed(1234)
train_index <- sample(seq_len(nrow(mlb)), size = 0.75*nrow(mlb))
mlb_train <- mlb[train_index, ]
mlb_test <- mlb[-train_index, ]
```

3.9.4.1   Step 3: Training a Model on the Data

To train the model in R, we will use the `rpart::rpart()` function, which provides an implementation for prediction using regression-tree modeling.

m <- rpart(dv~iv, data=mydata)
- *dv*: dependent variable
- *iv*: independent variable
- *mydata*: training data containing `dv` and `iv`.

We use two numerical features in the MLB data (01a_data.txt) `Age` and `Height` as features.

```
#install.packages("rpart")
library(rpart)
mlb.rpart <- rpart(Weight ~ Height + Age, data=mlb_train)
mlb.rpart
## n= 775
...
##      7) Age>=30.015 74  19803.910 222.1216 *
```

The output contains rich information, `split` indicates the method to split, *n* is the number of observations that fall in this segment, `yval` is the predicted value if the test data falls into the specific segment (tree node decision cluster).

3.9.4.2   Visualizing Regression Decision Trees

A useful way of displaying the `rpart` decision tree is by using the `rpart.plot()` function in the `rpart.plot` package (Fig. 3.15).

```
# install.packages("rpart.plot")
library(rpart.plot)
rpart.plot(mlb.rpart, digits=3)
```

More detailed graphs can be obtained by specifying additional options in the function call, or we can also use the `rattle::fancyRpartPlot()` method to display regression trees and explain the order and rules of node splits (Fig. 3.16).

```
rpart.plot(mlb.rpart, digits = 4, fallen.leaves = T, type=3, extra=101)
library(rattle)
fancyRpartPlot(mlb.rpart, cex = 0.8)
```

3.9.4.3   Step 4: Evaluating Model Performance

To evaluate the model performance, we can make predictions using the model prediction tree and the generic `predict()` method.

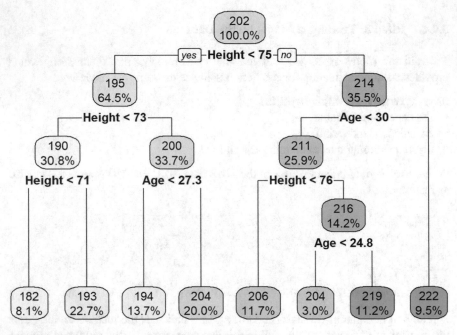

Fig. 3.15 Rpart regression-tree modeling of the MLB data

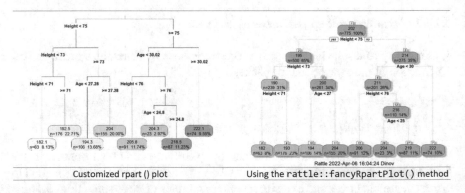

Fig. 3.16 Alternative rendering of the regression trees for the MLB data

```
mlb.p <- predict(mlb.rpart, mlb_test)
summary(mlb.p)
##    Min. 1st Qu.  Median    Mean 3rd Qu.    Max.
##   182.1   192.5   204.0   202.1   205.8   222.1
summary(mlb_test$Weight)
##    Min. 1st Qu.  Median    Mean 3rd Qu.    Max.
##   150.0   186.5   200.0   201.3   219.0   260.0
```

We can compare the five-number statistics for the predicted estimates to the observed `Weight` values. Note that the model cannot precisely identify extreme cases, such as the maximum. However, within the IQR, the predictions are relatively accurate. Correlation could also be used to measure the correspondence of two equal length numeric variables. Let's use `cor()` to examine the prediction accuracy.

```
cor(mlb.p, mlb_test$Weight) ## [1] 0.5508078
```

The predicted values (Weights) are moderately correlated with their true value counterparts. Chap. 9 provides additional strategies for model quality assessment.

3.9.4.4 Measuring Performance with Mean Absolute Error

To measure the distance between predicted value and the true value, we can use a measurement called *mean absolute error (MAE)*. MAE is calculated using the following formula

$$\text{MAE} = \frac{1}{n} \sum_{i=1}^{n} |\text{pred}_i - \text{obs}_i|,$$

where for each case i, `pred_i` and `obs_i` represent the ith predicted value and the ith observed value. Let's manually construct a MAE function in R and evaluate our model performance.

```
MAE <- function(obs, pred)  {   mean(abs(obs-pred)) }
MAE(mlb_test$Weight, mlb.p) ## [1] 13.91322
```

This implies that *on average*, the difference between the predicted value and the observed value is 15.1. Considering that the range of the `Weight` variable in our test dataset is [150, 260], the model performs well. For comparison, suppose we used the most primitive method for prediction – the *sample mean*. How much larger would the MAE be?

```
mean(mlb_test$Weight)
## [1] 201.2934
MAE(mlb_test$Weight, mean(mlb_test$Weight)) ## [1] 16.80094
```

This example illustrates that the predictive decision tree is better than using the *overall mean* strategy to predict every observation in the test dataset. However, it is not dramatically better. There might be room for further improvement.

We can also try to improve the performance of our regression-tree forecasting by using a *model tree*, instead of a regression tree. The `RWeka::M5P()` function implements the M5 algorithm and uses a similar syntax as `rpart::rpart()`.

m <- M5P(dv ~ iv, data=mydata)

```
#install.packages("RWeka")
# For RWeka installations see:
# http://stackoverflow.com/questions/41878226/using-rweka-m5p-in-rstudio-yields-
java-Lang-noclassdeffounderror-no-uib-cipr-ma
Sys.getenv("WEKA_HOME") # where does it point to? Maybe some obscure path?
# if yes, correct the variable:
Sys.setenv(WEKA_HOME="C:\\MY\\PATH\\WEKA_WPM")
library(RWeka)
mlb.m5 <- M5P(Weight ~ Height + Age, data=mlb_train)
mlb.m5
## M5 pruned model tree:
## (using smoothed linear models)
## Height <= 74.5 :
## |   Height <= 72.5 :
...
## |   |   Age >  34.155 : LM17 (23/70.498%)
...
## Number of Rules: 17
```

Instead of using segment averages to predict an outcome, the M5 model uses a
linear regression (LM1) as the terminal node. In some datasets with more variables,
M5P could give us multiple linear models under different terminal nodes. Much like
the general regression trees, M5 builds tree-based models. The difference is that
regression trees produce univariate forecasts (values) at each terminal node, whereas
the M5 model-based regression trees generate multivariate linear models at each
node. These model-based forecasts represent piece-wise linear functional models
that can be used to numerically estimate outcomes at every node based on very high
dimensional data (feature-rich spaces).

```
summary(mlb.m5)
mlb.p.m5 <- predict(mlb.m5, mlb_test)
summary(mlb.p.m5)
cor(mlb.p.m5, mlb_test$Weight) ## [1] -0.2677442
MAE(mlb_test$Weight, mlb.p.m5) ## [1] 69.12329
```

We can use summary(mlb.m5) to report some rough diagnostic statistics for
the model. Notice that the correlation and MAE for the M5 model are better
compared to the results of the previous rpart() model.

3.10   Practice Problems

3.10.1   How Is Matrix Multiplication Defined?

Validate that $(A_{k,n} \times B_{n,m})^t = (B^t_{m,n}) \times (A^t_{n,k})$, both using math notation (first principles) and using R functions for some example matrices.

3.10.2 Scalar Versus Matrix Multiplication

Demonstrate the differences between the scalar multiplication ($*$) and matrix multiplication ($\% * \%$).

3.10.3 Matrix Equations

Write a simple matrix solver ($b = Ax$, i.e., $x = A^{-1}b$) and validate its accuracy using the R command `solve(A,b)`. Solve this equation

$$2a - b + 2c = 5$$
$$-a - 2b + c = 3 .$$
$$a + b - c = 2$$

3.10.4 Least Square Estimation

Use the SOCR Knee Pain dataset, extract the RB $-$ Right-Back locations (x, y), and fit in a linear model for vertical location (y) in terms of the horizontal location (x). Display the linear model on top of the scatter plot of the paired data.

3.10.5 Matrix Manipulation

Create a matrix A with elements `seq(1, 15, length = 6)` and argument `nrow = 3`; add a row to this matrix; add two columns to A to obtain a new matrix $C_{4, 4}$. Then generate a diagonal matrix D with dim $= 4$ and elements `rnorm (4,0,1)`. Apply element wise addition, subtraction, multiplication, and division to the matrices C and D. Apply matrix multiplication to D and C. Obtain the inverse of C and compare the result to `ginv()`.

3.10.6 Matrix Transposition

Validate the multiplicative transpose formula, $(A_{k, n} \cdot B_{n, m})^T = (B_{n, m})^T \cdot (A_{k, n})^T$, both using math notation, as well as using R calls, e.g., you can try $A = $ `matrix(1: 6,nrow=3)`, $B = $ `matrix(2:7, nrow = 2)`.

3.10.7   Sample Statistics

Use the SOCR Data Iris Sepal Petal Classes to compute the sample mean and variance of each variable. Then calculate the sample covariance – use both math notation and R built-in functions.

3.10.8   Eigenvalues and Eigenvectors

Generate a random matrix with $A = \text{matrix}(\text{rnorm}(9,0,1), \text{nrow} = 3)$, compute the eigenvalues and eigenvectors for A. Then try to solve this equation $det(A - \lambda I) = 0$, where λ is a vector of length 3. Compare λ and the eigenvalues you computed above. Example of manual and automated calculations of eigenspectra (eigenvalues and eigenvectors).

```
A <- matrix(rnorm(9,0,1),nrow = 3);
A  # define a random design matrix, may generate complex solutions
# or define a specific (non-random) design matrix
A <- matrix(c(0,1/4,1/4,3/4,0,1/4,1/4,3/4,1/2), 3,3, byrow=T); A
##      [,1] [,2] [,3]
## [1,] 0.00 0.25 0.25
## [2,] 0.75 0.00 0.25
## [3,] 0.25 0.75 0.50
eigen_spectrum <- eigen(A); eigen_spectrum
## eigen() decomposition
## $values ## [1]  1.00 -0.25 -0.25
## $vectors
##             [,1]           [,2]          [,3]
## [1,] 0.3207501  1.068531e-08 -1.068531e-08
## [2,] 0.4490508 -7.071068e-01 -7.071068e-01
## [3,] 0.8339504  7.071068e-01  7.071068e-01
# compute the eigen-spectrum (eigenvalues, l, and eigenvectors, v), Av = lv
B <- A - eigen(A)$values*diag(3); B
##       [,1] [,2] [,3]
## [1,] -1.00 0.25 0.25
## [2,]  0.75 0.25 0.25
## [3,]  0.25 0.75 0.75
# compute B = (A - eigen_value × I)
det(A-eigen(A)$values * diag(3))  ## [1] -2.833371e-09
# verify that the det(A-eigen(A)$values * diag(3)) is not trivial (0)
A%*%eigen(A)$vector - eigen(A)$value*diag(3) # validate that Av = l v
##             [,1]           [,2]          [,3]
## [1,] -0.6792499 -2.671328e-09 2.671328e-09
## [2,]  0.4490502  4.267767e-01 1.767767e-01
## [3,]  0.8339504 -1.767767e-01 7.322330e-02
all.equal(A,eigen(A)$vector%*%diag(eigen(A)$values)%*%solve(eigen(A)$vector))
## [1] TRUE
# compare A = v*l*inv(v)
# Compare I==AV-lambda*v, mind the $*$ and $%*%$ scalar and matrix operators
all.equal(diag(3), A%*%eigen(A)$vector - eigen(A)$values * eigen(A)$vector)
## [1] "Mean relative difference: 1.534584"
```

3.10.9   Regression Forecasting Using Numerical Data

Use the Quality of Life data (Case06_QoL_Symptom_ChronicIllness) to fit several different Multiple Linear Regression models predicting clinically relevant outcomes, e.g., `Chronic Disease Score`.

- Summarize and visualize the data using `summary`, `str`, `pairs.panels`, `ggplot`, and `plot_ly()`
- Report paired correlations for numeric data and try to visualize these (e.g., heatmap, pairs plot, etc.)
- Examine potential dependencies of the predictors and the dependent response variables
- Fit a Multiple Linear Regression model, report the results, and explain the summary, residuals, effect-size coefficients, and the coefficient of determination, R^2
- Draw model diagnostic plots, at least QQ plot, residuals plot, and leverage plot (half norm plot)
- Predict outcomes for new data
- Try to improve the model performance using the `step` function based on AIC and BIC
- Fit a regression tree model and compare it with OLS model
- Try to use `M5P` to improve the model

Chapter 4
Linear and Nonlinear Dimensionality Reduction

Now that we have most of the R fundamentals covered and saw a model-based forecasting (multivariate linear regression), we can delve into more interesting ML/AI data analytic methods. *Dimension reduction* reduces the number of features when dealing with a very large number of variables. Linear and nonlinear dimension reduction can help us extract a set of "uncorrelated" principal variables, or salient features, reduce the complexity of the data, and facilitate supervised data clustering and unsupervised classification. Dimensionality reduction is related to feature selection (Chap. 11); however, it goes beyond simply picking some of the original variables. Rather, we are constructing new (uncorrelated) variables, which sometimes may be expressed as linear functions of the original features and sometimes can only be inferred as highly nonlinear transformations (maps) of the initial variable state space.

Dimensionality reduction techniques enable exploratory data analytics by reducing the complexity of the dataset, while still approximately preserving important process characteristics, such as retaining the distances between cases or subjects. If we are able to reduce the complexity down to a few dimensions and protect some of that information content in the transformed data, then we may visually inspect the data and try other lower-dimensional methods to untangle its intrinsic characteristics. All *dimensionality reduction* techniques carry some resemblance to *variable selection*, which we will see in Chap. 11. The *continuous* process of dimensionality reduction yields lower variability compared to the *discrete* feature selection process, e.g., see Wolfgang M. Hartmann's paper.[1]

In this chapter, we will (1) start with a synthetic example motivating reduction of a 2D dataset into 1D; (2) explain the notion of rotation matrices; (3) show examples of principal component analysis (PCA), singular value decomposition (SVD), independent component analysis (ICA), factor analysis (FA), t-distributed Stochastic Neighbor Embedding (t-SNE), and Uniform Manifold Approximation and

---

[1] https://doi.org/10.1007/11558958_113

© The Author(s), under exclusive license to Springer Nature Switzerland AG 2023
I. D. Dinov, *Data Science and Predictive Analytics*, The Springer Series in Applied Machine Learning, https://doi.org/10.1007/978-3-031-17483-4_4

Twin1$_{\text{Height}}$	Twin2$_{\text{Height}}$
$y[1, 1]$	$y[1, 2]$
$y[2, 1]$	$y[2, 2]$
$y[3, 1]$	$y[3, 2]$
$\vdots$	$\vdots$
$y[500, 1]$	$y[500, 2]$

Table 4.1 Data frame representation of the simulated 2D data of normalized twin heights

Projection (UMAP); and (4) present linear and nonlinear dimensionality reductions using handwritten digit recognition and a Parkinson's disease case-study.

4.1   Motivational Example: Reducing 2D to 1D

Let's consider a simple example of twin heights. Suppose we simulate 1000 2D points representing *normalized* individual heights, i.e., number of standard deviations from the mean height for pairs of twins. Each 2D point represents a pair of twin heights. We will simulate this scenario using the bivariate Normal distribution (Table 4.1).

```
library(MASS)
set.seed(1234)
n <- 1000
y=t(mvrnorm(n, c(0, 0), matrix(c(1, 0.95, 0.95, 1), 2, 2)))
```

$$
y^T_{2 \times 500} = \begin{bmatrix} y[1, \ ] = \text{Twin1}_{\text{Height}} \\ y[2, \ ] = \text{Twin2}_{\text{Height}} \end{bmatrix} \sim \text{BVN} \left(\mu = \begin{bmatrix} \text{Twin1}_{\text{Height}} \\ \text{Twin2}_{\text{Height}} \end{bmatrix}, \Sigma = \begin{bmatrix} 1 & 0.95 \\ 0.95 & 1 \end{bmatrix} \right).
$$

Next, we will compare the scatter plot of the original (raw) data to its linearly transformed counterpart. This case-study is intentionally oversimplified to build intuition about the core dimensionality reduction principles. In this motivational example, we focus only on two dimensions representing a small fraction of the typical high-dimensional information contained in many practical case-studies. Here is one example of such a real pediatric neuroimaging genetics study[2] examining regional changes in brain cortical thickness associated with functional disturbances in schizophrenia.

---

[2] https://doi.org/10.1093/cercor/bhh172

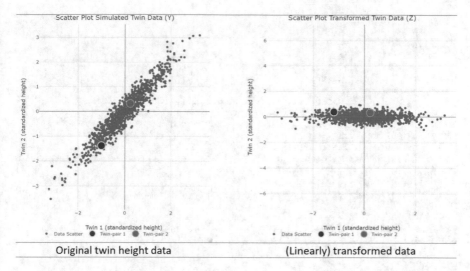

Fig. 4.1 Scatter plot of simulated (normalized) twin heights data—original (left) and transformed (right). The highlighted green and red points on the plots show the (bivariate) positions of the first couple of twin pairs

Tracking the distances between any two samples can be accomplished using the function stats::dist(), which computes the distance matrix (according to a user-specified distance metric, default = Euclidean) between the cases, i.e., *rows of the data frame*. For example, the distance between the first two pairs of twins, in terms of their normalized heights, is 2.100187.

```
d = dist(t(y))
as.matrix(d)[1, 2]   ## [1] 2.100187
```

To reduce the 2D data to a simpler 1D space, we can transform the data to a 1D matrix (a vector) approximately preserving the distances between the original 2D points. The 2D plots in the figure show the Euclidean distance between a couple of highlighted points. The length of this line represents the distance between the two points. In 2D, these lines connecting pairs of points tend to go along the direction of the main diagonal. If we rotate the plot, so that the diagonal is now aligned with the *x*-axis, we get the following *raw* and *transformed* data scatter plots (Fig. 4.1).

```
library(plotly)
# Plot raw (native) data
plot_ly() %>%
  add_markers(x = ~y[1, ], y = ~y[2, ], name="Data Scatter") %>%
  add_markers(x = y[1, 1], y = y[2, 1], marker=list(color = 'red', size = 20,
              line = list(color='yellow', width=2)), name="Twin-pair 1") %>%
  add_markers(x = y[1, 2], y = y[2, 2], marker=list(color = 'green', size=20,
              line = list(color='orange', width=2)), name="Twin-pair 2")%>%
  layout(title='Scatter Plot Simulated Twin Data (Y)',
         xaxis = list(title="Twin 1 (standardized height)"),
         yaxis = list(title="Twin 2 (standardized height)"),
         legend = list(orientation = 'h'))
# Transform and plot the mapped data
z1 = (y[1, ]+y[2, ])/2 # the sum (actually average)
z2 = (y[1, ]-y[2, ])   # the difference
z = rbind( z1, z2) # matrix z has the same dimension as y
thelim <- c(-3, 3)
plot_ly() %>%
  add_markers(x = ~z[1, ], y = ~z[2, ], name="Data Scatter") %>%
  add_markers(x = z[1, 1], y = z[2, 1], marker=list(color = 'red', size = 20,
              line = list(color='yellow', width=2)), name="Twin-pair 1") %>%
  add_markers(x = y[1, 2], y = y[2, 2], marker=list(color='green', size=20,
              line = list(color='orange', width=2)), name="Twin-pair 2") %>%
  layout(title='Scatter Plot Transformed Twin Data (Z)',
         xaxis = list(title="Twin 1 (standardized height)",
         scaleanchor = "y", scaleratio = 2), legend = list(orientation='h'),
         yaxis = list(title="Twin 2 (standardized height)", scaleanchor="x",
         scaleratio = 0.5))
```

As we saw in Chap. 3, matrix linear algebra notation can be used to represent this affine transformation of the data. Here we can see that to get the result z, we multiplied y by the matrix A

$$A = \begin{pmatrix} \dfrac{1}{2} & \dfrac{1}{2} \\ 1 & -1 \end{pmatrix} \Longrightarrow z = A \times y.$$

We can invert this transformation by multiplying the output (z) by the inverse matrix (rotation matrix?) A^{-1} as follows

$$A^{-1} = \begin{pmatrix} 1 & \dfrac{1}{2} \\ 1 & -\dfrac{1}{2} \end{pmatrix} \Longrightarrow y = A^{-1} \times z.$$

We can now try this example in R.

```
A <- matrix(c(1/2, 1, 1/2, -1), nrow=2, ncol=2); A   # define a matrix
##      [,1] [,2]
## [1,]  0.5  0.5
## [2,]  1.0 -1.0
A_inv <- solve(A); A_inv  # inverse
##      [,1] [,2]
## [1,]    1  0.5
## [2,]    1 -0.5
A %*% A_inv # Verify result
##      [,1] [,2]
## [1,]    1    0
## [2,]    0    1
```

This specific matrix transformation, $A : \mathbb{R}^2 \to \mathbb{R}^2$, does not preserve distances, i.e., it's not an *isometry* or a simple rotation in 2D. Is distance preservation important and how to construct distance-preserving transformations?

```
d=dist(t(y)); as.matrix(d)[1, 2]   # distance between first 2 points in Y
## [1] 2.100187
d1=dist(t(z)); as.matrix(d1)[1, 2] # distance between first 2 points in Z=A*Y
## [1] 1.541323
```

4.2   Matrix Rotations

One important question is how to identify transformations that preserve distances. In mathematics, transformations between metric spaces that are distance-preserving are called isometries, also known as congruencies or congruent transformations. First, let's test the distance-preserving property of the MA transformation we used above (Fig. 4.2)

$$\begin{vmatrix} A = \dfrac{Y_1 + Y_2}{2} \\ M = Y_1 - Y_2 \end{vmatrix}.$$

```
MA <- matrix(c(1/2, 1, 1/2, -1), 2, 2)
MA_z <- MA%*%y
d <- dist(t(y))
d_MA <- dist(t(MA_z))
plot_ly() %>%
  add_markers(x = ~as.numeric(d)[1:5000], y = ~as.numeric(d_MA)[1:5000],
         name="Transformed Twin Distances") %>%
  add_markers(x = ~as.numeric(d)[1], y = ~as.numeric(d_MA)[1],
         marker=list(color = 'red', size = 20,
         line = list(color = 'yellow', width = 2)), name="Twin-pair 1") %>%
  add_markers(x = ~as.numeric(d)[2], y = ~as.numeric(d_MA)[2],
         marker=list(color = 'green', size = 20,
         line = list(color = 'orange', width = 2)), name="Twin-pair 2") %>%
  add_trace(x = ~c(0,8), y = ~c(0,8), mode="lines",
         line = list(color="red", width=4), name="Preserved Distances") %>%
    layout(title='Preservation of Distances Between Twins (Transform=MA_z)',
         xaxis = list(title="Original Twin Distances", range = c(0, 8)),
         yaxis = list(title="Transformed Twin Distances", range = c(0, 8)),
         legend = list(orientation = 'h'))
```

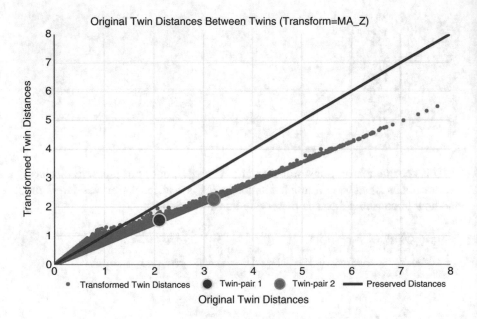

Fig. 4.2 Example of a distance-altering linear transformation, $A = \begin{pmatrix} \frac{1}{2} & \frac{1}{2} \\ 1 & -1 \end{pmatrix} : \mathbb{R}^2 \to \mathbb{R}^2$

Observe that this MA transformation, expressed as a matrix A, is not an isometry, i.e., it does not preserve pairwise distances. Here is one example of a couple of twin pairs $v_1 = \begin{bmatrix} v_{1,x} = 0 \\ v_{1,y} = 1 \end{bmatrix}$ and $v_2 = \begin{bmatrix} v_{2,x} = 1 \\ v_{2,y} = 0 \end{bmatrix}$, which are distance $d(v_1, v_2) = \sqrt{2}$ apart in their native space, but separated further by the transformation MA, $d(\text{MA}(v_1), \text{MA}(v_2)) = 2$.

```
MA; t(MA); solve(MA); t(MA) - solve(MA)
##      [,1] [,2]
## [1,]  0.5  0.5
## [2,]  1.0 -1.0
##      [,1] [,2]
## [1,]  0.5    1
## [2,]  0.5   -1
##      [,1] [,2]
## [1,]    1  0.5
## [2,]    1 -0.5
##      [,1] [,2]
## [1,] -0.5  0.5
## [2,] -0.5 -0.5
v1 <- c(0,1); v2 <- c(1,0); rbind(v1,v2)
##    [,1] [,2]
## v1    0    1
## v2    1    0
euc.dist <- function(x1, x2) sqrt(sum((x1 - x2) ^ 2))
euc.dist(v1,v2)
## [1] 1.414214
v1_t <- MA %*% v1; v2_t <- MA %*% v2
euc.dist(v1_t,v2_t)
## [1] 2
```

More generally, let's assume that the process Y is Bivariate Normally (BVN) distributed

$$Y = \begin{pmatrix} Y_1 \\ Y_2 \end{pmatrix} \sim \text{BVN}\left(\mu = \begin{pmatrix} \mu_1 \\ \mu_2 \end{pmatrix}, \quad \Sigma = \begin{pmatrix} \sigma_1^2 & \sigma_{12} \\ \sigma_{12} & \sigma_2^2 \end{pmatrix}\right), \quad \sigma_{12} = \rho\sigma_1\sigma_2,$$

$$\rho = \text{corr}(Y_1, Y_2).$$

Then, an affine transformation of Y is also Bivariate Normal

$$Z = AY + \eta \sim \text{BVN}\left(\eta + A\mu, A\Sigma A^T\right),$$

where BVN denotes bivariate normal distribution, $A = \begin{pmatrix} a & b \\ c & d \end{pmatrix}$, $Y = (Y_1, Y_2)^T$,

$\mu = (\mu_1, \mu_2)^T, \Sigma = \begin{pmatrix} \sigma_1^2 & \sigma_{12} \\ \sigma_{12} & \sigma_2^2 \end{pmatrix}$. This property can be verified by using calculus and change of variables transformations.

Thus, affine transformations preserve bivariate normality. However, in general, the linear transformation (A) is not guaranteed to be an isometry. The question now is under what additional conditions the transformation matrix A is guaranteed to be an isometry?

Notice that the squared distance between any pair of points $P_i, P_j \in \mathbb{R}^n$ is

$$d^2(P_i, P_j) = \sum_{k=1}^{n} \left(P_{jk} - P_{ik}\right)^2 - \|P\|^2 - P^T P,$$

where $P = (P_{j1} - P_{i1}, P_{j2} - P_{i2}, \cdots, P_{jn} - P_{in})^T$ is the n dimensional difference vector between the points. Thus, the only requirement we need for A to be an isometry is $(AY)^T(AY) = Y^T Y$, i.e., $A^T A = I$, which implies that A is an orthogonal (rotational) matrix, whose transpose is its inverse.

Let's use a two-dimension orthogonal matrix to illustrate this isometry property. Set $A = \frac{1}{\sqrt{2}}\begin{pmatrix} 1 & 1 \\ 1 & -1 \end{pmatrix}$. It's easy to verify that A is an orthogonal (2D rotation) matrix. The simplest way to test the isometry is to perform the linear transformation directly as follows (Fig. 4.3).

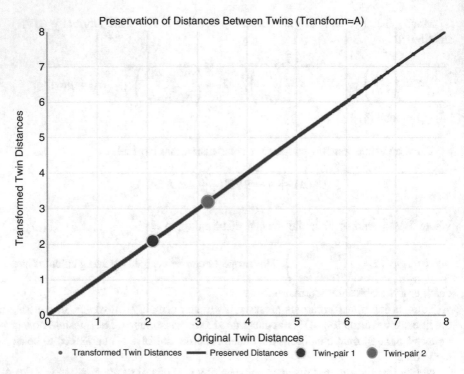

Fig. 4.3 Example of an isometry transformation, $A = \frac{1}{\sqrt{2}} \begin{pmatrix} 1 & 1 \\ 1 & -1 \end{pmatrix} : \mathbb{R}^2 \to \mathbb{R}^2$

```r
A <- 1/sqrt(2)*matrix(c(1, 1, 1, -1), 2, 2);    z <- A%*%y
d <- dist(t(y));    d2 <- dist(t(z))
plot_ly() %>%
  add_markers(x = ~as.numeric(d)[1:5000], y = ~as.numeric(d2)[1:5000],
       name="Transformed Twin Distances") %>%
  add_trace(x = ~c(0,8), y = ~c(0,8), mode="lines",
       line = list(color = "red", width=4), name="Preserved Distances") %>%
  add_markers(x = ~as.numeric(d)[1], y = ~as.numeric(d2)[1],
       marker=list(color='red',size=20, line=list(color='yellow', width=2)),
       name="Twin-pair 1") %>%
  add_markers(x = ~as.numeric(d)[2], y = ~as.numeric(d2)[2],
       marker=list(color = 'green', size = 20,
       line = list(color = 'orange', width = 2)), name="Twin-pair 2") %>%
  layout(title='Preservation of Distances Between Twins (Transform=A)',
       xaxis = list(title="Original Twin Distances", range = c(0, 8)),
       yaxis = list(title="Transformed Twin Distances", range = c(0, 8)),
       legend = list(orientation = 'h'))
```

We can observe that the distances between all twin-pair points computed from original data (x-axis) and the transformed data (y-axis) are identical. Thus, the transformation A is a rotation (isometry) of y. An alternative method is to simulate from the joint distribution of $Z = (Z_1, Z_2)^T$. As we have mentioned above, $Z = AY + \eta \sim \text{BVN}(\eta + A\mu, A\Sigma A^T)$, where

$$\eta = (0, 0)^T, \quad \Sigma = \begin{pmatrix} 1 & 0.95 \\ 0.95 & 1 \end{pmatrix}, \quad A = \frac{1}{\sqrt{2}} \begin{pmatrix} 1 & 1 \\ 1 & -1 \end{pmatrix}.$$

We can compute $A\Sigma A^T$ by hand or by using matrix multiplication in R:

```
sig <- matrix(c(1,0.95,0.95,1), nrow=2)
A%*%sig%*%t(A)
##        [,1] [,2]
## [1,] 1.95 0.00
## [2,] 0.00 0.05
```

The matrix $A\Sigma A^T$ represents the variance–covariance matrix, $\mathrm{cov}(z_1, z_2)$. We can simulate z_1, z_2 independently from $z_1 \sim N(0, 1.95)$ and $z_2 \sim N(0, 0.05)$. Note that *independence* and *uncorrelation* are equivalent for bivariate normal distribution, but not in general (Fig. 4.4).

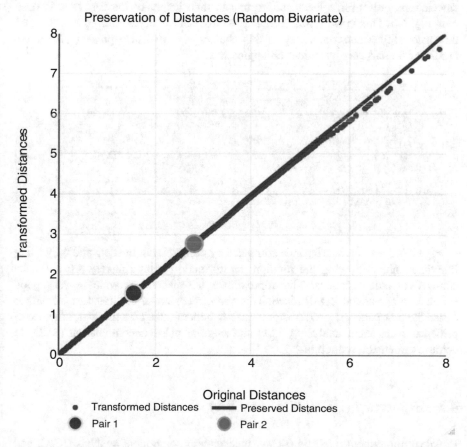

Fig. 4.4 Q–Q plot contrasting pairwise distances between points generated by pairs of independent Normal samples and pairs of Bivariate Normal random samples

To summarize, by plotting the raw and transformed distances and computing the pre- and post-transform distances between pairs of twins, we showed that the rotation transform is a mapping $A = \frac{1}{\sqrt{2}} \begin{pmatrix} 1 & 1 \\ 1 & -1 \end{pmatrix} : y \to z \equiv Ay$, while preserving the twin-pair distances. We applied this transformation and observed that the *distances between points were unchanged by the rotation A*. This rotation achieves the goals of

- Preserving the distances between points and
- Reducing the dimensionality of the data (see the plot on Fig. 4.5 illustrating the effects of reducing twin-pairs data from 2D to 1D)

To perform dimensionality reduction, we are now interested in *removing the second dimension* of the transformed data and recomputing the distances only using the first coordinate. In other words, in this simple 2D→1D simplification, we first use a linear transformation of the original twin pair heights, and then all subsequent calculations only utilize the resulting transformed height of the first twin in each pair, Fig. 4.5. This information compression from 2D to 1D is referred to as (linear) dimensionality reduction. Later in this chapter, we will also present alternative nonlinear dimensionality reduction approaches.

```
d4 = dist(z[1, ]) ### distance computed using just first dimension!!!
# take a smaller sample size to expedite the plotting
ind <-  sample(1:length(d4), 10000, replace = FALSE)
x1 <- d[ind]
y1 <- d4[ind]
plot_ly() %>%
  add_markers(x = ~x1, y = ~y1, name="Transformed Distances") %>%
  add_trace(x = ~c(0,8), y = ~c(0,8), mode="lines",
       line = list(color = "red", width = 4), name="Preserved Distances") %>%
  layout(title='Approximate Twin-Pair Distance Preservation in 1D',
       xaxis = list(title="(2D) Original Distances", range = c(0, 8)),
       yaxis = list(title="(1D) Rotation Matrix (A) Transformed Distances",
       range = c(0, 8)), legend = list(orientation = 'h'))
```

Figure 4.5 shows that distance computed by compressing the data and only using one dimension following the rotation transformation approximately preserves the actual twin pair distances. The approximate 1D distance provides a very good estimate of the actual 2D distance. This first dimension of the transformed data is called the first `principal component`. In general, this idea motivates the use of principal component analysis (PCA) and singular value decomposition (SVD) to achieve dimension reduction.

4.3   Summary (PCA, ICA, and FA)

Principal component analysis (PCA), independent component analysis (ICA), and factor analysis (FA) are similar linear strategies, seeking to identify a new basis (vectors representing the principal directions) that the data can be projected onto

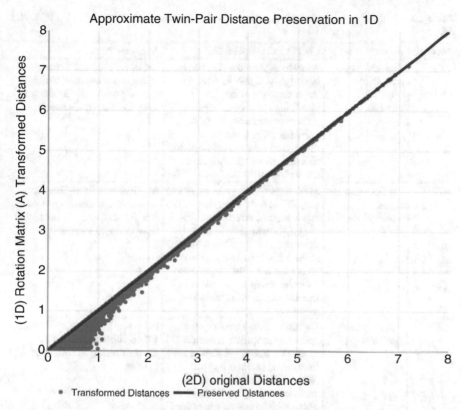

Fig. 4.5 Example of dimensionality reduction. Comparing the original 2D twin-pair distances (*x*-axis) against 1D distances (*y*-axis) computed using only using the first coordinate of the output of an isometry transformation of the original data, $A = \frac{1}{\sqrt{2}} \begin{pmatrix} 1 & 1 \\ 1 & -1 \end{pmatrix} : \mathbb{R}^2 \to \mathbb{R}^2$

maximizing certain (specific to each technique) objective function, Table 4.2. These basis functions, or vectors, are just linear combinations of the original features in the data.

The singular value decomposition (SVD) is a related approach that will be discussed later in this chapter. SVD provides a specific matrix factorization algorithm that can be employed in various techniques to decompose a data matrix $X_{m \times n}$ as $U\Sigma V^T$. The factors in this product include

- U, an $m \times m$ real or complex unitary matrix, i.e., isometry, $U^T U = U U^T = I$ with $|\det(U)| = 1$,
- Σ, an $m \times n$ rectangular diagonal matrix of *singular values*, representing non-negative values on the diagonal, and
- V is an $n \times n$ unitary matrix.

Table 4.2 Contrasting the assumptions, objective functions, and applications of PCA, ICA, and FA

Method	Assumptions	Cost function optimization	Applications
PCA	Gaussian signals, linear bivariate relations	Aims to explain the variance in the original signal. Minimizes the covariance of the data and yields high-energy orthogonal vectors in terms of the signal variance. PCA looks for an orthogonal linear transformation that maximizes the variance of the variables.	Relies on 1st and 2nd moments of the measured data, which makes it useful when data features are close to Gaussian
ICA	No Gaussian signal assumptions	Minimizes higher-order statistics (e.g., 3rd and 4th order skewness and kurtosis), effectively minimizing the *mutual information* of the transformed output. ICA seeks a linear transformation where the basis vectors are statistically independent, but neither Gaussian, orthogonal, nor ranked in order.	Applicable for non-Gaussian, very noisy, or mixture processes composed of simultaneous input from multiple sources
FA	Approximately Gaussian data	Objective function relies on second order moments to compute likelihood ratios. FA *factors* are linear combinations that maximize the shared portion of the variance underlying *latent variables*, which may use a variety of optimization strategies (e.g., maximum likelihood).	PCA-generalization used to test a theoretical model of latent factors causing the observed features

4.4   Principal Component Analysis (PCA)

Principal component analysis (PCA) is a mathematical tehnique that transforms a number of possibly correlated variables into a smaller number of uncorrelated variables through a process known as orthogonal transformation.

4.4.1   Principal Components

Let's consider the simplest situation where we have n observations $\{p_1, p_2, \cdots, p_n\}$ with 2 features $p_i = (x_i, y_i)$. When we plot the data, we use the x-axis and the y-axis for placing each of the corresponding feature values. However, we can also make a new coordinate system using the principal component vectors (Fig. 4.6).

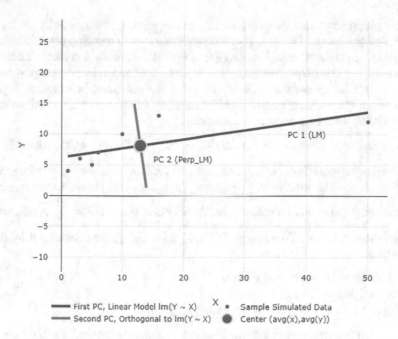

Fig. 4.6 2D scatter plot of simulated data with the corresponding two principal directions

```
ex <- data.frame(x=c(1, 3, 5, 6, 10, 16, 50), y=c(4, 6, 5, 7, 10, 13, 12))
yLM <- lm(y ~ x, data=ex)
perpSlope = - 1/(yLM$coefficients[2]) # slope of perpendicular line
newX <- data.frame(x = mean(ex$x))
newY <- predict.lm(yLM,newX)
point0 <- c(x=newX, y=newY) # (x,y) coordinates of point0 on LM line
point1 <- c(x=newX[1]-1, y=newY-perpSlope) # (x,y) coordinates of point1 on
perpendicular line
point2 <- c(x=newX[1]+1, y=newY+perpSlope) # (x,y) coordinates of point2 on
perpendicular line
modelLabels <- c('PC 1 (LM)', 'PC 2 (Perp_LM)')
modelLabels.x <- c(40, 20)
modelLabels.y <- c(10, 6)
modelLabels.color <- c("blue", "green")
plot_ly(ex) %>%
  add_lines(x = ~x, y = ~yLM$fitted, name="First PC, Linear Model lm(Y ~ X)",
            line = list(width = 4)) %>%
  add_markers(x = ~x, y = ~y, name="Sample Simulated Data") %>%
  add_lines(x = ~c(point1$x,point2$x), y = ~c(point1$y,point2$y),
            name="Second PC, Orthogonal to lm(Y ~ X)", line = list(width=4)) %>%
  add_markers(x = ~newX[1]$x, y = ~newY, name="Center (avg(x),avg(y))",
              marker = list(size = 20, color = 'green',
              line = list(color = 'yellow', width = 2))) %>%
layout(xaxis=list(title="X",scaleanchor="y"), #control the y:x aspect ratio
       yaxis = list(title="Y", scaleanchor  = "x"),
       legend = list(orientation = 'h'),
       annotations=list(text=modelLabels, x=modelLabels.x, y=modelLabels.y,
                        color = modelLabels.color, showarrow=FALSE ))
```

This graph illustrates the first PC, pc_1, as a minimum distance fit in the feature space, and the second PC, pc_2, as a minimum distance fit to a line perpendicular to the first PC. In higher dimensions, the third PC would similarly represent a minimum distance fit to a line perpendicular to the 2D plane determined by pc_1 and pc_2, and so forth. In our 2D space, two PCs are the most we can have; however, in higher-dimensional spaces, we need to consider how many PCs to estimate and utilize in the lower-dimensional data compression process.

In general, the formula for the first PC is $pc_1 = a_1^T X = \sum_{i=1}^{N} a_{i,1} X_i$, where X_i is a $n \times 1$ vector representing a column of the matrix X (having a total of n observations and N features). The weights $a_1 = \{a_{1,1}, a_{2,1}, \cdots, a_{N,1}\}$ are chosen to maximize the variance of pc_1. By this inductive rule, the kth PC is $pc_k = a_k^T X = \sum_{i=1}^{N} a_{i,k} X_i$, where the weight vectors (loadings) $a_k = \{a_{1,k}, a_{2,k}, \ldots, a_{N,k}\}$ are constrained by these conditions:

1. The variance of pc_k is maximized.
2. $\text{Cov}(pc_k, pc_l) = 0, \forall 1 \leq l < k$.
3. $a_k^T a_k = 1$ (the weight vectors are unitary).

Let's demonstrate how to find the loadings a_1 along the first PC. First, we need to express the variance of our first principal component using the variance covariance matrix of X

$$\text{Var}(pc_1) = E\left(pc_1^2\right) - \left(E(pc_1)\right)^2$$

$$= \sum_{i,j=1}^{N} a_{i,1} a_{j,1} E\left(x_i x_j\right) - \sum_{i,j=1}^{N} a_{i,1} a_{j,1} E(x_i) E(x_j) = \sum_{i,j=1}^{N} a_{i,1} a_{j,1} S_{i,j},$$

where $S_{i,j} = E(x_i x_j) - E(x_i) E(x_j)$.

This implies that $\text{Var}(pc_1) = a_1^T S a_1$, where $S = S_{i,j}$ is the covariance matrix of $X = \{X_1, \ldots, X_N\}$. Since a_1 maximizes $\text{Var}(pc_1)$ and the normalization constraint requires $a_1^T a_1 = 1$, we can rewrite a_1 as

$$a_1 = \max{}_{a_1} \left(a_1^T S a_1 - \lambda \left(a_1^T a_1 - 1\right)\right).$$

To maximize this quadratic function, we can take the derivative of this expression with respect to a_1 and set it to 0, which yields $(S - \lambda I_N) a_1 = 0$.

In Chap. 3, we showed that a_1 will correspond to the largest eigenvalue of S, the variance covariance matrix of X. Hence, pc_1 retains the largest amount of variation in the sample. Having the first PC, mathematical induction facilitates the derivation of

a_k, corresponding to the kth largest eigenvalue of S, $\forall k \geq 1$. In practice, PCA requires the mean for each column in the data matrix to be zero. That is, the sample mean of each column is shifted to zero. Let's use a subset ($N = 33$) of the Parkinson's Progression Markers Initiative (PPMI) data to manually demonstrate the relationship between S and PC loadings. First, we need to import the dataset into R and remove the patient ID column.

```
library(rvest)
wiki_url <- read_html("https://wiki.socr.umich.edu/index.php/SMHS_PCA_ICA_FA")
html_nodes(wiki_url, "#content")
summary(pd.sub)
pd.sub <- pd.sub[, -1]
```

Then, we need to center the pdsub by subtracting the average of all column means from each element in the column. Next, we cast pd.sub as a matrix and compute its variance covariance matrix, S. Finally, we can calculate the corresponding eigenvalues and eigenvectors of S.

```
mu <- apply(pd.sub, 2, mean)
mean(mu)      ## [1] 4.379068
pd.center <- as.matrix(pd.sub)-mean(mu)
S <- cov(pd.center)
eigen(S)
## eigen() decomposition
## $values
## [1] 1.315073e+02 1.178340e+01 6.096920e+00 1.424351e+00 6.094592e-02 8.035403e 03
## $vectors
##                [,1]          [,2]          [,3]         [,4]         [,5]          [,6]
## [1,] -0.007460885 -0.0182022093  0.016893318  0.02071859  0.97198980 -0.232667561
## [2,] -0.005800877  0.0006155246  0.004186177  0.01552971  0.23234862  0.972482080
## [3,]  0.080830361  0.0000389904 -0.027351225  0.99421646 -0.02352324 -0.009618592
## [4,]  0.229718933 -0.2817718053 -0.929463536 -0.06088782  0.01466136  0.003019008
## [5,]  0.282109618 -0.8926329596  0.344508308 -0.06772403 -0.01764367  0.006061772
## [6,]  0.927911126  0.3462292153  0.127908417 -0.05068855  0.01305167  0.002456374
```

The next step would be to calculate the PCs using the prcomp() function in R. Note that we will use the raw (uncentered) version of the data and have to specify the center=TRUE option to ensure the column means are trivial. We can save the model information into pca1 where pca1$rotation provides the loadings for each PC.

```
pca1 <- prcomp(as.matrix(pd.sub), center = T)
summary(pca1)
## Importance of components:
##                               PC1      PC2      PC3      PC4      PC5      PC6
## Standard deviation        11.4677   3.4327  2.46919  1.19346  0.2469  0.08964
## Proportion of Variance     0.8716   0.0781  0.04041  0.00944  0.0004  0.00005
## Cumulative Proportion      0.8716   0.9497  0.99010  0.99954  1.0000  1.00000
pca1$rotation
##                                              PC1           PC2           PC3
## Top_of_SN_Voxel_Intensity_Ratio      0.007460885  -0.0182022093   0.016893318
## Side_of_SN_Voxel_Intensity_Ratio     0.005800877   0.0006155246   0.004186177
## Part_IA                             -0.080839361  -0.0600389904  -0.027351225
## Part_IB                             -0.229718933  -0.2817718053  -0.929463536
## Part_II                             -0.282109618  -0.8926329596   0.344508308
## Part_III                            -0.927911126   0.3462292153   0.127908417
##                                              PC4           PC5           PC6
## Top_of_SN_Voxel_Intensity_Ratio      0.02071859  -0.97198980  -0.232667561
## Side_of_SN_Voxel_Intensity_Ratio     0.01552971  -0.23234862   0.972482080
## Part_IA                              0.99421646   0.02352324  -0.009618592
## Part_IB                             -0.06088782  -0.01466136   0.003019008
## Part_II                             -0.06772403   0.01764367   0.006061772
## Part_III                            -0.05068855  -0.01305167   0.002456374
```

We notice that the reported loadings are just the eigenvectors multiplied by -1. These loadings represent vectors in 6D space (we have 6 columns in the original data). The scale factor -1 just represents the opposite direction of the eigenvector. Alternatively, we can use the factoextra package to directly compute the eigenvalues corresponding to each PC.

```
# install.packages("factoextra")
library("factoextra")
eigen <- get_eigenvalue(pca1)
eigen
##           eigenvalue variance.percent cumulative.variance.percent
## Dim.1 1.315073e+02      87.159638589                    87.15964
## Dim.2 1.178340e+01       7.809737384                    94.96938
## Dim.3 6.096920e+00       4.040881920                    99.01026
## Dim.4 1.424351e+00       0.944023059                    99.95428
## Dim.5 6.094592e-02       0.040393390                    99.99467
## Dim.6 8.035403e-03       0.005325659                   100.00000
```

The eigenvalues of the S matrix correspond to the amount of the variation explained by each principal component (PC). We also reported information about the *variance* explained by each PC, relative to the corresponding PC loadings. The scree-plot has a clear "elbow" point at the second PC, suggesting that the first two PCs explain about 95% of the variation in the original dataset. Hence, we can effectively compress the original data into the first two PCs. In this case, the dimension of the data is substantially reduced (Fig. 4.7).

```
plot_ly(x = c(1:length(pca1$sdev)), y = pca1$sdev*pca1$sdev,
          name = "Scree", type = "bar") %>%
   layout(title="Scree Plot", xaxis = list(title="PC's"),
          yaxis = list(title="Variances (SD^2)"))
```

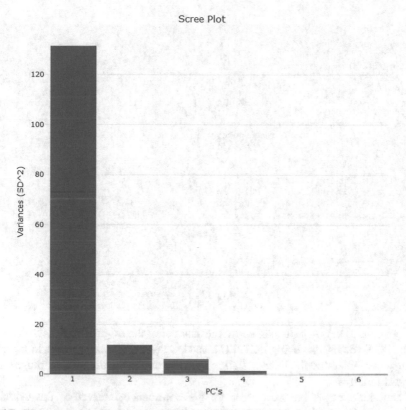

Fig. 4.7 PCA scree plot showing the rapid decay of the eigenvalue magnitudes

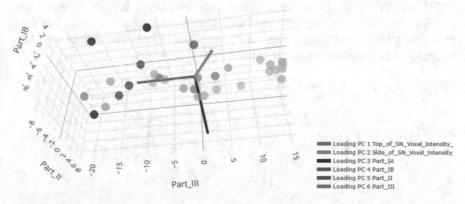

Fig. 4.8 3D projection of the 6D data along with the first three PCs

In the 3D loadings interactive plot below, you need to zoom-in to see the smaller projections (original features that have lower impact after the linear PC rotation) (Fig. 4.8).

```
# Scores
scores <- pca1$x
# Loadings
loadings <- pca1$rotation
# Visualization scale factor for loadings
scaleLoad <- 10
p <- plot_ly() %>%
  add_trace(x=scores[,1], y=scores[,2], z=scores[,3], type="scatter3d",
            mode="markers", name="",
            marker = list(color=scores[,2], colorscale = c("#FFE1A1",
            "#683531"), opacity = 0.7))
for (k in 1:ncol(loadings)) {
  # Project PCAs only on the last 3 original data dimensions (6,5,4)
  x <- c(0, loadings[6, k])*scaleLoad
  y <- c(0, loadings[5, k])*scaleLoad
  z <- c(0, loadings[4, k])*scaleLoad
  p <- p %>% add_trace(x=x, y=y, z=z, type="scatter3d", mode="lines",
                  name=paste0("Loading PC ", k, " ", colnames(pd.sub)[k]),
                  line=list(width=8), opacity=1)
}
p <- p %>% layout(legend = list(orientation = 'h'),
                  title="3D Projection of 6D Data along First 3 PCs",
                  scene = list( xaxis = list(title = rownames(loadings)[6]),
                      yaxis = list(title = rownames(loadings)[5]),
                      zaxis = list(title = rownames(loadings)[4]))); p
```

Dynamic 3D PCA plots can show the data using the original base (raw features) or the PCA vector base using PC1, PC2, and PC3 as the coordinate axes to represent the new variables and the lines radiating from the origin showing the loadings on the original features.

Next, let's run a bootstrap test for the confidence interval of the explained variance. This experiment confirms that the 95% confidence interval for the cumulative variance explained by the first three principal components is [0.8716, 0.9497, 0.99]. Note that this bootstrap confidence interval is lower than the 99% cumulative variance estimated earlier using all cases and only the first three PCs. This slightly lower aggregate variance estimate reflects the random stochastic sampling of cases (rows) from the entire dataset (Fig. 4.9).

```
set.seed(12)
num_boot = 1000
bootstrap_it = function(i) {  # define a bootstrap iteration function
  data_resample = pd.sub[sample(1:nrow(pd.sub), nrow(pd.sub), replace=TRUE),]
  p_resample = princomp(data_resample, cor = T)
  return(sum(p_resample$sdev[1:3]^2)/sum(p_resample$sdev^2))
}
pco = data.frame(per=sapply(1:num_boot, bootstrap_it))
quantile(pco$per, probs = c(0.025,0.975))  # specify 95% Confidence Interval
##      2.5%      97.5%
## 0.8124611 0.8985318
corpp = sum(pca1$sdev[1:3]^2)/sum(pca1$sdev^2)
plot_ly(x = pco$per, type = "histogram", name = "Data Histogram") %>%
    layout(title='Histogram of a Bootstrap Simulation <br />
                    Percent of Data Variability Captured by first 3 PCs',
            xaxis = list(title = "Percent of Variability"),
            yaxis = list(title = "Frequency Count"), bargap=0.1)
```

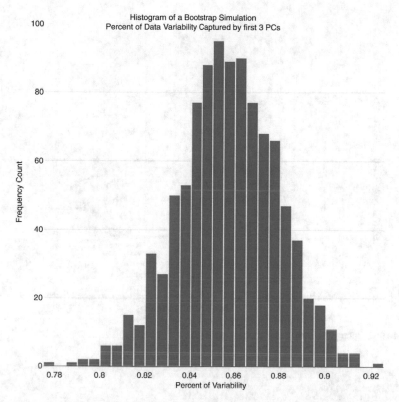

Fig. 4.9 Histogram of a bootstrap simulation indicating the empirical proportion of data variability accounted for by first three principal components alone

Suppose   we   want   to   fit   a   linear   model   to   predict
`Top_of_SN_Voxel_Intensity_Ratio`

$$\mathrm{Top}_{\{\text{SN Voxel (Intensity Ratio)}\}} \sim \mathrm{Side}_{\{\text{SN Voxel (Intensity Ratio)}\}} + \mathrm{Part}_{\mathrm{IA}}.$$

We can use `plot_ly()` to show a reduced 3D data scatterplot along with the (univariate) linear model (Fig. 4.10).

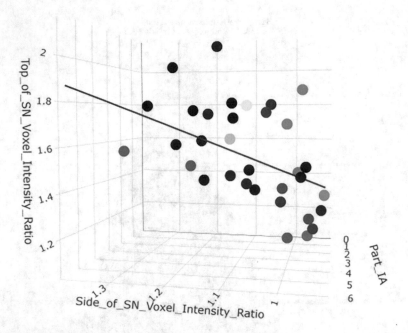

Fig. 4.10   Scatter plot with linear model (red line)

```
library(scatterplot3d)
#Fit linear model
lm.fit <- lm(Top_of_SN_Voxel_Intensity_Ratio ~
             Side_of_SN_Voxel_Intensity_Ratio + Part_IA, data = pd.sub)
# Get the ranges of the variable.names
summary(pd.sub$Side_of_SN_Voxel_Intensity_Ratio)
summary(pd.sub$Part_IA)
summary(pd.sub$Top_of_SN_Voxel_Intensity_Ratio)
# Get the model coefficients and define the model (x,y,z) grid values
cf = lm.fit$coefficients
pltx = seq(summary(pd.sub$Side_of_SN_Voxel_Intensity_Ratio)[1],
           summary(pd.sub$Side_of_SN_Voxel_Intensity_Ratio)[6],
           length.out = length(pd.sub$Side_of_SN_Voxel_Intensity_Ratio))
plty = seq(summary(pd.sub$Part_IA)[1], summary(pd.sub$Part_IA)[6],
           length.out = length(pd.sub$Part_IA))
pltz = cf[1] + cf[2]*pltx + cf[3]*plty
# Scatter Plot with the LM (sline)
plot_ly() %>%
  add_trace(x = ~pltx, y = ~plty, z = ~pltz, type="scatter3d", mode="lines",
        line = list(color = "red", width = 4),
        name="lm(Top_of_SN_Voxel_Intensity_Ratio ~
                 Side_of_SN_Voxel_Intensity_Ratio + Part_IA)") %>%
  add_markers(x = ~pd.sub$Side_of_SN_Voxel_Intensity_Ratio,
        y = ~pd.sub$Part_IA, z=~pd.sub$Top_of_SN_Voxel_Intensity_Ratio,
        color = ~pd.sub$Part_II, mode="markers") %>%
  layout(title="lm(Top_of_SN_Voxel_Intensity_Ratio ~
                 Side_of_SN_Voxel_Intensity_Ratio + Part_IA)",
    legend=list(orientation = 'h'), showlegend = F,
    scene = list(xaxis = list(title = 'Side_of_SN_Voxel_Intensity_Ratio'),
                 yaxis = list(title = 'Part_IA'),
                 zaxis = list(title='Top_of_SN_Voxel_Intensity_Ratio'))) %>%
  hide_colorbar()
```

$$\text{Top}_{\{\text{SN Voxel (Intensity Ratio)}\}} \sim \text{Side}_{\{\text{SN Voxel (Intensity Ratio)}\}} + \text{Part}_{\text{IA}}.$$

We can also plot in 3D a couple of different bivariate 2D plane models (e.g., based on PCA or lm.fit) of the trivariate relation between Top_of_SN_Voxel_Intensity_Ratio, Side_of_SN_Voxel_Intensity_Ratio, and Part_IA. Using plot_ly for interactive 3D visualizations, we first demonstrate displaying the lm() derived plane model and then show the PCA-derived planar model. Both models are superimposed on the 3D scatter plot of pd.sub$Side_of_SN_Voxel_Intensity_Ratio, pd.sub$Top_of_SN_Voxel_Intensity_Ratio, and pd.sub$Part_IA (Fig. 4.11).

```r
# 1. Using Linear Model.   Define the 3D features
x <- pd.sub$Side_of_SN_Voxel_Intensity_Ratio
y <- pd.sub$Top_of_SN_Voxel_Intensity_Ratio
z <- pd.sub$Part_IA
myDF <- data.frame(x, y, z)
### Fit a (bivariate-predictor) linear regression model
lm.fit <- lm(z ~ x+y)
coef.lm.fit <- coef(lm.fit)
### Reparameterize the 2D (x,y) grid, and define the corresponding model values z
on the grid
x.seq <- seq(min(x),max(x), length.out=100)
y.seq <- seq(min(y),max(y), length.out=100)
z.seq <- function(x,y) coef.lm.fit[1] + coef.lm.fit[2]*x + coef.lm.fit[3]*y
# define the values of z = z(x.seq, y.seq), as a Matrix of dimension
c(dim(x.seq), dim(y.seq))
z <- t(outer(x.seq, y.seq, z.seq))
# Setup Axes
axis_x <- seq(min(x), max(x), length.out=100)
axis_y <- seq(min(y), max(y), length.out=100)
#Sample points
library(reshape2)
lm_surface    <- expand.grid(x = axis_x, y = axis_y, KEEP.OUT.ATTRS = F)
lm_surface$z <- predict.lm(lm.fit, newdata = lm_surface)
lm_surface    <- acast(lm_surface, x ~ y, value.var = "z") # z ~ 0 + x + y
plot_ly(myDF, x = ~x, y = ~y, z = ~z,
         text = paste0("Part_II: ", pd.sub$Part_II), type="scatter3d",
         mode="markers", color=pd.sub$Part_II) %>%
  add_trace(x=~axis_x, y=~axis_y, z=~lm_surface, type="surface",
         color="gray", name="LM model", opacity=0.3) %>%
  layout(title="3D Plane Regression (Part_IA ~ Side_of_SN_Voxel +
         Top_of_SN_Voxel); Color=Part II", showlegend = F,
         scene = list(xaxis=list(title = "Side_of_SN_Voxel_Intensity_Ratio"),
                      yaxis=list(title = "Top_of_SN_Voxel_Intensity_Ratio"),
                      zaxis = list(title = "Part_IA"))) %>% hide_colorbar()
# 2. PCA Model.  Define the original 3D coordinates
x <- pd.sub$Side_of_SN_Voxel_Intensity_Ratio
y <- pd.sub$Top_of_SN_Voxel_Intensity_Ratio
z <- pd.sub$Part_IA
myDF <- data.frame(x, y, z)
### Fit (compute) the 2D PCA space (dimensionality reduction)
pca1 <- prcomp(as.matrix(cbind(pd.sub$Side_of_SN_Voxel_Intensity_Ratio,
pd.sub$Top_of_SN_Voxel_Intensity_Ratio, pd.sub$Part_IA)), center = T);
summary(pca1)
```

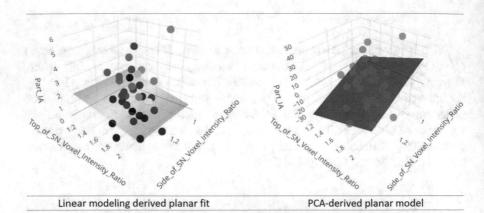

| Linear modeling derived planar fit | PCA-derived planar model |

Fig. 4.11 Alternative bivariate plane models superimposed on the 3D data scatter plot

```
## Importance of components:
##                       PC1     PC2     PC3
## Standard deviation    1.5218 0.27556 0.09958
## Proportion of Variance 0.9643 0.03162 0.00413
## Cumulative Proportion  0.9643 0.99587 1.00000
# Compute the Normal to the 2D PC plane
normVec = c(pca1$rotation[2,1]*pca1$rotation[3,2]-
            pca1$rotation[3,1]*pca1$rotation[2,2],
          pca1$rotation[3,1]*pca1$rotation[1,2]-
            pca1$rotation[1,1]*pca1$rotation[3,2],
          pca1$rotation[1,1]*pca1$rotation[2,2]-
            pca1$rotation[2,1]*pca1$rotation[1,2])
# Compute the 3D point of gravitational balance (Plane has to go through it)
dMean <- apply( cbind(pd.sub$Side_of_SN_Voxel_Intensity_Ratio,
pd.sub$Top_of_SN_Voxel_Intensity_Ratio, pd.sub$Part_IA), 2, mean)
d <- as.numeric((-1)*normVec %*% dMean)  # constrain model plane through mean
# Reparameterize the 2D (x,y) grid, and define the corresponding model
# values z on the grid. Recall z=-(d + ax+by)/c, where normVec=(a,b,c)
x.seq <- seq(min(x),max(x),length.out=100)
y.seq <- seq(min(y),max(y),length.out=100)
z.seq <- function(x,y) -(d + normVec[1]*x + normVec[2]*y)/normVec[3]
# define the values of z = z(x.seq, y.seq), as a Matrix of dimension
c(dim(x.seq), dim(y.seq))
# z <- t(outer(x.seq, y.seq, z.seq))/10; range(z)
z <- t(outer(x.seq, y.seq, z.seq)); range(z)  ## [1] -31.19195  29.19934
# Draw the 2D plane embedded in 3D, and then add points with "add_trace"
plot_ly(x=~x.seq, y=~y.seq, z=~z,
    colors = c("blue", "red"),type="surface", opacity=0.7) %>%
    add_trace(data=myDF,x=x, y=y, z=(pd.sub$Part_IA-mean(pd.sub$Part_IA))*10,
        mode="markers", showlegend=F, type="scatter3d",
        marker=list(color="green", opacity=0.9, symbol=105)) %>%
    layout(scene = list(aspectmode = "manual", aspectratio=list(x=1,y=1,z=1),
        xaxis = list(title = "Side_of_SN_Voxel_Intensity_Ratio"),
        yaxis = list(title = "Top_of_SN_Voxel_Intensity_Ratio"),
        zaxis = list(title = "Part_IA")) ) %>% hide_colorbar()
```

As we saw earlier in the PCA vs. ICA vs. FA summary Table 4.1, classical PCA assumes that the bivariate relations are intrinsically linear. Nonlinear PCA is a generalization that allows us to incorporate nominal and ordinal variables, as well as to handle and identify nonlinear relationships between variables in the dataset. More details about nonparametric inference and nonlinear principal components analysis are provided in this chapter.[3] In essence, nonlinear PCA assigns values to categories representing the numeric variables, which maximize the association (e.g., correlation) between the quantified variables (i.e., optimal scaling to quantify the variables according to their analysis levels). The Bioconductor *pcaMethods* package provides the functionality for nonlinear PCA.[4]

4.5 Independent Component Analysis (ICA)

ICA aims to find basis vectors representing independent components of the original data. For example, this may be achieved by maximizing the norm of the 4th order normalized kurtosis, which iteratively projects the signal on a new basis vector, computes the objective function (e.g., the norm of the kurtosis) of the result, slightly adjusts the basis vector (e.g., by gradient ascent), and recomputes the kurtosis again. At the end, this iterative optimization process generates a basis vector corresponding to the highest (residual) kurtosis representing the next independent component.

The process of independent component analysis is to maximize the statistical independence of the estimated components. Assume that each variable X_i is generated by a sum of n independent components

$$X_i = a_{i,1}s_1 + \cdots + a_{i,n}s_n.$$

Here, X_i is generated by $s_1, \cdots, s_n$ using the corresponding weights $a_{i,\,1}, \cdots a_{i,\,n}$. Finally, we can rewrite X in matrix format $X = As$, where $X = (X_1, \cdots, X_n)^T$, $A = (a_1, \cdots, a_n)^T$, $a_i = (a_{i,\,1}, \cdots, a_{i,\,n})$ and $s = (s_1, \cdots, s_n)^T$. Note that s is obtained by maximizing the independence of the components. This procedure is done by maximizing a relevant objective function. ICA does not assume that all of its components (s_i) are Gaussian and independent of each other. In the example below, we will create a correlated matrix X and utilize the fastICA() function in R to derive the ICA representation.

```
fastICA(X, n.comp, alg.typ, fun, rownorm, maxit, tol)
```

- **X**: data matrix
- **n.comp**: number of components
- **alg.type**: components extracted simultaneously(alg.typ == "parallel") or one at a time(alg.typ == "deflation")

---

[3] https://doi.org/10.1037/1082-989X.12.3.336
[4] https://doi.org/10.18129/B9.bioc.pcaMethods

- **fun**: functional form of F to approximate to neg-entropy
- **rownorm**: whether rows of the data matrix X should be standardized beforehand
- **maxit**: maximum number of iterations
- **tol**: a positive scalar giving the tolerance at which the un-mixing matrix is considered to have converged.

```
S <- matrix(runif(10000), 5000, 2)
S[1:10, ]
##              [,1]       [,2]
##  [1,] 0.3160720 0.30788753
…
## [10,] 0.1673277 0.47129195
A <- matrix(c(1, 1, -1, 3), 2, 2, byrow = TRUE)
X <- S %*% A  # In R, "*" & "%*%" indicate "scalar" & matrix multiplication
cor(X)
##              [,1]       [,2]
## [1,]  1.0000000 -0.4512668
## [2,] -0.4512668  1.0000000
```

Before we fit the ICA model, note that the correlation between two variables is − 0.45.

```
# install.packages("fastICA")
library(fastICA)
a <- fastICA(X, 2, alg.typ = "parallel", fun = "logcosh", alpha = 1,
             method = "C", row.norm = FALSE, maxit = 200, tol = 0.0001)
```

To visualize the correlation of the original preprocessed data (X) and the independence of the corresponding ICA components $S = \text{fastICA}(X)\$S$, we can draw the following composite scatter plot (Fig. 4.12).

```
plot_ly() %>%
  add_markers(x = a$X[ , 1], y =~a$X[ , 2], name="Pre-processed data",
              marker = list(color="green", opacity=0.9, symbol=105)) %>%
  add_markers(x = a$S[ , 1], y = a$S[ , 2], name="ICA components",
              marker = list(color="blue", opacity=0.99, symbol=5))  %>%
  layout(title='Scatter Plots of the Original (Pre-processed) Data and
                the corresponding ICA Transform',
         xaxis = list(title="Twin 1 (standardized height)", scaleanchor="y"),
         yaxis = list(title="Twin 2 (standardized height)", scaleanchor="x"),
         legend = list(orientation - 'h'))
```

Finally, we can confirm that the correlation of two ICA components is nearly 0.

```
cor(a$S)
## [,1] [,2]
## [1,] 1.00000e+00 2.05627e-15
## [2,] 2.05627e-15 1.00000e+00
```

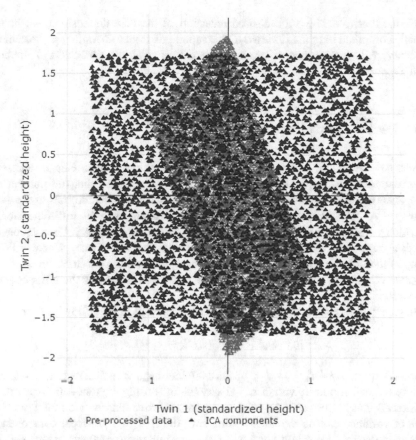

Fig. 4.12 Scatter plots of the original (simulated) data in green and the corresponding ICA transformed data in blue color

Let's look at a more interesting example, based on the pd.sub dataset, which includes six variables whose paired correlations are relatively high. After fitting the ICA model, the first two components are nearly independent.

```
cor(pd.sub)
a1 <- fastICA(pd.sub, n.comp=2, alg.typ="parallel", fun="logcosh", alpha=1,
               method = "C", row.norm = FALSE, maxit = 200, tol = 0.0001)
par(mfrow = c(1, 2))
cor(a1$X)
##             [,1]        [,2]        [,3]        [,4]        [,5]        [,6]
## [1,]  1.00000000  0.5474722 -0.1014419 -0.2696630 -0.04358545 -0.3392179
## [2,]  0.54747225  1.0000000 -0.2157587 -0.4438992 -0.37663875 -0.5226128
## [3,] -0.10144191 -0.2157587  1.0000000  0.4913169  0.50378157  0.5845831
## [4,] -0.26966299 -0.4438992  0.4913169  1.0000000  0.57987562  0.6735584
## [5,] -0.04358545 -0.3766388  0.5037816  0.5798756  1.00000000  0.6390134
## [6,] -0.33921790 -0.5226128  0.5845831  0.6735584  0.63901337  1.0000000
cor(a1$S)
##              [,1]         [,2]
## [1,] 1.000000e+00 1.868184e-15
## [2,] 1.868184e-15 1.000000e+00
```

Notice that to achieve the desired reduction of the data dimensions, we intentionally computed only the first two ICA components from the original six variables. Of course, all six components can be computed by using the fastICA() method option *n.comp* = 6.

4.6   Factor Analysis (FA)

Similar to ICA and PCA, FA tries to find special principal components to represent the observed data. As a generalization of PCA, FA requires that the number of components is smaller than the original number of variables (or columns of the data matrix). FA optimization relies on iterative perturbations with full-dimensional Gaussian noise and maximum-likelihood estimation where every observation in the data represents a sample point in a higher-dimensional space. Whereas PCA assumes the noise is spherical, factor analysis allows the noise to have an arbitrary diagonal covariance matrix and estimates the subspace as well as the noise covariance matrix.

In factor analysis, the centered data can be expressed in the following form

$$x_i - \mu_i = l_{i,1}F_1 + \cdots + l_{i,k}F_k + \epsilon_i = LF + \epsilon_i,$$

where $i \in 1, \cdots, p, j \in 1, \cdots, k, k < p$, and ϵ_i are independently distributed error terms with zero mean and finite variance. Let's try FA in R using the function factanal (). Recall that in our previous PCA using the pd.sub dataset, we found out that 95% of variance can be explained using only the first two principal components. This suggests that we might need two factors in this factor analysis, which can be confirmed by examining the *scree* plot. This analysis yields the number of components (noc), the number of (acceleration) factors (naf) to retain in an exploratory factor analysis, the number of components using the Kaiser rule (nkaiser), and the number of factors based on parallel analysis (nparallel).

The Kaiser rule selects only the top components corresponding to eigenvalues over $\bar{\lambda} = 1$, the eigenvalue equal to the information accounted for by an average single item. Suppose λ_i is the ith eigenvalue and LS_i is a location statistic, such as the sample mean or a sample centile. Then, the Kaiser rule is computed as

$$n_{\{\text{Kaiser}\}} = \sum_i (\lambda_i \geq \bar{\lambda}),$$

where $\bar{\lambda} = 1$ when using a correlation matrix. The parallel analysis strategy estimates the number of components as $n_{\{\text{parallel}\}} = \sum_i (\lambda_i \geq LS_i)$. And the number of factors based on acceleration factors is estimated as a numerical solution determining the elbow on the scree plot by determining the location of the fastest change of the slope of the scree graph. At each eigenvalue index, position i, the acceleration factor is calculated as the slope change $a_i = (\lambda_{i+1} - \lambda_i) - (\lambda_i - \lambda_{i-1})$. This slope change expression only includes the eigenvalues as they are all consecutive and equally spaced one unit apart along the x-axis. Having the index $i_o = \arg\max_i a_i$ corresponding to the largest acceleration value of a, the number of factors is identified as $n_{\{AF\}} = i_0 - 1$. The optimal coordinates (OC) corresponds to an extrapolation of the preceding eigenvalue based on a linear regression model fitting the eigenvalue index and the last eigenvalue coordinates. The optimal coordinates estimation is based on fitting a series of linear models and determining whether observed eigenvalues exceed the model predicted values. The equation for the ith position connects the points at indices $i + 1$ and k, the total number of features (dimensions). If the observed eigenvalue at index i exceeds the extrapolated model predicted value, this corresponds to an increase that may be an elbow in the scree plot. Optimizing for the largest value of i such that the corresponding eigenvalue exceeds the model predicted value for that index, we can identify the elbow point and deduce the corresponding $n_{\{OC\}}$ number of factors (Fig. 4.13).

```
library(nFactors)
ev <- eigen(cor(pd.sub)) # get eigenvalues
ap <- parallel(subject=nrow(pd.sub), var=ncol(pd.sub), rep=100, cent=0.05)
nS <- nScree(x=ev$values, aparallel=ap$eigen$qevpea)
summary(nS)
plot_ly() %>%
  add_trace(y = nS$Analysis$Eigenvalues, type="scatter", name='Eigenvalues',
            mode='lines+markers',marker=list(opacity=0.99,size=20,symbol=5)) %>%
  add_trace(y = nS$Analysis$Par.Analysis, type="scatter",
            name = 'Parallel Analysis (centiles of random eigenvalues)',
            mode='lines+markers',marker=list(opacity=0.99,size=20,symbol=2)) %>%
  add_trace(y = nS$Analysis$Acc.factor, type="scatter",
            name = 'Acceleration Factor', mode = 'lines+markers',
            marker = list(opacity=0.99, size=20, symbol=15)) %>%
  layout(title='Scree plot', legend = list(orientation = 'h'),
         xaxis = list(title="Components)", scaleanchor = "y"),
         yaxis = list(title="Eigenvalues)", scaleanchor = "x"))
## Report For a nScree Class
## Details: components
##   Eigenvalues Prop Cumu Par.Analysis Pred.eig   OC Acc.factor      AF
## 1           3    1    1            1        1               NA (< AF)
## 2           1    0    1            1        1 (< OC)         1
## 3           1    0    1            1        0               1
## 4           0    0    1            1        0               0
## 5           0    0    1            0      NA                0
## 6           0    0    1            0      NA               NA
## Number of factors retained by index
##       noc naf nparallel nkaiser
## 1       2   1         2       2
```

Note that three out of four Cattell's Scree test rules in the summary suggest we should use two factors. Thus, we can specify the parameter `factors=2` in the call to the function `factanal()`. In addition, we can use `varimax` rotation of the factor axes maximizing the variance of the squared loadings of factors (columns) on the original variables (rows), which effectively differentiates the original variables by the extracted factors. Oblique `promax` and `Procrustes rotation` (projecting the loadings to a target matrix with a simple structure) are two alternative and commonly used matrix rotations that may be specified.

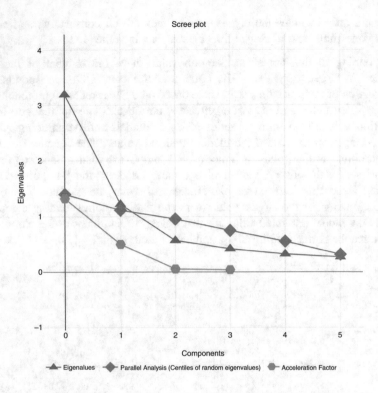

Fig. 4.13 Scree plots with alternative strategies for determining the optimal elbow point

```
fit <- factanal(pd.sub, factors=2, rotation="varimax")
fit
## Call:
## factanal(x = pd.sub, factors = 2, rotation = "varimax")
## Uniquenesses:
##  Top_of_SN_Voxel_Intensity_Ratio Side_of_SN_Voxel_Intensity_Ratio
##                            0.018                            0.534
##                          Part_IA                          Part_IB
##                            0.571                            0.410
##                          Part_II                         Part_III
##                            0.392                            0.218
## Loadings:
##                                  Factor1 Factor2
## Top_of_SN_Voxel_Intensity_Ratio          0.991
## Side_of_SN_Voxel_Intensity_Ratio -0.417   0.540
## Part_IA                           0.650
## Part_IB                           0.726  -0.251
## Part_II                           0.779
## Part_III                          0.825  -0.318
##                 Factor1 Factor2
## SS loadings       2.412   1.445
## Proportion Var    0.402   0.241
## Cumulative Var    0.402   0.643
## Test of the hypothesis that 2 factors are sufficient.
## The chi square statistic is 1.35 on 4 degrees of freedom.
## The p-value is 0.854
```

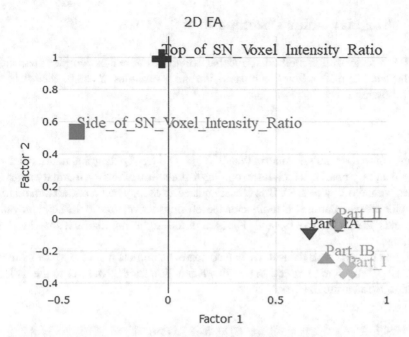

Fig. 4.14 FA plot projecting all features into the 2D plane spanned by *factor 1* (*x*-axis) and *factor 2* (*y*-axis)

Here, the relatively large p-value, 0.854, suggests that we failed to reject the null-hypothesis that two factors are sufficient for the FA model representation of these data. We can also visualize the loadings for all the variables onto the derived pair of factors (Fig. 4.14).

```
load <- fit$loadings
df <- as.data.frame(load[]);  Features <- rownames(df)
X <- df$Factor1; Y <- df$Factor2
df1 <- data.frame(Features, X, Y)
cols <- palette(rainbow(6))   # as.numeric(as.factor(Features))
cols <- cols[2:7] # this is necessary as cols has 8 rows (not 6, as does df1)
plot_ly(df1, x = ~X, y = ~Y, text = ~Features, color = cols) %>%
  add_markers(marker = list(opacity=0.99, size=20, color=cols,
              symbol=~as.numeric(as.factor(Features)))) %>%
  add_text(textfont = list(family= "Times", size= 20, color= cols),
           textposition="top right") %>%
  layout(title = '2D FA', xaxis = list(title = 'Factor 1',
         zeroline = TRUE,range = c(-0.5, 1)),
         yaxis = list(title = 'Factor 2'), showlegend = FALSE)
```

4.7   Singular Value Decomposition (SVD)

SVD is a factorization method applicable to matrices of real or complex elements. If we have a data matrix X with n observation and p variables, X can be factorized into the following form

$$X = UDV^T,$$

where U is a $n \times p$ unitary matrix that $U^TU = I$, D is a $p \times p$ diagonal matrix, and V^T is a $p \times p$ unitary matrix, which is the conjugate transpose of the $n \times n$ unitary matrix, V. Thus, we have $V^TV = I$. SVD is closely related to PCA when a correlation matrix is used for the calculations. U represents the left singular vectors, D the singular values, U yields the PCA scores, and V contains the right singular vectors, i.e., PCA loadings.

Using the pd.sub dataset, we can compare the outputs from the svd() function and the princomp() function (another R function for PCA). Prior to the SVD, we need to scale the data matrix.

```
# SVD output
df <- nrow(pd.sub)-1
zvars <- scale(pd.sub)
z.svd <- svd(zvars)
z.svd$d/sqrt(df)
## [1] 1.7878123 1.1053808 0.7550519 0.6475685 0.5688743 0.5184536
z.svd$v
##              [,1]        [,2]         [,3]         [,4]        [,5]         [,6]
## [1,]   0.2555204  0.71258155 -0.37323594  0.10487773 -0.4773992  0.22073161
## [2,]   0.3855208  0.47213743  0.35665523 -0.43312945  0.5581867  0.04564469
## [3,]  -0.3825033  0.37288211  0.70992668  0.31993403 -0.2379855 -0.22728693
## [4,]  -0.4597352  0.09803466 -0.11166513 -0.79389290 -0.2915570 -0.22647775
## [5,]  -0.4251107  0.34167997 -0.46424927  0.26165346  0.5341197 -0.36505061
## [6,]  -0.4976933  0.06258370  0.03872473 -0.01769966  0.1832789  0.84438182
#PCA output
pca2 <- princomp(pd.sub, cor=T)
pca2
## Call:
## princomp(x = pd.sub, cor = T)
## Standard deviations:
##     Comp.1     Comp.2     Comp.3     Comp.4     Comp.5     Comp.6
## 1.7878123 1.1053808 0.7550519 0.6475685 0.5688743 0.5184536
##  6  variables and  33 observations.
loadings(pca2)
## Loadings:
##                                Comp.1 Comp.2 Comp.3 Comp.4 Comp.5 Comp.6
## Top_of_SN_Voxel_Intensity_Ratio   0.256  0.713  0.373  0.105  0.477  0.221
## Side_of_SN_Voxel_Intensity_Ratio  0.386  0.472 -0.357 -0.433 -0.558
## Part_IA                          -0.383  0.373 -0.710  0.320  0.238 -0.227
## Part_IB                          -0.460         0.112 -0.794  0.292 -0.226
## Part_II                          -0.425  0.342  0.464  0.262 -0.534 -0.365
## Part_III                         -0.498                      -0.183  0.844
##
##                 Comp.1 Comp.2 Comp.3 Comp.4 Comp.5 Comp.6
## SS loadings      1.000  1.000  1.000  1.000  1.000  1.000
## Proportion Var   0.167  0.167  0.167  0.167  0.167  0.167
## Cumulative Var   0.167  0.333  0.500  0.667  0.833  1.000
```

When the correlation matrix is used in the calculation ($\texttt{cor=T}$), the V matrix of SVD contains the corresponding PCA loadings.

4.7.1   SVD Summary

Intuitively, the SVD matrix decomposition approach, $X = UDV^T$, represents a centered data into three geometric transformations: (1) a rotation or reflection (U), (2) a diagonal matrix of scaling factors (D), and (3) another rotation or reflection matrix (V). Here, we assume that the data X stores samples/cases in rows and variables/features in columns. If these are reversed, then the interpretations of the U and V matrices are reversed accordingly.

- The columns of V represent the directions of the principal axes, the columns of UD are the principal components, and the singular values in D are related to the eigenvalues of the data variance–covariance matrix (Σ) via $\lambda_i = \frac{d_i^2}{n-1}$, where the eigenvalues $\{\lambda_i\}$ capture the magnitudes of the data variances in the respective PC directions.
- The standardized scores are given by the columns of $\sqrt{n-1}\,U$, and the corresponding loadings are given by columns of $\frac{1}{n-1}VD$. However, these "loadings" *are not* the principal directions. The requirement for X to be centered is needed to ensure that the covariance matrix $\text{Cov}(X) = \frac{1}{n-1}X^T X$.
- Alternatively, to perform PCA on the *correlation matrix* (instead of the covariance matrix), the columns of X need to be *scaled* (centered and standardized).
- To reduce the data dimensionality from p to k, where $k < p$, we multiply the first k columns of U by the $k \times k$ upper-left corner of the matrix D to get an $n \times k$ matrix $U_k D_k$ containing the first k PCs.
- Multiplying the first k PCs by their corresponding principal directions V_k^T reconstructs the original data from the first k PCs, $X_k = U_k D_k V_k^T$, with the lowest possible reconstruction error.
- Typically we have more subjects/cases (n) than variables/features ($p < n$). The dimensions of the rotation matrices are $U_{n \times n}$ and $V_{p \times p}$, and the last $n - p > 0$ columns of U may be trivial (zeros). When $n \ll p$, it's useful to drop the zero columns of U to avoid dealing with unnecessarily large (trivial) matrices.

4.8   t-Distributed Stochastic Neighbor Embedding (t-SNE)

The t-SNE technique represents a recent machine learning strategy for nonlinear dimensionality reduction that is useful for embedding (e.g., scatter-plotting) of high-dimensional data into lower-dimensional (1D, 2D, 3D) spaces. For each object (point in the high-dimensional space), the method models *similar objects* using nearby and *dissimilar objects* using remote distant objects. The two steps in t-SNE include (1) construction of a probability distribution over pairs of the original high-dimensional objects where similar objects have a high probability of being paired and correspondingly, dissimilar objects have a small probability of being selected; and (2) defining a similar probability distribution over the points in the derived low-dimensional embedding minimizing the Kullback–Leibler divergence[5] between the original high- and projected low-dimensional data distributions relative to the locations of the objects in the embedding map. Either Euclidean or non-Euclidean distance measures between objects may be used as similarity metrics.

4.8.1   t-SNE Formulation

Suppose we have a sample of high-dimensional data, $\{x_1, x_2, \cdots, x_N\}$, where each observation x_i represents a vector of measurements along multiple features. In step 1, for each pair, (x_i, x_j), t-SNE estimates the probabilities $p_{i,j}$ that are proportional to their corresponding similarities, $p_{j|i}$:

$$p_{j|i} = \frac{\exp\left(\frac{-\left\|x_i - x_j\right\|^2}{2\sigma_i^2}\right)}{\sum\limits_{k \neq i} \exp\left(\frac{-\left\|x_i - x_j\right\|^2}{2\sigma_i^2}\right)}.$$

The similarity between x_j and x_i may be thought of as the conditional probability, $p_{j|i}$. That is, assuming ND Gaussian distributions centered at each point x_i, neighbors are selected based on a probability distribution (proportion of their probability density), which represents the chance that x_i may select x_j as its closest neighbor, $p_{i,j} = \frac{p_{j|i} + p_{i|j}}{2N}$.

The *perplexity* (hyper-parameter perp) of a discrete probability distribution, p, is defined as an exponential function of the entropy, $H(p)$, over all discrete events

$$\text{perp}(x) = 2^{H(p)} = 2^{-\sum\limits_{x} p(x) \log_2 p(x)}.$$

t-SNE performs a binary search for the value σ_i that produces a predefined value perp. The simple interpretation of the perplexity at a data point x_i, $2^{H(p_i)}$, is as a smooth measure of the effective number of (close) points in the x_i neighborhood. The performance of t-SNE may vary with changes in the perplexity hyper-parameter, which is typically specified by the user, e.g., in the range $5 \leq \text{perp} \leq 50$.

Then, the precision (variance, σ_i) of the local Gaussian kernels may be chosen to ensure that the *perplexity* of the conditional distribution equals a specified perplexity. This allows adapting the kernel bandwidth to the sample data density—smaller σ_i values are fitted in denser areas of the sample data space, and correspondingly, larger σ_i are fitted in sparser areas. A particular value of σ_i yields a probability distribution, p_i, over all the other data points, which has an increasing entropy as σ_i increases.

---

[5] https://doi.org/10.1109/TIT.2014.2320500

t-SNE learns a mapping $f: \{x_1, x_2, \cdots, x_N\} \rightarrow \{y_1, y_2, \cdots, y_d\}$, where $x_i \in \mathbb{R}^N$ and $y_i \in \mathbb{R}^d$ ($N \ll d$) that resembles closely the *original similarities*, $p_{i,j}$ and represents the *derived similarities*, $q_{i,j}$ between pairs of embedded points y_i, y_j, defined by

$$q_{i,j} = \frac{\left(1 + \|y_i - y_j\|^2\right)^{-1}}{\sum_{k \neq i} \left(1 + \|y_i - y_j\|^2\right)^{-1}}.$$

The `t-distributed` reference in t-SNE acronym refers to the heavy-tailed *Student t distribution* ($t_{df=1}$), which coincides with Cauchy distribution with density $f(z) = \frac{1}{1+z^2}$. It is used to model and measure similarities between closer points in the embedded low-dimensional space, as well as dissimilarities of objects that map far apart in the embedded space.

The rationale for using *Student t distribution* for mapping the points is based on the fact that the volume of an ND ball of radius r, B^N, is proportional to r^N. Specifically, $V_N(r) = \frac{\pi^{\frac{N}{2}}}{\Gamma(\frac{N}{2}+1)} r^N$, where $\Gamma(z) = \int_0^\infty x^{z-1} e^{-x} dx, \forall \operatorname{Re}(z) > 0$ is the Euler's gamma function, which is an extension of the factorial function to noninteger arguments. For large N, when we select uniformly random points inside B^N, most points will be expected to be close to the ball surface (boundary), S^{N-1}, and only a small proportion would be expected near the B^N center. In fact, half the volume of B^N is included in a thin hyper-area *inside* B^N and *outside* a ball of radius $r_1 = \frac{1}{\sqrt{2}} \approx r \approx r$. You can picture this with $N = 2$, $\{x \in \mathbb{R}^2 \mid \|x\| \leq r\}$, representing a disk in a 2D plane.

When reducing the dimensionality of a dataset, if we use the Gaussian distribution for the mapping embedding into the lower-dimensional space, there will be a distortion of the distribution of the distances between neighboring objects. This is simply because the *distribution* of the distances is much different between the original (high-dimensional) and the map-transformed low-dimensional spaces. t-SNE tries to (approximately) preserve the distances in the two spaces to avoid imbalances that may lead to excessive attraction-repulsion forces. Using Student t distribution with $df = 1$ (aka Cauchy distribution) for mapping the points preserves (to some extent) the distance similarity distribution, because of the heavier tails of t compared to the Gaussian distribution. For a given similarity between a pair of data points, the two corresponding map points will need to be much further apart in order for their similarity to match the data similarity.

A t-SNE minimization process with respect to the objects y_i using gradient descent of a (nonsymmetric) objective function, *Kullback–Leibler divergence* between the distributions Q and P, is used to determine the object locations y_i in the map, i.e.,

$$\mathrm{KL}\left(P \| Q\right) = \sum_{i \neq j} p_{i,j} \log\left(\frac{p_{i,j}}{q_{i,j}}\right).$$

The minimization of the KL objective function by gradient descent may be analytically represented by

$$\frac{\partial \text{KL}\left(P\|Q\right)}{\partial y_i} = \sum_j \left(p_{i,j} - q_{i,j}\right) f\left(\|x_i - x_j\|\right) u_{i,j},$$

where $f(z) = \frac{z}{1+z^2}$ and $u_{i,j}$ is a unit vector from y_j to y_i. This gradient represents the aggregate sum of all spring forces applied to map point x_i.

This optimization leads to an embedding mapping that "preserves" the object (data point) similarities of the original high-dimensional inputs into the lower-dimensional space. Note that the data similarity matrix $(p_{i,j})$ is fixed, whereas its counterpart, the map similarity matrix $(q_{i,j})$ depends on the embedding map. Of course, we want these two distance matrices to be as close as possible, implying that similar data points in the original space yield similar map-points in the reduced dimension.

4.8.2   t-SNE Example: Hand-Written Digit Recognition

Later, in Chaps. 6 and 14, we will present the Optical Character Recognition (OCR) and analysis of hand-written notes (unstructured text). Below, we show a simple example of generating a 2D embedding of the hand-written digits dataset using t-SNE (Fig. 4.15).

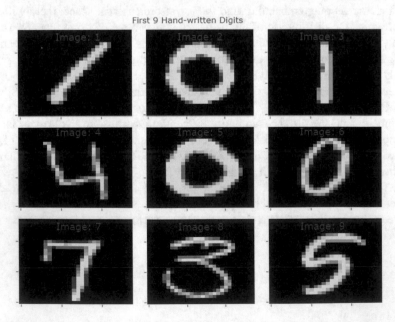

Fig. 4.15 A collage of the first nine hand-written digits (out of 42,000 images)

```r
# install.packages("tsne"); library (tsne)
# install.packages("Rtsne")
library(Rtsne)
# Download the hand-written digits data
pathToZip <- tempfile()
download.file("https://www.socr.umich.edu/people/dinov/2017/Spring/DSPA_HS650/data/DigitRecogni
zer_TrainingData.zip", pathToZip)
train <- read.csv(unzip(pathToZip))
dim(train)    ## [1] 42000    785
unlink(pathToZip)
# identify the Label-nomenclature; digits 0,1,2,...,9; and map to diff colors
colMap <- function(x)  {    # reindexing by ranking the observed values
  cols <- rainbow(length(x))[order(order(x))]
}
train.labels<-train$label
train$label<-as.factor(train$label)
train.labels.colors <- colMap(train.labels)
names(train.labels.colors) <- train$label # unique(train$label)
# May need to check and increase the RAM allocation
memory.limit()        ## [1] 32643
memory.limit(50000) ## [1] 50000
# Remove the labels (column 1) and Scale the image intensities to [0; 1]
train  <- data.matrix(train[, -1]); dim(train)  ## [1] 42000    784
train <- t(train/255)
# Visualize some of the images
library("imager")


# first convert the CSV data (one row per image, 42,000 rows)
array_3D <- array(train[ , ], c(28, 28, 42000))
mat_2D   <- matrix(array_3D[,,1], nrow = 28, ncol = 28)
# We can use plot_ly to display the image as heatmap
plot_ly(z=~t(mat_2D[, ncol(mat_2D):1]), type="heatmap", showscale=FALSE) %>%
  layout(xaxis=list(title="x", scaleanchor="y"), yaxis=list(title="Y",
          scaleanchor="x"), legend=list(orientation='h'))
N <- 42000
img_3D <- as.cimg(array_3D[,,], 28, 28, N)
# plot the k-th image (1<=k<=N)
k <- 5; plot(img_3D, k)
k <- 6; plot(img_3D, k)
k <- 7; plot(img_3D, k)
# plot a collage of the first 9 images
NoAx <- list(title="", zeroline=FALSE, showline=FALSE,
                showticklabels=FALSE, showgrid=FALSE)
pl_list <- list()
annot   <- list()
for (k in 1:9) {
  ## Transpose and Flip vertically the 2D images to display correctly
  pl_list[[k]] <- plot_ly(z=(apply(t(img_3D[,, k, 1]), 2, rev)),
              type="heatmap", showscale=FALSE, name=paste0("Image: ",k)) %>%
    layout(title=paste0("Image: ", k), legend=list(orientation='h'),
              xaxis=NoAx, yaxis=NoAx)
  annot[[k]] <- list(x =0.1+ 0.4*((k-1)%%3) , y=1.37-(0.37*floor((k-1)/3+1)),
                  text = paste0("Image: ", k), showarrow = F,
                  xref='paper', yref='paper', font=list(size=20))
}
pl_list %>% subplot(nrows = 3) %>%
    layout(title= "First 9 Hand-written Digits", annotations = annot)
```

Next, we can apply t-SNE to project the high-dimensional image data $(28 \times 28 = 784$ features) in 2D and 3D space, respectively. Clustering of congruent labels (manual 0–9 classes) into isolated groups suggests that t-SNE can identify affinities in the imaging data that can be exploited to preserve distances in the lower-dimensional projection spaces (Fig. 4.16).

```
# Run the t-SNE, tracking the execution time (artificially reducing
# the sample-size to get reasonable calculation time)
execTime_tSNE <- system.time(tsne_digits <- Rtsne(t(train)[1:10000 , ],
    dims = 2, perplexity=30, verbose=TRUE, max_iter = 500)); execTime_tSNE
## Done in 8.40 seconds (sparsity = 0.012259)!
## Learning embedding...
## Iteration 50: error is 97.574505 (50 iterations in 1.53 seconds)
…
## Iteration 500: error is 2.284485 (50 iterations in 1.40 seconds)
## Fitting performed in 14.91 seconds.
##    user  system elapsed
##   41.36    0.81   42.82 # Full dataset(42K*1K) execution may take longer
# 2D t-SNE Plot
df <- data.frame(tsne_digits$Y[1:1000, ], train.labels.colors[1:1000])
plot_ly(df, x = ~X1, y = ~X2, mode = 'text') %>%
  add_text(text = names(train.labels.colors)[1:1000],
           textfont = list(color = df$train.labels.colors.1.1000.)) %>%
 layout(title="t-SNE 2D Embedding",xaxis=list(title=""),yaxis=list(title=""))
# 3D t_SNE plot
execTime_tSNE <- system.time(tsne_digits3D <- Rtsne(t(train)[1:10000 , ], dims =
3, perplexity=30, verbose=TRUE, max_iter = 500)); execTime_tSNE
df3D <- data.frame(tsne_digits3D$Y[1:1000, ], train.labels.colors[1:1000])
plot_ly(df3D, x=~df3D[,1], y=~df3D[,2], z=~df3D[,3], mode='markers+text') %>%
  add_text(text = names(train.labels.colors)[1:1000],
           textfont = list(color = df$train.labels.colors.1.1000.)) %>%
  layout(title = "t-SNE 3D Embedding",
         scene = list(xaxis = list(title=""),  yaxis=list(title=""),
         zaxis=list(title="")))
```

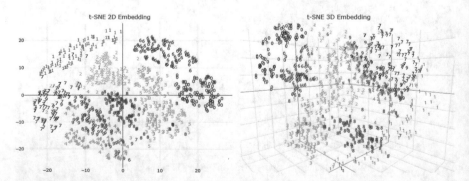

Fig. 4.16 t-SNE dimensionality reduction showing the projections of the first 1000 image samples. Clustering of images within each digit-class label suggests the method identifies intrinsic image affinities that can be used to protect distances between samples in low-dimensions

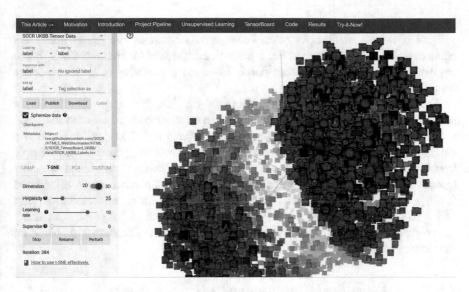

Fig. 4.17 Screenshot of the SOCR t-SNE dimensionality reduction webapp providing an interactive demonstration of PCA, t-SNE, and UMAP

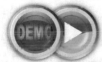   This hands-on interactive SOCR t-SNE Dimensionality Reduc-

tion Activity[6] provides an interactive demonstration of t-SNE utilizing TensorBoard and the UK Biobank data that can be accessed directly with any modern web-browser. This webapp shows PCA, t-SNE, and UMAP dimensionality reduction for a dataset with 208 neuroimaging derived features of about 10,000 participants, Fig. 4.17. The webapp also allows users to input their own data and perform dimensionality reduction on the fly.

4.9   Uniform Manifold Approximation and Projection (UMAP)

In 2018, McInnes and Healy proposed the Uniform Manifold Approximation and Projection (UMAP) technique for dimensional reduction.[7]

Similar to t-SNE, UMAP first constructs a high-dimensional graph representation of initial data and employs graph-layout algorithms to project the original high-dimensional data into a lower-dimensional space. The iterative process aims to preserve the *graph structure* as much as possible. The initial high-dimensional

---

[6] https://socr.umich.edu/HTML5/SOCR_TensorBoard_UKBB
[7] https://doi.org/10.48550/arXiv.1802.03426

graph representation uses *simplicial complexes*, as weighted graphs where edge weights represent likelihoods of the connectivity between two graph points are connected, i.e., neighborhoods. For a given point, the UMAP connectedness metric computes the distance with other points based on the overlap of their respective neighborhoods.

The parameter controlling the neighborhood size (i.e., radius) governs the within and between cluster size tradeoffs. Choosing too small a radius may lead to small and rather isolated clusters. Selecting too large a radius may cluster all points into a single group. For local radius selection, UMAP preprocessing utilizes the distances between each point and its nth nearest neighbor. A "fuzzy" simplicial complex (graph) is constructed by iterative minimization of the connectivity likelihood function as the radius increases. Assuming that each point is connected to at least one of its closest neighbors, UMAP ensures that local and global graph structure is (somewhat protected and) preserved during the optimization process (e.g., based on stochastic gradient descent).

4.9.1   Mathematical Formulation

UMAP relies on local approximations of patches on the manifold to construct local fuzzy simplicial complex (topological) representations of the high-dimensional data. For each low-dimensional representation of the projection of the data, UMAP tries to generate an analogous equivalent simplicial complex representation. The iterative UMAP optimization process aims to preserve the topological layout in the low-dimensional space by minimizing the cross-entropy between the high- and low-dimensional topological representations.

The DSPA Appendix 3 (Shapes and Manifolds) includes examples of how to generate some of geometric and topological primitives, including 0, 1, and 2 simplicial complexes. The figure below shows the first few such primitives—a point, line, triangle, and tetrahedron (Fig. 4.18).

Fig. 4.18 Examples of simplicial complexes, 0 (points), 1 (lines), 2 (triangles), and 3 (tetrahedra) cells

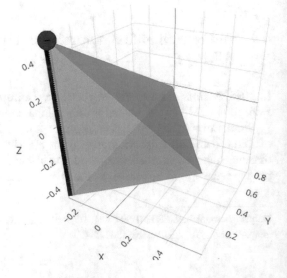

```r
library(plotly)
p <- plot_ly(type = 'mesh3d',
        # Define all (4) zero-cells (points or vertices), P_i(x,y,z), 0<=i<4
            x = c(0,           1/sqrt(3), -1/(2*sqrt(3)), -1/(2*sqrt(3))),
            y = c(sqrt(2/3),   0,          0,              0),
            z = c(0,           0,         -1/2,            1/2),
        # Next define all triples (i,j,k) of vertices that form a 2-cell face.
        # All Tetrahedra have 4 faces
            i = c(0, 0, 0, 1),
            j = c(1, 2, 3, 2),
            k = c(2, 3, 1, 3),
        # Define the appearance of the 4 faces (2-cells)
            facecolor = toRGB(viridisLite::viridis(4)),
            showscale = TRUE,
            opacity=0.8
)
traceEdge <- list(x1 = c(-1/(2*sqrt(3)), -1/(2*sqrt(3))),
    y1 = c(0, 0), z1 = c(-1/2, 1/2), type = "scatter3d",
    line = list(color = "rgb(1, 1, 1)",   #dark color for line traces
                width = 20), mode = "lines", opacity = 1)
# emphasize one of the faces by stressing the three 1-cells (edges)
p <- add_trace(p, x=~traceEdge$x1, y=~traceEdge$y1, z=~traceEdge$z1,
                type="scatter3d", mode=traceEdge$mode,
                opacity=traceEdge$opacity,
                line = list(color=traceEdge$line$color,
                            width=traceEdge$line$width), showlegend=F)
# add one 0-cell (point)
p <- add_trace(p, x=-1/(2*sqrt(3)), y=0, z=1/2, type="scatter3d",
        mode="markers", marker=list(size=16, color="blue", opacity=1.0)) %>%
    layout(title = "Simplicial Complexes (0,1,2,3) Cells", showlegend = FALSE,
        scene = list(xaxis = list(title = "X"),yaxis = list(title = "Y"),
        zaxis = list(title = "Z")))
p
```

For a given finite set of data observations, we are trying to represent the topological space that the observed data is sampled from. This topological formulation can be approximated as patches of open covers modeled by simplicial complexes. Locally, the data may be assumed to lie in a metric space where distances between data points can be measured. This leads to neighborhood approximations that can locally be represented as nD balls centered at each data point. This topological space covering may not represent a complete and open cover as all data samples are finite and small. Biased or incomplete samples may lead to poor approximations of the topology of the problem state-space. Zero-cells (0-simplexes, points) are fit for each observed data point, 1-cells (lines) are fit for each pair of data in the same neighborhood, and so on. More information about simplex trees is available in this chapter *The Simplex Tree: An Efficient Data Structure for General Simplicial Complexes.*[8] Let's show an example of a simplicial tree decomposition of 10 data points using the R package *simplextree* (Fig. 4.19).

---

[8] https://doi.org/10.1007/978-3-642-33090-2_63

Fig. 4.19 Simulated
simplicial tree
decomposition of 2D data
using 0, 1, and 2 cells

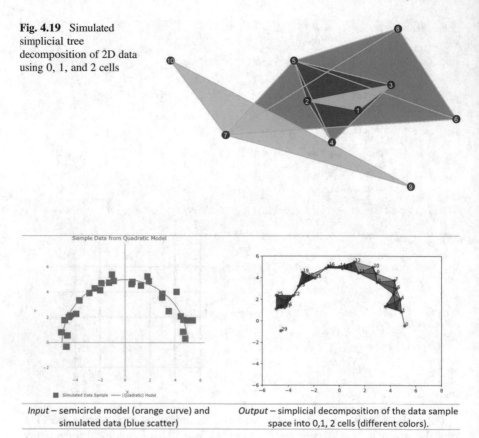

Input – semicircle model (orange curve) and
simulated data (blue scatter)

Output – simplicial decomposition of the data sample
space into 0,1, 2 cells (different colors).

Fig. 4.20 Simulation of 2D simplicial decomposition of the data-space topological structure

```
# install.packages("simplextree")
library(simplextree)
simplicialTreeExample <- simplex_tree(list(1:3, 2:5, 5:8, 7:8, c(7,9,10)))
plot(simplicialTreeExample, color_pal=rainbow(simplicialTreeExample$dimension+1))
```

The next example will provide more intuition by using a quadratic model to
generate 2D spatial data. We will approximate the topological space that the data are
likely sampled from using a simplicial decomposition. Finally, we will display the
structure of the estimated simplicial complex. This example is also interesting as it
shows dynamic integration between R and Python, a topic that will be expanded later
in Chap. 10. Specifically, we will start with data generation in R, then go into python
to generate the simplicial complex for the data, and finally will display the results
(Fig. 4.20).

```r
# 1. Generate some data
n <- 30 # number of points to generate
# Generate the space of model parameter
theta = seq(length.out=n, from=0, to=pi)
a <- 0.0; b <- 0.0; r <- 5.0
# Simulate data from half circle
x = a + r*cos(theta) + rnorm(n, 0, 0.4)
y = b + r*sin(theta) + rnorm(n, 0, 0.4)
x1 = a + r*cos(theta)
y1 = b + r*sin(theta)
df <- as.data.frame(cbind(x,y))
plot_ly() %>%
  add_trace(x=x, y=y, type="scatter", name = 'Simulated Data Sample',
            mode='markers', marker=list(opacity=0.99, size=20, symbol=1)) %>%
  add_trace(x=x1, y = y1, type="scatter", name = '(Quadratic) Model',
            mode = 'lines') %>%
 layout(title='Sample Data from Quadratic Model',legend=list(orientation='h')
        xaxis = list(title="X)", scaleanchor = "y"),
        yaxis = list(title="Y)", scaleanchor = "x"))
# install.packages("reticulate")
library(reticulate)
# specify the path of the Python version that you want to use
py_path = "C:/Users/user/Anaconda3/"    # manual
# py_path = Sys.which("python3")          # automated
use_python(py_path, required = T)
Sys.setenv(RETICULATE_PYTHON - "C:/Users/user/Anaconda3/")
# 2. Simplicial decomposition
# this block of code is run in Rstudio, but inside a ```{python} …``` chunk
import matplotlib
import matplotlib.pyplot as plt
import numpy as np
import os
os.environ['QT_QPA_PLATFORM_PLUGIN_PATH'] =
'C:/Users/user/Anaconda3/Library/plugins/platforms'
print(r.df[1:6])     # Access R data from python environment
# Functions to build a Vietoris-Rips simplicial complex from point data
def euclidianDist(a,b):
  return np.linalg.norm(a - b) #Euclidean distance metric
# Build neighborhood graph; raw_data is a numpy array
def buildGraph(raw_data, epsilon = 3.1, metric=euclidianDist):
  #initialize node set, reference indices from original data array
  nodes = [x for x in range(raw_data.shape[0])]
  edges = [] #initialize empty edge array
  #initialize weight array, weights in this case are edge distances
```

```python
    weights = []
    for i in range(raw_data.shape[0]): #iterate through each data point
        #inner loop to calculate pairwise point distances
        for j in range(raw_data.shape[0]-i):
            a = raw_data[i]
            #each simplex is a set (no order), hence [0,1] = [1,0]
            b = raw_data[j+i]
            if (i != j+i):
                dist = metric(a,b)
                if dist <= epsilon:
                    edges.append({i,j+i}) #add edge
                    weights.append([len(edges)-1,dist]) #store index and weight
    return nodes,edges,weights

def lower_nbrs(nodeSet, edgeSet, node):
    return {x for x in nodeSet if {x,node} in edgeSet and node > x}

def rips(graph, k):
    nodes, edges = graph[0:2]
    VRcomplex = [{n} for n in nodes]
    for e in edges: #add 1-simplexes (edges)
        VRcomplex.append(e)
    for i in range(k):
        for simplex in [x for x in VRcomplex if len(x)==i+2]: #skip 0-cells
            #for each u in simplex
            nbrs = set.intersection(*[lower_nbrs(nodes, edges, z) for z in
simplex])
            for nbr in nbrs:
                VRcomplex.append(set.union(simplex,{nbr}))
    return VRcomplex

def drawComplex(origData, ripsComplex, axes=[-6,8,-6,6]):
  plt.clf()
  plt.axis(axes)
  plt.scatter(origData[:,0],origData[:,1]) #plotting just for clarity
  for i, txt in enumerate(origData):
      plt.annotate(i, (origData[i][0]+0.05, origData[i][1])) #add labels

  #add lines for edges
  for edge in [e for e in ripsComplex if len(e)==2]:
      #print(edge)
      pt1,pt2 = [origData[pt] for pt in [n for n in edge]]
      #plt.gca().add_line(plt.Line2D(pt1,pt2))
      line = plt.Polygon([pt1,pt2], closed=None, fill=None, edgecolor='r')
      plt.gca().add_line(line)

  #add triangles
  for triangle in [t for t in ripsComplex if len(t)==3]:
      pt1,pt2,pt3 = [origData[pt] for pt in [n for n in triangle]]
      line = plt.Polygon([pt1,pt2,pt3], closed=False, color="blue",alpha=0.3,



              fill=True, edgecolor=None)
      plt.gca().add_line(line)
  plt.show()
# 3. Visualize the simplicial complex
newData = np.array(r.df)
graph = buildGraph(raw_data=newData, epsilon=1.7)
ripsComplex = rips(graph=graph, k=3)
drawComplex(origData=newData, ripsComplex=ripsComplex)
```

The 2D simplicial complex construction above illustrates a weighted graph representation of the 2D data using 0, 1, and 2 cells. In general, similar decomposition using higher-order simplexes can be obtained, with increasing computational complexity. This simplex graph helps with the lower-dimensional projections in the UMAP algorithm as the simplicial decomposition captures the intrinsic topological structure of the data.

Our aim is to generate a low-dimensional representation of the data that has similar (or homologous) topological structure as that of the higher-dimensional simplicial decomposition. Ideally, each UMAP projection should be a low-dimensional representation of the data into the desired embedding space (e.g., $\mathbb{R}^2$ or $\mathbb{R}^3$). We will measure distances on the manifolds using some metric, e.g., standard Euclidean distance. In particular, we focus on distances to the nearest neighbors, where neighborhoods are defined as balls centered at specific data points of a min_dist diameter, a user-specified hyper-parameter.

The lower-dimensional projections are driven by iteratively solving optimization problems of finding the low-dimensional simplicial graph that closely resembles the fuzzy topological structure of the previous graph (or the original simplicial decomposition). The simplexes are represented as graphs with weighted edges that can be thought of as probabilities that compare the homologous 0-simplexes, 1-simplexes, and so on. These probabilities can be modeled as Bernoulli processes. This is because the corresponding simplexes either exist or don't exist and the probability is the univariate parameter of the Bernoulli distribution, which can be estimated using the cross entropy measure.

For example, if $S1$ the set of all possible 1-simplexes, let's denote by $\omega(e)$ and $\omega'(e)$ the weight functions of the 1-simplex e in the high-dimensional space and the corresponding lower-dimensional counterpart, respectively. Then, the cross entropy measure for the 1-simplexes is

$$
\sum_{e \in E} \left[\underbrace{\omega(e) \log\left(\frac{\omega(e)}{\omega'(e)}\right)}_{\text{attractive force}} + \underbrace{(1 - \omega(e)) \log\left(\frac{1 - \omega(e)}{1 - \omega'(e)}\right)}_{\text{repulsive force}} \right].
$$

The iterative optimization process would minimize the objective function composed of all cross entropies for all simplicial complexes using a strategy like stochastic gradient descent. The optimization process balances the push–pull interaction between the *attractive forces* between the points favoring larger values of $\omega'(e)$ (that correspond to small distances between the points), and the *repulsive forces* between the ends of e when $\omega(e)$ is small (that correspond to small values of $\omega'(e)$.

If X and Y are some topological spaces, a map $f : X \rightarrow Y$ is called a *homeomorphism* if it is a continuous bijection with a continuous inverse, $f^{-1} : Y \rightarrow X, f \circ f^{-1} \equiv I$. In 2D, there exists a homeomorphism between a circle and an ellipse; however, no homeomorphism maps a circle onto an open interval.

Homeomorphisms consider only the open subsets of the embedding space and they are not affected by the metric on the space. Any pair of n-simplices are homeomorphic. As high-dimensional data may be considered as point clouds in a high-dimensional space, we can study the embedding manifolds as simplicial complexes by decomposing them into their topological building blocks—*simplices*. A simplicial complex X is a collection of simplices in $\mathbb{R}^N$ where for any simplex in X, all of its faces (lower-order simplices) are also in X and the intersection of any two simplices is either empty or a face in both of them. All simplicial complexes X can be described, up to homeomorphism, by listing the vertices of each simplex in X. Common vertices allow us to understand which simplices share faces.

There is a generalization of simplices defined by their vertices to abstract simplicial complexes, where X is a series of sets $\{X_i\}_{i \geq 0}$, such that the elements of X^n (the n-simplices) are $(n + 1)$-element sets that satisfy the condition $\forall x_{i=1}^n \in X^n$, all n-element subsets of this set are in X^{n-1}. Different simplices can share common elements, e.g., vertices, edges, faces. For instance, a square in $\mathbb{R}^2$ can be describe by explicating the 0-, 1- and 2-cells

$$S_0 = \{\{a\}, \{b\}, \{c\}, \{d\}\}; S_1 = \{\{a,\ b\}, \{a,\ c\}, \{a,\ d\}, \{b,\ c\}, \{c,\ d\}\}, S_2 = \{\{a,\ b,\ c\}, \{a,\ c,\ d\}\}.$$

The simplex vertex order is important for defining face-maps. An ordered n-simplex can be represented as $[x_0, x_1, \cdots, x_n]$. We can characterize an n-simplex in a simplicial complex by the collection of its $n + 1$ face-maps, the i-th face-map sends the simplex to the face excluding the i-th vertex from the original simplex, i.e.,

$$f_i : [x_0, x_1, \cdots, x_i, \cdots, x_n] \to [x_0, x_1, \cdots, x_{i-1}, x_{i+1}, \cdots, x_n].$$

Fuzzy sets are sets where element participation in the set is represented by continuous membership functions, i.e., set membership is not binary (in or out) but rather probabilistic. Hence, a fuzzy set is a set of objects A and a function $\mu : A \to [0, 1]$ where $\mu(a) = 1$ indicates a definitive membership of a in the fuzzy set. Fuzzy simplicial sets have the property that the membership strength of the face of a simplex is at least the membership strength of the simplex.

Suppose we start with a Riemannian manifold (M, g) embedded in $\mathbb{R}^n$. Given a point $p \in M$, consider a ball B, $p \in B \subseteq M$, whose volume with respect to the locally constant metric g is $V(B) = \frac{\pi^{n/2}}{\Gamma(1+n/2)}$. Then the distance of the shortest path in M from p to another point $q \in B$ is $\frac{1}{r} d_{\mathbb{R}^N}(p, q)$, where r is the radius of B in M and $d_{\mathbb{R}^N}(p, q)$ is the chosen $\mathbb{R}^N$ distance between p and q in $\mathbb{R}^N$.

To convert between metric spaces and fuzzy simplicial sets, consider a fixed data point x_i in the dataset D. We can approximate the distance from x_i to any other point x_j in D by $d_{x_i}(x_i, x_j) = \frac{1}{r_i} d_{\mathbb{R}^N}(x_i, x_j)$. This gives us a partly defined metric space, using the (observed) distances between x_i and x_j, $\forall j$, even though we may not know the distances between x_j and x_k for $j, k \neq i$. Denote by ρ_i the distance between x_i and its nearest neighbor in D in $\mathbb{R}^N$ and assume M is locally connected, i.e., x_i must be connected to its nearest neighbor $\forall j \neq i$. Then,

$$
d_{x_i}(x_i, x_j) = \begin{cases} \dfrac{1}{r_i} d_{\mathbb{R}^N}(x_i, x_j), & \text{if } j = i \text{ or } k = i \\ \infty, & \text{otherwise} \end{cases}.
$$

By this definition, x_i and its nearest neighbor are distance 0 apart, and $\forall j, k \neq i$, the unknown distances of x_j and x_k relative to x_i are set this to infinity. With this formulation, we lose the exact metric characterization of the state space and instead utilize the extended *pseudo-metric space* consisting of the set X and the function $d : X \times X \rightarrow \mathbb{R} \cup \{\infty\}$, which has pseudo-metric properties: (1) $d(x, y) \geq 0$, (2) $d(x, x) = 0$, (3) $d(x, y) = d(y, x)$, and (4) either $d(x, z) = \infty$ or $d(x, z) \leq d(x, y) + d(y, z)$. The pseudo-metric permits infinite distances as well as the posibility that $d(x, y) = 0$ for $x \neq y$.

The most commonly used objective function in UMAP is cross entropy of pairs of fuzzy sets represented via symmetric weight matrices

$$
C_{\text{UMAP}} = \sum_{i,j} \left[\underbrace{v_{i,j} \log\left(\frac{v_{i,j}}{w_{i,j}}\right)}_{\text{attractive force}} + \underbrace{(1 - v_{i,j}) \log\left(\frac{1 - v_{i,j}}{1 - w_{i,j}}\right)}_{\text{repulsive force}} \right],
$$

where $v_{i,\,j}$ are *symmetrized input weights* (affinities), weights of the corresponding fuzzy simplices in the native high-dimensional space. For 1-simpex, these are effectively graph edge weights. The associated UMAP *unsymmetrized input weights* are $v_{i|j} = e^{-(r_{i,j} - \rho_i)/\sigma_i}$, where $r_{i,\,j}$ are the input distances, ρ_i is the distance to the nearest neighbor (suppressing zero distances for duplicate neighbors), and σ_i (perplexity parameters) are estimated using the number of nearest neighbors (hyperparameter k) via the restriction $\sum_j v_{i|j} = \log(2k)$.

The relation between symmetrized and unsymmetrized input weights is given by

$$
v_{i,j} = (v_{j|i} + v_{i|j}) - v_{j|i} v_{i|j} \quad (\text{element} - \text{wise}),
$$
$$
V_{\text{symm}} = V + V^T - V \circ V^T \quad (\text{matrix} - \text{wise}),
$$

where the Hadamard element-wise product is $\circ$ and V^T is the transpose matrix. The symmetrization corresponds to a fuzzy set union.

The corresponding *output weights* in the lower-dimensional projection space are

$$
w_{i,j} = \frac{1}{1 + a d_{i,j}^{2b}},
$$

where the parameters a and b typically in the range $[0.5, 5]$ are estimated using nonlinear least squares subject to the distances $d_{i,j}$ that control the tightness of the lower-dimensional compression function.

The attractive and repulsive UMAP gradient expressions for stochastic gradient descent (SGD, Chap. 13) are

$$\underbrace{\frac{\partial C_{\text{UMAP}}^{+}}{\partial y_i}}_{\text{attractive}} = \frac{-2abd_{i,j}^{2(b-1)}}{1 + ad_{i,j}^{2b}} \left(y_i - y_j\right),$$

$$\underbrace{\frac{\partial C_{\text{UMAP}}^{-}}{\partial y_i}}_{\text{repulsive}} = \frac{2b}{\left(\epsilon + d_{i,j}^2\right)\left(1 + ad_{i,j}^{2b}\right)} \left(y_i - y_j\right),$$

where the correction $\epsilon \sim 0.001$ avoids singularities. Note that in the repulsive SGD expression, the exact gradient also contains a term $1 - v_{i,j}$, which can be ignored as for most pairs of edges (paired distances) $v_{i,j} = 0$.

4.9.2 Hand-Written Digits Recognition

Let's use again the MNIST digits dataset[9] and apply UMAP projection from the original 784-dimensional space into 2D. The R package umap provides functionality to use UMAP for dimensional reduction of high-dimensional data. Let's demonstrate UMAP projecting the hand-written digits dataset in 2D and using the projection for prediction and forecasting using new testing/validation data (Fig. 4.21).

```
library(plotly)                  # install.packages('plotly')
library(umap)                    # install.packages('umap')
# https://rdrr.io/cran/man/umap/umap.defaults.html
custom.settings = umap.defaults
custom.settings$n_neighbors = 5
custom.settings$n_components=3
# custom.settings
execTime_UMAP <- system.time(umap_digits3D <- umap(t(train)[1:10000 , ],
                             umap.config=custom.settings)); execTime_UMAP
cols <- palette(rainbow(10))
# 2D UMAP Plot
dfUMAP <- data.frame(umap_digits3D$layout[1:1000, ], train.labels.colors[1:1000])
plot_ly(dfUMAP, x = ~X1, y = ~X2, mode = 'text') %>%
  add_text(text=names(train.labels.colors)[1:1000],
          textfont=list(color=dfUMAP$train.labels.colors.1.1000.)) %>%
  layout(title="UMAP (748D->2D) Embedding", xaxis = list(title = ""),
          yaxis = list(title = ""))
```

---

[9]https://doi.org/10.1109/MSP.2012.2211477

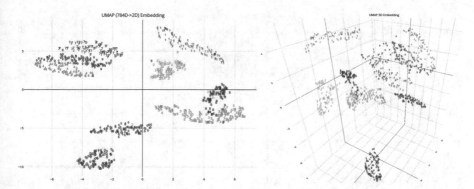

Fig. 4.21 UMAP dimensionality reduction showing the projections of the first 1,000 image samples. Similarly to the t-SNE result in Figure 4.16, image clustering in 2D (left) and 3D (right) suggests UMAP identifies intrinsic image affinities that can be used to protect distances between samples in low-dimensions.

4.9.3 Apply UMAP for Class-Prediction Using New Data

We can use again the MNIST hand-written digits dataset, or even the simpler iris dataset, to show the UMAP protocol for predicting the image-to-digit, or flower-to-species (taxa) mappings. In the MNIST data, we will use a set of 1000 new 2D images for prediction. If using the iris data, we can simulate new iris flower features by introducing random (additive) noise $N(0, 0.1)$ to the original iris data (Fig. 4.22).

```r
# Use next 1,000 images as prospective new data to classify into 0-9 labels
umapData_1000 <- train[ , 10001:11000]
str(umapData_1000)
# Prediction/Forecasting
umapData_1000_Pred <- predict(umap digits3D, t(umapData_1000))
# mind transpose of data (case * Feature)
# 2D UMAP Plot
dfUMAP <- data.frame(x=umap_digits3D$layout[1:1000, 1],
          y=umap_digits3D$layout[1:1000, 2], col=train.labels.colors[1:1000])
plot_ly(dfUMAP, x = ~x, y = ~y, mode = 'text') %>%
    # Add training data UMAP projection scatter Digits
    add_text(text=names(train.labels.colors)[1:1000],
            textfont=list(color=~col, size=15), showlegend=F) %>%
    # Add 1,000 testing hand-written digit cases onto the 2D UMAP projection
    # pane as colored scatter points
    add_markers(x=umapData_1000_Pred[ , 1], y=umapData_1000_Pred[ , 2],
                name =train.labels[10001:11000],
                marker = list(color=train.labels.colors[10001:11000])) %>%
    layout(title="UMAP Prediction: Projection of 1,000 New Images in 2D",
            xaxis = list(title = ""),  yaxis = list(title = ""))
```

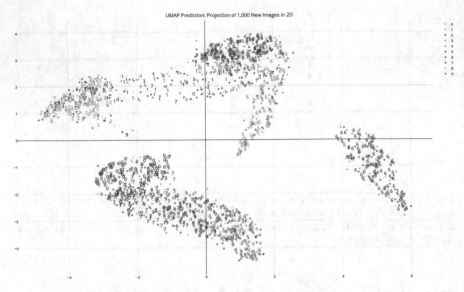

Fig. 4.22 Results of the forecasting and prediction of the image-to-digit mapping using the 2D UMAP simplicial decomposition projections, instead of the original 784 image features

4.10 UMAP Parameters

The UMAP configuration allows specifying a number of parameters controlling the UMAP projection embedding of the function `umap()`. These hyper-parameters include

- *n_neighbors*: integer; number of nearest neighbors.
- *n_components*: integer; dimension of target (output) space.
- *metric*: character or function determining how distances between data points are computed. String-labeled metric, e.g., *euclidean*, *manhattan*, *cosine*, *pearson*, *pearson2*. The triangle inequality may not be satisfied by some metrics and the internal *knn* search may not be optimal.
- *n_epochs*: integer; number of iterations performed during layout optimization.
- *input*: character, use either "data" or "dist"; determines whether the primary input argument to `umap()` is treated as a data matrix or as a distance matrix.
- *init*: character or matrix. The default string "spectral" computes an initial embedding using eigenvectors of the connectivity graph matrix. An alternative is the string "random," which creates an initial layout based on random coordinates. This setting can also be set to a matrix, in which case layout optimization begins from the provided coordinates.
- *min_dist*: numeric; determines how close points appear in the final layout.
- *set_op_ratio_mix_ratio*: numeric in range [0,1]; determines the knn-graph used to create a fuzzy simplicial graph.

- *local_connectivity*: numeric; used during construction of fuzzy simplicial set.
- *bandwidth*: numeric; used during construction of fuzzy simplicial set.
- *alpha*: numeric; initial value of "learning rate" of layout optimization.
- *gamma*: numeric; determines, together with alpha, the learning rate of layout optimization.
- *negative_sample_rate*: integer; determines how many non-neighbor points are used per point and per iteration during layout optimization.
- *a*: numeric; contributes to gradient calculations during layout optimization. When left at NA, a suitable value will be estimated automatically.
- *b*: numeric; contributes to gradient calculations during layout optimization.
- *spread*: numeric; used during automatic estimation of a/b parameters.
- *random_state*: integer; seed for random number generation used during umap().
- *transform_state*: integer; seed for random number generation used during `pre-dict()`.
- *knn.repeat*: number of times to restart knn search.
- *verbose*: logical or integer; determines whether to show progress messages.
- *umap_learn_args*: vector of arguments to python package umap-learn.

4.10.1   Stability, Replicability, and Reproducibility

Replicability is a milder condition that requires obtaining homologous results across multiple studies examining the same phenomenon aiming at answering the same scientific questions, each study using its own independent (yet homologous) input data.

Reproducibility is a stronger condition that requires obtaining consistent computational results using a *fixed* protocol including input data, computational steps, scientific methods, software code, compiler, and other experimental conditions.

As most UMAP implementations involve stochastic processes that employ random number generation, there may be variations in the output results from repeated runs of the algorithm. To stabilize these outputs and ensure result reproducibility we can use seed-setting, `umapData.umap.1234 = umap(umapData, random_state=1234)`.

4.10.2   UMAP Interpretation

Below is a summary of key UMAP interpretation points.

- The choice of the hyper-parameters will affect the output: choosing optimal parameter values may be difficult and is always data dependent. The stability of running UMAP repeatedly with a range of hyper-parameters may provide a more sensible interpretation of the lower-dimensional MAP projection.

- The sizes of the lower-dimensional UMAP cluster should not be over-interpreted, since UMAP relies only on local graph neighborhood distances (not global) to construct the initial high-dimensional graph representation.
- Similarly, between-cluster distances are not representative of dissimilarities between the cluster elements.
- Initial random noise in the data will not be preserved as random variation in the UMAP projections and some spurious clustering may be present that may not be signal related.

4.11 Dimensionality Reduction Case Study (Parkinson's Disease)

Let's demonstrate the use of some of these dimensionality reduction methods to a real biomedical case-study involving a large cohort of Parkinson's disease volunteers.[10]

4.11.1 Step 1: Collecting Data

The data we will be using in this case study are the clinical, genetic, and imaging data for Parkinson's disease in the SOCR website. Let's start with importing the data into R.

```
# Loading required package: xml2
wiki_url <- read_html("https://wiki.socr.umich.edu/index.php/SOCR_Data_PD_BiomedBigMetadata")
html_nodes(wiki_url, "#content")
pd_data <- html_table(html_nodes(wiki_url, "table")[[1]])
head(pd_data); summary(pd_data)
```

4.11.2 Step 2: Exploring and Preparing the Data

Before we show various dimension reduction procedures, let's perform some light preprocessing, e.g., modify the factor variable Dx, diagnosis and remove the patient pseudo-identifiers and time variables.

---

[10] https://www.ppmi-info.org/

```
pd_data$Dx <- gsub("PD", 1, pd_data$Dx)
pd_data$Dx <- gsub("HC", 0, pd_data$Dx)
pd_data$Dx <- gsub("SWEDD", 0, pd_data$Dx)
pd_data$Dx <- as.numeric(pd_data$Dx)
attach(pd_data)
pd_data<-pd_data[, -c(1, 33)]
```

4.11.3   PCA

Next, we fit a PCA model using one of several CPA functions available in R. Here we will use the `princomp()` function and the correlation rather than the covariance matrix for these calculations. We can also use another PCA function that we saw previously `prcomp()` (Fig. 4.23).

```
pca.model <- princomp(pd_data, cor=TRUE)
summary(pca.model) # pc loadings (i.e., eigenvector columns)
## Importance of components:
##                          Comp.1      Comp.2      Comp.3     Comp.4     Comp.5
## Standard deviation     1.39495952  1.28668145  1.28111293  1.2061402  1.18527282
## Proportion of Variance 0.06277136  0.05340481  0.05294356  0.0469282  0.04531844
## Cumulative Proportion  0.06277136  0.11617617  0.16911973  0.2160079  0.26136637
##                          Comp.6      Comp.7      Comp.8     Comp.9     Comp.10
## Standard deviation     1.15961464  1.135510    1.10882348  1.0761943  1.06687730
## Proportion of Variance 0.04337762  0.041593    0.03966095  0.0373611  0.03671701
## Cumulative Proportion  0.30474399  0.346337    0.38599794  0.4233590  0.46007604
##                          Comp.11     Comp.12     Comp.13    Comp.14    Comp.15
## Standard deviation     1.05784209  1.04026215  1.03067437  1.0259684  0.99422375
## Proportion of Variance 0.03609774  0.03490791  0.03426741  0.0339552  0.03188648
## Cumulative Proportion  0.49617378  0.53108169  0.56534910  0.5993043  0.63119070
##                          Comp.16     Comp.17     Comp.18    Comp.19    Comp.20
## Standard deviation     0.97385632  0.96688855  0.92687735  0.92376374 0.89853718
## Proportion of Variance 0.03059342  0.03015721  0.02771296  0.02752708 0.02604416
## Cumulative Proportion  0.66178421  0.69194141  0.71965437  0.74710145 0.77322561
##                          Comp.21     Comp.22     Comp.23    Comp.24    Comp.25
## Standard deviation     0.88924412  0.87005195  0.86433816  0.84794183 0.82232529
## Proportion of Variance 0.02550823  0.02441905  0.02409937  0.02319372 0.02181351
## Cumulative Proportion  0.79873384  0.82315289  0.84725226  0.87044598 0.89225949
##                          Comp.26     Comp.27     Comp.28    Comp.29    Comp.30
## Standard deviation     0.80703739  0.78546699  0.77505522  0.76624322 0.68806884
## Proportion of Variance 0.02100998  0.01990188  0.01937770  0.01893963 0.01527222
## Cumulative Proportion  0.91326947  0.93317135  0.95254911  0.97148875 0.98676096
##                          Comp.31
## Standard deviation     0.64063259
## Proportion of Variance 0.01323904
## Cumulative Proportion  1.00000000
plot(pca.model)
```

Below we show a couple of bivariate plots depicting the PCA projections of the Parkinson's disease data in a 2D plane spanned by the first two principal directions (Figs. 4.24 and 4.25).

```
biplot(pca.model)
fviz_pca_biplot(pca.model, axes = c(1, 2), geom = "point",
  col.ind = "black", col.var = "steelblue", label = "all",
  invisible = "none", repel = F, habillage = pd_data$Sex,
  palette = NULL, addEllipses = TRUE, title = "PCA - Biplot")
```

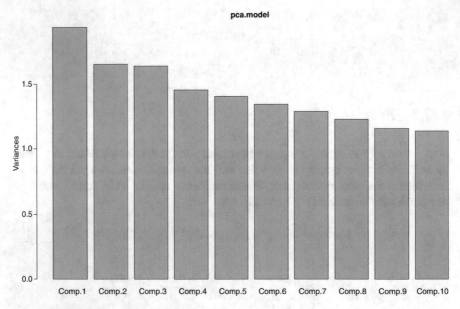

Fig. 4.23 PPMI/Parkinson's disease data scree plot

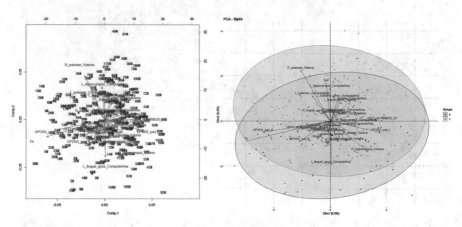

Fig. 4.24 A pair of alternative 2D plots of the PCA projections along the first two principal directions

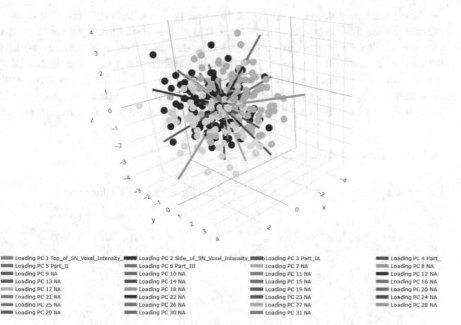

Loading PC 1 Top_of_SN_Voxel_Intensity_	Loading PC 2 Side_of_SN_Voxel_Intensity_	Loading PC 3 Part_IA	Loading PC 4 Part_
Loading PC 5 Part_II	Loading PC 6 Part_III	Loading PC 7 NA	Loading PC 8 NA
Loading PC 9 NA	Loading PC 10 NA	Loading PC 11 NA	Loading PC 12 NA
Loading PC 13 NA	Loading PC 14 NA	Loading PC 15 NA	Loading PC 16 NA
Loading PC 17 NA	Loading PC 18 NA	Loading PC 19 NA	Loading PC 20 NA
Loading PC 21 NA	Loading PC 22 NA	Loading PC 23 NA	Loading PC 24 NA
Loading PC 25 NA	Loading PC 26 NA	Loading PC 27 NA	Loading PC 28 NA
Loading PC 29 NA	Loading PC 30 NA	Loading PC 31 NA	

Fig. 4.25 A 3D scatter plot with line segments depicting the factor loadings along the 31 principal directions

```
plot_ly(x = c(1:length(pca.model$sdev)), y = pca.model$sdev*pca.model$sdev,
        name = "Scree", type = "bar") %>%
  layout(title="Scree Plot", xaxis = list(title="PC's"),
         yaxis = list(title="Variances (SD^2)"))
# Scores
scores <- pca.model$scores
# Loadings
loadings <- pca.model$loadings
# Visualization scale factor for loadings
scaleLoad <- 10
p <- plot_ly() %>%
  add_trace(x=scores[,1], y=scores[,2], z=scores[,3], type="scatter3d",
mode="markers", name=pd_data$Dx,
            marker = list(color=pd_data$Dx, colorscale = c("gray", "red"),
opacity = 0.7), showlegend=F)
for (k in 1:nrow(loadings)) {
  x <- c(0, loadings[k,1])*scaleLoad
  y <- c(0, loadings[k,2])*scaleLoad
  z <- c(0, loadings[k,3])*scaleLoad
  p <- p %>% add_trace(x=x, y=y, z=z, type="scatter3d", mode="lines",
  name=paste0("Loading PC ", k, " ", colnames(pd.sub)[k]), line=list(width=8),
opacity=1)
}
p <- p %>%
  layout(legend = list(orientation = 'h'),
         title=paste0("3D Projection of ", length(pca.model$sdev),
                      "D PD Data along First 3 PCs (Colored by Dx)"))
p
```

Albeit the two cohorts (normal controls and patients, DX, red and gray colored markers in the 3D scene) are slightly separated in the second principal direction, we can see in this real-world example that PCs do not necessarily correspond to a definitive "elbow" plot suggesting an optimal number of components. In our PCA model, each PC explains about the same amount of variation. Thus, it is hard to tell how many PCs, or factors, we need to select. This would be an *ad hoc* decision in this case. We can understand this better after understanding the following FA model.

4.11.4   Factor Analysis (FA)

Let's set up a Cattel's Scree test to determine the number of factors first.

```
ev <- eigen(cor(pd_data)) # get eigenvalues
ap <- parallel(subject=nrow(pd_data), var=ncol(pd_data), rep=100, cent=.05)
nS <- nScree(x=ev$values, aparallel=ap$eigen$qevpea)
summary(nS)
##      Eigenvalues Prop Cumu Par.Analysis Pred.eig    OC Acc.factor      AF
## 1             2    0    0            1        2 (< OC)        NA (< AF)
## 2             2    0    0            1        2                0
## 3             2    0    0            1        1                0
## 4             1    0    0            1        1                0
## 5             1    0    0            1        1                0
## 6             1    0    0            1        1                0
## 7             1    0    0            1        1                0
## 8             1    0    0            1        1                0
## 9             1    0    0            1        1                0
## 10            1    0    0            1        1                0
## 11            1    0    0            1        1                0
## 12            1    0    1            1        1                0
## 13            1    0    1            1        1                0
## 14            1    0    1            1        1                0
## 15            1    0    1            1        1                0
## 16            1    0    1            1        1                0
## 17            1    0    1            1        1                0
## 18            1    0    1            1        1                0
## 19            1    0    1            1        1                0
## 20            1    0    1            1        1                0
## 21            1    0    1            1        1                0
## 22            1    0    1            1        1                0
## 23            1    0    1            1        1                0
## 24            1    0    1            1        1                0
## 25            1    0    1            1        1                0
## 26            1    0    1            1        1                0
## 27            1    0    1            1        1                0
## 28            1    0    1            1        1                0
## 29            1    0    1            1        1                0
## 30            0    0    1            1       NA                0
## 31            0    0    1            1       NA               NA
## Number of factors retained by index
##   noc naf nparallel nkaiser
## 1   1   1        14      14
```

Although the Cattel's Scree test suggests that we should use 14 factors, the real fit shows 14 is not enough. Previous PCA results suggest we need around 20 PCs to obtain a cumulative variance of 0.6. After a few trials, we find that 19 factors can pass the chi-square test for a sufficient number of factors at 0.05 level.

```
fa.model<-factanal(pd_data, 19, rotation="varimax")
fa.model
## Uniquenesses:
##        L_caudate_ComputeArea                L_caudate_Volume
##                 0.840                              0.005
##        R_caudate_ComputeArea                R_caudate_Volume
##                 0.868                              0.849
...
## Loadings:
##                           Factor1 Factor2 Factor3 Factor4 Factor5 Factor6
## L_caudate_ComputeArea
## L_caudate_Volume                                                   0.980
## R_caudate_ComputeArea
## R_caudate_Volume
## L_putamen_ComputeArea
## L_putamen_Volume
## R_putamen_ComputeArea
## R_putamen_Volume
## L_hippocampus_ComputeArea
## L_hippocampus_Volume
## R_hippocampus_ComputeArea    -0.102

##            Factor1 Factor2 Factor3 Factor4 Factor5 Factor6 Factor7 Factor8
## SS loadings  1.282   1.029   1.026   1.019   1.013   1.011   0.921   0.838
## Propor. Var  0.041   0.033   0.033   0.033   0.033   0.033   0.030   0.027
## Cumul. Var   0.041   0.075   0.108   0.140   0.173   0.206   0.235   0.263
...
## Test of the hypothesis that 19 factors are sufficient.
## The chi square statistic is 54.51 on 47 degrees of freedom.
## The p-value is 0.211
```

This data matrix has relatively low correlation. Thus, it is not suitable for ICA (Fig. 4.26).

```
cor(pd_data)[1:10, 1:10]
##                          L_caudate_ComputeArea L_caudate_Volume
## L_caudate_ComputeArea             1.000000000       0.05794916
## L_caudate_Volume                  0.057949162       1.00000000
## R_caudate_ComputeArea            -0.060576361       0.01076372
...
## L_hippocampus_Volume             -0.026338163       1.00000000
# generate some random categorical labels for all N observations
class <- pd_data$Dx
df <- as.data.frame(pd_data[1:5], class=class)
plot_ly(df) %>%
    add_trace(type = 'splom', dimensions = list(
        list(label=colnames(pd_data)[1], values=~L_caudate_ComputeArea),
        list(label=colnames(pd_data)[2], values=~L_caudate_Volume),
        list(label=colnames(pd_data)[3], values=~R_caudate_ComputeArea),
        list(label=colnames(pd_data)[4], values=~R_caudate_Volume),
        list(label=colnames(pd_data)[5], values=~L_putamen_ComputeArea)),
      text=~class, marker = list(line =
      list(width = 1, color = 'rgb(230,230,230)'))) %>%
    layout(title= 'Parkinsons Disease (PD) Data Pairs Plot',
        hovermode='closest', dragmode= 'select',
        plot_bgcolor='rgba(240,240,240, 0.95)')
```

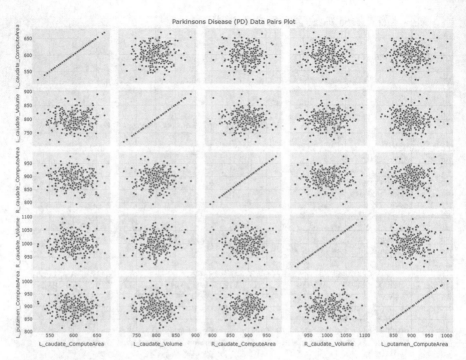

Fig. 4.26 Low bivariate correlations are evident in the pairs plot for a sample of Parkinson's disease data features

4.11.5   t-SNE

Next, let's try the t-Distributed Stochastic Neighbor Embedding method on the Parkinson's disease (PD) data (Fig. 4.27).

```
# install.packages("Rtsne")
library(Rtsne)
# If working with post-processed PD data above: remove duplicates (after
stripping time)
# pd_data <- unique(pd_data[,])
# If working with raw PD data: reload it
pd_data <- html_table(html_nodes(wiki_url, "table")[[1]])
# Run the t-SNE, tracking the execution time (artificially reducing the sample-
size to get reasonable calculation time)
execTime_tSNE <- system.time(tsne_PD <- Rtsne(pd_data, dims = 3,
        perplexity=30, verbose=TRUE, max_iter = 1000)); execTime_tSNE
## Performing PCA
## Read the 1128 x 35 data matrix successfully!
## OpenMP is working. 1 threads.
## Using no_dims = 3, perplexity = 30.000000, and theta = 0.500000
## Computing input similarities...
## Building tree...
## Done in 0.18 seconds (sparsity = 0.111894)!
## Learning embedding...
```

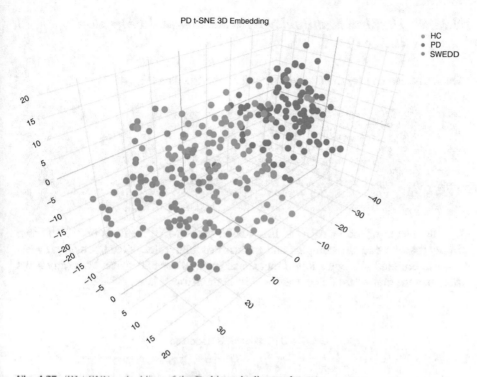

Fig. 4.27 3D t-SNE embedding of the Parkinson's disease dataset

```
## Iteration 50: error is 71.955791 (50 iterations in 0.31 seconds)
…
## Iteration 250: error is 69.312742 (50 iterations in 0.14 seconds)
## Iteration 300: error is 1.040695 (50 iterations in 0.25 seconds)
…
## Iteration 1000: error is 0.610235 (50 iterations in 0.57 seconds)
## Fitting performed in 7.66 seconds.
# Plot the result 2D map embedding of the data
table(pd_data$Dx)
##    HC    PD SWEDD
##   400   400   328
# Either use the DX label column to set the colors col=as.factor(pd_data$Dx)
# Or to set the colors explicitly
CharToColor = function(input_char){
    mapping = c("HC"="blue", "PD"="red", "SWEDD"="green")
    mapping[input_char]
}
pd_data$Dx.col = sapply(pd_data$Dx, CharToColor)
df3D <- data.frame(tsne_PD$Y, pd_data$Dx.col)
plot_ly(df3D, x = ~df3D[, 1], y = ~df3D[, 2], z= ~df3D[, 3],
        type="scatter3d", mode = 'markers',
        color = pd_data$Dx.col, name=pd_data$Dx) %>%
  layout(title = "PD t-SNE 3D Embedding", scene=list(xaxis=list(title=""),
               yaxis=list(title=""), zaxis=list(title=""))))
```

4.11.6   *Uniform Manifold Approximation and Projection (UMAP)*

Similarly, we can try the UMAP method on the PD data (Fig. 4.28).

```
execTime_UMAP <- system.time(umap_PD_3D <- umap(pd_data[, -c(27, 34)]))
execTime_UMAP
cols <- palette(rainbow(3))
# 2D UMAP Plot
dfUMAP <- data.frame(umap_PD_3D$layout, df3D$pd_data.Dx.col)
plot_ly(dfUMAP, x = ~X1, y = ~X2, mode = 'text') %>%
add_text(text=pd_data$Dx,textfont=list(color=dfUMAP$df3D.pd_data.Dx.col)) %>%
  layout(title="UMAP PD (32D->2D) Embedding",
         xaxis = list(title = ""),  yaxis = list(title = ""))
```

The results of the PCA, ICA, FA, t-SNE, and UMAP methods on the PD data imply that the data are complex and intrinsically high dimensional, which prevents explicit embeddings into a low-dimensional (e.g., 2D or 3D) space. More advanced methods to interrogate this dataset will be demonstrated later.

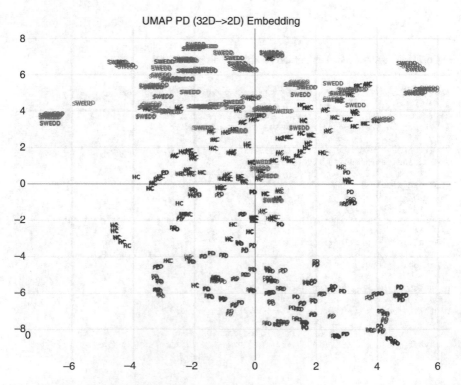

Fig. 4.28   2D UMAP embedding of the Parkinson's disease dataset indicating the three class labels (HC, SWEDD, and PD)

4.12   Practice Problems

4.12.1   Parkinson's Disease Example

Use principal component analysis (PCA), singular value decomposition (SVD), independent component analysis (ICA), and factor analysis (FA) to reduce the dimensionality of the PD data presented earlier or the irritable bowel syndrome (IBS), ulcerative colitis, and Crohn's disease data available online.[11] Interpret each of the results.

4.12.2   Allometric Relations in Plants example

Load Allometric Relations in Plants data[12] and perform proper type conversion, e.g., convert "Province" and "Born". Perform principal component analysis.

* Generate a data summary
* Apply `factoextra` and compare it to the results of `prcomp`
* Report the rotations (scores)
* Show the scree plot
* Select the number of PCs and employ a bootstrap test
* Perform SVD and ICA and compare the results of PCA.

  – Use these three variables "L,""M,""D" to perform ICA and show pair-plots of before-ICA and after-ICA scatter in the data. `plot_ly()`, and `scatter3dplot()` may be helpful, which you saw in Chaps. 2 and 3.

* Perform factor analysis

  – Use `require(nFactors)` to determine the number of the factors and show a scree plot as stated in notes;
  – Use `factanal()` to apply FA and compare the rotation "varimax" and "promax"
  – Report the loadings and consider an appropriate visualization method

* Interpret the findings in the context of the case-study.

---

[11] https://wiki.socr.umich.edu/index.php/SOCR_Data_April2011_NI_IBS_Pain

[12] https://wiki.socr.umich.edu/index.php/SOCR_Data_Dinov_032708_AllometricPlanRels

4.12.3 3D Volumetric Brain Study

Use the 3D brain tumor segmentation (BraTS) image dataset.[13] Split it into training and testing sets. The complete brain MR dataset contains 257 3D volumes of dimensions $240(x) \times 240(y) \times 155(z)$. For each case, there is a categorical (phenotypic) label and there are four different imaging modalities including T1 (T1-weighted), T1C (contrast-enhanced T1-weighted), T2 (T2-weighted), and fluid attenuation inversion recovery (FLAIR). This chapter[14] may be of interest.

Consider each *voxel* (3D generalization of a pixel) in the 3D brain volume as a feature. Use both t-SNE and UMAP to reduce the high-dimensional data ($240 \times 240 \times 155 = 8,928,000$) to 2D or 3D. Color-code the lower-dimensional projections by the categorical labels associated with disease (clinical phenotypes). Is there clearly identifiable patterns suggestions discrimination between clinical class labels? Compare your findings against the SCOR PCA/t-SNE/UMAP interactive webapp using the default UKBB dataset.[15]

---

[13] https://www.med.upenn.edu/cbica/brats2020/data.html

[14] https://doi.org/10.1016/j.bspc.2021.102458

[15] https://socr.umich.edu/HTML5/SOCR_TensorBoard_UKBB

Chapter 5
Supervised Classification

In this chapter, we will present various progressively supervised machine learning, classification, and clustering techniques. There are two categories of machine learning techniques—unsupervised and supervised (human-guided). In general, supervised *classification* methods aim to identify or predict predefined classes and label new objects as members of specific classes. In contrast, unsupervised *clustering* approaches attempt to group objects into subsets, without knowing a priori labels, and determine relationships between objects.

In the context of machine learning and artificial intelligence, classification and clustering apply mostly for supervised and unsupervised problems, respectively. In Chap. 8, we will discuss **unsupervised clustering** and **classification** methods where the outcomes (groupings with common characteristics) are automatically derived based on intrinsic affinities and associations in the data without human indication of clustering, see Table 5.1. Unsupervised learning is purely based on input data (X) without corresponding output labels. The goal is to model the underlying structure, affinities, or distribution in the data in order to learn more about its intrinsic characteristics. It is called unsupervised learning because there are no *a priori* correct answers and there is no human guidance. Algorithms are left to their own devices to discover and present the interesting structure in the data. *Clustering* (discover the inherent groupings in the data) and *association* (discover association rules that describe the data) represent the core unsupervised learning problems. The **k-means** clustering and the **Apriori association rule** provide solutions to unsupervised learning problems.

In this chapter, we start with *supervised classification* methods, which utilize user-provided labels representative of specific classes associated with concrete observations, cases or units. These training classes/outcomes are used as references for the classification. Many problems can be addressed by decision-support systems utilizing combinations of supervised and unsupervised classification processes. Supervised learning involves input variables (X) and an outcome variable (Y) to learn mapping functions from the input to the output: $Y = f(X)$. The goal is to approximate the mapping function so that when it is applied to new (validation)

Table 5.1 Examples of different types of unsupervised learning techniques

Unsupervised clustering approaches

Bayesian		Hierarchical		Partitioning based			
Decision based	Nonparametric	Divisive (top-down)	Agglomerative (bottom-up)	Spectral	K-means centroid	Graph-theoretic	Model based
Bayesian classifier has high computational requirements. As there are a priori given labels, some prior is needed/specified to train the classifier, which is in turn used to label new data. Then, the newly labeled samples are subsequently used to train a new (supervised) classifier, i.e., decision-directed unsupervised learning. If the initial classifier is not appropriate, the process may diverge	Chinese restaurant process (CRP), infinite Hidden Markov Model (HMM)	Principal Direction Divisive Partitioning (PDDP)	Start with each case in a separate cluster and repeatedly join the closest pairs into clusters, until a stopping criterion is matched: (1) there is only a single cluster for all cases, (2) predetermined number of clusters is reached, (3) the distance between the closest clusters exceeds a threshold	SpecC	kmeans, hkmeans	Growing Neural Gas	mclust

Table 5.2 Examples of common types of supervised and unsupervised learning techniques

Inference	Outcome	Supervised	Unsupervised
Classification and prediction	Binary	Classification-Rules, OneR, kNN, naïve Bayes, Decision-Tree, C5.0, AdaBoost, XGBoost, LDA/QDA, Logit/Poisson, SVM	*Apriori*, Association-Rules, k-Means, naïve Bayes
Classification and prediction	Categorical	Regression Modeling & Forecasting	*Apriori*, Association-Rules, k-Means, naïve Bayes
Regression modeling	Real quantitative	(MLR) Regression Modeling, LDA/QDA, SVM, Decision-Tree, NeuralNet	Regression Modeling Tree, *Apriori*/Association-Rules

data (Z) it (accurately) predicts the (expected) outcome variables (Y). It is called supervised learning because the learning process is supervised by initial training labels guiding and correcting the learning until the algorithm achieves an acceptable level of performance.

Regression (output variable is a real value) and *classification* (output variable is a category) problems represent the two types of supervised learning. Examples of supervised machine learning algorithms include *Linear regression* and *Random Forest*; both provide solutions for regression-type problems, but *Random forest* also provides solutions to classification problems.

Just like the categorization of exploratory data analytics that we discussed in Chap. 3 is challenging, so is systematic codification of complementary machine learning techniques. Table 5.2 attempts to provide a rough representation of common machine learning methods. However, it is not really intended to be a gold-standard protocol for choosing the best analytical method. Before you settle on a specific strategy for data analysis, you should always review the data characteristics in light of the assumptions of each technique and assess the potential to gain new knowledge or extract valid information from applying a specific technique.

Many of these will be discussed in later chapters. In this chapter, we will present step-by-step the *k-nearest neighbor (kNN)* algorithm. Specifically, we will demonstrate (1) data retrieval and normalization, (2) splitting the data into *training* and *testing* sets, (3) fitting models on the training data, (4) evaluating model performance on testing data, (5) improving model performance, and (6) determining optimal values of k.

In Chap. 9, we will present detailed strategies and evaluation metrics to assess the performance of all clustering and classification methods.

5.1   k-Nearest Neighbor Approach

Classification tasks could be very difficult for datasets with a large number of complex and heterogeneous features and a broad range of target classes. In those scenarios, where the items of similar class type tend to be homogeneous, nearest neighbor classification may be appropriate because assigning unlabeled cases to their most similarly labeled neighbors may be fairly easy to accomplish.

Such classification methods can help us understand the intrinsic process mechanisms and apply them to characterize new unlabeled observations by examining the class labels of their neighbors. Such topological neighborhoods classification techniques are *distribution-free*, i.e., they have no prior distribution assumptions. However, this nonparametric approach makes the methods rely heavily on the training instances, which explains their *lazy algorithms* designation.

The k-Nearest Neighbor (kNN) algorithm involves the following steps:

1. Create a training dataset that has classified examples labeled by nominal variables and different features in ordinal or numerical variables.
2. Create a *testing* dataset containing unlabeled examples with similar features as the *training* data.
3. Given a predetermined number k, match each *test case* with the k closest *training* records that are "nearest" to the test case, according to a certain similarity or distance measure.
4. Assign a *test case* class label according to the majority vote of the k nearest training cases.

Mathematically, for a given k, a specific similarity metric d, and a new testing case x, the kNN classifier performs two steps (k is typically *odd* to avoid ties):

- Runs through the whole training dataset (y) computing $d(x, y)$. Let A represent the k closest points to x in the training data y.
- Estimates the conditional probability for each class, which corresponds to the fraction of points in A with that given class label. If $I(z)$ is an indicator function
$I(z) = \begin{cases} 1 & z = \text{true} \\ 0 & \text{otherwise} \end{cases}$, then the testing data input x gets assigned to the class with the largest probability, $P(y = j \mid X = x)$:

$$P(y = j \mid X = x) = \frac{1}{k} \sum_{i \in A} I\left(y^{(i)} = j\right).$$

5.2 Distance Function and Dummy Coding

How do we measure the similarity between records? We can think of similarity measures as distance metrics between the pairs of records or cases. There are many distance functions to choose from. Traditionally, we use *Euclidean distance* as our similarity metric.

If we use a line to connect the two points representing the testing and the training records in n dimensional space, the length of the line is the Euclidean distance. If a, b both have n features, the coordinates for them are $(a_1, a_2, \cdots, a_n)$ and $(b_1, b_2, \cdots, b_n)$. The Euclidean distance is

$$\text{dist}(a, b) = \sqrt{(a_1 - b_1)^2 + (a_2 - b_2)^2 + \cdots + (a_n - b_n)^2}.$$

When we have nominal features, it requires some care before applying a quantitative distance measure, such as the Euclidean distance. We could create dummy variables as indicators of all the nominal feature levels. The dummy variable would equal one when we have the feature and zero otherwise. Here are two examples:

$$\text{Gender} = \begin{cases} 0 & X = \text{male} \\ 1 & X = \text{female} \end{cases}, \text{Cold} = \begin{cases} 0 & \text{Temp} \geq 37F \\ 1 & \text{Temp} < 37F \end{cases}.$$

These dichotomous examples can easily be generalized to account for multiple nominal categories. In such situations, we create a new dummy variable for each categorical level and then compute the (Euclidean) distance using the pairwise differences between the binary dummy variables, also called *one-hot-encoding* features.

5.2.1 *Estimation of the Hyperparameter* k

The parameter k could not be too large or too small. If our k is too large, the test record tends to be classified as the most popular class in the training records, rather than the most similar one. On the other hand, if the k is too small, outliers, noise, or mislabeled training data cases might lead to errors in predictions. The common practice is to calculate the square root of the number of training cases and use that number as an (initial) estimate of k. A more robust way would be to choose several k values and select the one with the optimal (best) classifying performance.

5.2.2   Rescaling of the Features

Different features might have different scales. For example, we can have a measure of pain scaling from 1 to 10 or 1 to 100. Some similarity or distance measures assume the same measuring unit in all feature dimensions. This requires that the data may need to be transferred into the same scale. Re-scaling can make each feature contribute to the distance in a relatively equal manner, avoiding potential bias.

5.2.3   Rescaling Formulas

There are many alternative strategies to rescale a dataset. Here are two examples

- min–max normalization

$$X_{new} = \frac{X - \min(X)}{\max(X) - \min(X)}.$$

After re-scaling the data, X_{new} would range from 0 to 1, representing the distance between each value and its minimum as a percentage. Larger values indicate further distance from the minimum, 100% means that the value is at the maximum.

- z-score standardization

$$X_{new} = \frac{X - \bar{\mu}}{\hat{\sigma}} = \frac{X - \text{Mean}(X)}{\text{SD}(X)}.$$

This is based on the properties of normal distribution that we have talked about in Chap. 2. After z-score standardization, the re-scaled feature will have unbounded range. This is different from the min–max normalization which always has a finite range from 0 to 1. Following z-score standardization, the transformed features are *uniteless* and may resemble standard normal distribution.

5.2.4   Case Study: Youth Development

Step 1: *Collecting Data*

The data we are using for this case study are the "Boys Town Study of Youth Development," which is the second case study, CaseStudy02_Boystown_Data.csv available in the supporting canvas website. The variables in this dataset include:

- **ID**: Case subject identifier
- **Sex**: dichotomous variable (1 = male, 2 = female)

- **GPA**: Interval-level variable with range of 0–5 (0—"A" average, 1—"B" average, 2—"C" average, 3—"D" average, 4—"E", 5—"F")
- **Alcohol use**: Interval level variable from 0 to 11 (drink everyday—never drinked)
- **Attitudes on drinking in the household**: Alcatt—Interval level variable from 0 to 6 (totally approve—totally disapprove)
- **DadJob**: 1—yes, dad has a job and 2—no
- **MomJob**: 1—yes and 2—no
- **Parent closeness** (example: In your opinion, does your mother make you feel close to her?)

  - Dadclose: Interval level variable 0–7 (usually never)
  - Momclose: interval level variable 0–7 (usually never)

- **Delinquency**:

  - larceny (how many times have you taken things >$50?): Interval level data 0–4 (never—many times)
  - vandalism: Interval level data 0–7 (never—many times)

Step 2: *Exploring and Preparing the Data*

First, we need to import the data and perform some data manipulations. Prior to using the Euclidean distance, we will generate dummy variables (one-hot-encoding preprocessing) for sex, dadjob, and momjob.

```
library(class)
library(gmodels)
boystown<-
  read.csv("https://umich.instructure.com/files/399119/download?download_frd=1", sep=" ")
boystown$sex <- boystown$sex-1
boystown$dadjob <- -1*(boystown$dadjob-2)
boystown$momjob <- -1*(boystown$momjob-2)
str(boystown)
## 'data.frame':    200 obs. of  11 variables:
## $ id        : int  1 2 3 4 5 6 7 8 9 10 ...
## $ sex       : num  0 0 0 0 1 1 0 0 1 1 ...
## $ gpa       : int  5 0 3 2 3 3 1 5 1 3 ...
## $ Alcoholuse: int  2 4 2 2 6 3 2 6 5 2 ...
## $ alcatt    : int  3 2 3 1 2 0 0 3 0 1 ...
## $ dadjob    : num  1 1 1 1 1 1 1 1 1 1 ...
## $ momjob    : num  0 0 0 0 1 0 0 0 1 1 ...
## $ dadclose  : int  1 3 2 1 2 1 3 6 3 1 ...
## $ momclose  : int  1 4 2 2 1 2 1 2 3 2 ...
## $ larceny   : int  1 0 0 3 1 0 0 0 1 1 ...
## $ vandalism : int  3 0 2 2 2 0 5 1 4 0 ...
```

The str() function reports that we have 200 observations and 11 variables. However, the ID variable is not important in this case study, so we can delete it, and we can focus on academic performance, *GPA*, recidivism, *vandalism* and *larceny, alcohol use*, or other outcome variables. One concrete example involves trying to predict *recidivism* and use knn to classify participants in two categories.

Let's focus on a specific outcome variable representing two or more infractions of *vandalism* and *larceny*, which can be considered as "**Recidivism.**" Participants with one or no infractions can be labeled as "Controls." First we can use PCA to explore the data and then construct the new derived *recidivism* variable and split the data into training and testing sets.

```
# First explore the data by running a PCA
rawData <- boystown[ , -1]; head(rawData)
pca1 <- prcomp(as.matrix(rawData), center = T)
summary(pca1)
## Importance of components:
##                            PC1    PC2    PC3    PC4    PC5    PC6     PC7
## Standard deviation      1.9264 1.6267 1.4556 1.3887 1.3023 1.2495 0.95092
## Proportion of Variance  0.2463 0.1756 0.1406 0.1280 0.1126 0.1036 0.06001
## Cumulative Proportion   0.2463 0.4219 0.5625 0.6905 0.8031 0.9067 0.96672
##                            PC8     PC9    PC10
## Standard deviation      0.46931 0.44030 0.29546
## Proportion of Variance  0.01462 0.01287 0.00579
## Cumulative Proportion   0.98134 0.99421 1.00000
pca1$rotation
##                     PC1            PC2           PC3           PC4          PC5
## sex          0.017329782  -0.041942445   0.038644169   0.028574405  -0.01345929
## gpa          0.050811919   0.251727224  -0.552866390   0.482012801  -0.12517612
## Alcoholuse  -0.955960402  -0.171043716  -0.004495945   0.207154515   0.09577419
## alcatt      -0.087619514   0.345341205  -0.639579077  -0.330797550   0.46933240
## dadjob       0.007936535  -0.001870547  -0.017028011   0.006888380  -0.01469275
## momjob       0.030397552  -0.003518869   0.008763667  -0.001482878  -0.02342974
## dadclose     0.052947782  -0.689075136  -0.246264250  -0.452876476   0.21528193
## momclose    -0.055904765  -0.273643927  -0.435005164  -0.092086033  -0.75752753
## larceny      0.063455041  -0.005344755  -0.108928362   0.033669839  -0.07405310
## vandalism   -0.254240056   0.486423422   0.147159970  -0.632255411  -0.35813577
##                     PC6           PC7           PC8          PC9         PC10
## sex          0.026402404   0.02939770  -0.996267983   0.036561664  -0.001236127
## gpa         -0.599548626  -0.13874602  -0.035498809   0.004136514   0.019965416
## Alcoholuse  -0.015534060   0.05830281  -0.002438336   0.032626941  -0.008177261
## alcatt       0.362724708   0.01546912  -0.045913748   0.019571649   0.001150003
## dadjob       0.001537909  -0.04457354   0.001761749   0.050310596  -0.997425089
## momjob       0.006536869  -0.01490905   0.037550689   0.997051461   0.051468175
## dadclose    -0.456556766  -0.04166384  -0.008660225   0.005147468   0.001021197
```

```
## momclose     0.381040880  -0.06639096   0.008710480  -0.018261764   0.020666371
## larceny     -0.084351462   0.98381408   0.026413939   0.013630662  -0.039663208
## vandalism   -0.383715180  -0.00198434  -0.042593385   0.003164270  -0.004956997
Y <- ifelse (boystown$vandalism + boystown$larceny > 1, "Recidivism", "Control")
# more than 1 vandalism or larceny conviction
X <- boystown[, -c(1, 10, 11)]   # covariates exclude ID, vandalism & larceny
boystown_z <- as.data.frame(lapply(X, scale))
bt_train <- boystown_z[1:150, ]
bt_test  <- boystown_z[151:200, ]
bt_train_labels <- Y[1:150]
bt_test_labels  <- Y[151:200]
table(bt_train_labels)
## bt_train_labels
##    Control Recidivism
##        46        104
```

Let's look at the proportions for the two categories in both the training and testing sets.

```
round(prop.table(table(bt_train_labels)), digits=2)
## bt_train_labels
##    Control Recidivism
##       0.31       0.69
round(prop.table(table(bt_test_labels)), digits=2)
## bt_test_labels
##    Control Recidivism
##        0.2        0.8
```

We can see that most of the participants have incidents related to recidivism (~70–80%).

The remaining eight features use different measuring scales. If we use these features directly, variables with larger scale may have a greater impact on the classification performance. Therefore, re-scaling may be useful to level the playing field.

Step 3: *Normalizing Data*

First let's create a new min–max function and validate its performance using some simulated data.

```
normalize<-function(x) {  return((x-min(x))/(max(x)-min(x)))  }
normalize(c(1, 2, 3, 4, 5))    # some test examples
## [1] 0.00 0.25 0.50 0.75 1.00
normalize(c(1, 3, 6, 7, 9))
## [1] 0.000 0.250 0.625 0.750 1.000
```

After confirming the function transforms the simulated data as expected, we can use `lapply()` to apply the normalization transformation to each element in a "list" of predictors.

```
boystown_n <- as.data.frame(lapply(bt_train, normalize))
# alternatively we can use "scale", as we showed above
# boystown_z <- as.data.frame(lapply(X, scale))
```

In practice, we may also compare the summary statistics derived from alternative normalization approaches before deciding on one specific preprocessing strategy.

Step 4: *Data Preparation—Creating Training and Test Datasets*

We have 200 observations in this dataset. The more data we use to train the algorithm, the more precise and lest variable the prediction is expected to be. We can use 3/4 of the data for training and the remaining 1/4 for testing. For simplicity, we will just take the first 75% cases as training and the remaining 25% as testing. Alternatively, we can use a randomization strategy to split the data into testing and training sets.

```
# may want to use random split of the raw data into training and testing
# subset_int <- sample(nrow(boystown_n),floor(nrow(boystown_n)*0.75))
# 75% training + 25% testing
# bt_train<- boystown_n [subset_int, ]; bt_test<-boystown_n[-subset_int, ]
# Note that the object boystown_n already excludes the outcome variable
(Delinquency), index 11!
bt_train <- boystown_z[1:150, ]
bt_test  <- boystown_z[151:200, ]
```

Then let's extract the *recidivism* labels or classes for the training and testing sets.

```
bt_train_labels <- Y[1:150]
bt_test_labels  <- Y[151:200]
```

Step 5: *Training a Model on the Data*

Next, we will use the class::knn() method for k-nearest neighborhood classification.

```
#install.packages('class', repos = "http://cran.us.r-project.org")
library(class)
```

The function knn() has the following invocation protocol:

```
p <- knn(train, test, class, k)
```

- train: data frame containing numeric training data (features)
- test: data frame containing numeric testing data (features)
- class/cl: class for each observation in the training data
- k: predetermined integer indicating the number of nearest neighbors.

We can first test with $k = 7$, which is less than the square root of our number of observations: $\sqrt{200} \approx 14$.

```
bt_test_pred <- knn(train=bt_train, test=bt_test, cl=bt_train_labels, k=7)
```

Step 6: *Evaluating Model Performance*

We utilize the CrossTable() function, see Chap. 2, to evaluate the kNN model. We have two classes in this example. The goal is to create a 2×2 table that shows the matched true and predicted classes as well as the unmatched ones. However chi-square values are not needed, and by using option prop. chisq=False, we can suppress their reporting.

```
# install.packages("gmodels", repos="http://cran.us.r-project.org")
library(gmodels)
CrossTable(x=bt_test_labels, y=bt_test_pred, prop.chisq = F)
##    Cell Contents
## |-------------------------|
## |                       N |
## |           N / Row Total |
## |           N / Col Total |
## |         N / Table Total |
## |-------------------------|
## Total Observations in Table:  50
##                 | bt_test_pred
## bt_test_labels  |   Control | Recidivism |  Row Total |
## ----------------|-----------|------------|------------|
##        Control  |         0 |         10 |         10 |
##                 |     0.000 |      1.000 |      0.200 |
##                 |     0.000 |      0.213 |            |
##                 |     0.000 |      0.200 |            |
## ----------------|-----------|------------|------------|
##     Recidivism  |         3 |         37 |         40 |
##                 |     0.075 |      0.925 |      0.800 |
##                 |     1.000 |      0.787 |            |
##                 |     0.060 |      0.740 |            |
## ----------------|-----------|------------|------------|
##   Column Total  |         3 |         47 |         50 |
##                 |     0.060 |      0.940 |            |
## ----------------|-----------|------------|------------|
```

In this table, the highlighted cell values in the first row first column and the second row-second column contain the number of cases that have predicted classes matching the true class labels. The other two cells (along the minor diagonal) represent the counts for unmatched cases. The *accuracy* of this classifier is calculated by: $\frac{\text{cell}[1, 1] + \text{cell}[2, 2]}{\text{total}} = \frac{37}{50} = 0.72$. Note that this value may slightly fluctuate each time you run the classifier, due to the stochastic nature of the algorithm.

Step 7: *Improving Model Performance*

The normalization strategy may play a role in the classification performance. We can try alternative standardization methods—standard z-score centralization and min–max normalization. Let's try standardization prior to training the kNN and predicting and assessing the accuracy of the results.

```
bt_test_pred <- knn(train=bt_train, test=bt_test, cl=bt_train_labels,
                    prob=T, k=14) # retrieve Probabilities
bt_test_predBin <- ifelse(attributes(bt_test_pred)$prob > 0.6,
                    "Recidivism", "Control")  # Binarize the probabilities
CT <- CrossTable(x=bt_test_labels, y=bt_test_predBin, prop.chisq = F)
```

In this case, the kNN performance using the z-score and the min–max normalization strategies are pretty similar. Albeit, in general, there may be marginal differences, e.g., a few more cases may be correctly labeled based on one of the standardization or normalization approaches.

Step 8:   *Testing Alternative Values of k*

Originally, we used the square root of 200 as our *k*. However, this might not be the best *k* in this study. We can test different *k*'s for their predicting performances.

```
bt_test_pred <- knn(train=bt_train, test=bt_test, cl=bt_train_labels, prob=T,
k=18)          # retrieve Probabilities
bt_test_predBin <- ifelse(attributes(bt_test_pred)$prob > 0.6, "Recidivism",
"Control")     # Binarize the probabilities
CT <- CrossTable(x=bt_test_labels, y=bt_test_predBin, prop.chisq = F)
print(paste0("Prediction accuracy of model 'bt_test_pred' (k=18) is ",
(CT$prop.tbl[1,1]+CT$prop.tbl[2,2]) ))
## [1] "Prediction accuracy of model 'bt_test_pred' (k=18) is 0.82"
```

The choice of the hyperparameter *k* in kNN clustering is very important and it can be fine-tuned using the e1071::tune.knn() of the caret::train() methods. Note that using the tune.knn() method without explicit control over the class-probability cutoff does not generate good results. Specifying that probability exceeding 0.6 corresponds to *recidivism* significantly improves the kNN performance using caret::train() and caret::predict() methods.

```
# install.packages("e1071")
library(e1071)
knntuning = tune.knn(x= bt_train, y = as.factor(bt_train_labels), k = 1:30)
knntuning
## - sampling method: 10-fold cross validation
## - best parameters:
##   k = 11
summary(knntuning)
library(caret)
knnControl <- trainControl(method = "cv", ## cross validation
    number = 10,   ## 10-fold
    summaryFunction=twoClassSummary, classProbs=TRUE, verboseIter=FALSE)
knn_model <- train(x=bt_train, y=bt_train_labels , metric = "ROC",
                   method = "knn", tuneLength = 20, trControl = knnControl)
print(knn_model)
## Resampling: Cross-Validated (10 fold)
## Summary of sample sizes: 135, 135, 134, 136, 136, 135, ...
## Resampling results across tuning parameters:
##   k    ROC        Sens   Spec
##   5    0.2924091  0.025  0.8854545
##   7    0.3630455  0.045  0.9245455
...
##  43    0.5879318  0.000  1.0000000
## ROC was used to select the optimal model using the largest value.
## The final value used for the model was k = 31.
library(dplyr)
summaryPredictions <- predict(knn_model, newdata = bt_test, type = "prob")
summaryPredictionsLabel <- ifelse (summaryPredictions$Recidivism > 0.6,
                         "Recidivism", "Control")
testDataPredSummary <- as.data.frame(cbind(trueLabels=bt_test_labels,
                         controlProb=summaryPredictions$Control,
                         recidivismProb=summaryPredictions$Recidivism,
                         knnPredLabel=summaryPredictionsLabel))
print(paste0("Accuracy = ", 2*as.numeric(table(testDataPredSummary$trueLabels
                         == testDataPredSummary $knnPredLabel)[2]), "%"))
## [1] "Accuracy = 78%"
```

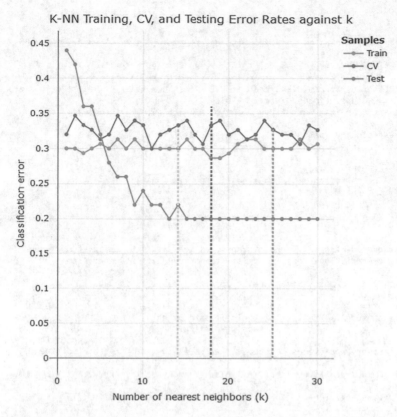

Fig. 5.1 Optimization of the kNN hyperparameter (k) using training, testing and cross-validation errors

It's useful to visualize the `error rate` against the value of k. This can help us select the optimal k parameter that minimizes the cross-validation (CV) error. Here, we will demonstrate a simple protocol for manually generating repeated folds from the data, which will be used to assess the performance of the kNN algorithm. More details and the general statistical cross-validation protocol will be presented later in Chap. 9 (Fig. 5.1).

```r
library(class)
library(ggplot2)
library(reshape2)
# define a function that generates CV folds
cv_partition <- function(y, num_folds = 10, seed = NULL) {
  if(!is.null(seed)) {    set.seed(seed)    }
  n <- length(y)
  # split() divides the data into the folds defined by gl().
  # gl() generates factors according to the pattern of their levels
  folds <- split(sample(seq_len(n), n), gl(n = num_folds, k = 1, length = n))
  folds <- lapply(folds, function(fold) {
    list(training = which(!seq_along(y) %in% fold), test = fold)
  })
  names(folds) <- paste0("Fold", names(folds))
  return(folds)
}
# Generate 10-folds of the data
folds = cv_partition(bt_train_labels, num_folds = 10)
# Define a training set_CV_error calculation function
train_cv_error = function(K) {
  # Train error
  knn_model <- train(x=bt_train, y=bt_train_labels , metric = "ROC",
                 method = "knn", tuneLength = 20, trControl = knnControl)
  summaryPredictions <- predict(knn_model, newdata = bt_train, type = "prob")
  summaryPredictionsLabel <- ifelse (summaryPredictions$Recidivism > 0.6,
                                  "Recidivism", "Control")
  train_error = mean(summaryPredictionsLabel != bt_train_labels)
  # CV error
  cverrbt = sapply(folds, function(fold) {
      knn_model <- train(x=bt_train[fold$training,],
                 y=bt_train_labels[fold$training], metric = "ROC",
                 method = "knn", tuneLength = 20, trControl = knnControl)
      summaryPredictions <- predict(knn_model, newdata=bt_train[fold$test,],
                              type = "prob")
      summaryPredictionsLabel <- ifelse (summaryPredictions$Recidivism > 0.6,
                              "Recidivism", "Control")
      mean(summaryPredictionsLabel != bt_train_labels[fold$test])
    }
  )


  cv_error = mean(cverrbt)
  #Test error
  knn.test = knn(train = bt_train, test = bt_test, cl = bt_train_labels, k=K)
  test_error = mean(knn.test != bt_test_labels)
  return(c(train_error, cv_error, test_error))
}
k_err = sapply(1:30, function(k) train_cv_error(k))
df_errs = data.frame(t(k_err), 1:30)
colnames(df_errs) = c('Train', 'CV', 'Test', 'K')
dataL <- melt(df_errs, id="K")
# Plot results
library(plotly)
plot_ly(dataL, x = ~K, y = ~value, color = ~variable, type = "scatter",
              mode = "markers+lines") %>%
  add_segments(x=25, xend=25, y=0.0, yend=0.33, type="scatter", name="k=9",
              line=list(color="darkgray", width = 2, dash = 'dot'),
              mode = "lines", showlegend=FALSE) %>%
  add_segments(x=14, xend=14, y=0.0, yend=0.33, type= "scatter", name="k=14",
              line=list(color="lightgray", width = 2, dash = 'dot'),
              mode = "lines", showlegend=FALSE) %>%
  add_segments(x=18, xend=18, y=0.0, yend=0.36, type="scatter",  name="k=18",
              line=list(color="gray", width = 2, dash = 'dot'),
              mode = "lines", showlegend=FALSE) %>%
  layout(title='K-NN Training, CV, and Testing Error Rates against k',
          legend=list(title=list(text='<b> Samples </b>')),
                  xaxis=list(title='Number of nearest neighbors (k)'),
                  yaxis=list(title='Classification error'))
```

Table 5.3 Confusion matrix

Confusion matrix	Reference negative	Reference positive
kNN fails to reject	TN	FN
kNN rejects	FP	TP
Metrics	Specificity = TN/(TN + FP)	Sensitivity = TP/(TP + FN)

Step 9S: *Quantitative Assessment*

Recall the fundamentals of hypothesis testing inference, which relies on estimation of the confusion matrix, Table 5.3.

Suppose we want to evaluate the kNN model ($k = 12$) in terms of its prediction of *recidivism*. We can manually compute and report some of the accuracy metrics for the kNN model ($k = 12$).

```
bt_test_pred <- knn(train=bt_train, test=bt_test,  cl=bt_train_labels,
                    prob=T, k=12) # retrieve Probabilities
bt_test_predBin <- ifelse(attributes(bt_test_pred)$prob > 0.6,
                    "Recidivism", "Control")   # Binarize the probabilities
CT <- CrossTable(x=bt_test_labels, y=ht_test_predBin, prop.chisq = F)
mod12_TN <  CT$prop.row[1, 1]
mod12_FP <- CT$prop.row[1, 2]
mod12_FN <- CT$prop.row[2, 1]
mod12_TP <- CT$prop.row[2, 2]
# Sensitivity and Specificity
mod12_sensi <- mod12_TN/(mod12_TN+mod12_FP)
mod12_speci <- mod12_TP/(mod12_TP+mod12_FN)
print(paste0("kNN model k=12 Sensitivity=", mod12_sensi))
## [1] "kNN model k=12 Sensitivity=0.2"
print(paste0("kNN model k=12 Specificity=", mod12_speci))
## [1] "kNN model k=12 Specificity=0.875"
table(bt_test_labels, bt_test_predBin)
```

Therefore, model12, corresponding to $k = 12$, yields a marginal accuracy on the testing cases. Another strategy for model validation and improvement involves the use of the caret::confusionMatrix() method, which reports several complementary metrics quantifying the performance of the prediction model. Let's examine deeper the performance of model12 to predict *recidivism* (Fig. 5.2).

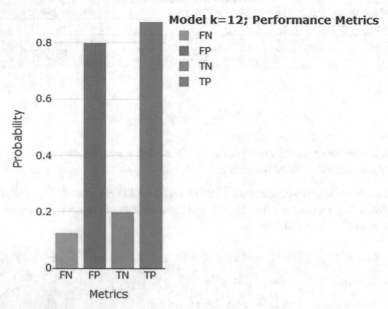

Fig. 5.2 Barplot of the confusion matrix for the kNN model (k = 12)

```
# install.packages("caret")
library("caret")
# Model 12: bt_test_predBin
confusionMatrix(as.factor(bt_test_labels), as.factor(bt_test_predBin))
## Confusion Matrix and Statistics
##
##                 Reference
## Prediction    Control Recidivism
##    Control        2          8
##    Recidivism     5         35
##                  Accuracy : 0.74
##                    95% CI : (0.5966, 0.8537)
##       No Information Rate : 0.86
##       P-Value [Acc > NIR] : 0.9927
##                     Kappa : 0.0845
##    Mcnemar's Test P-Value : 0.5791
##               Sensitivity : 0.2857
##               Specificity : 0.8140
##            Pos Pred Value : 0.2000
##            Neg Pred Value : 0.8750
##                Prevalence : 0.1400
##            Detection Rate : 0.0400
##      Detection Prevalence : 0.2000
##         Balanced Accuracy : 0.5498
```

```
plot_ly(x = c("TN", "FN", "FP", "TP"),
        y = c(mod12_TN, mod12_FN, mod12_FP, mod12_TP),
        name = c("TN", "FN", "FP", "TP"), type = "bar",
        color=c("TN", "FN", "FP", "TP")) %>%
  layout(title="Confusion Matrix",
    legend=list(title=list(text='<b> Model k=12; Performance Metrics </b>')),
    xaxis=list(title='Metrics'), yaxis=list(title='Probability'))
```

5.2.5   Case Study: Predicting Galaxy Spins

Let's now use the SOCR Case-Study 22 (22_SDSS_GalaxySpins_Case_Study) to train a kNN classifier on 49,122 (randomly selected galaxies, out of a total 51,122) training cases and test the accuracy of predicting the Galactic Spin (L = left or R = right hand spin) on the remaining (randomly chosen testing 2000) galaxies. We will first evaluate and report the classifier performance, and then, compare and improve the performance of several independent classifiers that will be described later, e.g., kNN, naïve Bayesian, LDA.

In addition, we will graph the training, testing and CV error rates for different hyperparameters and justify an "optimal" choice for $k = k_o$ (Fig. 5.3).

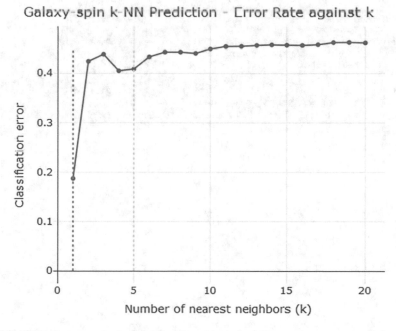

Fig. 5.3 kNN hyperparameter tuning using the galaxy-spin data

```r
# Load necessary R Libraries
library(e1071); library(caret); library(class); library(gmodels)
# Loading Galaxy data
galaxy_data <-
 read.csv("https://umich.instructure.com/files/6105118/download?download_frd=1", sep=",")
dim(galaxy_data)  ## [1] 51122     12
galaxy_data <- galaxy_data[ , -1]   # drop the Galaxy ID from covariates
str(galaxy_data)
## 'data.frame':    51122 obs. of  11 variables:
##  $ RA    : num   236 237 238 238 238 ...
##  $ DEC   : num   -0.493 -0.482 -0.506 -0.544 -0.527 ...
##  $ HAND  : chr   "R" "L" "L" "L" ...
##  $ UZS   : num   17.4 19.2 19.4 19.5 17.8 ...
##  $ GZS   : num   16.2 18 17.5 18.3 16.6 ...
##  $ RZS   : num   15.6 17.4 16.6 17.9 16.2 ...
##  $ IZS   : num   15.2 17 16.2 17.6 15.8 ...
##  $ ZZS   : num   14.9 16.7 15.8 17.3 15.6 ...
##  $ ELLIPS: num   0.825 0.961 0.411 0.609 0.505 ...
##  $ PHIS  : num   154 100.2 29.2 109.4 39.6 ...
##  $ RSS   : num   0.0547 0.0977 0.0784 0.076 0.0796 ...
# randomly save 2k galaxies for validation purposes
subset_int <- sample(nrow(galaxy_data), 2000)
# training data, dropping the label
galaxy_data_train<- galaxy_data[-subset_int,-3]; dim(galaxy_data_train)
galaxy_data_test <- galaxy_data[subset_int, -3]; dim(galaxy_data_test)
# Labels
galaxy_train_labels <- as.factor(galaxy_data[-subset_int, 3])
galaxy_test_labels  <- as.factor(galaxy_data[subset_int, 3])
gd_test_pred1<-knn(train=galaxy_data_train, test=galaxy_data_test,
                   cl=galaxy_train_labels, k=1)
gd_test_pred10<-knn(train=galaxy_data_train, test=galaxy_data_test,
                    cl=galaxy_train_labels, k=10)
gd_test_pred20<-knn(train=galaxy_data_train, test=galaxy_data_test,
                    cl=galaxy_train_labels, k=20)
gd_test_pred50<-knn(train=galaxy_data_train, test=galaxy_data_test,
                    cl=galaxy_train_labels, k=50)
ct_1<-CrossTable(x=galaxy_test_labels, y=gd_test_pred1, prop.chisq = F)
                    cl=galaxy_train_labels, k=20)
gd_test_pred50<-knn(train=galaxy_data_train, test=galaxy_data_test,
                    cl=galaxy_train_labels, k=50)
ct_1<-CrossTable(x=galaxy_test_labels, y=gd_test_pred1, prop.chisq = F)
```

```
##      Cell Contents
## |-------------------------|
## |                       N |
## |             N / Row Total |
## |             N / Col Total |
## |           N / Table Total |
## |-------------------------|
## Total Observations in Table:  2000
##                   | gd_test_pred1
## galaxy_test_labels |          L |          R | Row Total |
## -------------------|------------|------------|------------|
##                  L |        997 |         22 |       1019 |
##                    |      0.978 |      0.022 |      0.509 |
##                    |      0.973 |      0.023 |            |
##                    |      0.498 |      0.011 |            |
## -------------------|------------|------------|------------|
##                  R |         28 |        953 |        981 |
##                    |      0.029 |      0.971 |      0.490 |
##                    |      0.027 |      0.977 |            |
##                    |      0.014 |      0.476 |            |
## -------------------|------------|------------|------------|
##       Column Total |       1025 |        975 |       2000 |
##                    |      0.512 |      0.487 |            |
## -------------------|------------|------------|------------|
# Alternatively we can use the tuning function
knn.tune = tune.knn(x= galaxy_data_train, y = galaxy_train_labels, k = 1:20,
                    tunecontrol=tune.control(sampling = "fix") , fix=10)
summary(knn.tune)    #Summarize the resampling results set
# plot(knn.tune)
df <- as.data.frame(cbind(x=knn.tune$performance$k,
                          y=knn.tune$performance$error))
plot_ly(df, x = ~x, y = ~y, type = "scatter", mode = "markers+lines") %>%
  add_segments(x=1, xend=1, y=0.0, yend=0.45, type = "scatter",
               line=list(color="gray", width = 2, dash = 'dot'),
               mode = "lines", showlegend=FALSE) %>%
  add_segments(x=5, xend=5, y=0.0, yend=0.45, type = "scatter",
               line=list(color="lightgray", width = 2, dash = 'dot'),
               mode = "lines", showlegend=FALSE) %>%
  layout(title='Galaxy-spin k-NN Prediction - Error Rate against k',
         xaxis=list(title='Number of nearest neighbors (k)'),
         yaxis=list(title='Classification error'))
```

5.3   Probabilistic Learning—Naïve Bayes Classification

In the previous section, we described the types of machine learning methods and presented a lazy learning classification of numerical data using k-nearest neighbors. What about nominal features or textual data? In this section, we will begin to explore some classification techniques for categorical data. Specifically, we will present the naïve Bayes algorithm, review its assumptions, discuss Laplace estimation, and apply the classifier on a Head and Neck Cancer Medication case study. Later, in Chap. 7, we will also discuss text mining and natural language processing of unstructured text data.

5.3.1 Overview of the Naïve Bayes Method

It may be useful to first review the basics of probability theory and Bayesian inference. Bayes classifiers use training data to calculate an observed probability of each class based on all the features. The probability links feature values to classes like a map. When labeling the test data, we utilize the feature values in the test data and the "map" to classify our test data with the most likely class. This idea seems simple, but the corresponding algorithmic implementations might be very sophisticated.

The best scenario of accurately estimating the probability of an outcome-class map is when all features simultaneously contribute to the Bayes classifier. The naïve Bayes algorithm is frequently used for text classifications. The maximum *a posteriori* assignment to the class label is based on obtaining the conditional probability density function for each feature given the value of the class variable.

5.3.2 Model Assumptions

The method name, *naïve* Bayes, suggests the dependence of the technique on some simple ("*naïve*") assumptions. Its most important assumption is that all the features are expected to be *equally important* and *independent*. This rarely happens with real world data. However, sometimes even when these assumptions are violated, naïve Bayes still performs fairly well, particularly when the number of features p is large. This is why the naïve Bayes algorithm is often used as a powerful text classifier.

There is an interesting theory explaining the relations between QDA (Quadratic Discriminant Analysis), LDA (Linear Discriminant Analysis), and naïve Bayes classification.[1]

5.3.3 Bayes Formula

Let's first define the set-theoretic Bayes formula. Assume that B_i's are mutually exclusive events, for all $i = 1, 2, \cdots, n$, where n represents the number of features. If A and B are two events, the Bayes conditional probability formula is expressed as follows:

$$\text{Posterior Probability} = \frac{\text{likelihood} \times \text{Prior Probability}}{\text{Marginal Likelihood}}.$$

Symbolically,

---

[1] https://doi.org/10.48550/arXiv.1906.02590

$$P(A|B) = \frac{P(B|A)P(A)}{P(B)}.$$

When $B_i's$ represent a partition of the event space, $S = \cup_i B_i$ and $B_i \cap B_j = \varnothing, \forall i \neq j,$ we have:

$$P(A|B) = \frac{P(B|A) \times P(A)}{P(B|B_1) \times P(B_1) + P(B|B_2) \times P(B_2) + \cdots + P(B|B_n) \times P(B_n)}.$$

Now, let's represent the Bayes formula in terms of classification using observed features. Having observed n features, F_i, for each of K possible `class` outcomes, C_k. Using the Bayes' theorem and decomposing the conditional probability, the Bayesian classifier may be reformulated as a more tractable estimate

$$P(C_k \mid F_1, \cdots, F_n) = \frac{P(F_1, \cdots, F_n|C_k)P(C_k)}{P(F_1, \cdots, F_n)}.$$

In the above expression, only the numerator depends on the class label, C_k, as the values of the features F_i are observed (or imputed) making the denominator constant. Let's focus on the numerator. The numerator essentially represents the `joint probability` model

$$P(F_1, \cdots, F_n|C_k)P(C_k) = \underbrace{P(F_1, \cdots, F_n, C_k)}_{\text{jointmodel}}.$$

Repeatedly using the chain rule and the definition of conditional probability simplifies this to

$$
\begin{aligned}
P(F_1, \cdots, F_n, C_k) &= P(F_1|F_2, \cdots, F_n, C_k) \times P(F_2, \cdots, F_n, C_k) = \\
&= P(F_1|F_2, \cdots, F_n, C_k) \times P(F_2|F_3, \cdots, F_n, C_k) \times P(F_3, \cdots, F_n, C_k) = \\
&= P(F_1|F_2, \cdots, F_n, C_k) \times P(F_2|F_3, \cdots, F_n, C_k) \times P(F_3|F_4, \cdots, F_n, C_k) \\
&\quad \times P(F_4, \cdots, F_n, C_k) \\
&= \cdots = \\
&= P(F_1|F_2, \cdots, F_n, C_k) \times P(F_2|F_3, \cdots, F_n, C_k) \\
&\quad \times P(F_3|F_4, \cdots, F_n, C_k) \times \cdots \times P(F_n|C_k)
\end{aligned}
$$

Note that the "naïve" qualifier in the method name, *naïve Bayes classifier*, is attributed to the oversimplification of the conditional probability. Assuming each feature F_i is conditionally statistically independent of every other feature $F_j, \forall j \neq i,$ given the category C_k, we get

$$P(F_i|F_{i+1},\cdots,F_n,C_k)=P(F_i|C_k).$$

This reduces the joint probability model to

$$P(F_1,\cdots,F_n,C_k)=P(F_1|C_k)\times P(F_2|C_k)\times P(F_3|C_k)\times\cdots\times P(F_n|C_k)\times P(C_k).$$

Therefore, the joint model is simplified to

$$P(F_1,\cdots,F_n,C_k)=P(C_k)\prod_{i=1}^{n}P(F_i|C_k).$$

Essentially, we express the probability of class level L given an observation, represented as a set of *independent features* F_1, $F_2,\cdots$, F_n. Then, the posterior probability that the observation is in class L is equal to

$$P(C_L|F_1,\cdots,F_n)=\frac{P(C_L)\prod_{i=1}^{n}P(F_i|C_L)}{\prod_{i=1}^{n}P(F_i)},$$

where the denominator, $\prod_{i=1}^{n}P(F_i)$, is a scaling factor that represents the marginal probability of observing all features jointly.

For a given case $X=(F_1,F_2,\cdots,F_n)$, i.e., given vector of observed *features*, the naïve Bayes classifier assigns the *most likely class* $\widehat{C}$ by calculating $\dfrac{P(C_L)\prod_{i=1}^{n}P(F_i|C_L)}{\prod_{i=1}^{n}P(F_i)}$ for all class labels L, and then assigning the class $\widehat{C}$ corresponding to the *maximum posterior probability*. Analytically, the ultimate class label assignment $\widehat{C}$ is defined by

$$\widehat{C}=\arg\max_{L}\frac{P(C_L)\prod_{i=1}^{n}P(F_i|C_L)}{\prod_{i=1}^{n}P(F_i)}.$$

As the denominator is static for L, the posterior probability above is maximized when the numerator is maximized, i.e., $\widehat{C}=\arg\max_{L}P(C_L)\prod_{i=1}^{n}P(F_i|C_L)$.

The contingency table below illustrates schematically how the Bayesian, marginal, conditional, and joint probabilities may be calculated for a finite number of features (columns) and classes (rows).

Features \classes	F_1	F_2	$\cdots$	F_n	Total
C_1	$\cdots$	$\cdots$	$\cdots$	$\cdots$	Marginal $P(C_1)$
C_2	$\cdots$	$\cdots$	$\cdots$	Joint $P(C_2, F_n)$	$\cdots$
$\vdots$	$\vdots$	$\vdots$	$\vdots$	$\vdots$	$\vdots$
C_L	Conditional $P(F_1 \mid C_L) = \frac{P(F_1, C_L)}{P(C_L)}$	$\cdots$	$\cdots$	$\cdots$	$\cdots$
Total		Marginal $P(F_2)$	$\cdots$	$\cdots$	N

In the online DSPA2 Appendix, we provide additional technical details, code, and applications of Bayesian simulation, modeling, and inference.

5.3.4 The Laplace Estimator

If at least one $P(F_i \mid C_L) = 0$, then $P(C_L \mid F_1, \cdots, F_n) = 0$, which yields that the probability of assigning this class is trivial. However, $P(F_i \mid C_L) = 0$ could happen by random chance, e.g., when selecting the training data, reflecting the possibility that some classes may not be present in the training observations.

One of the solutions to this scenario is *Laplace estimation*, also known as *Laplace smoothing*, which can be accomplished in two ways. One is to add a small positive value ϵ to each count in the frequency table, which ensures that each class-feature combination in the training data is nontrivial, i.e., $P(F_i \mid C_L) > 0$ for all i, L, and we avoid degenerate cases.

Another strategy is to add some small value, ϵ, to the numerator and denominator when calculating the posterior probability. Note that these small perturbations of the denominator should be larger than the changes in the numerator to avoid trivial (0) posterior for another class.

5.3.5 Case Study: Head and Neck Cancer Medication

Step 1: Collecting Data

We utilize the inpatient Head and Neck Cancer Medication data for this case study, which is the case study 14 in our data archive, which includes the following variables

- **PID:** coded patient ID
- **ENC_ID:** coded encounter ID

- **Seer_stage:** SEER cancer stage ($0 =$ In situ, $1 =$ Localized, $2 =$ Regional by direct extension, $3 =$ Regional to lymph nodes, $4 =$ Regional (both codes 2 and 3), $5 =$ Regional, NOS, $7 =$ Distant metastases/systemic disease, $8 =$ Not applicable, $9 =$ Unstaged, unknown, or unspecified)[2]
- **Medication_desc:** description of the chemical composition of the medication
- **Medication_summary:** brief description about medication brand and usage
- **Dose:** the dosage in the medication summary
- **Unit:** the unit for dosage in the Medication_summary
- **Frequency:** the frequency of use in the Medication_summary
- **Total_dose_count:** total dosage counts according to the Medication_summary

Step 2: Exploring and Preparing the Data

Let's first load and summarize the cancer dataset and change the `seer_stage` (cancer stage indicator) variable into a factor variable.

```
hn_med<-
    read.csv("https://umich.instructure.com/files/1614350/download?download_frd=1",
             stringsAsFactors = FALSE)
str(hn_med)
## 'data.frame':      662 obs. of  9 variables:
hn_med$seer_stage <- factor(hn_med$seer_stage)
str(hn_med$seer_stage)
```

Data Preparation—Processing Text Data for Analysis

As you can see, the `medication_summary` contains a great amount of text. We should do some text mining to prepare the data for analysis. In R, the `tm` package is a good choice for text mining.

```
# install.packages("tm", repos = "http://cran.us.r-project.org")
library(tm)
```

The first step in text mining is to convert text features (text elements) into a `corpus` object, which is a collection of text documents.

```
hn_med_corpus <- Corpus(VectorSource(hn_med$MEDICATION_SUMMARY))
print(hn_med_corpus)
```

After we construct the `corpus` object, the report indicates that we have 662 documents where each document represents an encounter (e.g., notes on medical treatment) for a patient.

---

[2]https://seer.cancer.gov/tools/ssm

```
inspect(hn_med_corpus[1:3])
## [1] (Zantac) 150 mg tablet oral two times a day
## [2] 5,000 unit subcutaneous three times a day
## [3] (Unasyn) 15 g IV every 6 hours
hn_med_corpus[[1]]$content
## [1] "(Zantac) 150 mg tablet oral two times a day"
hn_med_corpus[[2]]$content
## [1] "5,000 unit subcutaneous three times a day"
hn_med_corpus[[3]]$content
## [1] "(Unasyn) 15 g IV every 6 hours"
```

There are unwanted punctuations and other symbols in the corpus document that we want to remove. We use the `tm_map()` function for the cleaning.

```
corpus_clean <- tm_map(hn_med_corpus, tolower)
corpus_clean <- tm_map(corpus_clean, removePunctuation)
corpus_clean <- tm_map(corpus_clean, removeNumbers)
corpus_clean <- tm_map(corpus_clean, stripWhitespace)
```

The above lines of code changed all the characters to lowercase, removed all punctuations and extra white spaces (typically created by deleting punctuations), and removed numbers (we could also convert the corpus to plain text).

```
inspect(corpus_clean[1:3])
corpus_clean[[1]]$content
hn_med_dtm <- DocumentTermMatrix(corpus_clean)
```

The `DocumentTermMatrix()` function can successfully tokenize the medication summary into words. It can count frequent terms in each document in the corpus object.

Data Preparation—Creating Training and Test Datasets
Just like in the kNN method, we need to separate the dataset into training and test subsets. We have to subset the raw data with other features, the corpus object and the document term matrix.

```
set.seed(12345)      # 80% training + 20% testing
subset_int <- sample(nrow(hn_med),floor(nrow(hn_med)*0.8))
hn_med_train <- hn_med[subset_int, ]
hn_med_test <- hn_med[-subset_int, ]
hn_med_dtm_train <- hn_med_dtm[subset_int, ]
hn_med_dtm_test <-hn_med_dtm[-subset_int, ]
corpus_train <- corpus_clean[subset_int]
corpus_test  <- corpus_clean[-subset_int]
```

Let's examine the distribution of *seer stages* in the training and test datasets.

```
prop.table(table(hn_med_train$seer_stage))
prop.table(table(hn_med_test$seer_stage))
```

We can binarize (dichotomize) the seer_stage into two categories:

- *No stage* or *early stage* cancer (seer in [0;4]) and
- *Later stage* cancer (seer in [5;9])

Of course, other binarizations are possible as well. Note that a %in% b is an intuitive interface to match and acts as a binary operator returning a logical vector (T = True or F = False) indicating if there is a match between the left and right operands.

```
hn_med_train$stage <- hn_med_train$seer_stage %in% c(5:9)
hn_med_train$stage <- factor(hn_med_train$stage, levels=c(F, T),
                      labels = c("early_stage", "later_stage"))
hn_med_test$stage <- hn_med_test$seer_stage %in% c(5:9)
hn_med_test$stage <- factor(hn_med_test$stage, levels=c(F, T),
                      labels = c("early_stage", "later_stage"))
prop.table(table(hn_med_train$stage))
prop.table(table(hn_med_test$stage))
```

Visualizing Text Data—Word Clouds

A word cloud can help us visualize text data. More frequent words would have larger fonts in the figure, while less common words are appearing in smaller fonts. There is a wordcloud package in R that is commonly used for creating such word cloud figures (Fig. 5.4).

```
# install.packages("wordcloud", repos = "http://cran.us.r-project.org")
library(wordcloud)
wordcloud(corpus_train, min.freq=40,random.order=FALSE,colors=brewer.pal(5,"Dark2"))
early <- subset(hn_med_train, stage=="early_stage")
later <- subset(hn_med_train, stage=="later_stage")
wordcloud(early$MEDICATION_SUMMARY, max.words = 20, colors=brewer.pal(3, "Dark2"))
wordcloud(later$MEDICATION_SUMMARY, max.words = 20, colors=brewer.pal(3, "Dark2"))
```

The random.order=FALSE option makes more frequent words appear in the center of the word cloud. The min.freq=40 option sets the cutoff word frequency to be at least 40 times in the corpus object. Therefore, the words must appear in at least 40 medication summaries to be shown on the graph. This Figure shows the differences between the medical summaries of the early and later cancer stage patients.

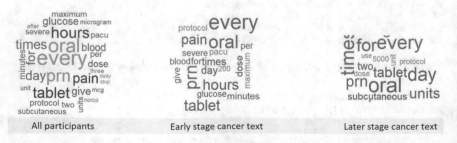

Fig. 5.4 Wordclouds of the preprocessed cancer medication summary (unstructured text)

Data Preparation—Creating Indicator Features for Frequent Words

For simplicity, we utilize the medication summary as the only feature to classify cancer stages. You may recall that earlier in the kNN section we used the native data features to obtain kNN classifications. *Now, we are going to enrich the data by adding frequencies of words as new text-derived data features.*

```
summary(findFreqTerms(hn_med_dtm_train, 5))
hn_med_dict <- as.character(findFreqTerms(hn_med_dtm_train, 5))
hn_train <- DocumentTermMatrix(corpus_train, list(dictionary=hn_med_dict))
hn_test  <- DocumentTermMatrix(corpus_test, list(dictionary=hn_med_dict))
```

This example limits the document term matrix to words that have appeared in at least five different documents. This creates (about) 118 new features.

The naïve Bayes classifier trains on data with categorical features, as it uses frequency tables for learning the data affinities. To create the combinations of *class* and *feature values* comprising the frequency-table (matrix), all features must be categorical. For instance, numeric features have to be converted (binned) into categories. Thus, we need to transform our *word count features* into categorical data. One way to achieve this is to change the count into an indicator of whether this word appears in the document describing the patient encounter. We can create a simple function to convert the presence of a specific word (column) in an encounter document (row) to a binary "Yes" (present) or "No" (absent).

```
convert_counts <- function(wordFreq) {
  wordFreq <- ifelse(wordFreq > 0, 1, 0)
  wordFreq <- factor(wordFreq, levels = c(0, 1), labels = c("No", "Yes"))
  return(wordFreq)
}
```

We employ hard-thresholding here x <- ifelse(x>0, 1, 0), which binarizes a feature x by comparing it to 1. Now let's apply this function convert counts() on each column (MARGIN=2) of the training and testing datasets.

```
hn_train <- apply(hn_train, MARGIN = 2, convert_counts)
hn_test <- apply(hn_test, MARGIN = 2, convert_counts)
# Check the structure of hn_train & hn_train: # head(hn_train); dim(hn_train)
```

So far, we successfully created indicators for words that appeared at least in five different documents in the training data. These new dummy variables enrich the smaller features set we used earlier and may improve subsequent supervised or unsupervised modeling, prediction, inference, or classification.

Step 3: *Training a Model on the Data*

We will use the e1071 package for demonstrating the naïve Bayes classification of the cancer data.

```
# install.packages("e1071", repos = "https://cran.us.r-project.org")
library(e1071)
hn_classifier <- naiveBayes(hn_train, hn_med_train$stage)
```

The function `naiveBayes()` has following invocation protocol

```
m <- naiveBayes(train, class, laplace=0)
```

- *train*: data frame containing numeric training data (features)
- *class*: factor vector with the class for each row in the training data.
- *laplace*: positive double controlling Laplace smoothing; default is 0 and disables Laplace smoothing.

Then, we can use the classifier to make predictions using the method `predict` `()`. Recall that when we presented the AdaBoost example in Chap. 2, we saw the general machine learning and artificial intelligence protocol, from *training*, to *prediction* and *assessment*.

For most supervised and unsupervised methods, the generic function `predict` `()` has the following invocation syntax

```
p <- predict(m, test, type="class")
```

- *m*: classifier, in our case `naiveBayes()`
- *test*: test data frame or matrix
- *type*: either `"class"` or `"raw"` specifies whether the predictions should be the most likely class value or the raw predicted probabilities.

```
hn_test_pred <- predict(hn_classifier, hn_test)
```

Step 4: *Evaluating Model Performance*

Similar to the approach in the earlier kNN method, we can use *cross table* to compare the predicted (naïve Bayes) vs. the true classes using the testing data (Fig. 5.5).

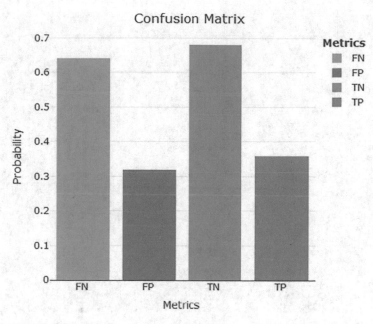

Fig. 5.5 Barplot of the confusion matrix corresponding to the naïve Bayesian classifier for the cancer dataset

```
library(gmodels)
CT <- CrossTable(hn_test_pred, hn_med_test$stage)
##    Cell Contents
## |-------------------------|
## |                       N |
## | Chi-square contribution |
## |           N / Row Total |
## |           N / Col Total |
## |         N / Table Total |
## |-------------------------|
## Total Observations in Table:  133
##              | hn_med_test$stage
## hn_test_pred | early_stage | later_stage |  Row Total |
## -------------|-------------|-------------|------------|
##  early_stage |          64 |          30 |         94 |
##              |       0.019 |       0.039 |            |
##              |       0.681 |       0.319 |      0.707 |
##              |       0.719 |       0.682 |            |
##              |       0.481 |       0.226 |            |
## -------------|-------------|-------------|------------|
##  later_stage |          25 |          14 |         39 |
##              |       0.046 |       0.093 |            |
##              |       0.641 |       0.359 |      0.293 |
##              |       0.281 |       0.318 |            |
##              |       0.188 |       0.105 |            |
## -------------|-------------|-------------|------------|
## Column Total |          89 |          44 |        133 |
```

```
##                        |        0.669 |        0.331 |              |
## -------------|-------------|-------------|-------------|
CT
##                   y
## x                     early_stage later_stage
##    early_stage                64          30
##    later_stage                25          14
## $prop.tbl
##                   y
## x                     early_stage later_stage
##    early_stage         0.4812030   0.2255639
##    later_stage         0.1879699   0.1052632
mod_TN <- CT$prop.row[1, 1]
mod_FP <- CT$prop.row[1, 2]
mod_FN <- CT$prop.row[2, 1]
mod_TP <- CT$prop.row[2, 2]
# caret::confusionMatrix(hn_test_pred, hn_med_test$stage)
# CT$prop.row
library(plotly)
plot_ly(x = c("TN", "FN", "FP", "TP"),
        y = c(mod_TN, mod_FN, mod_FP, mod_TP),
        name = c("TN", "FN", "FP", "TP"), type = "bar",
        color=c("TN", "FN", "FP", "TP")) %>%
  layout(title="Confusion Matrix",
             legend=list(title=list(text='<b> Metrics </b>')),
             xaxis=list(title='Metrics'), yaxis=list(title='Probability'))
```

It may be worth quickly looking forward to Chap. 9, where we present a summary table containing commonly used measures for evaluating the performance of binary tests, classifiers, or predictions. In this case, the *prediction accuracy* of the naïve Bayes classifier, assessed on the testing dataset, is:

$$\text{ACC} = \frac{\text{TP} + \text{TN}}{\text{TP} + \text{FP} + \text{FN} + \text{TN}} = \frac{78}{133} = 0.59.$$

Step 5: *Improving Model Performance*

By slightly altering the data preprocessing protocol and changing the parameter laplace=5, the accuracy goes to acc $= \frac{87}{133} = 0.65$. Although there is a small difference in accuracy, in general, such protocol alterations may increase or decrease the rate of true *later stage* patient identification using testing and validation data.

```
hn_med_dict <- as.character(findFreqTerms(hn_med_dtm_train, 5))
hn_train <- DocumentTermMatrix(corpus_train, list(dictionary=hn_med_dict))
hn_test  <- DocumentTermMatrix(corpus_test, list(dictionary=hn_med_dict))
# View(as.data.frame(inspect(hn_train)))
traindf <- data.frame(stage=hn_med_train$stage, as.matrix(hn_train))
testdf <- data.frame(stage=hn_med_test$stage, as.matrix(hn_test))
# Training and Testing data, transform predictors/features to factors
for (cols in names(traindf)) traindf[[cols]] <- factor(traindf[[cols]])
for (cols in names(testdf)) testdf[[cols]] <- factor(testdf[[cols]])
set.seed(1234)
hn_classifier1 <- naiveBayes(hn_train, hn_med_train$stage,
                             laplace = 5, type = "class")
hn_test_pred1 <- predict(hn_classifier1, hn_test)
caret::confusionMatrix(hn_test_pred1, testdf$stage)
```

Step 6: *Compare Naïve Bayesian vs. LDA*

The naïve Bayes with normality assumption is a special case of discriminant analysis. It might be interesting to compare the prediction results of *naïve Bayes* and linear discriminate analysis (*LDA*) classification. LDA assumes the predictors are jointly approximately normally distributed.

```
library(MASS)
library("dplyr")
binarizeFunction <- function(x) { ifelse(x=="Yes", 1,0) }
# A function to Convert Categorical variables to numeric
cat2Numeric <- function (dfInput) {
  df = as.data.frame(lapply( as.data.frame(dfInput), factor)) %>%
                        mutate_all(binarizeFunction)
  return(df)
}
# define the numeric DF of predictors (X) and outcome (Y=stage)
df_hn_train = data.frame(cat2Numeric(hn_train),
                         stage = as.numeric(hn_med_train$stage))
df_hn_test = data.frame(cat2Numeric(hn_test),
                        stage = as.numeric(hn_med_test$stage))
# Remove the multicollinearity - this should be done via VIF assessment,
#       but for now, just take the first few predictors
df_hn_train <- df_hn_train[ , c(1:34, 40:50, 60:70, 109)]
# Fit LDA
set.seed(1234)
hn_lda <- lda(data=df_hn_train, stage ~ .)
hn_pred = predict(hn_lda, df_hn_test)
CrossTable(hn_pred$class, df_hn_test$stage)
##    Cell Contents
## |-------------------------|
```

```
##  |                       N |
##  | Chi-square contribution |
##  |           N / Row Total |
##  |           N / Col Total |
##  |         N / Table Total |
##  |-------------------------|
## Total Observations in Table:  133
##                 | df_hn_test$stage
## hn_pred$class |         1 |         2 | Row Total |
## --------------|-----------|-----------|-----------|
##             1 |        83 |        33 |       116 |
##               |     0.372 |     0.753 |           |
##               |     0.716 |     0.284 |     0.872 |
##               |     0.933 |     0.750 |           |
##               |     0.624 |     0.248 |           |
## --------------|-----------|-----------|-----------|
##             2 |         6 |        11 |        17 |
##               |     2.541 |     5.139 |           |
##               |     0.353 |     0.647 |     0.128 |
##               |     0.067 |     0.250 |           |
##               |     0.045 |     0.083 |           |
## --------------|-----------|-----------|-----------|
##  Column Total |        89 |        44 |       133 |
##               |     0.669 |     0.331 |           |
## --------------|-----------|-----------|-----------|
```

There are differences in the performance of the naïve Bayesian (acc $= \frac{87}{133} = 0.65$) and the LDA classifiers (acc $= \frac{94}{133} = 0.7$) in terms of the overall accuracy. LDA has a lower type II error ($\frac{33}{133} = 0.25$), compared to naïve Bayesian with parameter laplace $= 5$ ($\frac{40}{133} = 0.30$). This may be clinically important to avoid missing the critically important later-stage cancer patients. In later chapters, we will step deeper into the space of classification problems and see more sophisticated approaches, especially for difficult problems like cancer forecasting.

5.4   Decision Trees and Divide-and-Conquer Classification

When classification models need to be *apparent* and directly mechanistically interpreted, kNN and naïve Bayes methods we saw earlier may not be useful, as they do not yield explicit classification rules. In some cases, we need to derive direct and clear rules for our classification decisions. Just like a driving ability test, credit scoring, or grading rubrics, mechanistic understanding of the derived labeling, prediction, or decision-making is often beneficial. For instance, we can assign credit, or deduct a penalty, for each driving operation task. These rules facilitate the critical decision to issue a driver license to applicants that are qualified, ready, and able to safely operate a specific type of a motor vehicle.

In this section, we will see a simple motivational example of decision trees based on the Iris data and describe decision tree divide-and-conquer methods. Also, we will examine certain measures quantifying classification accuracy, show strategies for pruning decision trees, work through a Quality of Life in Chronic Disease case study, and review the *One Rule* and *RIPPER* algorithms.

5.4.1   Motivation

Decision tree learners enable classification via tree structures modeling the relationships among all features and potential outcomes in the data. All decision trees begin with a trunk representing all points that are part of the same cohort. Iteratively, the trunk is split into narrower and narrower branches by forking-decisions based on the intrinsic data structure. At each step, splitting the data into branches may include binary or multinomial classification. The final decision is obtained when the tree branching process terminates. The terminal (leaf) nodes represent the action to be taken as the result of the series of branching decisions. For predictive models, the leaf nodes provide the expected forecasting results given the series of events in the decision tree. There are a number of R packages available for decision tree classification including rpart, C5.0, party, etc.

5.4.1.1   Hands-On Example: Iris Data

Let's start by seeing a simple example using the Iris dataset, which we saw in Chap. 2. The data features or attributes include `Sepal.Length`, `Sepal.Width`, `Petal.Length`, and `Petal.Width`, and classes are represented by the `Species taxa` (setosa, versicolor, and virginica).

```
# install.packages("party")
library("party")
str(iris)
## 'data.frame':    150 obs. of  5 variables:
##  $ Sepal.Length: num  5.1 4.9 4.7 4.6 5 5.4 4.6 5 4.4 4.9 ...
##  $ Sepal.Width : num  3.5 3 3.2 3.1 3.6 3.9 3.4 3.4 2.9 3.1 ...
##  $ Petal.Length: num  1.4 1.4 1.3 1.5 1.4 1.7 1.4 1.5 1.4 1.5 ...
##  $ Petal.Width : num  0.2 0.2 0.2 0.2 0.2 0.4 0.3 0.2 0.2 0.1 ...
##  $ Species     : Factor w/ 3 levels "setosa","versicolor",..: 1 1 1 1 ...
head(iris); table(iris$Species)
##   Sepal.Length Sepal.Width Petal.Length Petal.Width Species
## 1          5.1         3.5          1.4         0.2  setosa
## 2          4.9         3.0          1.4         0.2  setosa
...
##     setosa versicolor  virginica
##         50         50         50
```

The `ctree(Species ~ Sepal.Length + Sepal.Width + Petal.Length + Petal.Width, data=iris)` function will build a conditional-inference decision tree model of the outcome iris species (Fig. 5.6).

```
iris_ctree <- ctree(Species ~ Sepal.Length + Sepal.Width + Petal.Length +
                    Petal.Width, data=iris)
print(iris_ctree)
##    Conditional inference tree with 4 terminal nodes
## Response:  Species
## Inputs:  Sepal.Length, Sepal.Width, Petal.Length, Petal.Width
## Number of observations:  150
## 1) Petal.Length <= 1.9; criterion = 1, statistic = 140.264
##   2)* weights = 50
## 1) Petal.Length > 1.9
##   3) Petal.Width <= 1.7; criterion = 1, statistic = 67.894
##     4) Petal.Length <= 4.8; criterion = 0.999, statistic = 13.865
##       5)* weights = 46
##     4) Petal.Length > 4.8
##       6)* weights = 8
##   3) Petal.Width > 1.7
##     7)* weights = 46
plot(iris_ctree, cex=2)  # party::plot.BinaryTree()
```

Similarly, we can demonstrate a classification of the *iris taxa* via the method `rpart()` (Fig. 5.7).

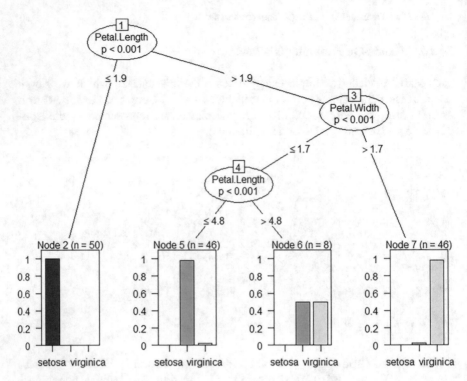

Fig. 5.6 Decision tree classification graph for the iris dataset illustrating explicit rules for deriving flower labels using a set of sepal and petal morphometric measures

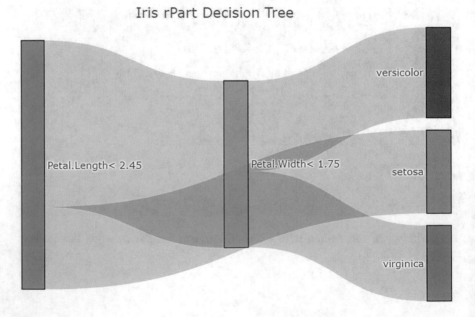

Fig. 5.7 Sankey chart of a simple decision tree illustrating an explicit classification graph for the iris flowers dataset. At run time, this interactive SVG plot provides additional information using mouse events and actions

```
library(rpart)
library(rpart.utils)
library(plotly)
iris_rpart <- rpart(Species ~ . , method="class", data=iris)
# Set the Graph/Tree Node names
treeFrame <- iris_rpart$frame
# Identify Leaf nodes
isLeave <- treeFrame$var == "<leaf>"
nodes <- rep(NA, length(isLeave))
# Get 3 Isis taxa labels: "setosa", "versicolor", "virginica" for all nodes
ylevel <- attr(iris_rpart, "ylevels")
nodes[isLeave] <- ylevel[treeFrame$yval][isLeave]
nodes[!isLeave] <- labels(iris_rpart)[-1][!isLeave[-length(isLeave)]]
# Get all Tree Graph Connections (source --> target)
treeFrame <- iris_rpart$frame
treeRules <- rpart.utils::rpart.rules(iris_rpart)


targetPaths <- sapply(as.numeric(row.names(treeFrame)),
                function(x) { strsplit(unlist(treeRules[x]),split=",") } )
lastStop <- sapply(1:length(targetPaths),
              function(x) { targetPaths[[x]][length(targetPaths[[x]])] } )
oneBefore <- sapply(1:length(targetPaths),
              function(x) { targetPaths[[x]][length(targetPaths[[x]])-1] } )
# Initialize the tree edges
target=c()
source=c()
values=treeFrame$n
for(i in 2:length(oneBefore)) {
  tmpNode=oneBefore[[i]]
  q = which(lastStop==tmpNode)
  q=ifelse(length(q)==0, 1, q)
  source = c(source, q)
  target = c(target, i)
}
source=source-1
target=target-1
# Display the sankey tree
plot_ly(type = "sankey", orientation = "h",
        node = list(label = nodes, pad = 15, thickness = 30),
        line = list(color="black", width=1)),
        link = list(source = source, target = target, value=values[-1])) %>%
  layout(title = "Iris rPart Decision Tree", font = list(size = 12))
```

5.4.2 Decision Tree Overview

Decision tree algorithms represent upside down trees with lots of branches where a series of logical decisions are encoded as branches between nodes of the tree. The classification begins at the root node (containing all cases) and goes through many branches until it gets to the terminal nodes. This iterative process splits the data into different classes by a rigid criterion.

5.4.2.1 Divide and Conquer

Decision trees involve recursive partitioning that use data features and attributes to split the data into groups (nodes) of similar classes. To make classification trees using data features, we need to observe the pattern between the data features and potential classes using training data. We can draw scatter plots and separate groups that are clearly bundled together. Each of the groups is considered a segment of the data. After getting the approximate range of each feature value within each group, we can make the decision tree. Here is a common schematic illustrating a second-order data tensor as a data frame or an array with rows and columns indexing cases and features

$$X = [X_1, X_2, X_3, \cdots, X_k] = \left.\begin{pmatrix} x_{1,1} & x_{1,2} & \cdots & x_{1,k} \\ x_{2,1} & x_{2,2} & \cdots & x_{2,k} \\ \vdots & \vdots & \ddots & \vdots \\ x_{n,1} & x_{n,2} & \cdots & x_{n,k} \end{pmatrix}\right\}\ \text{cases}$$

$$\underbrace{\hphantom{xxxxxxxxxxxxxxxxxxxxxx}}_{\text{features/attributes}}$$

The decision tree algorithms use a top-down recursive divide-and-conquer approach (sometimes they may also use bottom up or mixed splitting strategies) to divide and evaluate the splits of a dataset D (input). The best split decision corresponds to the split with the *highest information gain*, reflecting a partition of the data into K subsets (using divide-and-conquer). The iterative algorithm terminates when some stopping criteria are reached. Examples of stopping conditions used to terminate the recursive process include:

- All the samples belong to the same class, that is, they have the same label, and the sample is already `pure`.
- Stop when the majority of the points are already of the same class (relative to some error threshold).
- There are no remaining attributes on which the samples may be further partitioned.

One objective criterion for splitting or clustering data into groups is based on the *information gain measure*, or *impurity reduction*, which can be used to select the test attribute at each node in the decision tree. The attribute with the highest information gain (i.e., greatest entropy reduction) is selected as the test attribute for the current node. This attribute minimizes the information needed to classify the samples in the resulting partitions. There are three main measures to evaluate the impurity reduction—*Misclassification error, Gini index*, and *Entropy*.

For a given table containing pairs of attributes and their class labels, we can assess the homology of the classes in the table. A table is pure (homogeneous) if it only contains a single class. If a data table contains several classes, then we say that the table is impure or heterogeneous. This degree of impurity or heterogeneity can be quantitatively evaluated using impurity measures like entropy, Gini index, and misclassification error.

5.4.2.2   Entropy

The Entropy is an information measure of the amount of disorder or uncertainty in a system. Suppose we have a data set $D = (X_1, X_2, \cdots, X_n)$ that includes n features (variables) and suppose each of these features can take on any of k possible values (states). Then the cardinality of the entire system is k^n as each of the features are assumed to have k independent states, thus the total number of different datasets that can be expected is $\underbrace{k \times k \times k \times \cdots \times k}_{n} = k^n$. Suppose $p_1, p_2, \cdots, p_k$ represent the proportions of each class (by the law of total probability, $\sum_i p_i = 1$) present in the child node that results from a split in a decision tree classifier. Then the entropy measure is defined by

$$\text{Entropy}(D) = -\sum_i p_i \log_2 p_i.$$

If each of the $1 \leq i \leq k$ states for each feature is equally likely to be observed with probability $p_i = \frac{1}{k}$, then the entropy is *maximized*

$$\text{Entropy}(D) = -\sum_{i=1}^{k} \frac{1}{k} \log \frac{1}{k} = \sum_{i=1}^{k} \frac{1}{k} \log k = k \frac{1}{k} \log k = \log k = O(1).$$

In the other extreme, the entropy is *minimized* when the probability of one class is unitary and all other classes are associated with trivial likelihoods. Note that by L'Hopital's Rule[3] $\lim_{x \to 0} (x \log(x)) = \lim_{x \to 0} \frac{\frac{1}{x}}{-\frac{1}{x^2}} = \lim_{x \to 0} x = 0$ for a single class classification where the probability of one class is unitary ($p_{i_o} = 1$) and the other ones are trivial ($p_{i \neq i_o} = 0$)

$$\text{Entropy}(D) = p_{i_o} \times \log p_{i_o} + \sum_{i \neq i_o} p_i \log p_i = 1 \times \log 1$$

$$+ \lim_{x \to 0} \sum_{i \neq i_o} x \log(x) = 0 + 0 = 0.$$

In classification settings, higher entropy (i.e., more disorder) corresponds to a sample that has a *mixed collection of labels*. Conversely, lower entropy corresponds to a classification where we have mostly pure partitions. In general, the entropy of a sample $D = \{X_1, X_2, \cdots, X_n\}$ is defined by

$$H(D) = -\sum_{i=1}^{k} P(c_i|D) \log P(c_i|D),$$

---

[3] https://doi.org/10.5951/MT.56.4.0257

where $P(c_i|D)$ is the probability of a data point in D being labeled with class c_i, and k is the number of classes (clusters). $P(c_i|D)$ can be estimated from the observed data by

$$P(c_i|D) = \frac{P(D|c_i)P(c_i)}{P(D)} = \frac{|\{x_j \in D|x_j \text{ has label } y_j = c_i\}|}{|D|}.$$

When the observations are evenly split among all k classes then $P(c_i|D) = \frac{1}{k}$ and the entropy is maximized (chaotic system)

$$H(D) = -\sum_{i=1}^{k} \frac{1}{k} \log \frac{1}{k} = \log k = O(1).$$

At the other extreme, if all the observations are from one class, then the entropy is minimized (static system)

$$H(D) = -1 \times \log(1) = 0.$$

Also note that the base of the log function is somewhat irrelevant, and it can be used to normalize (scale) the range of the entropy $\left(\log_b(x) = \frac{\log_2(x)}{\log_2(b)}\right)$. The Information gain is the expected reduction in entropy caused by knowing the value of an attribute.

5.4.2.3   Misclassification Error and Gini Index

Similar to the Entropy measure, the Misclassification error and the Gini index are also applied to evaluate information gain. The Misclassification error is defined by the formula

$$ME = 1 - \max_k (p_k),$$

and the Gini index is expressed as

$$GI = \sum_k p_k(1 - p_k) = 1 - \sum_k p_k^2.$$

5.4.2.4   C5.0 Decision Tree Algorithm

The C5.0 algorithm is a popular implementation of decision trees.[4,5] To begin with, let's consider the term purity. If the segments of data contain a single class, they

---

[4]https://doi.org/10.1007/BF00116251

[5]https://doi.org/10.1016/j.compag.2018.12.013

are considered `pure`. The `entropy` represents a mathematical formalism measuring purity for data segments.

$$\text{Entropy}(S) = -\sum_{i=1}^{c} p_i \log_2(p_i),$$

where `entropy` is the measurement, c is the number of total class levels, and p_i refers to the proportion of observations that fall into each class (i.e., probability of a randomly selected data point to belong to the ith class level. For two possible classes, the `entropy` ranges from 0 to 1. For n classes, the entropy ranges from 0 to $\log_2(n)$, where the minimum entropy corresponds to data that is purely homogeneous (completely deterministic/predictable) and the maximum entropy represents completely disordered data (stochastic or extremely noisy). You might wonder: *what is the benefit of using entropy?* The answer reflects the fact that the smaller the entropy, the more information is contained in the corresponding decision node split. Hence, systems (data) with high entropy indicate significant information content (randomness) and processes with low entropy indicate highly-compressible data with informative structure embedded in it.

If we only have one class in the segment then the entropy is trivial, Entropy $(S) = (-1) \times \log_2(1) = 0$. Let's try another example. If we have a segment of data that contains two classes, the first class contains 80% of the data and the second class contains the remaining 20%. Then, we have the following `entropy`: Entropy $(S) = 0.8\log_2(0.8) - 0.2\log_2(0.2) - 0.7219281$. For a two-class problem, the relationship between class-proportions and entropy is illustrated in the following graph. Assume x is the proportion for one of the classes (Fig. 5.8).

```
N <- 1000
set.seed(1234)
x <- runif(N)
x_ind <- sort(x)
y <- -x_ind*log2(x_ind)-(1-x_ind)*log2(1-x_ind)
modelLabels <- c('High-Structure/Low-Entropy', 'Low-Structure/High-Entropy',
                 'High-Structure/Low-Entropy')
modelLabels.x <- c(0.03, 0.5, 0.97)
modelLabels.y <- c(0.5, 0.7, 0.5)
modelLabels.col <- c("blue", "red", "blue")
plot_ly() %>%
   add_lines(x = ~x_ind, y = ~y, name="Entropy", line = list(width = 4)) %>%
   add_segments(x=0.8, xend=0.8, y=0.001, yend = 0.7219281, showlegend=F) %>%
   add_markers(x = 0.8, y = 0.7219281, name="(x=0.8,Entropy=0.72)",
               marker = list(size = 20, color = 'green',
               line = list(color = 'yellow', width = 2))) %>%
   layout(title="Binary Class Entropy",
       xaxis=list(title="Proportion of Class 1 Observations",
       scaleanchor="y"),  # control the y:x axes aspect ratio
       yaxis = list(title="Entropy", scaleanchor = "x",
       range=c(-0.1, 1.1)), legend = list(orientation = 'h'),
       annotations = list(text=modelLabels, x=modelLabels.x,
       y=modelLabels.y, textangle=90,
       font=list(size=15, color=modelLabels.col), showarrow=FALSE))
```

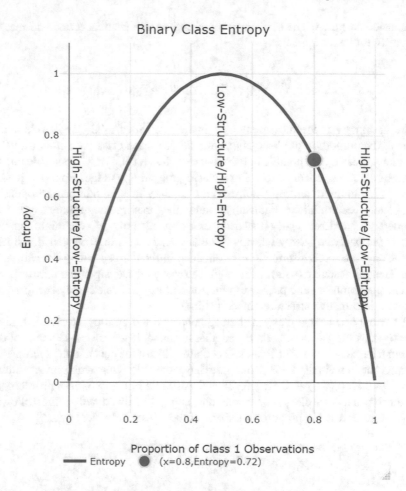

Fig. 5.8 Interpretation of the binary-class entropy

The closer the binary proportion split is to 0.5, the greater the entropy. The more homogeneous the split (one class becomes the majority), the lower the entropy. **Decision trees** aim to find splits in the data that reduce the entropy, i.e., increasing the homogeneity of the elements within all classes.

This measuring mechanism could be used to measure and compare the information we get using different features as data partitioning characteristics. Let's consider this scenario. Suppose S and S_1 represent the entropy of the system before and after the splitting/partitioning of the data according to a specific data feature attribute (F). Denote the entropies of the original and the derived partition by Entropy(S) and Entropy(S_1), respectively. The **information we gained** from partitioning the data using this specific feature (F) is calculated as a change in the entropy

$$\text{Gain}(F) = \text{Entropy}(S) - \text{Entropy}(S_1).$$

Note that smaller entropy Entropy(S_1) corresponds with better classification and more information gained. A more complicated case would be that the partitions create multiple segments. Then, the entropy for each partition method is calculated by the following formula

$$\text{Entropy}(S) = \sum_{i=1}^{n} w_i \text{Entropy}(P_i) = \sum_{i=1}^{n} w_i \left(-\sum_{j=1}^{c} p_i \log_2(p_i) \right),$$

where w_i is the proportion of examples falling in that segment and P_i is segment i. Thus, the total entropy of a partition method is calculated as the weighted sum of entropies for each segment created by this method. When we get the maximum reduction in entropy using a specific feature (F), then the Gain(F) = Entropy(S), since Entropy(S_1) = 0. On the contrary, if we gain no information using a split for this feature, we have Gain$(F) = 0$.

5.4.2.5   Pruning the Decision Tree

While constructing a decision tree, we can classify those observations using as many splits as we want. This eventually might overclassify (overfit) the data. An extreme example of this would be that we make each observation as a separate class, which is meaningless. So, how do we meaningfully control the size of the decision tree? One possible solution is to make a cutoff for the number of decisions that a decision tree process could make. Similarly, we can control the minimum number of points in each segment. This method is called *early stopping*, or *prepruning* the decision tree. However, this might terminate the decision procedure ahead of some important pending partition.

Another solution *postpruning* can be applied when we begin with growing a big decision tree and subsequently reduce the branches based on error rates with corresponding penalty at the decision nodes. This is often more effective than the prepruning solution. The `C5.0 algorithm` uses the *postpruning* method to control the size of the decision tree. It first grows an overfitting large tree that contains all the possibilities of partitioning. Then, it cuts out nodes and branches with little effect on classification errors.

5.4.3   Case Study 1: Quality of Life and Chronic Disease

Step 1: *Collecting Data*

We'll use the Quality of life and chronic disease dataset, `Case06_QoL_Symptom_ChronicIllness.csv`, which has 41 variables. Two of the important variables include

- **Charlson Comorbidity Index**: ranging from 0 to 10. A score of 0 indicates no comorbid conditions. Higher scores indicate a greater level of comorbidity.
- **Chronic Disease Score**: A summary score based on the presence and complexity of prescription medications for select chronic conditions. A high score in decades the patient has severe chronic diseases. A value of "-9" indicates a missing observation.

Step 2: *Exploring and Preparing the Data*
Let's load the data first.

```
qol <-
  read.csv("https://umich.instructure.com/files/481332/download?download_frd=1")
str(qol)
## 'data.frame':      2356 obs. of  41 variables:
## $ ID                : int  171 171 172 179 180 180 181 182 183 186 ...
## $ INTERVIEWDATE     : int  0 427 0 0 0 42 0 0 0 0 ...
## $ LANGUAGE          : int  1 1 1 1 1 1 1 1 1 2 ...
## $ AGE               : int  49 49 62 44 64 64 52 48 49 78 ...
## ...
## $ CHARLSONSCORE     : int  2 2 3 1 0 0 2 8 0 1 ...
## $ CHRONICDISEASESCORE: num  1.6 1.6 1.54 2.97 1.28 1.28 1.31 1.67 2.21...
```

Most of the coded variables like QOL_Q_01(health rating) have ordinal values (1 = excellent, 2 = very good, 3 = good, 4 = fair, 5 = poor, 6 = no answer), and we can use the table() function to see their distributions. We also have some numerical variables in the dataset like CHRONICDISEASESCORE, which can be examined using summary().

Our outcome of interest CHRONICDISEASESCORE has some missing data. A simple way to address this is just to remove those observations with missing values. However, we could also try to impute the missing values using various imputation methods mentioned in Chap. 2.

```
table(qol$QOL_Q_01)
##   1   2   3   4   5   6
##  44 213 801 900 263 135
qol <- qol[!qol$CHRONICDISEASESCORE==-9, ]
summary(qol$CHRONICDISEASESCORE)
##    Min. 1st Qu.  Median    Mean 3rd Qu.    Max.
##   0.000   0.880   1.395   1.497   1.970   4.760
```

Let's create two classes using the variable CHRONICDISEASESCORE. We classify the patients with CHRONICDISEASESCORE < mean (CHRONICDISEASESCORE) as having minor disease and the rest as having severe disease. This dichotomous classification (qol$cd) may not be perfect, and we will talk about alternative classification strategies in the practice problems section at the end of this chapter.

```
qol$cd <- qol$CHRONICDISEASESCORE>1.497
qol$cd <- factor(qol$cd, levels=c(F, T),
                 labels = c("minor_disease", "severe_disease"))
```

Data Preparation—Creating Random Training and Test Datasets

To make the qol data more organized, we can order the data by the variable ID.

```
qol <- qol[order(qol$ID), ]
# Remove ID (col=1) # the clinical Diagnosis (col=41) will be handled later
qol <- qol[ , -1]
```

Then, we can subset the *training* and *testing* datasets. Here is an example of a *nonrandom split* of the entire data into training (2114) and testing (100) sets.

```
qol_train <- qol[1:2114, ]
qol_test <- qol[2115:2214, ]
```

Alternatively, here is an example of *random assignments* of cases into training and testing sets (80–20% split).

```
set.seed(1234)
train_index <- sample(seq_len(nrow(qol)), size = 0.8*nrow(qol))
qol_train <- qol[train_index, ]
qol_test <- qol[-train_index, ]
```

We can quickly inspect the distributions of the training and testing data to ensure they are not vastly different. We can see that the classes are split fairly equal in training and test datasets.

```
prop.table(table(qol_train$cd))
##
## minor_disease severe_disease
## 0.5324675 0.4675325
prop.table(table(qol_test$cd))
##
## minor_disease severe_disease
## 0.4853273 0.5146727
```

Step 3: *Training a Model on the Data*

We will demonstrate using the C5.0() function from the C50 package. The function C5.0() has the following invocation protocol:

```
model <- C5.0(train, class, trials=1, costs=NULL)
```

- *train*: data frame containing numeric training data (features)
- *class*: factor vector with the class for each row in the training data
- *trials*: an optional number to control the boosting iterations (default = 1)
- *costs*: an optional matrix to specify the costs of false positive and false negative classification, or prediction.

In the `qol` dataset (ID column is already removed), column 41 is the class vector (qol$cd) and column 40 is the numerical version of vector 41 (qol $CHRONICDISEASESCORE). We need to delete these two columns to create our training data that only contains feature variables that will be used for predicting the outcome.

```
# install.packages("C50")
library(C50)
summary(qol_train[,-c(40, 41)])
...
##          SEX          QOL_Q_01         QOL_Q_02         QOL_Q_03
##   Min.   :1.000   Min.   :1.000   Min.   :1.000   Min.   :1.000
##   1st Qu.:1.000   1st Qu.:3.000   1st Qu.:3.000   1st Qu.:3.000
##   Median :1.000   Median :4.000   Median :3.000   Median :4.000
##   Mean   :1.423   Mean   :3.678   Mean   :3.417   Mean   :3.705
##   3rd Qu.:2.000   3rd Qu.:4.000   3rd Qu.:4.000   3rd Qu.:4.000
##   Max.   :2.000   Max.   :6.000   Max.   :6.000   Max.   :6.000
...
set.seed(1234)
qol_model <- C5.0(qol_train[,-c(40, 41)], qol_train$cd)
qol_model
## Classification Tree
## Number of samples: 1771
## Number of predictors: 39
## Tree size: 5
## Non-standard options: attempt to group attributes
summary(qol_model)
## Decision tree:
## CHARLSONSCORE <= 0: minor_disease (645/169)
## CHARLSONSCORE > 0:
## :...CHARLSONSCORE > 5: minor_disease (29/9)
##     CHARLSONSCORE <= 5:
##     :...AGE > 47: severe_disease (936/352)
##         AGE <= 47:
##         :...MSA_Q_08 <= 1: minor_disease (133/46)
##             MSA_Q_08 > 1: severe_disease (28/8)
## Evaluation on training data (1771 cases):
##     (a)   (b)    <- classified as
##     ----  ----
##     583   360    (a): class minor_disease
##     224   604    (b): class severe_disease
## Attribute usage:
## 100.00% CHARLSONSCORE
##   61.94% AGE
##    9.09% MSA_Q_08
# plot(qol_model, subtree = 17) # ?C50::plot.C5.0
```

The output of `qol_model` indicates that we have a tree with 25 terminal nodes. The result of `summary(qol_model)` suggests that the classification error for the decision tree is 28% in the training data.

Step 4: *Evaluating Model Performance*

Now we can make predictions using the decision tree that we just built. The predict() function we will use is the same one we showed for naïve Bayes classification, as well as earlier in Chap. 2. In general, predict() is extended by each specific type of regression, classification, clustering or forecasting machine learning technique. For example, randomForest::predict. randomForest() is invoked by

```
predict(RF_model, newdata, type="response", norm.votes=TRUE,
 predict.all=FALSE, proximity=FALSE, nodes=FALSE, cutoff, ...),
```

where type represents the type of prediction output to be generated—"response" (equivalent to "class"), "prob" or "votes." Thus, the predicted values are either predicted "response" class labels, a matrix of class probabilities, or vote counts.

This time we are going to introduce the confusionMatrix() function under package caret as the evaluation method. When we combine it with a table() function, the output of the evaluation is very straight forward.

```
# See docs for predict # ?C50::predict.C5.0
qol_pred <- predict(qol_model, qol_test[ ,-c(40, 41)])
# removing the last 2 clinical outcomes columns CHRONICDISEASESCORE and cd
# install.packages("caret")
library(caret)
confusionMatrix(table(qol_pred, qol_test$cd))
## qol_pred         minor_disease severe_disease
##    minor_disease            143             71
##    severe_disease            72            157
##
##               Accuracy : 0.6772
##                 95% CI : (0.6315, 0.7206)
##    No Information Rate : 0.5147
##    P-Value [Acc > NIR] : 3.001e-12
##                  Kappa : 0.3538
##  Mcnemar's Test P-Value : 1
##            Sensitivity : 0.6651
##            Specificity : 0.6886
##         Pos Pred Value : 0.6682
##         Neg Pred Value : 0.6856
##             Prevalence : 0.4853
##         Detection Rate : 0.3228
##   Detection Prevalence : 0.4831
##      Balanced Accuracy : 0.6769
```

The confusion matrix shows prediction accuracy is about 68%; however, this may vary (see the corresponding confidence interval).

Step 5: *Trial Option*

Recall that the C5.0 function has an option, trials, that is, an integer specifying the number of boosting iterations. The default value of one indicates that a single model is used, and we can specify a larger number of iterations, for instance, trials=6.

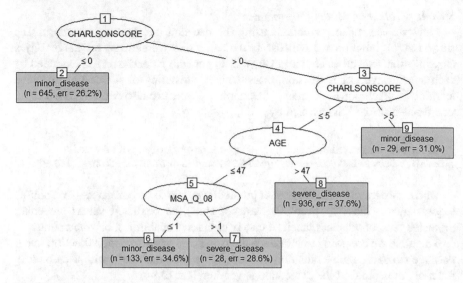

Fig. 5.9 Constructing a chronic disease prediction decision tree using the C5.0 algorithm

```
set.seed(1234)          # try alternative trials value options
qol_boost6 <- C5.0(qol_train[ , -c(40, 41)], qol_train$cd, trials=6)
qol_boost6
## Call:
## C5.0.default(x = qol_train[, -c(40, 41)], y = qol_train$cd, trials = 6)
## Classification Tree
## Number of samples: 1771
## Number of predictors: 39
## Number of boosting iterations: 6
## Average tree size: 4.7
```

The size of the tree may vary with each repeated experiment and depends on the parameter settings. Since this is a fairly small tree, we can visualize it by the function `plot()`. We also use the option `type="simple"` to make the tree look more condensed. We can also zoom in and display just a specific branch of the tree by using the `subtree` parameter (Fig. 5.9).

```
plot(qol_boost6, type="simple")   # C50::plot.C5.0
```

Caution: The plotting of decision trees will fail if you have columns that start with numbers or special characters (e.g., "*5variable*," "*!variable*"). In general, avoid spaces, special characters, and other nonterminal symbols in column/row names.

The next step is to demonstrate prediction and testing of the accuracy of a fitted decision tree model.

```
qol_boost_pred6 <- predict(qol_boost6, qol_test[ ,-c(40, 41)])
confusionMatrix(table(qol_boost_pred6, qol_test$cd))
## Confusion Matrix and Statistics
## qol_boost_pred6  minor_disease severe_disease
##   minor_disease            145             69
##   severe_disease            70            159
##                 Accuracy : 0.6862
##                   95% CI : (0.6408, 0.7292)
##      No Information Rate : 0.5147
##      P-Value [Acc > NIR] : 1.747e-13
##                    Kappa : 0.3718
##  Mcnemar's Test P-Value : 1
##              Sensitivity : 0.6744
##              Specificity : 0.6974
##           Pos Pred Value : 0.6776
##           Neg Pred Value : 0.6943
##               Prevalence : 0.4853
##           Detection Rate : 0.3273
##     Detection Prevalence : 0.4831
##        Balanced Accuracy : 0.6859
```

The reported accuracy is about 69%. However, this result may vary each time we run the experiment (mind the reported confidence interval). In some studies, the *trials* option provides significant improvement to the overall accuracy. A good choice for this option is `trials=10`.

Loading the Misclassification Error Matrix

Suppose we want to reduce the *false-negative rate*, which corresponds to misclassifying a severe case as mild. False negatives (failure to detect severe disease cases) may be more costly than false-positive errors (misclassifying mild disease cases as severe). Misclassification errors can be expressed as a matrix, which can be *loaded* to penalize specific types of erroneous predictions.

```
error_cost<-matrix(c(0, 1, 4, 0), nrow = 2)
error_cost
##      [,1] [,2]
## [1,]    0    4
## [2,]    1    0
```

Let's build a decision tree with the option `cpsts=error_cost`.

```
set.seed(1234)
qol_cost <- C5.0(qol_train[-c(40, 41)], qol_train$cd, costs=error_cost)
qol_cost_pred <- predict(qol_cost, qol_test)
confusionMatrix(table(qol_cost_pred, qol_test$cd))
## Confusion Matrix and Statistics
## qol_cost_pred    minor_disease severe_disease
##   minor_disease             73             14
##   severe_disease           142            214
##                Accuracy : 0.6479
##                  95% CI : (0.6014, 0.6923)
##             Sensitivity : 0.3395
##             Specificity : 0.9386
```

Although the overall accuracy decreased, the false negative cell labels were reduced from 69 (without specifying a cost matrix) to 14 (when specifying a nontrivial (loaded) cost matrix). This comes at the cost of increasing the rate of false-positive labeling (minor disease cases misclassified as severe).

Model Visualization

There are multiple choices to plot trees fitted by `rpart` or `C5.0`.

```
library("rpart")
set.seed(1234)              # here we use rpart::cp=*complexity parameter*=0.01
qol_model <- rpart(cd ~ ., data=qol_train[, -40], cp=0.01)
qol_model
## n= 1771
## 1) root 1771 828 minor_disease (0.5324675 0.4675325)
##   2) CHARLSONSCORE< 0.5 645 169 minor_disease (0.7379845 0.2620155) *
##   3) CHARLSONSCORE>=0.5 1126 467 severe_disease (0.4147425 0.5852575)
##     6) AGE< 47.5 165  66 minor_disease (0.6000000 0.4000000) *
##     7) AGE>=47.5 961 368 severe_disease (0.3829344 0.6170656) *
```

Alternatively, we can visually plot the decision tree model using different rendering methods (Fig. 5.10).

```
library(rpart.plot)
rpart.plot(qol_model, type = 4,extra = 1, clip.right.labs = F)
library("rattle")
fancyRpartPlot(qol_model, cex=1, caption="rattle::fancyRpartPlot (QoL Data)")
```

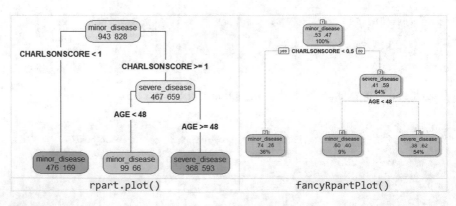

Fig. 5.10 Alternative renderings of the (chronic disease prediction) decision tree model

Parameter Tuning

```
qol_pred <- predict(qol_model, qol_test, type = 'class')
confusionMatrix(table(qol_pred, qol_test$cd))
## qol_pred          minor_disease severe_disease
##    minor_disease            143             74
##    severe_disease            72            154
##                 Accuracy : 0.6704
##                   95% CI : (0.6245, 0.7141)
##      No Information Rate : 0.5147
##      P-Value [Acc > NIR] : 2.276e-11
##                    Kappa : 0.3405
###  Mcnemar's Test P-Value : 0.934
##              Sensitivity : 0.6651
##              Specificity : 0.6754
##           Pos Pred Value : 0.6590
##           Neg Pred Value : 0.6814
##               Prevalence : 0.4853
##           Detection Rate : 0.3228
##     Detection Prevalence : 0.4898
##        Balanced Accuracy : 0.6703
```

These rpart results are consistent with their counterparts reported using C5.0.
Using the method rpart.control(), we can tune the parameters to further improve the
results (Fig. 5.11).

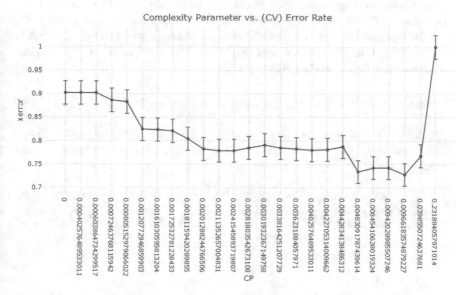

Fig. 5.11 Optimizing the chronic disease decision tree model—complexity parameter value
(horizontal axis) vs. cross-validation error rate (vertical axis)

```
set.seed(1234)
control = rpart.control(cp = 0.000, xxval = 100, minsplit = 2)
qol_model= rpart(cd ~ ., data = qol_train[ , -40], control = control)
data <- as.data.frame(qol_model$cptable)
data$CP <- as.factor(data$CP)
plot_ly(data=data, x=~CP, y=~xerror, type='scatter', mode='lines+markers',
        name = 'Test', error_y = ~list(array = xstd, color = 'gray')) %>%
  layout(title="Complexity Parameter vs. (CV) Error Rate")
```

Now, we can prune the tree according to the optimal cp, *complexity parameter* to which the rpart object will be trimmed. Instead of using the *real error* (e.g., $1 - R^2$, RMSE) to capture the discrepancy between the observed labels and the model-predicted labels, we will use the xerror which averages the discrepancy between observed and predicted classifications using *cross-validation*, see Chap. 9. We can compare the *full* (qol_model) and *pruned* (selected_tr) decision trees by contrasting the outputs of summary(qol_model) and summary(selected_tr).

```
set.seed(1234)
selected_tr <- prune(qol_model,
        cp=qol_model$cptable[which.min(qol_model$cptable[,"xerror"]),"CP"])
fancyRpartPlot(selected_tr,cex=1,caption="rattle::fancyRpartPlot (QoL Data)")
```

```
qol_pred_tune <- predict(selected_tr, qol_test,type = 'class')
confusionMatrix(table(qol_pred_tune, qol_test$cd))
```

The results are roughly the same as those obtained via C5.0. Even though there is no substantial classification improvement, the tree-pruning process generates a graphical representation of the decision-making protocol (selected_tr) that is expected to be much simpler and more intuitive compared to the original (un-pruned) tree (qol_model) (Fig. 5.12).

```
fancyRpartPlot(qol_model,cex=0.1,caption="rattle::fancyRpartPlot (QoL Data)")
```

We can compare different impurity indices by using different specifications, *split* = *"entropy," "error,"* or *"gini,"* and applying alternative information gain criteria.

```
set.seed(1234)
qol_model = rpart(cd ~ ., data=qol_train[, -40], parms=list(split="entropy"))
fancyRpartPlot(qol_model, cex=1, caption="rattle::fancyRpartPlot (QoL data)")
```

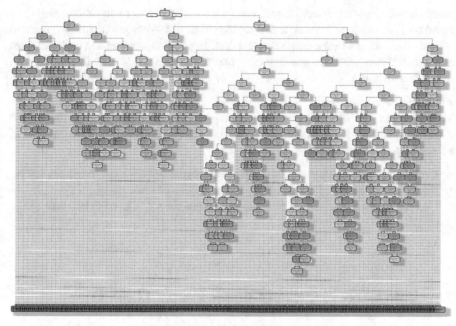

rattle::fancyRpartPlot (QoL Data)

Fig. 5.12 In this quality of life and chronic disease dataset, as well as in other high-dimensional cases, rendering the complete decision tree model may or may not be useful. Such complex trees could represent significant overfitting, may be unstable with respect to repeated experiments, and may yield widely varying predictions on validation data

5.4.4 Classification Rules

In addition to the classification trees we saw above, we can explore *classification rules* that utilize if-else logical statements to assign classes to unlabeled data. Below we review three classification rule strategies.

Separate and Conquer
Separate and conquer repeatedly splits the data (and subsets of the data) by rules that cover a subset of examples. This procedure is very similar to the *divide-and-conquer* approach. However, a notable difference is that each rule can be independent, yet each decision node in a tree must be linked to past decisions.

The One Rule Algorithm
To understand the One Rule (OneR) algorithm, we need to know about its "sibling"—no rule (ZeroR) method. ZeroR rule means that we assign the mode class to unlabeled test observations regardless of its feature value. The One Rule (OneR) algorithm is an improved version of ZeroR that uses a single rule for

classification. In other words, OneR splits the training dataset into several segments based on feature values. Then, it assigns the mode of the classes in each segment to related observations in the unlabeled test data. In practice, we first test multiple rules and pick the rule with the smallest error rate to be our One Rule. Remember, the rules are subjective.

The RIPPER Algorithm

The *Repeated Incremental Pruning to Produce Error Reduction* algorithm is a combination of the ideas behind decision tree and classification rules. It consists of a three-step process:

* *Grow*: add conditions to a rule until it cannot split the data into more segments.
* *Prune*: delete some of the conditions that have large error rates.
* *Optimize*: repeat the above two steps until we cannot add or delete any of the conditions.

5.5   Case Study 2: QoL in Chronic Disease (Take 2)

Let's take another look at the same dataset as Case Study 1—this time applying *classification rules*. Naturally, we skip over the first two data handling steps and go directly to step three.

(Continuing) Step 3: *Training a Model on the Data*

Let's start by using the OneR() function in the RWeka package. Before installing the package, you might want to check that the Java program in your computer is up to date. Also, its version has to match the version of R (i.e., 64 bit R needs 64 bit Java). The function OneR() has the following invocation syntax.

```
model <- OneR(class~predictors, data=mydata)
```

* *class*: factor vector with the class for each row **mydata**.
* *predictors*: feature variables in **mydata**. If we want to include x_1, x_2 as predictors and y as the class label variable, we do $y \sim x_1 + x_2$. When using a model specification to include all covariates, e.g., $y \sim .$, we effectively include all of the column variables as predictors of the outcome feature.
* *mydata*: the dataset where the features and labels could be found.

```
# install.packages("RWeka")
library(RWeka)
set.seed(1234)
qol_1R <- OneR(cd~., data=qol[ , -40])
qol_1R
## CHARLSONSCORE:
## < -4.5   -> severe_disease
## < 0.5    -> minor_disease
## < 5.5    -> severe_disease
## < 8.5    -> minor_disease
## >= 8.5   -> severe_disease
## (1453/2214 instances correct)
```

Note that 1, 453 out of 2, 214 cases are correctly classified, 66%, by the "one rule".

Step 4: *Evaluating Model Performance*

```
summary(qol_1R)
## Correctly Classified Instances 1453 65.6278 %
## Incorrectly Classified Instances 761 34.3722 %
## Kappa statistic 0.3206
## Mean absolute error 0.3437
## Root mean squared error 0.5863
## Relative absolute error 68.8904 %
## Root relative squared error 117.3802 %
## Total Number of Instances 2214
## === Confusion Matrix ---
## a b <-- classified as
## 609 549 | a = minor_disease
## 212 844 | b = severe_disease
```

We obtain a rule that correctly specifies 66% of the patients, which is in line with the prior decision tree classification results. Due to algorithmic stochasticity, it's normal that these results may vary each time you run the algorithm, albeit we used set.seed(1234) to ensure some result reproducibility.

Step 5: *Alternative Model1*

Another possible option for the classification rules would be the RIPPER rule algorithm that we discussed earlier in the chapter. In R, we use the Java-based function JRip() to invoke this algorithm. The JRip() function uses a similar invocation protocol as OneR().

```
model <- JRip(class~predictors, data=mydata)
```

```
set.seed(1234)
qol_jrip1 <- JRip(cd~., data=qol[ , -40])
qol_jrip1
## JRIP rules:
## (CHARLSONSCORE >= 1) and (RACE_ETHNICITY >= 4) and (AGE >= 49) =>
cd=severe_disease (448.0/132.0)
## (CHARLSONSCORE >= 1) and (AGE >= 53) => cd=severe_disease (645.0/265.0)
##  => cd=minor_disease (1121.0/360.0)
## Number of Rules : 3
summary(qol_jrip1)
## Correctly Classified Instances        1457                65.8085 %
## Incorrectly Classified Instances       757                34.1915 %
## Kappa statistic                       0.3158
## Mean absolute error                   0.4459
## Root mean squared error               0.4722
## Relative absolute error              89.3711 %
## Root relative squared error          94.5364 %
## Total Number of Instances             2214
## === Confusion Matrix ===
##    a    b   <-- classified as
##  761  397 |   a = minor_disease
##  360  696 |   b = severe_disease
```

This JRip() classifier uses only three rules and has a relatively similar accuracy, 66%. Classification using real world data is rarely perfect (close to 100% accuracy) since most observed data includes a blend of normal and pathological variation, intrinsic, extrinsic, and nonmechanistic errors.

Step 5: *Alternative Model2*

Another idea is to use a meta-tree approach to repeat the generation of trees multiple times, predict according to each tree's performance, and finally ensemble those weighted votes into a combined classification result. This is precisely the idea behind random forest classification, which will be discussed later in Chap. 9 (Fig. 5.13).

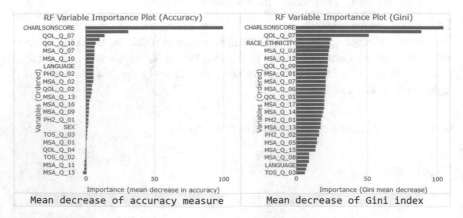

Fig. 5.13 Variable importance plots of the most salient features in the chronic disease dataset derived from a meta decision tree approach (randomForest)

```
# install.packages("randomForest")
require(randomForest)
set.seed(12)
rf.fit <- randomForest(cd ~ . , data=qol_train[ , -40], importance=TRUE,
                       ntree=2000,mtry=26)
# Accuracy
imp_rf.fit <- importance(rf.fit)
x <- rownames(imp_rf.fit)
y <- imp_rf.fit[,3]
plot_ly(x = ~y, y = ~reorder(x,y),  name = "Var.Imp", type = "bar") %>%
  layout(title="RF Variable Importance Plot (Accuracy)",
         xaxis=list(title="Importance (mean decrease in accuracy)"),
         yaxis = list(title="Variables (Ordered)"))
# Gini Index
y <- imp_rf.fit[,4]
plot_ly(x = ~y, y = ~reorder(x,y),  name = "Var.Imp", type = "bar") %>%
  layout(title="RF Variable Importance Plot (Gini)",
         xaxis=list(title="Importance (Gini mean decrease)"),
         yaxis = list(title="Variables (Ordered)"))
```

We can compare two random forest models, each representing different parameter settings (Fig. 5.14).

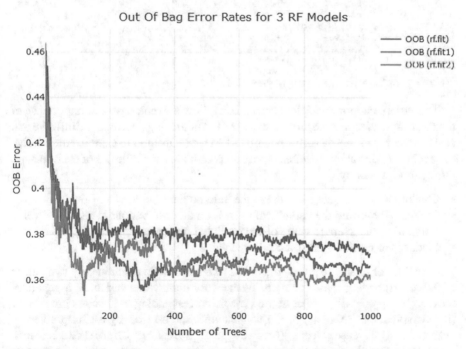

Fig. 5.14 Error convergence of three random forest meta-algorithm models (vertical axis) across number of trees grown (horizontal axis) using out-of-bag chronic disease data

```
rf.fit1 <- randomForest(cd ~ . , data=qol_train[ , -40], importance=TRUE,
                        ntree=2000, mtry=26)
rf.fit2 <- randomForest(cd ~ . , data=qol_train[ , -40], importance=TRUE,
                        nodesize=5, ntree=5000, mtry=26)
plot_ly(x = c(1:1000), y = rf.fit$err.rate[1:1000,1], name = 'OOB (rf.fit)',
        type = 'scatter', mode = 'lines', line = list(width = 2)) %>%
  add_trace(x=c(1:1000), y=rf.fit1$err.rate[1:1000,1], name='OOB (rf.fit1)',
        type = 'scatter', mode = 'lines', line = list(width = 2)) %>%
  add_trace(x=c(1:1000), y=rf.fit2$err.rate[1:1000,1], name='OOB (rf.fit2)',
        type = 'scatter', mode = 'lines', line = list(width = 2)) %>%
  layout(title = "Out Of Bag Error Rates for 3 RF Models",
        xaxis=list(title="Number of Trees"), yaxis=list (title="OOB Error"))
```

```
qol_pred2 <- predict(rf.fit2, qol_test, type = 'class')
confusionMatrix(table(qol_pred2, qol_test$cd))
## qol_pred2          minor_disease severe_disease
##   minor_disease             142             71
##   severe_disease             73            157
##
##                Accuracy : 0.6749
##                  95% CI : (0.6291, 0.7184)
##     No Information Rate : 0.5147
##     P-Value [Acc > NIR] : 5.956e-12
##                   Kappa : 0.3492
##  Mcnemar's Test P-Value : 0.9336
##             Sensitivity : 0.6605
##             Specificity : 0.6886
##          Pos Pred Value : 0.6667
##          Neg Pred Value : 0.6826
##              Prevalence : 0.4853
##          Detection Rate : 0.3205
##    Detection Prevalence : 0.4808
##       Balanced Accuracy : 0.6745
```

The variable importance plots (`varplot`) show the rank orders of importance of the most salient features according to a specific metric (e.g., accuracy, Gini). We can also use the `randomForest::partialPlot()` method to examine the relative impact of the top salient features (continuous or binary variables). For each feature, this method works by

- Creating a test data set identical to the training data
- Sequentially setting the variable of interest for all observations to a selected value
- Computing the average value of the predicted response for each test set
- Plotting the results against the selected value

Note that for binary features, `partialPlot()` would result in only two values of the corresponding mass function. Whereas for continuous variables, it generates the marginal probability effect of the variable corresponding to the class probability (for classification problems) or the continuous response (for regression problems). Using the QoL case study, (`Case06_QoL_Symptom_ChronicIllness.csv`), this example shows the partial plots of the *top six* rank-ordered features of the QoL dataset chosen by the random forest model.

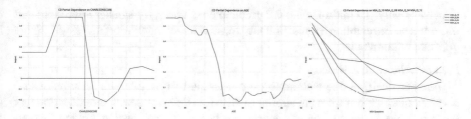

Fig. 5.15 Random forest-derived partial dependence of the outcome, chronic disease (CD), on a set of six covariates

These graphs explicate some of the hidden, or latent, effects of individual covariates and sets of covariates on the model outcome prediction (Fig. 5.15).

```
imp <- randomForest::importance(rf.fit)
impvar <- rownames(imp)[order(imp[, 1], decreasing=TRUE)]
p <- vector("list", 6)
for (i in 1:6) {   # seq_along(impvar))
    # plot the marginal probabilities for all features
    p[[i]] <- partialPlot(rf.fit, qol_train, impvar[i], xlab=impvar[i],
            main=paste("Partial Dependence of 'CD'\n on ", impvar[i]), plot=F)
}
plot_ly(x=p[[1]]$x, y=p[[1]]$y, name=impvar[1], type='scatter', mode='lines',
        line = list(width = 2)) %>%
    layout(title = paste0("CD Partial Dependence on ",impvar[1]),
            xaxis = list(title = impvar[1]), yaxis = list (title = "Impact"))
plot_ly(x=p[[2]]$x, y=p[[2]]$y, name=impvar[2], type='scatter', mode='lines',
        line = list(width = 2)) %>%
    layout(title = paste0("CD Partial Dependence on ",impvar[2]),
            xaxis = list(title = impvar[2]), yaxis = list (title = "Impact"))
plot_ly(x=p[[3]]$x, y=p[[3]]$y, name=impvar[3], type='scatter', mode='lines',
        line = list(width = 2)) %>%
    add_trace(x = p[[4]]$x, y = p[[4]]$y, name = impvar[4], type = 'scatter',
            mode = 'lines', line = list(width = 2)) %>%
    add_trace(x = p[[5]]$x, y = p[[5]]$y, name = impvar[5], type = 'scatter',
            mode = 'lines', line = list(width = 2)) %>%
    add_trace(x = p[[6]]$x, y = p[[6]]$y, name = impvar[6], type = 'scatter',
            mode = 'lines', line = list(width = 2)) %>%
    layout(title = paste0("CD Partial Dependence on ",impvar[3], " ",
            impvar[4], " ",impvar[5], " ",impvar[6]),
            xaxis = list(title="MSA Questions"), yaxis = list (title="Impact"))
```

In random forest (RF) classification, the node size (`nodesize`) refers to the smallest node that can be split, i.e., nodes with fewer cases than the `nodesize` are never subdivided. Increasing the node size leads to smaller trees, which may compromise previous predictive power. On the flip side, increasing the tree size (`maxnodes`) and the number of trees (`ntree`) tends to increase the predictive accuracy. However, there are tradeoffs between increasing node-size and tree-size simultaneously. To optimize the RF predictive accuracy, try smaller node sizes and more trees. Ensembling (forest) results from a larger number of trees will likely generate better results.

Step 6: *Alternative Model3*

Another decision tree technique we can test is Extra-Trees (*extremely randomized trees*). Extra-trees are similar to Random Forests with the exception that at each node, Random Forest chooses the best-cutting threshold for the feature, whereas Extra-Tree selects a uniformly random cut, so that the feature with the biggest gain (or best classification score) is chosen. The R extraTrees package provides one implementation of Extra-Trees where single random cuts are extended to several random cuts for each feature. This extension improves performance as it reduces the probability of making very poor cuts and still maintains the designed extra-tree stochastic cutting. Below, we compare the results of four alternative chronic disease classification methods—random forest, SVM, kNN, and extra-tree (Fig. 5.16).

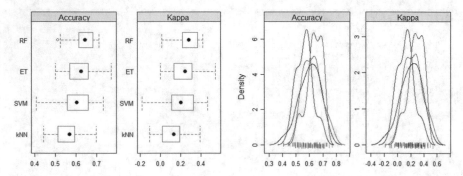

Fig. 5.16 Comparing the performance of four different chronic disease prediction models (RF, ET, SVM, kNN) using accuracy and kappa value

```
library(caret)
library(extraTrees)
control <- trainControl(method="repeatedcv", number=10, repeats=3)
## Run all subsequent models in parallel
library(doParallel)
cl <- makePSOCKcluster(4)
registerDoParallel(cl)
system.time({
  rf.fit  <- train(cd~., data=qol_test[,-40],method="rf", trControl=control);
  knn.fit <- train(cd~., data=qol_test[,-40],method="knn",trControl=control);
  svm.fit <- train(cd~., data=qol_test[,-40], method="svmRadial",
                   trControl=control);
  et.fit  <- train(cd~., data=qol_test[ , -40], method="extraTrees",
                   trControl=control)
})
##   user  system elapsed
##   4.14    0.06   55.16
stopCluster(cl) # close multi-core cluster
results <- resamples(list(RF=rf.fit, kNN=knn.fit, SVM=svm.fit, ET=et.fit))
# summary of model differences
summary(results)
## Models: RF, kNN, SVM, ET
## Number of resamples: 30
## Accuracy
##          Min.    1st Qu.    Median      Mean    3rd Qu.      Max. NA's
## RF   0.5111111 0.6136364 0.6444444 0.6388259 0.6818182 0.7111111      0
## kNN  0.4444444 0.5111111 0.5681818 0.5640044 0.5909091 0.6976744      0
## SVM  0.4090909 0.5555556 0.6046512 0.6009385 0.6590909 0.7333333      0
## ET   0.5000000 0.5681818 0.6250000 0.6231196 0.6590909 0.7727273      0
## Kappa
##          Min.    1st Qu.    Median      Mean    3rd Qu.      Max. NA's
## RF    0.01394422 0.22164160 0.2842914 0.2752858 0.3665764 0.4202180    0
## kNN  -0.10837438 0.01834335 0.1345719 0.1270165 0.1885143 0.3943662    0
## SVM  -0.17938144 0.11067194 0.2078785 0.2022046 0.3251449 0.4674556    0
## ET    0.00000000 0.13636364 0.2461288 0.2449171 0.3146395 0.5407098    0
# plot summaries
scales <- list(x=list(relation="free"), y=list(relation="free"))
bwplot(results, scales=scales)               # Box plots of
densityplot(results, scales=scales, pch = "|") # Density plots of accuracy
dotplot(results, scales=scales)              # Dot plots of accuracy, Kappa
splom(results) # contrast pair-wise model scatterplots of prediction accuracy
```

5.6 Practice Problems

5.6.1 Iris Species

The classification of the iris flowers represents an easy example of the naïve Bayesian classifier.

```
data(iris)
nbc_model <- naiveBayes(Species ~ ., data = iris)
## alternatively:
nbc_model <- naiveBayes(iris[, c("Sepal.Length", "Sepal.Width",
                         "Petal.Length", "Petal.Width")], iris[,"Species"])
predicted.nbcvalues <- predict(nbc_model, iris[,c("Sepal.Length",
                               "Sepal.Width", "Petal.Length", "Petal.Width")])
table(predicted.nbcvalues, iris[, "Species"])
## predicted.nbcvalues setosa versicolor virginica
##           setosa        50          0         0
##           versicolor     0         47         3
##           virginica      0          3        47
```

5.6.2   Cancer Study

In the cancer case study we presented earlier, we classified the patients with seer_stage of "not applicable"(seer_stage=8) and "unstaged, unknown or unspecified" (seer_stage=9) as no cancer or early cancer stages. Let's remove these two categories and replicate the naïve Bayes classifier case study again.

```
hn_med1 <- hn_med[!hn_med$seer_stage %in% c(8, 9), ]
str(hn_med1); dim(hn_med1)
## 'data.frame':    580 obs. of  9 variables:
##  $ PID        : int  10000 10008 10029 10063 10103 1012 10135 10143 ...
##  $ ENC_ID     : int  46836 46886 47034 47240 47511 3138 47739 47769 ...
##  $ seer_stage : Factor w/ 9 levels "0","1","2","3",..: 2 2 5 2 2 2 2 2 ...
##  $ MEDICATION_DESC   : chr   "ranitidine" "heparin injection"
"ampicillin/sulbactam IVPB UH" "fentaNYL injection UH" ...
##  $ MEDICATION_SUMMARY: chr   "(Zantac) 150 mg tablet oral two times a day"
"5,000 unit subcutaneous three times a day" "(Unasyn) 15 g IV every 6 hours"
##  $ DOSE       : chr   "150" "5000" "1.5" "50" ...
##  $ UNIT       : chr   "mg" "unit" "g" "microgram" ...
##  $ FREQUENCY  : chr   "two times a day" "three times a day"  ...
##  $ TOTAL_DOSE_COUNT  : int  5 3 11 2 2 2 6 1 24 2 ...
## [1] 580    9
```

Now we have only 580 observations. We can either use the first 480 of them as the training dataset and the last 100 as the test dataset, or select 80–20 (training-testing) split, and evaluate the prediction accuracy when laplace=1. Also, we can use the same code for creating the classes in training and test dataset. Since the seer_stage=8 or 9 is not in the data, we classify seer_stage=0, 1, 2 or 3 as "early_stage" and seer_stage=4, 5 or 7 as "later_stage."

```
hn_med_train1$stage <-hn_med_train1$seer_stage %in% c(4, 5, 7)
hn_med_train1$stage <-factor(hn_med_train1$stage, levels=c(F, T),
                        labels = c("early_stage", "later_stage"))
hn_med_test1$stage <-hn_med_test1$seer_stage %in% c(4, 5, 7)
hn_med_test1$stage <-factor(hn_med_test1$stage, levels=c(F, T),
                        labels = c("early_stage", "later_stage"))
prop.table(table(hn_med_train1$stage))
## early_stage later_stage
##   0.7392241   0.2607759
prop.table(table(hn_med_test1$stage))
## early_stage later_stage
##   0.7413793   0.2586207
```

To test the naïve Bayes classifier, we can use the document term matrices constructed from a corpus of high-frequency terms that have appeared in at least five documents in the training dataset.

```
##                              | hn_med_test1$stage
## hn_test_pred1               | early_stage | later_stage
## early_stage                 |      85     | 29
## later_stage                 |       1     | 1
```

$$ACC = \frac{TP + TN}{TP + FP + FN + TN} = \frac{86}{116} = 0.74.$$

Note that this is a degenerate classifier as using laplace $= 15$ yields a single class prediction, later_stage.

5.6.3 Baseball Data

Use the MLB Data (01a_data.txt) to predict the Player's Position (or perhaps the player's Team) using naiveBayes classifier. Compute and report the agreement between predicted and actual labels (for the player's position). Below is some example code (Fig. 5.17).

```
mydata <-
    read.table('https://umich.instructure.com/files/330381/download?download_frd=1',
            as.is=T, header=T)  # 01a_data.txt
sample_size <- floor(0.75 * nrow(mydata))
## set the seed to make your partition reproductible
set.seed(123)
train_ind <- sample(seq_len(nrow(mydata)), size - sample_size)
train <- mydata[train_ind, ]
# TESTING DATA
test <- mydata[-train_ind, ]
library("e1071")
nbc_model <- naiveBayes(train[ , c("Weight", "Height", "Age")],
as.factor(train$Position), laplace = 15)
nbc_model
predicted.nbcvalues <- predict(nbc_model, as.data.frame(test))
# report results
tab <- table(predicted.nbcvalues, test$Position)
tab_df <- tidyr::spread(as.data.frame(tab), key = Var2, value = Freq)
sum(diag(table(predicted.nbcvalues, test$Position)))  ## [1] 74
plot_ly(x = colnames(tab), y = colnames(tab),
      z = as.matrix(tab_df[, -1]), type = "heatmap")
```

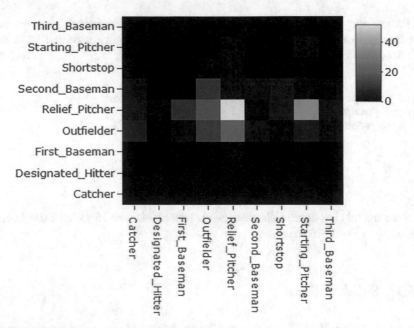

Fig. 5.17 Heatmap of the actual (vertical columns) and predicted (horizontal rows) MLB data positions based on multi-class naïve Bayesian classifier

5.6.4 Medical Specialty Text-Notes Classification

Let's demonstrate text-classification using a clinical transcription text dataset,[6] which consists of an index and five data elements—description, medical_specialty (prediction outcome target), sample_name, transcription, and keywords. Our task is to derive computed phenotypes automatically classifying the 40 different medical specialties using the clinical transcription text (Figs. 5.18 and 5.19).

```
dataCT <-
    read.csv('https://umich.instructure.com/files/21152999/download?download_frd=1',
            header=T)
str(dataCT)
## 'data.frame':     4999 obs. of  6 variables:
##  $ Index        : int  0 1 2 3 4 5 6 7 8 9 ...
##  $ description  : chr  " A 23-year-old white female presents with
complaint of allergies." " Consult for laparoscopic gastric bypass." " ...
##  $ keywords     : chr  "allergy / immunology, allergic rhinitis,
allergies, asthma, nasal sprays, rhinitis, nasal, erythematous, allegr" ...
# 1. EDA
library(dplyr)
mySummary <- dataCT %>% count(medical_specialty, sort = TRUE)
mySummary
plot_ly(dataCT, x = ~medical_specialty) %>% add_histogram()
```

---

[6]https://umich.instructure.com/courses/38100/files/folder/Case_Studies/35_MedicalSpecialty_NotesText_Classification_Dataset

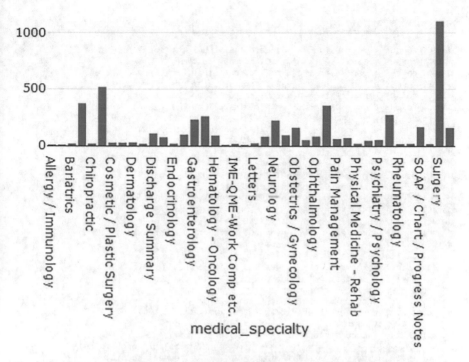

Fig. 5.18 Histogram plot of the medical specialty histogram using the clinical transcription text dataset

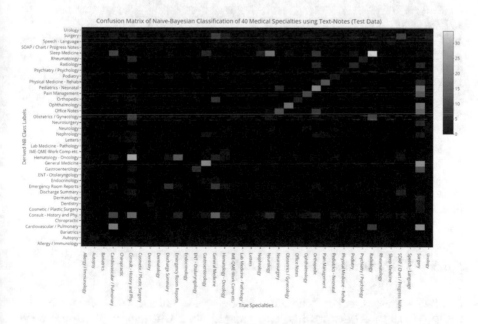

Fig. 5.19 Heatmap of the actual (vertical columns) and predicted (horizontal rows) medical specialties based on multiclass naïve Bayesian classifier

```
# 2. Preprocess the medical clinical notes (transcription)
# library(tm)
dataCT_corpus <- Corpus(VectorSource(dataCT$transcription))
dataCT_corpus_clean <- tm_map(dataCT_corpus, tolower)
dataCT_corpus_clean <- tm_map(dataCT_corpus_clean, removePunctuation)
dataCT_corpus_clean <- tm_map(dataCT_corpus_clean, removeNumbers)
dataCT_corpus_clean <- tm_map(dataCT_corpus_clean, stripWhitespace)
dataCT_corpus_dtm <- DocumentTermMatrix(dataCT_corpus_clean)
set.seed(1234)
subset_train <- sample(nrow(dataCT),floor(nrow(dataCT)*0.8))  # 80% training +
20% testing
dataCT_train <- dataCT[subset_train, ]
dataCT_test <- dataCT[-subset_train, ]
dataCT_corpus_dtm_train <- dataCT_corpus_dtm[subset_train, ]
hn_med_dtm_test <- dataCT_corpus_dtm[-subset_train, ]
dataCT_corpus_train <- dataCT_corpus_clean[subset_train]
dataCT_corpus_test <- dataCT_corpus_clean[-subset_train]
dataCT_train$MedSpecFac <- factor(dataCT_train$medical_specialty)
dataCT_test$MedSpecFac <- factor(dataCT_test$medical_specialty)
# prop.table(table(dataCT_test$medical_specialty))
prop.table(table(dataCT_test$MedSpecFac))
summary(findFreqTerms(dataCT_corpus_dtm_train, 5))
##      Length     Class      Mode
##      12630 character character
dataCT_corpus_dict <- as.character(findFreqTerms(dataCT_corpus_dtm_train, 5))
dataCT_train1 <- DocumentTermMatrix(dataCT_corpus_train,
                                    list(dictionary=dataCT_corpus_dict))
dataCT_test1 <- DocumentTermMatrix(dataCT_corpus_test,
                                    list(dictionary=dataCT_corpus_dict))
dataCT_train1 <- apply(dataCT_train1, MARGIN = 2, convert_counts)
dataCT_test1 <- apply(dataCT_test1, MARGIN = 2, convert_counts)
dataCT_classifier <- naiveBayes(dataCT_train1, dataCT_train$MedSpecFac,
                                laplace = 0)
dataCT_pred <- predict(dataCT_classifier, dataCT_test1)
# table(dataCT_pred)
# report results
tab <- table(dataCT_pred, dataCT_test$MedSpecFac)
tab_df <- tidyr::spread(as.data.frame(tab), key = Var2, value = Freq)
# gmodels::CrossTable(dataCT_pred, dataCT_test$MedSpecFac)
sum(diag(table(dataCT_pred, dataCT_test$MedSpecFac)))   ## [1] 51
plot_ly(x = colnames(tab), y = colnames(tab), z = as.matrix(tab_df[, -1]),
         type = "heatmap") %>%
  layout(title="Confusion Matrix of Naive-Bayesian Classification of 40 Medical
Specialties using Text-Notes (Test Data)",
         xaxis=list(title='True Specialties'),
         yaxis=list(title='Derived NB Class Labels'))
```

Later, in Chap. 14, we will extend this example and demonstrate a more powerful *binary* and *multinomial* (categorical) classification of the medical specialty unit based on the clinical notes, using deep neural networks.

5.6.5   Chronic Disease Case Study

In the previous QoL chronic disease case study, we classified the CHRONICDISEASESCORE into two groups. What will happen if we use three groups? Let's separate CHRONICDISEASESCORE evenly into three groups. Recall the `quantile()` function that we talked about in Chap. 2. We can use it to get the cut-points for classification. Then, a `for` loop will help us split the variable `CHRONICDISEASESCORE` into three categories.

```
quantile(qol$CHRONICDISEASESCORE, probs = c(1/3, 2/3))
## 33.33333% 66.66667%
##      1.06      1.80
for(i in 1:2214){
  if(qol$CHRONICDISEASESCORE[i]>0.7&qol$CHRONICDISEASESCORE[i]<2.2) {
    qol$cdthree[i]=2
  } else if (qol$CHRONICDISEASESCORE[i]>=2.2) {
    qol$cdthree[i]=3
  } else { qol$cdthree[i]=1  }
}
qol$cdthree <- factor(qol$cdthree, levels=c(1, 2, 3),
              labels = c("minor_disease", "mild_disease", "severe_disease"))
table(qol$cdthree)
##  minor_disease   mild_disease severe_disease
##            379           1431            404
```

After labeling the three categories in the new variable `cdthree`, our job of preparing the class variable is done. Let's follow along the earlier sections in the chapter to figure out how well the tree classifiers and rule classifiers perform in the three-category case. First, try to build a tree classifier using `C5.0()` with 10 boost trials. One small tip is that in the training dataset, we cannot have column 40 (`CHRONICDISEASESCORE`), 41 (`cd`) and now 42 (`cdthree`) because they all contain class outcome-related variables.

```
# qol_train1<-qol[1:2114, ]   # qol_test1<-qol[2115:2214, ]
train_index <- sample(seq_len(nrow(qol)), size = 0.8*nrow(qol))
qol_train1<-qol[train_index, ]
qol_test1<-qol[-train_index, ]
prop.table(table(qol_train1$cdthree))
##  minor_disease   mild_disease severe_disease
##      0.1693958      0.6453981      0.1852061
prop.table(table(qol_test1$cdthree))
##  minor_disease   mild_disease severe_disease
##      0.1783296      0.6501129      0.1715576
set.seed(1234)
qol_model1<-C5.0(qol_train1[, -c(40, 41, 42)], qol_train1$cdthree, trials=10)
qol_model1
## Classification Tree
## Number of samples: 1771
## Number of predictors: 39
## Number of boosting iterations: 10
## Average tree size: 230.3
## Non-standard options: attempt to group attributes
qol_pred1 <- predict(qol_model1, qol_test1)
confusionMatrix(table(qol_test1$cdthree, qol_pred1))
```

We can see that the prediction accuracy with three categories is way lower than the one we did with two categories. We can also try to build a rule classifier with `OneR()`.

```
set.seed(1234)
qol_1R1<-OneR(cdthree~., data=qol[ , -c(40, 41)])
qol_1R1
## INTERVIEWDATE:
## < 3.5    -> mild_disease
## < 28.5  -> severe_disease
## < 282.0 -> mild_disease
## < 311.5 -> severe_disease
## >= 311.5    -> mild_disease
## (1436/2214 instances correct)
summary(qol_1R1)
qol_pred1<-predict(qol_1R1, qol_test1)
confusionMatrix(table(qol_test1$cdthree, qol_pred1))
```

The `OneRule` classifier is purely based on the value of the feature `INTERVIEWDATE`. The internal classification accuracy is 65% and equal to the external (validation data) prediction accuracy. Although the latter assessment is a bit misleading as the majority of external validation data are classified in only one class – *mild_disease*. Finally, let's revisit the `JRip()` classifier with the same three-class labels according to `cdthree`.

```
set.seed(1234)
qol_jrip1<-JRip(cdthree~., data=qol[ , -c(40, 41)])
qol_jrip1
## JRIP rules:
## (CHARLSONSCORE <= 0) and (AGE <= 50) and (MSA_Q_06 <= 1) and (QOL_Q_07 >= 1)
and (MSA_Q_09 <= 1) => cdthree=minor_disease (35.0/11.0)
## (CHARLSONSCORE >= 1) and (QOL_Q_10 >= 4) and (QOL_Q_07 >= 9) =>
cdthree=severe_disease (54.0/20.0)
## (CHARLSONSCORE >= 1) and (QOL_Q_02 >= 5) and (MSA_Q_09 <= 4) and (MSA_Q_04 >=
3) => cdthree=severe_disease (64.0/30.0)
## (CHARLSONSCORE >= 1) and (QOL_Q_02 >= 4) and (PH2_Q_01 >= 3) and (QOL_Q_10 >=
4) and (RACE_ETHNICITY >= 4) => cdthree=severe_disease (43.0/19.0)
##  => cdthree=mild_disease (2018.0/653.0)
## === Confusion Matrix ===
##
##    a    b    c   <-- classified as
##   24  342   13 |   a = minor_disease
##   10 1365   56 |   b = mild_disease
##    1  311   92 |   c = severe_disease
qol_pred1 <- predict(qol_jrip1, qol_test1)
confusionMatrix(table(qol_test1$cdthree, qol_pred1))
```

In terms of the predictive accuracy on the testing data (`qol_test1$cdthree`), we can see from these outputs that the `RIPPER` algorithm performed better (67%) compared to the `C5.0` decision tree (60%) and similarly to the `OneR` algorithm (65%). This suggests that simple algorithms might outperform complex methods for certain real-world case studies. Later, in Chap. 9, we will provide more details about optimizing and improving classification and prediction performance. These supervised classification techniques can be further tested with other data from the list of our case studies.[7]

---

[7] https://umich.instructure.com/courses/38100/files/

Chapter 6
Black Box Machine Learning Methods

Next, we are going to cover several powerful black box machine learning and artificial intelligence techniques. These techniques have complex mathematical formulations; however, efficient algorithms and reliable software packages have been developed to utilize them for various practical applications. We will (1) describe neural networks as analogs of biological neurons; (2) develop hands-on a neural network that can be trained to compute the square-root function; (3) describe support vector machine (SVM) classification; (4) present the random forest (RF) as an ensemble ML technique; and (5) analyze several case studies, including optical character recognition (OCR), the Iris flowers, Google Trends and the stock market, and quality of life in chronic disease.

Later, in Chap. 14, we will provide more details and additional examples of deep neural network learning. For now, let's start by exploring the *mechanics* inside black box machine learning approaches.

6.1 Neural Networks

6.1.1 From Biological to Artificial Neurons

An Artificial Neural Network (ANN) model mimics the biological brain response to multisource (sensory-motor) stimuli (inputs). ANN simulates the brain using a network of interconnected neuron cells to create a massive parallel processor. Indeed, ANNs rely on graphs of artificial nodes, not brain cells, to model intrinsic process characteristics using observational data.

The basic ANN component is a *cell node*. Suppose we have n inputs $x = \{x_i\}_{i=1}^{n}$ to a node, feeding information outputted by prior upstream network nodes, and one output, propagating the information downstream through the network. The first step in fitting an ANN involves estimation of the weight coefficients for each input feature. These weights, $\{w_i\}_{i=1}^{n}$, correspond to the relative importance of each input. Within the node, the weighted signals are pulled by the "neuron cell" and this aggregated sum is passed on according to an *activation function*, $f(\cdot)$. The last step is generating an output y at the end of each node. A typical output will have the following mathematical relationship to the inputs. The weights $\{w_i\}_{i \geq 1}$ control the weight-averaging of the inputs, $\{x_i\}$, used to assess the activation function. The constant factor weight w_o and the corresponding *bias term b* allows us to shift or offset the entire activation function (left or right)

$$\underbrace{y(x)}_{\text{output}} = \overbrace{f}^{\text{activation}} \left(w_o \underbrace{b}_{\text{bias}} + \sum_{i=1}^{n} \overbrace{w_i}^{\text{weights}} \underbrace{x_i}_{\text{inputs}} \right).$$

There are three important components for building a neural network:

- *Activation function*: transforms weighted and aggregated inputs into an output.
- *Network topology*: describes the number of "neuron cells," the number of layers, nodes per layer, and manner in which the cells are connected.
- *Training algorithm*: optimization strategy to estimate the network weights $\{w_i\}$.

Let's unpack at each of these components one by one.

6.1.2   Activation Functions

There are many alternative activation functions. One example is a threshold activation function that results in an output signal only when a specified input threshold has been attained

$$f(x) = \begin{cases} 0 & x < 0 \\ 1 & x \geq 0 \end{cases}.$$

This is the simplest form of an activation function. It may be rarely used in real-world situations. A most commonly used alternative is the sigmoid activation function, $f(x) = \frac{1}{1+e^{-x}}$, where the *Euler number e* is defined by the limit $e = \lim_{n \to \infty}(1 + \frac{1}{n})^n \approx 2.71828....$ The output signal is no longer binary but can be any real number ranging from 0 to 1. Many other activation functions might be useful in different ANN models (Fig. 6.1).

Depending on the specific problem, we can choose a proper activation function based on the needs for a corresponding codomain or function range. For example, with hyperbolic tangent activation function, we can only have outputs ranging from -1 to 1 regardless of what input we have. With linear functions the output may range from $-\infty$ to $+\infty$. And the Gaussian activation function yields an ANN model called *Radial Basis Function* network.

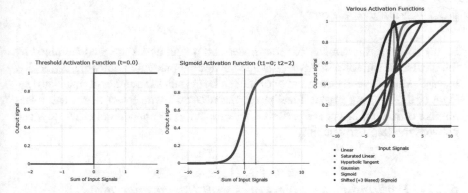

Fig. 6.1   Examples of node-specific activation functions

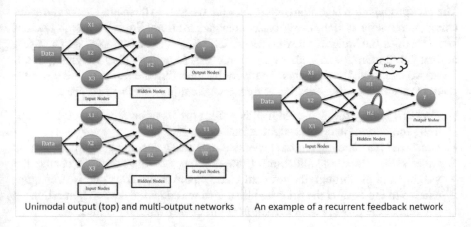

Unimodal output (top) and multi-output networks   An example of a recurrent feedback network

Fig. 6.2   Schematics of alternative two-layer networks

6.2   Network Topology

The number of layers: The x's, or features, in the dataset are called *input nodes* while
the predicted values are called the *output nodes*. Multilayer networks include
multiple hidden layers. Figure 6.2 shows a two-layer neural network.

When we have multiple layers, the information flow could be complicated. The
arrows in the previous figure suggest a feed forward network. In such networks, we
can also have multiple outcomes modeled simultaneously. Alternatively, in a recurrent network (feedback network), information can also travel backwards in loops
(or delays). Such network cycles may capture short-term memory, which dramatically increases the power of recurrent networks. More details and examples of
recurrent neural networks (RNNs) are presented in Chap. 12.

6.2.1   Network Layers

In any network, the number of input nodes and output nodes are predetermined by the predictive variables in the dataset and the desired prediction outcome. Typically, researchers can specify the number of hidden layers and the number of nodes in each layer of the network model. Ideally, simpler networks with fewer nodes and lower number of hidden layers are preferred for simplicity, computational efficiency, and network model interpretability.

6.2.2   Training Neural Networks with Backpropagation

The backpropagation algorithm determines the weights in the neural network model using the strategy of optimizing back-propagating errors. First, we assign random weight values (all weights must be nontrivial, i.e., $\neq 0$). For example, we can use a normal distribution, or any other random process, to assign initial weights (priors). Then, we can adjust the weights iteratively by repeating the process until a certain convergence or stopping criterion is met. Each iteration contains two phases.

- *Forward phase*: run the (training) data from the input layer to the output layer using the current iteration weight estimates.
- *Backward phase*: compare the generated outputs against the corresponding true target values (training validation). If the difference is significant, we change the weights and go through the forward phase again. If the error rate is decreased, relative to the error at the prior iteration, then we adopt the new weight estimates and repeat the process until certain iteration-ending criterion is met.

In the end, we pick a set of weights minimizing the total aggregate error to be the final weights of the specific neural network model.

6.2.3   Case Study 1: Google Trends and the Stock Market— Regression

Step 1: Collecting data
In this case study, we are going to use the Google Trends and stock market dataset; a documentation file with the meta-data and CSV-formatted data is available on the supporting Case Studies Canvas Site.[1] These daily data (between 2008 and 2009) can be used to examine the associations between Google search trends and market conditions, e.g., real estate or stock market indices.

---

[1] https://umich.instructure.com/courses/38100/files/folder/Case_Studies

Variables:

- **Index**: Time Index of the Observation
- **Date**: Date of the observation (Format: YYYY-MM-DD)
- **Unemployment**: The Google Unemployment Index tracks queries related to "unemployment, social, social security, unemployment benefits" and so on.
- **Rental**: The Google Rental Index tracks queries related to "rent, apartments, for rent, rentals," etc.
- **RealEstate**: The Google Real Estate Index tracks queries related to "real estate, mortgage, rent, apartments" and so on.
- **Mortgage**: The Google Mortgage Index tracks queries related to "mortgage, calculator, mortgage calculator, mortgage rates."
- **Jobs**: The Google Jobs Index tracks queries related to "jobs, city, job, resume, career, monster" and so forth.
- **Investing**: The Google Investing Index tracks queries related to "stock, finance, capital, yahoo finance, stocks," etc.
- **DJI_Index**: The Dow Jones Industrial (DJI) index. These data are interpolated from five records per week (Dow Jones stocks are traded on week-days only) to 7 days per week to match the constant 7-day records of the Google Trends data.
- **StdDJI**: The standardized-DJI Index computed by: $StdDJI = 3 + (DJI-11091)/1501$, where $m = 11{,}091$ and $s = 1501$ are the approximate mean and standard deviation of the DJI for the period (2005–2011).
- **30-Day Moving Average Data Columns**: The eight variables below are the 30 day moving averages of the eight corresponding (raw) variables above: *Unemployment30MA, Rental30MA, RealEstate30MA, Mortgage30MA, Jobs30MA, Investing30MA, DJI_Index30MA*, and *StdDJI_30MA*.
- **180-Day Moving Average Data Columns**: The eight variables below are the 180-day moving averages of the eight corresponding (raw) variables: *Unemployment180MA, Rental180MA, RealEstate180MA, Mortgage180MA, Jobs180MA, Investing180MA, DJI_Index180MA*, and *StdDJI_180MA*.

Let us use the Google Real Estate Index, `RealEstate`, as the dependent variable we want to predict using the other covariates in the dataset.

Step 2: Exploring and preparing the data
First, we load the dataset into R.

```
google <-
  read.csv("https://umich.instructure.com/files/416274/download?download_frd=1",
          stringsAsFactors = F)
```

We'll remove the first two columns since the goal now is to model and predict Real Estate or other economic indices.

```
google <- google[, -c(1, 2)]
str(google)
## 'data.frame':    731 obs. of  24 variables:
##  $ Unemployment     : num  1.54 1.56 1.59 1.62 1.64 1.64 1.71 1.85  ...
##  $ Rental           : num  0.88 0.9 0.92 0.92 0.94 0.96 0.99 1.02  ...
##  $ RealEstate       : num  0.79 0.81 0.82 0.82 0.83 0.84 0.86 0.89  ...
##  $ Mortgage         : num  1 1.05 1.07 1.08 1.1 1.11 1.15 1.22 1.23 ...
##  $ Jobs             : num  0.99 1.05 1.1 1.14 1.17 1.2 1.3 1.41 1.43 ...
##  $ Investing        : num  0.92 0.94 0.96 0.98 0.99 0.99 1.02 1.09  ...
##  $ DJI_Index        : num  13044 13044 13057 12800 12827 ...
##  $ StdDJI           : num  4.3 4.3 4.31 4.14 4.16 4.16 4.16 4 4.1 ...
##  $ Unemployment_30MA : num  1.37 1.37 1.38 1.38 1.39 1.4 1.4 1.42 ...
##  $ Rental_30MA      : num  0.72 0.72 0.73 0.73 0.74 0.75 0.76 0.77 ...
##  $ RealEstate_30MA  : num  0.67 0.67 0.68 0.68 0.68 0.69 0.7 0.7 0.71 ...
##  $ Mortgage_30MA    : num  0.98 0.97 0.97 0.97 0.98 0.98 0.98 0.99 ...
##  $ Jobs_30MA        : num  1.06 1.06 1.05 1.05 1.05 1.05 1.05 1.06 ...
##  $ Investing_30MA   : num  0.99 0.98 0.98 0.98 0.98 0.97 0.97 0.97 ...
##  $ DJI_Index_30MA   : num  13405 13396 13390 13368 13342 ...
##  $ StdDJI_30MA      : num  4.54 4.54 4.53 4.52 4.5 4.48 4.46 4.44 ...
##  $ Unemployment_180MA: num  1.44 1.44 1.44 1.44 1.44 1.44 1.44 1.44  ...
##  $ Rental_180MA     : num  0.87 0.87 0.87 0.87 0.87 0.87 0.86 0.86  ...
##  $ RealEstate_180MA : num  0.89 0.89 0.88 0.88 0.88 0.88 0.88 0.88  ...
##  $ Mortgage_180MA   : num  1.18 1.18 1.18 1.18 1.17 1.17 1.17 1.17  ...
##  $ Jobs_180MA       : num  1.24 1.24 1.24 1.24 1.24 1.24 1.24 1.24  ...
##  $ Investing_180MA  : num  1.04 1.04 1.04 1.04 1.04 1.04 1.04 1.04  ...
##  $ DJI_Index_180MA  : num  13493 13492 13489 13486 13482 ...
##  $ StdDJI_180MA     : num  4.6 4.6 4.6 4.6 4.59 4.59 4.59 4.58 4.58  ...
```

As we can see from the structure of the data, these indices have different ranges. We should `rescale` the data to make all features unitless, and therefore, comparable. In Chap. 5, we learned that normalizing these features using our own `normalize()` function could fix the problem of heterogeneity of measuring units across features. We can use `lapply()` to apply the `normalize()` function to each feature (column in the data frame).

```
normalize <- function(x) { return((x - min(x)) / (max(x) - min(x)))  }
google_norm <- as.data.frame(lapply(google, normalize))
summary(google_norm$RealEstate)
```

The last step clearly normalizes all feature vectors into the range [0, 1]. The next step would be to split the `google` dataset into *training* and *testing* sets. This time, we will use the `sample()` and `floor()` functions to separate training and testing sets (75:25). The `sample()` function creates a set of (random) indicators for row indices. We can subset the original dataset with random rows using these indicators. The `floor()` function takes a number x and returns the closest integer to x.

```
sample(row, floor(size))
```

- *row*: rows in the dataset that you want to select from. If you want to select all the rows, you can use *nrow(data)* or 1 : *nrow(data)* (for a single number or a vector).
- *size*: how many rows you want for your subset.

```
sub <- sample(nrow(google_norm), floor(nrow(google_norm)*0.75))
google_train <- google_norm[sub, ]
google_test <- google_norm[-sub, ]
```

Following this data preprocessing, we can move forward with the neural network training phase.

Step 3: Training a model on the data

Here, we use the function `neuralnet::neuralnet()`, Fig. 6.3, which returns a NN object containing:

- *call*; the matched call.
- *response*; extracted from the data argument.
- *covariate*; the variables extracted from the data argument.

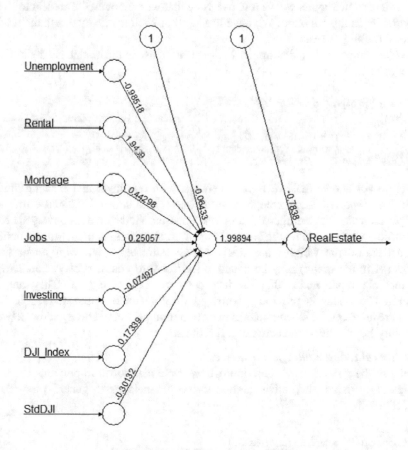

Error: 0.600307   Steps: 985

Fig. 6.3 A simple single-layer network predicting the Real Estate index from other market covariates

- *model.list*; a list containing the covariates and the response variables extracted from the formula argument.
- *err.fct* and *act.fct*; the error and activation functions.
- *net.result*; a list containing the overall result of the neural network for every repetition.
- *weights*; a list containing the fitted weights of the neural network for every repetition.
- *result.matrix*; a matrix containing the reached threshold, needed steps, error, AIC, BIC, and weights for every repetition. Each column represents one repetition.

`model <- neuralnet(target ~ predictors, data=mydata, hidden=1)`, where:

- *target*: variable we want to predict.
- *predictors*: predictors we want to use. Note that we cannot use "." to denote all the variables in this function. We have to add all predictors one by one to the model.
- *data*: training dataset.
- *hidden*: number of hidden nodes that we want to use in the model. By default, it is set to one.

```
# install.packages("neuralnet")
library(neuralnet)
google_model <-
   neuralnet(RealEstate~Unemployment+Rental+Mortgage+Jobs+
             Investing+DJI_Index+StdDJI, data=google_train)
plot(google_model)  # neuralnet::plot.nn
```

Figure 6.3 shows that we have a network with one layer and a single hidden node. The reported `Error` represents the aggregate sum of squared errors and `Steps` indicates the number of iterations until the ANN model converged. Note that these outputs could be different when you run exact same model-fitting optimization because the weights are stochastically estimated. Also, *bias nodes* (blue singletons in the graph) may be added to feedforward neural networks acting like intermediate input nodes that produce constant values, e.g., 1. They are not connected to nodes in previous layers, yet they generate biased activation. Bias nodes are not required but are helpful in some neural networks as they allow network flexibility by offsetting the activation functions.

Step 4: Evaluating model performance
Similar to the `predict()` function that we have mentioned in previous chapters, `compute()` is an alternative method that could help us to generate the model predictions.

```
prediction <- compute(m, test)
```

- *m*: a trained neural networks model.
- *test*: the test dataset. This dataset should only contain the same type of predictors in the neural network model.

Our model used `Unemployment`, `Rental`, `Mortgage`, `Jobs`, `Investing`, `DJI_Index`, `StdDJI` as predictors. Therefore, we need to reference these corresponding column numbers in the test dataset, i.e., columns 1, 2, 4, 5, 6, 7, 8, respectively.

```
google_pred <- compute(google_model, google_test[, c(1:2, 4:8)])
pred_results <- google_pred$net.result
cor(pred_results, google_test$RealEstate)
##           [,1]
## [1,] 0.9761242
```

As mentioned in Chap. 3, we can use the testing data to estimate the correlation between predicted results and observed Real Estate Index and evaluate the algorithmic performance. For real datasets, a correlation exceeding 0.9 is a very good indicator of the performance of the NN model. Could this be improved further?

Step 5: *Improving model performance*
This time we will include 4 hidden nodes in the single-layer NN model. Let's see what results we can get from this more complicated model (Fig. 6.4).

```
google_model2 <-
        neuralnet(RealEstate~Unemployment+Rental+Mortgage+Jobs+
                  Investing+DJI_Index+StdDJI, data=google_train, hidden = 4)
plot(google_model2)
```

Although the graph looks more complicated than the previous neural network, we have a smaller `Error`, i.e., sum squared error. Neural network models may be used both for *classification* and *regression*, which we will see in the next part. Let's first plot the regression between the observed and predicted outcomes (Fig. 6.5).

```
google_pred2 <- compute(google_model2, google_test[, c(1:2, 4:8)])
pred_results2 <- google_pred2$net.result
cor(pred_results2, google_test$RealEstate)
##           [,1]
## [1,] 0.9877632
plot_ly() %>%
  add_markers(x=pred_results2, y=google_test$RealEstate,
            name="Data Scatter", type="scatter", mode="markers") %>%
  add_trace(x = c(0,1), y = c(0,1), type="scatter", mode="lines",
          line = list(width = 4), name="Ideal Agreement") %>%
  layout(title=paste0('Scatterplot (Normalized) Observed vs. Predicted Real
Estate Values, Cor(Obs,Pred)=',
                  round(cor(pred_results2, google_test$RealEstate), 2)),
        xaxis = list(title="NN (hidden=4) Real Estate Predictions"),
        yaxis = list(title="(Normalized) Observed Real Estate"),
        legend = list(orientation = 'h'))
```

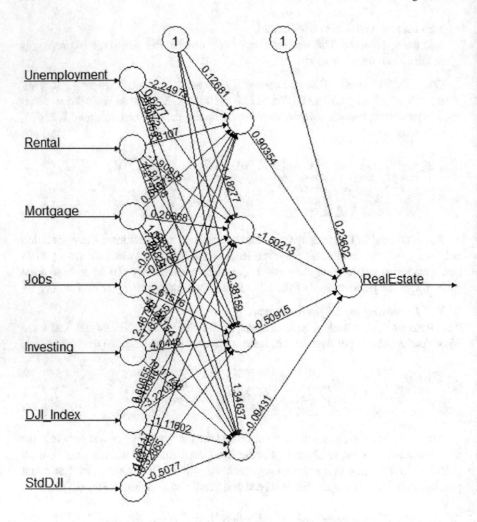

Error: 0.337411   Steps: 1932

Fig. 6.4 A four-node single-layer network predicting the Real Estate index from other market covariates

We get an even higher correlation. This is almost an ideal result. The predicted and observed RealEstate indices have a strong linear relationship. Nevertheless, too many hidden nodes might sometimes decrease the correlation between predicted and observed values, which will be examined in the practice problems later in this chapter.

Step 6: Adding additional layers
We observe an even lower Error by using three hidden layers, each with 4, 3, 3 nodes, respectively. However, this enhanced neural network may complicate the

Scatterplot (Normalized) Observed vs. Predicted Real Estate Values, Cor(Obs,Pred)=0.99

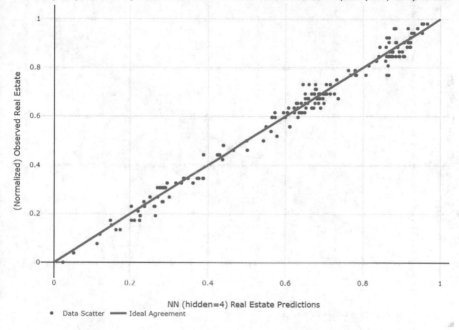

                              NN (hidden=4) Real Estate Predictions
           •   Data Scatter   ▬▬▬ Ideal Agreement

Fig. 6.5 Scatterplot of single-layer ANN-predicted Real Estate values (horizontal axis) vs. the (normalized) observed Real Estate values. The high correlation between these suggests an excellent performance of the network model prediction

interpretation of the results (or may overfit the network to intrinsic noise in the data) (Fig. 6.6).

```
google_model2 <-
        neuralnet(RealEstate~Unemployment+Rental+Mortgage+Jobs+
              Investing+DJI_Index+StdDJI, data=google_train, hidden = c(4,3,3))
google_pred2 <- compute(google_model2, google_test[, c(1:2, 4:8)])
pred_results2 <- google_pred2$net.result
cor(pred_results2, google_test$RealEstate)
## [1,] 0.9876618
plot_ly() %>%
  add_markers(x=pred_results2, y=google_test$RealEstate,
            name="Data Scatter", type="scatter", mode="markers") %>%
  add_trace(x = c(0,1), y = c(0,1), type="scatter", mode="lines",
        line = list(width = 4), name="Ideal Agreement") %>%
  layout(title=paste0('Scatterplot (Normalized) Observed vs. Predicted Real
Estate Values, Cor(Obs,Pred)=',
                    round(cor(pred_results2, google_test$RealEstate), 2)),
        xaxis = list(title="NN (hidden=(4,3,3)) Real Estate Predictions"),
        yaxis = list(title="(Normalized) Observed Real Estate"),
        legend = list(orientation = 'h'))
```

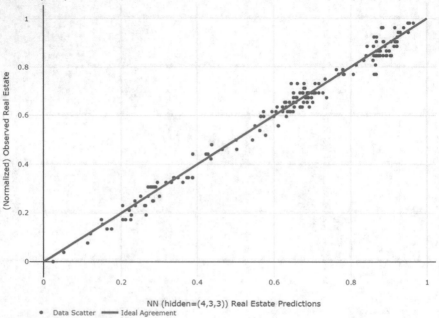

Fig. 6.6 Scatterplot of a multilayer ANN-predicted Real Estate values (horizontal axis) vs. the (normalized) observed Real Estate values. The high correlation between these suggests an excellent performance of the network model prediction

6.2.4   *Simple NN Demo—Learning to Compute* $\sqrt{}$

Neural networks can be used at the interface of experimental, theoretical, computational, and data sciences. Here is one powerful example, data science applications to string theory.[2] We will demonstrate the foundation of the neural network prediction to estimate a basic mathematical function square-root, $\sqrt{} : \mathbb{R}^+ \to \mathbb{R}^+$. First, let's generate and plot the data.

```
# generate random training data: X_i ~ Uniform (0,100)
rand_data <- abs(runif(1000, 0, 100))
# create a 2 column data-frame (input=data, output=sqrt_data)
sqrt_df <- data.frame(rand_data, sqrt_data=sqrt(rand_data))
s <- seq(from=0, to=100, length.out=1000)
plot_ly(x = ~s, y = ~sqrt(s), type="scatter", mode = "lines") %>%
  layout(title='Square-root Function',
          xaxis = list(title="Input (x)", scaleanchor="y"),
          yaxis = list(title="Output (y=sqrt(x))", scaleanchor="x"),
          legend = list(orientation = 'h'))
```

---

[2]https://doi.org/10.1016/j.physrep.2019.09.005

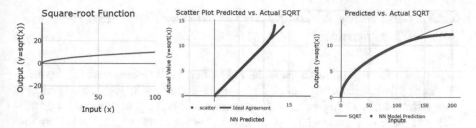

Fig. 6.7 Performance of a single-layer (10 modes) ANN for predicting the square-root function

Next, we fit the NN model and examine the NN-prediction results using the testing data (Fig. 6.7).

```
# Train the neural net
set.seed(1234)
net.sqrt <- neuralnet(sqrt_data ~ rand_data, sqrt_df,hidden=10,threshold=0.1)
# generate testing data seq(from=0.1, to=N, step=0.1)
N <- 200 # out of range [100: 200] is also included in the testing!
test_data <- seq(0, N, 0.1); test_data_sqrt <- sqrt(test_data)
test_data.df <- data.frame(rand_data=test_data, sqrt_data=sqrt(test_data));
 # try to predict the square-root values using 10 hidden nodes
 # Compute or predict for test data input, test_data.df
pred_sqrt <- predict(net.sqrt, test_data.df)
plot_ly(x = ~pred_sqrt[,1], y = ~test_data_sqrt, type = "scatter",
mode="markers", name="scatter") %>%
  add_trace(x = c(0,14), y = c(0,14), mode="lines", line = list(width = 4),
name="Ideal Agreement") %>%
  layout(title='Scatter Plot Predicted vs. Actual SQRT',
          xaxis = list(title="NN Predicted", scaleanchor="y"),
          yaxis = list(title="Actual Value (y=sqrt(x))", scaleanchor="x"),
          legend = list(orientation = 'h'))
compare_df <-data.frame(pred_sqrt, test_data_sqrt); # compare_df
plot_ly(x = ~test_data, y = ~test_data_sqrt, type="scatter", mode="lines",
name="SQRT") %>%
  add_trace(x = ~test_data, y = ~pred_sqrt, mode="markers", name="NN Model
Prediction") %>%
  layout(title='Predicted vs. Actual SQRT',
          xaxis = list(title="Inputs"),
          yaxis = list(title="Outputs (y=sqrt(x))"),
          legend = list(orientation = 'h'))
```

We observe that within the training domain, the NN, net.sqrt, actually learns and predicts pretty well the square-root function. Of course, there will be expected variation subject to changes in the training domain, parameter settings, and repeated experiments, as we randomly generate the training data (rand_data) and fitting the NN model (net.sqrt) is also stochastic.

6.2.5 Case Study 2: Google Trends and the Stock Market—Classification

In practice, NN may be more useful as a classifier. Let's demonstrate this by using the Stock Market data. We mark the samples according to their RealEstate categorization. Those higher than 75 percentile will be labeled 0, those lower than 0.25 percentile will get labeled 2, and those in between will get labeled 1. Note that even in the classification setting, the responses still must be numeric.

```
google_class = google_norm
id1 = which(google_class$RealEstate>quantile(google_class$RealEstate,0.75))
id2 = which(google_class$RealEstate<quantile(google_class$RealEstate,0.25))
id3 = setdiff(1:nrow(google_class),union(id1,id2))
google_class$RealEstate[id1]=0
google_class$RealEstate[id2]=1
google_class$RealEstate[id3]=2
summary(as.factor(google_class$RealEstate))
##   0   1   2
## 179 178 374
```

We divide the data into training and testing sets and generate three derived one-hot-encoding features (dummy variables), which correspond to the three RealEstate outcome labels (categories).

```
set.seed(2017)
train = sample(1:nrow(google_class),0.7*nrow(google_class))
google_tr = google_class[train,]
google_ts = google_class[-train,]
train_x = google_tr[,c(1:2,4:8)]
train_y = google_tr[,3]
colnames(train_x)
## "Unemployment" "Rental" "Mortgage" "Jobs" "Investing" "DJI_Index" "StdDJI"
test_x = google_ts[ , c(1:2,4:8)]
test_y = google_ts[3]
train_y_ind = model.matrix(~factor(train_y)-1)
colnames(train_y_ind) = c("High","Median","Low")
train = cbind(train_x, train_y_ind)
```

We specify nonlinear output and report intermediate results every 5000 iterations.

```
nn_single <- neuralnet(High+Median+Low~Unemployment+Rental+Mortgage+
                Jobs+Investing+DJI_Index+StdDJI,
              data = train, hidden=4, linear.output=FALSE,
              lifesign='full', lifesign.step=5000)
```

Below is the prediction function using this neural network model to forecast the RealEstate class label.

```
pred = function(nn, dat) {
    yhat = compute(nn, dat)$net.result
    yhat = apply(yhat, 1, which.max)-1
    return(yhat)
}
mean(pred(nn_single, google_ts[,c(1:2,4:8)]) != as.factor(google_ts[,3]))
## [1] 0.01818182
```

Finally, report the *confusion matrix* illustrating the agreement/disagreement between the three observed `RealEstate` class labels and their (NN) predicted counterparts.

```
table(pred(nn_single, google_ts[,c(1:2,4:8)]), as.factor(google_ts[,3]))
##       0   1   2
##  0   51   0   0
##  1    0  54   2
##  2    2   0 111
```

Next, we can inspect the structure of the resulting neural network model.

```
plot(nn_single)
```

Similarly, we can change `hidden` to utilize multiple hidden layers; however, a more complicated model won't necessarily guarantee an improved performance.

```
nn_single =
        neuralnet(High+Median+Low~Unemployment+Rental+Mortgage+
                Jobs+Investing+DJI_Index+StdDJI,
                data = train, hidden=c(4,5), linear.output=FALSE,
                lifesign='full', lifesign.step=5000)
mean(pred(nn_single, google_ts[,c(1:2,4:8)]) != as.factor(google_ts[,3]))
## [1] 0.02727273
```

6.3 Support Vector Machines (SVM)

Recall that in Chap. 5 we presented lazy machine learning methods, which assign class labels using geometrical distances of different features. In multidimensional feature spaces, we can utilize spheres, centered according to the training dataset, to assign testing data labels. What kinds of shapes may be embedded in higher-dimensional spaces to help with the classification process?

6.3.1 Classification with Hyperplanes

In higher dimensions, the easiest shape would be an $(n-1)D$ hyperplane embedded in nD, which splits the entire space into two parts. Support vector machines (SVM) can use hyperplanes to split the data into separate groups, or classes. Obviously, this may be useful for datasets that are *linearly separable*. As an example, consider lines, $(n-1)D$ planes, embedded in R^2. Assuming that we have only two features, will you choose line A or line B as the better `hyperplane` separating the data? Or even another plane C?

6.3.1.1   Finding the Maximum Margin

To answer the above question, we need to search for the *Maximum Margin Hyperplane (MMH)*. That is the hyperplane that creates greatest separation between the two closest observations. We define support vectors as the points from each class that are closest to MMH. Each class must have at least one observation as a support vector. Using support vectors alone is insufficient for finding the MMH. Although some mathematical calculations are involved, the fundamental of the SVM process is fairly simple. Let's look at linearly separable data and nonlinearly separable data individually.

6.3.1.2   Linearly Separable Data

If the dataset is linearly separable, we can find the outer boundaries of our two groups of data points. These boundaries are called convex hulls (red lines in the following graph). The MMH (green solid line) is just the line that is perpendicular to the shortest line (orange, dash) between the two convex hulls. We can illustrate this with a simple 2D example (Fig. 6.8).

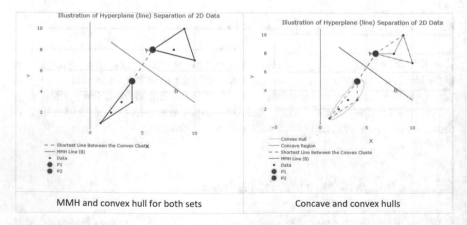

Fig. 6.8 Hypothetical linear space partitioning in 2D. Mind the difference between convex hull and concave hull of a set of points

```r
# install.packages("alphahull")
library(alphahull)
convexSplinePolygon <- function(boundaryVertices, vertexNumber, k=3)  {
    # Wrap k vertices around each end.
    n <- dim(boundaryVertices)[1]
    if (vertexNumber < n) {  print("vertexNumber< n!!!");  stop()    }
    if (k >= 1) { data <- rbind(boundaryVertices[(n-k+1):n, ],
                                boundaryVertices, boundaryVertices[1:k, ])
    } else { data <- boundaryVertices    }
    # Spline-interpolate the x and y coordinates
    data.spline <- spline(1:(n+2*k), data[ , 1], n=vertexNumber)
    x <- data.spline$x
    x1 <- data.spline$y
    x2 <- spline(1:(n+2*k), data[,2], n=vertexNumber)$y
    # Keep only the middle part
    cbind(x1, x2)[k < x & x <= n+k, ]
}
# Concave hull (alpha-convex hull)
group1 <- list(x=A[6:9], y=B[6:9])
# check and remove any duplicate points to prevent ahull() function errors
group2 <- lapply(group1, "[",
                       which(!duplicated(as.matrix(as.data.frame(group1)))))
concaveHull1 <- ahull(group2, alpha=6)
# Convex hull
group3 <- list(x=A[1:5], y=B[1:5])
# points(group3, pch=19)
convHull2 <- lapply(group3, "[", chull(group3))
library(sp)
SpP = SpatialPolygons(list(Polygons(list(Polygon(group2)),ID="s1")))
x1 <- SpP@polygons[[1]]@Polygons[[1]]@coords[,1]
y1 <- SpP@polygons[[1]]@Polygons[[1]]@coords[,2]
df1 <- convexSplinePolygon(as.matrix(as.data.frame(convHull2)), 100)
plot_ly() %>%
  add_trace(x=df1[,1], y=df1[,2], type="scatter", mode="lines",
            name="Convex Hull", line=list(color="lightblue")) %>%
  add_lines(x = x1, y = y1, type="scatter", mode="lines",
            name="Concave Region", line=list(color="orange")) %>%
  add_segments(x = df1[1,1],  xend=df1[dim(df1)[1],1], y = df1[1,2],
            yend = df1[dim(df1)[1],2], type="scatter",
            mode="lines", name="", line=list(color="gray"), showlegend=F) %>%
  add_segments(x = x1[3],  xend=x1[4], y=y1[3], yend = y1[4], type="scatter",
            mode="lines", name="Concave Region", line=list(color="orange"),
            showlegend=F) %>%
```

```
  add_lines(x = c(6,4), y = c(8,5), name=
"Shortest Line Between the Convex Clusters (A)", line=list(dash='dash'))  %>%
  add_lines(x = c(10,2), y=c(3,8.7), mode="lines", name="MMH Line (B)")  %>%
  add_segments(x=1, xend=4, y=1, yend = 5, line=list(color="gray",
            dash='dash'), showlegend=F) %>%
  add_segments(x=1, xend=4, y=1, yend = 3, line=list(color="gray",
            dash='dash'), showlegend=F) %>%
  add_segments(x=4, xend=4, y=3, yend = 5, line=list(color="gray",
            dash='dash'), showlegend=F) %>%
  add_segments(x=6, xend=10, y=8, yend = 7, line=list(color="gray",
            dash='dash'), showlegend=F) %>%
  add_segments(x=6, xend=10, y=8, yend = 7, line=list(color="gray",
            dash='dash'), showlegend=F) %>%
  add_segments(x=10, xend=9, y=7, yend = 10, line=list(color="gray",
            dash='dash'), showlegend=F) %>%
  add_markers(x = A, y = B, type="scatter", mode="markers", name="Data",
            marker=list(color="blue")) %>%
  add_markers(x = 4, y = 5, name="P1",
            marker = list(size = 20, color = 'blue',
            line = list(color = 'yellow', width = 2))) %>%
  add_segments(x=6, xend=9, y=8, yend = 10, line=list(color="gray",
            dash='dash'), showlegend=F) %>%
  add_markers(x = 6, y = 8, name="P2",
            marker = list(size = 20, color = 'blue',
            line = list(color = 'yellow', width = 2))) %>%
  layout(title="Illustration of Hyperplane (line) Separation of 2D Data",
        xaxis=list(title="X", scaleanchor="y"),  # control y:x aspect ratio
        yaxis = list(title="Y", scaleanchor = "x"),
        legend = list(orientation = 'h'),
        annotations = list(text=modelLabels,  x=modelLabels.x,
                y=modelLabels.y, textangle=c(-40,0),
                font=list(size=15, color=modelLabels.col), showarrow=FALSE))
```

An alternative way to linearly separate the data into (two) clusters is to find two parallel planes that can separate the data into two groups, and then increase the distance between the two planes as much as possible. We can use vector notation to mathematically define planes. In an n-dimensional space, a plane could be expressed by the following equation

$$\vec{w} \cdot \vec{x} + b = 0,$$

where $\vec{w}$ (weights) is the plane normal vector, $\vec{x}$ is the vector of unknowns (coordinates of points on the plane), both have n coordinates, and b is a constant scalar that completely determines the plane (as it specifies a point the plane goes through).

To clarify this notation let's look at the situation in a 3D space where we can express (embed) 2D Euclidean planes using a point (x_o, y_o, z_o) and normal-vector (a, b, c) form. This is just a linear equation, where $d = -(ax_o + by_o + cz_0)$,

$$ax + by + cz + d = 0,$$

or equivalently

$$w_1 x_1 + w_2 x_2 + w_3 x_3 + b = 0.$$

We can see that it is equivalent to the vector notation. Using the vector notation, we can specify two hyperplanes as follows

$$\vec{w} \cdot \vec{x} + b \geq +1$$

and

$$\vec{w} \cdot \vec{x} + b \leq -1$$

We require that all the observations in the first class fall above the first plane and all observations in the other class fall below the second plane. The distance between two planes is calculated by

$$\frac{2}{\| \vec{w} \|},$$

where $\| \cdot \|$ is the Euclidean norm. To maximize the distance, we need to minimize the Euclidean norm. To sum up, we are going to find $\min \frac{\| \vec{w} \|}{2}$ subject to the following constraint

$$y_i \left(\vec{w} \cdot \vec{x_i} - b \right) \geq 1, 0 \leq i \leq n,$$

where for each data point index i, $y_i = \pm 1$ correspond to $w \cdot x_i - b \geq 1$ and $w \cdot x_i - b \leq -1$, respectively.

We will see more about *constrained and unconstrained optimization* later in Chap. 13. For each nonlinear programming problem, the *primal problem*, there is related nonlinear programming problem, also known as the *Lagrangian dual problem*. Under certain assumptions for convexity and suitable constraints, the primal and dual problems have equal optimal objective values. Primal optimization problems are typically described as:

$$\min_x f(x)$$
$$\text{subject to}$$
$$g_i(x) \leq 0$$
$$h_j(x) = 0$$

Then the Lagrangian dual problem is defined as a parallel nonlinear programming problem

$$\min_{u,v} \; \theta(u, v)$$

$$\text{subject to} \; ,$$

$$u_i \geq 0, \quad \forall i$$

where

$$\theta(u, v) = \inf_x \left(f(x) + \sum_i u_i g_i(x) + \sum_j v_j h_j(x) \right).$$

Chapter 13 provides additional technical details about optimization duality. Suppose the Lagrange primal problem is

$$L_p = \frac{1}{2} \|w\|^2 - \sum_{i=1}^{n} \alpha_i \left[y_i \left(w_0 + x_i^t w \right) - 1 \right], \text{where } \alpha_i \geq 0.$$

To optimize that objective function, we can set the partial derivatives equal to zero:

$$\frac{\partial}{\partial w} \; : \; w = \sum_{i=1}^{n} \alpha_i y_i x_i,$$

$$\frac{\partial}{\partial b} \; : \; 0 = \sum_{i=1}^{n} \alpha_i y_i.$$

Substituting into the Lagrange primal, we obtain the Lagrange dual problem

$$L_D = \sum_{i=1}^{n} \alpha_i - \frac{1}{2} \sum_{i=1}^{n} \alpha_i \alpha_i' y_i y_i' x_i^t x_i' = \sum_{i=1}^{n} \alpha_i - \frac{1}{2} \sum_{i=1}^{n} \sum_{j=1}^{n} y_i \alpha_i (x_i \cdot x_j) y_j \alpha_j.$$

Then, we maximize L_D subject to $\alpha_i \geq 0$ and $\sum_{i=1}^{n} \alpha_i y_i = 0$. For each $i \in \{1, \cdots, n\}$, this iterative optimization results in adjusting the coefficient α_i in the gradient direction $\frac{\partial f}{\partial \alpha_i}$.

Hence, the resulting coefficient vector $(\alpha_1', \cdots, \alpha_n')$ is projected onto the nearest vector of coefficients which satisfies the given constraints. Repeating this process drives the coefficient vector to a local optimum.

By the Karush–Kuhn–Tucker optimization conditions,[3] we have $\widehat{\alpha} \left[y_i \left(\widehat{b} + x_i^t \widehat{w} \right) - 1 \right] = 0.$

---

[3] https://doi.org/10.1016/j.ejor.2005.09.007

This implies that if $y_i \widehat{f}(x_i) > 1$, then $\widehat{\alpha}_i = 0$. The **support** of a function $(f(x_i) = \widehat{b} + x_i^t \widehat{w})$ is the smallest subset of the domain containing only arguments (x) which are not mapped to zero $(f(x) \neq 0)$. In our case, the solution $\widehat{w}$ is defined in terms of a linear combination of the **support points**

$$\widehat{f}(x) = w^t x = w = \sum_{i=1}^{n} \alpha_i y_i x_i.$$

That's where the name of support vector machines (SVM) comes from.

6.3.1.3 Nonlinearly Separable Data

For nonlinearly separable data, we can linearize the problem in a higher dimensional space. Still, we use a separating hyperplane, but allow some of the points to be misclassified into the wrong class. To penalize for misclassification, we add a regularization term after the fidelity term (Euclidean norm) and then minimize the additive mixture of the two terms. Therefore, the solution will optimize the following *regularized* objective (cost) function

$$\min \left(\frac{\| \vec{w} \|}{2} + C \sum_{i=1}^{n} \xi_i \right)$$

subject to

$$y_i \left(\vec{w} \cdot \vec{x}_i - b \right) \geq 1, \forall \vec{x}_i, \xi_i \geq 0,$$

where the hyperparameter C controls the error term (regularization) penalty and ξ_i is the distance between the misclassified observation i and the plane.

We have the following Lagrange primal problem:

$$L_p = \frac{1}{2} \|w\|^2 + C \sum_{i=1}^{n} \xi_i - \sum_{i=1}^{n} \alpha_i \left[y_i \left(b + x_i^t w \right) - (1 - \xi_i) \right] - \sum_{i=1}^{n} \gamma_i \xi_i,$$

where

$$\alpha_i, \gamma_i \geq 0.$$

Similar to what we did earlier in the linearly separable case, we can use the derivatives of the primal problem to solve the dual problem. Notice the inner product in the final expression. We can replace this inner product with a kernel function that maps the feature space into a higher dimensional space (e.g., using a polynomial kernel) or an infinite dimensional space (e.g., using a Gaussian kernel).

6.3.1.4   Using Kernels for Nonlinear Spaces

An alternative way to solve for the nonlinear separable is called the *kernel trick*, which involves adding new dimensions (or features) to embed the original nonlinearly separable problem into a linearly separable problem in a higher dimensional space. The solution of the quadratic optimization problem in this case involves the use of a *regularized* objective function

$$\min_{w,b} \left(\frac{\| \vec{w} \|}{2} + C \sum_{i=1}^{n} \xi_i \right),$$

subject to

$$y_i \left(\vec{w} \cdot \phi\left(\vec{x}_i \right) - b \right) \geq 1 - \xi_i, \forall \vec{x}_i, \xi_i \geq 0.$$

Again, the hyperparameter C controls the regularization penalty and ξ_i are the slack variables introduced by lifting the initial low-dimensional (nonlinear) problem to a new higher dimensional linear problem. The quadratic optimization of this (primal) higher-dimensional problem is similarly transformed into a Lagrangian dual problem:

$$L_p = \max_{\alpha} \min_{w,b} \left\{ \frac{1}{2} \|w\|^2 + C \sum_{i=1}^{n} \alpha_i \left(1 - w^T \phi\left(\vec{x}_i \right) + b \right) \right\},$$

where

$$0 \leq \alpha_i \leq C, \forall i.$$

The solution to the Lagrange dual problem provides estimates of α_i and we can predict the *class label* of a new (testing) sample x_{test} via

$$y_{\text{test}} = \text{sign}(w^t \phi(x_{\text{test}}) + b) = \text{sign} \left(\sum_{i=1}^{n} \alpha_i y_i \underbrace{\phi\left(\vec{x}_{i,\text{test}} \right)^t \phi\left(\vec{x}_{j,\text{test}} \right)}_{\text{kernel, } K\left(\vec{x}_i, \ \vec{x}_j \right) = \phi\left(\vec{x}_{i,\text{test}} \right) \cdot \phi\left(\vec{x}_{j,\text{test}} \right)} + b \right).$$

Below is one example where the 2D data (mtcars, $n = 32$, $k = 10$, cars fuel consumption) doesn't appear to be linearly separable in its native 2D (*weight* × *horsepower*) space where the binary colors correspond to *V-shaped* or *Straight* engine types.

```
library(plotly)
mtcars$vs[which(mtcars$vs == 0)] <- 'V-Shaped Engine'
mtcars$vs[which(mtcars$vs == 1)] <- 'Straight Engine'
mtcars$vs <- as.factor(mtcars$vs)
p_2D <- plot_ly(mtcars, x = ~wt, y = ~hp/10, color = ~vs,
                colors = c('blue', 'red'), name=~vs) %>%
  add_markers() %>%
  add_segments(x = 1, xend = 6, y = 8, yend = 18, colors="gray",
               opacity=0.2, showlegend = FALSE) %>%
  layout(xaxis = list(title = 'Weight'), yaxis = list(title = 'Horsepower'),
         legend = list(orientation = 'h'),
         title="(mtcars) Automobile Weight vs. Horsepower Relation") %>%
  hide_colorbar()
p_2D
```

However, the data can be lifted in 3D where it is more clearly linearly separable
(by engine type) via a 2D plane (Fig. 6.9).

```
# Compute the Normal to the 2D PC plane
normVec = c(1, 1.3, -3.0)
# Compute the 3D point of gravitational balance (Plane has to go through it)
dMean <- c(3.2, -280, 2)
d <- as.numeric((-1)*normVec %*% dMean)  # force 2D plane through the mean
x=mtcars$wt; y=mtcars$hp; z=mtcars$qsec; w=mtcars$vs  # define x, y, z dims
w.col = ifelse(mtcars$vs=="Straight Engine", "blue", "red")
w.name = ifelse(mtcars$vs=="Straight Engine", "Straight", "V-shape")
# Reparametrize the 2D (x,y) grid, and define the corresponding model values z on
the grid. Recall z=-(d + ax+by)/c, where normVec=(a,b,c)
x.seq <- seq(min(x),max(x),length.out=100)
y.seq <- seq(min(y),max(y),length.out=100)
z.seq <- function(x,y) -(d + normVec[1]*x + normVec[2]*y)/normVec[3]
# define the values of z = z(x.seq, y.seq), as a Matrix of dimension
c(dim(x.seq), dim(y.seq))
z1 <- t(outer(x.seq, y.seq, z.seq))/10; range(z1)  # 10 correction
## [1] 14.53043 26.92413
# Draw the 2D plane embedded in 3D, and then add points with "add_trace"
myPlotly <- plot_ly(x=~x.seq, y=~y.seq, z=~z1,
                    colors="gray", type="surface", opacity=0.5, showlegend=FALSE) %>%
  add_trace(data=mtcars, x=x, y=y, z=mtcars$qsec, mode="markers",
            type="scatter3d", marker=list(color=w.col,opacity=0.9,symbol=105)) %>%
  layout(showlegend = FALSE, scene = list(
         aspectmode = "manual", aspectratio = list(x=1, y=1, z=1),
         xaxis = list(title = "Weight", range = c(min(x),max(x))),
         yaxis = list(title = "Horsepower", range = c(min(y),max(y))),
         zaxis = list(title = "1/4 mile time", range = c(14, 23)))
  ) %>% hide_colorbar()
myPlotly
```

To translate this simple example to the more general case, we transform our data
using kernel functions. In general, kernel functions can be expressed as

$$K\left(\overrightarrow{x_i}, \overrightarrow{x_j}\right) = \phi\left(\overrightarrow{x_i}\right) \cdot \phi\left(\overrightarrow{x_j}\right),$$

where ϕ is a mapping of the data into another space.

The *linear kernel* would be the simplest one and corresponds to the *dot product* of
the features.

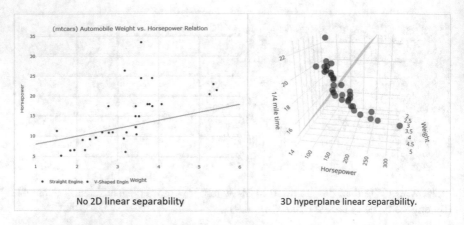

Fig. 6.9 Demonstration of higher-dimensional embedding using the automobile fuel efficiency data. Note the lack of linear separability in 2D projection space (left), and the improved hyperplane vehicle engine type separability in the 3D embedding (right)

$$K\left(\overrightarrow{x_i}, \overrightarrow{x_j}\right) = \overrightarrow{x_i} \cdot \overrightarrow{x_j}.$$

The *polynomial kernel* of degree d transforms the data by adding a simple nonlinear transformation of the data

$$K\left(\overrightarrow{x_i}, \overrightarrow{x_j}\right) = \left(\overrightarrow{x_i} \cdot \overrightarrow{x_j} + 1\right)^d.$$

The *sigmoid kernel* is very similar to the neural networks approach. It uses a sigmoid activation function.

$$K\left(\overrightarrow{x_i}, \overrightarrow{x_j}\right) = \tanh\left(k\,\overrightarrow{x_i} \cdot \overrightarrow{x_j} - \delta\right).$$

The *Gaussian radial basis function (RBF) kernel* is similar to an RBF neural network and may be a good place to start, in general.

$$K\left(\overrightarrow{x_i}, \overrightarrow{x_j}\right) = \exp\left(\frac{-\parallel \overrightarrow{x_i} - \overrightarrow{x_j} \parallel^2}{2\sigma^2}\right).$$

6.3.2 Case Study 3: Optical Character Recognition (OCR)

In Chap. 4, we saw machine learning strategies for handwritten digit recognition. We now want to expand that to character recognition. The following example illustrates management and transferring of handwritten notes (text) and converting them to typeset or printed text representing the characters in the original notes (unstructured image data).

Fig. 6.10 An example of
the preprocessed gridded
handwritten letters
(classification input)

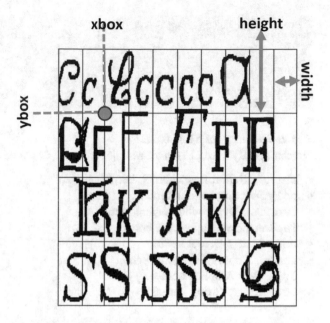

Protocol

- Divide the image (typically optical image of handwritten notes on paper) into a fine grid where each cell contains 1 glyph (symbol, letter, number).
- Match the glyph in each cell to 1 of the possible characters in a dictionary.
- Combine individual characters together into words to reconstitute the digital representation of the optical image of the handwritten notes.

In this example, we use an optical document image (data) that has already been pre-partitioned into rectangular grid cells containing one character of the 26 English letters, A through Z.

The resulting gridded dataset is distributed by the UCI Machine Learning Data Repository.[4] The dataset is available in the supporting website and contains 20,000 examples of 26 English capital letters printed using 20 different randomly reshaped and morphed fonts (Fig. 6.10).

Step 1: Prepare and explore the data
Load the data and split it into training and testing sets.

---

[4] https://archive.ics.uci.edu/ml

```
# read in data and examine its structure
hand_letters <-
 read.csv("https://umich.instructure.com/files/2837863/download?download_frd=1",
    header = T)
str(hand_letters)
# divide into training (3/4) and testing (1/4) data
hand_letters_train <- hand_letters[1:15000, ]
hand_letters_test  <- hand_letters[15001:20000, ]
```

Step 2: Training an SVM model

We can specify vanilladot as a linear kernel or choose an alternative kernel

- rbfdot Radial Basis kernel, i.e., "Gaussian"
- polydot Polynomial kernel
- tanhdot Hyperbolic tangent kernel
- laplacedot Laplacian kernel
- besseldot Bessel kernel
- anovadot ANOVA RBF kernel
- splinedot Spline kernel
- stringdot String kernel

```
# begin by training a simple linear SVM
library(kernlab)
set.seed(123)
hand_letter_classifier <- ksvm(as.factor(letter) ~ .,
                               data=hand_letters_train, kernel="vanilladot")
hand_letter_classifier  # check the basic information about the model
...
## Training error : 0.129733
```

Step 3: Evaluating model performance(Fig. 6.11)

```
# predictions on testing dataset
hand_letter_predictions <- predict(hand_letter_classifier, hand_letters_test)
head(hand_letter_predictions)
# table(hand_letter_predictions, hand_letters_test$letter)
# look only at agreements vs. disagreements
# construct a vector of TRUE/FALSE indicating correct/incorrect predictions
agreement <- hand_letter_predictions == hand_letters_test$letter table(agreement)
## agreement
## FALSE   TRUE
##   780   4220
prop.table(table(agreement))
## agreement
## FALSE   TRUE
## 0.156 0.844
tab <- table(hand_letter_predictions, hand_letters_test$letter)
tab_df <- tidyr::spread(as.data.frame(tab), key = Var2, value = Freq)
sum(diag(table(hand_letter_predictions, hand_letters_test$letter))) #  4220
plot_ly(x = colnames(tab), y = colnames(tab), z = as.matrix(tab_df[, -1]),
        type = "heatmap")
```

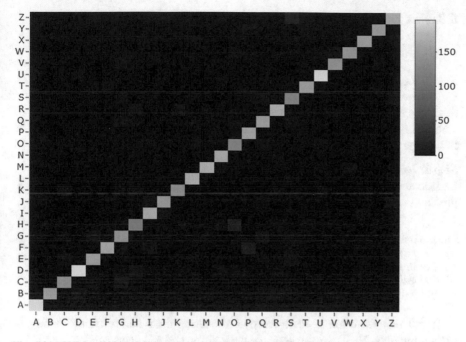

Fig. 6.11 SVM validation on the handwritten letters — classification output labels vs. true labels

Step 4: Improving model performance

Replacing the `vanilladot` linear kernel with `rbfdot` Radial Basis Function kernel, i.e., "Gaussian" kernel, may improve the SVM optical character recognition (OCR) prediction.

```
hand_letter_classifier_rbf <- ksvm(as.factor(letter) ~ .,
                           data = hand_letters_train, kernel = "rbfdot")
hand_letter_predictions_rbf <- predict(hand_letter_classifier_rbf,
                                       hand_letters_test)
agreement_rbf <- hand_letter_predictions_rbf == hand_letters_test$letter
table(agreement_rbf)
## FALSE   TRUE
##   361   4639
prop.table(table(agreement_rbf))
## agreement_rbf
##   FALSE    TRUE
##  0.0722  0.9278
```

Note the improvement of the automated (SVM) classification accuracy (0.928) for `rbfdot` compared to the previous (`vanilladot`) result (0.844).

6.3.3   Case Study 4: Iris Flowers

Let's have another look at the *iris data* that we saw in Chap. 2.

Step 1: Collecting data
SVM requires all features to be numeric and each feature has to be scaled into a relatively small interval. We are using Edgar Anderson's Iris Data in R for this case study. This dataset measures the length and width of sepals and petals from three Iris flower species.

Step 2: Exploring and preparing the data
Let's load the data first and examine the variable Species, which we would like to predict.

```
data(iris)
str(iris)
table(iris$Species)
## setosa versicolor virginica
## 50 50 50
```

Recall that we often need to remove measuring units before fitting models or classifying data. Next, we can separate the training and test dataset using the $75%$–$25%$ rule (Fig. 6.12).

```
sub<-sample(nrow(iris), floor(nrow(iris)*0.75))
iris_train<-iris[sub, ]
iris_test<-iris[-sub, ]
library(e1071)
iris.svm_1 <- svm(Species~Petal.Length+Petal.Width, data=iris_train,
                kernel="linear", cost=1)
iris.svm_2 <- svm(Species~Petal.Length+Petal.Width, data=iris_train,
                kernel="radial", cost=1)
par(mfrow=c(2,1))
plot(iris.svm_1, iris[,c(5,3,4)], symbolPalette = rainbow(4),
    color.palette = terrain.colors)
legend("center", "Linear")
plot(iris.svm_2, iris[,c(5,3,4)], symbolPalette = rainbow(4),
    color.palette = terrain.colors)
legend("center", "Radial", )
```

Step 3: Training a model on the data
We are going to use kernlab for this case study; however, many other packages like e1071 and klaR also provide SVM modeling, regression, and classification. The function ksvm() invocation syntax is

```
model <- ksvm(target~predictors, data=mydata, kernel="rbfdot", c=1)
```

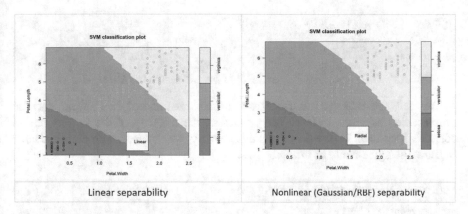

Fig. 6.12 Iris flower SVM classification—2D linear and nonlinear (RBF) kernel separation

- *target*: the outcome variable that we want to predict.
- *predictors*: features that the prediction is based on. In this function we can use the "." to represent all the variables in the dataset again.
- *data*: the training dataset including *target outputs* and *covariate predictors*.
- *kernel*: is the kernel mapping we want to use. By default, it is the radial basis function (rbfdot).
- *C* is a number that specifies the cost of misclassification.

```
# install.packages("kernlab")
library(kernlab)
iris_clas <- ksvm(Species~., data=iris_train, kernel="vanilladot")
iris_clas
## Number of Support Vectors : 25
## Objective Function Value : -0.9366 -0.2491 -15.1783
## Training error : 0.026786
```

Here, we used all the variables other than the Species in the dataset as predictors. In this model, we used the kernel vanilladot, a linear kernel, and obtained a training error of about 0.03.

Step 4: Evaluating model performance
Given any prefit model, we have already used the predict() function to make predictions. Here, we have a categorical (factor) outcome, so we need the command table() to show us how well the predictions and actual data match.

```
iris.pred<-predict(iris_clas, iris_test)
table(iris.pred, iris_test$Species)
## iris.pred   setosa versicolor virginica
##   setosa        15          0         0
##   versicolor     0         10         2
##   virginica      0          0        11
```

We can see that only a few cases of Iris versicolor flowers may be misclassified as virginica. The species of the majority of the flowers are all correctly identified. To see the results more clearly, we can use the proportional table to show the agreements of the categories.

```
agreement<-iris.pred==iris_test$Species
prop.table(table(agreement))
## agreement
##      FALSE       TRUE
## 0.05263158 0.94736842
```

Here, the double-equal operator == generates Boolean true or false results from comparing the testing data predicted species class labels to their true taxa label counterparts. Over 90% of predictions are correct. Nevertheless, is there any chance that we can improve the outcome? What if we try a Gaussian kernel?

Step 5: RBF kernel function
Linear kernel is the simplest one but usually not the best one. Let's try the *RBF (Radial Basis "Gaussian" Function)* kernel instead.

```
iris_clas1<-ksvm(Species~., data=iris_train, kernel="rbfdot")
iris_clas1
## Objective Function Value : -6.2592 -6.6136 -16.5963
## Training error : 0.017857
iris.pred1 <- predict(iris_clas1, iris_test)
table(iris.pred1, iris_test$Species)
## iris.pred1   setosa versicolor virginica
##   setosa        15          0         0
##   versicolor     0         10         2
##   virginica      0          0        11
agreement<-iris.pred1==iris_test$Species
prop.table(table(agreement))
## agreement
##      FALSE       TRUE
## 0.05263158 0.94736842
```

The model performance did not drastically improve, compared to the previous *linear* kernel case (repeated runs might yield slightly different results). This is because the Iris dataset has a mostly linear feature space separation. In practice, we could try alternative kernel functions and see which one fits the dataset the best.

6.3.4   Parameter Tuning

We can tune the SVM using the function `tune.svm()` in the package `e1071`.

```
costs = exp(-5:8)
tune.svm(Species~., kernel = "radial", data = iris_train, cost = costs)
```

Further, we can draw a cross-validation (**cv**) plot to gauge the model performance (Fig. 6.13).

```
# install.packages("sparsediscrim")
set.seed(2017)
library(sparsediscrim)
library (reshape); library(ggplot2)
folds = cv_partition(iris$Species, num_folds = 5)
train_cv_error_svm = function(costC) {
  #Train
  ir.svm = svm(Species~., data=iris, kernel="radial", cost=costC)
  train_error = sum(ir.svm$fitted != iris$Species) / nrow(iris)
  #Test
 test_error=sum(predict(ir.svm,iris_test)!=iris_test$Species)/nrow(iris_test)
  #CV error
  ire.cverr = sapply(folds, function(fold) {
    svmcv = svm(Species~.,data = iris, kernel="radial", cost=costC,
                subset = fold$training)
    svmpred = predict(svmcv, iris[fold$test,])
    return(sum(svmpred != iris$Species[fold$test]) / length(fold$test))
  })
  cv_error = mean(ire.cverr)
  return(c(train_error, cv_error, test_error))
}
costs = exp(-5:8)
ir_cost_errors = sapply(costs, function(cost) train_cv_error_svm(cost))
df_errs = data.frame(t(ir_cost_errors), costs)
colnames(df_errs) = c('Train', 'CV', 'Test', 'Logcost')
dataL <- melt(df_errs, id="Logcost")
plot_ly(dataL, x = ~log(Logcost), y = ~value, color = ~variable,
        colors = c('blue', 'red', "green"), type="scatter", mode="lines") %>%
  layout(xaxis = list(title = 'log(Cost)'),
      yaxis = list(title = 'Classifier Error'), legend=list(orientation='h'),
      title="SVM CV-Plot of Model Performance (Iris Data)") %>%hide_colorbar()
```

6.3.5   Improving the Performance of Gaussian Kernels

Now, let's attempt to improve the performance of a Gaussian kernel by tuning.

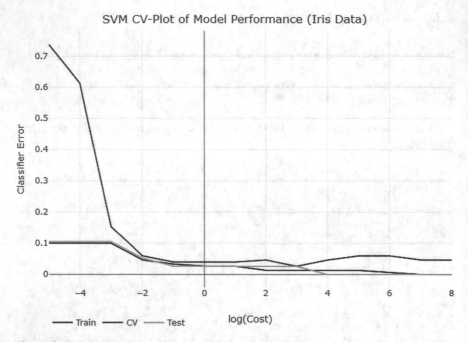

Fig. 6.13 Training, testing, and cross-validation errors during parameter tuning of the SVM classifier on the Iris flowers data

```
set.seed(2020)
gammas = exp(-5:5)
tune_g = tune.svm(Species~., kernel = "radial", data = iris_train,
                  cost = costs, gamma = gammas)
tune_g
## Parameter tuning of 'svm':
## - sampling method: 10-fold cross validation
## - best parameters:
##     gamma      cost
##   0.04978707 2.718282
## - best performance: 0.03636364
```

We observe that the model achieves a better prediction now.

```
iris.svm_g <- svm(Species~., data=iris_train,
                  kernel="radial", gamma=0.0183, cost=20)
table(iris_test$Species, predict(iris.svm_g, iris_test))
##              setosa versicolor virginica
##   setosa         15          0         0
##   versicolor      0         10         0
##   virginica       0          2        11
agreement<-predict(iris.svm_g, iris_test)==iris_test$Species
prop.table(table(agreement))
```

Chapter 14 will provide additional details about deep neural networks learning.

6.4 Ensemble Meta-Learning

Meta-learning involves building and ensembling multiple learners relying either on single or multiple learning algorithms. Meta-learners combine the outputs of several techniques and report consensus results that are more reliable, in general. For example, to decrease the *variance* (bagging) or *bias* (boosting), the *random forest* method attempts in two steps to correct the general decision trees' trend to overfit the model to the training set

1. Step 1: producing a distribution of simple ML models on subsets of the original data
2. Step 2: combine the distribution into one "aggregated" model

Before stepping into the details, let's briefly summarize the basics of algorithmic performance inprovement using bias-variance tradeoff.

- *Bagging* (stands for Bootstrap Aggregating) is the way to *decrease the variance* of your prediction by generating additional data for training from your original dataset using combinations with repetitions to produce multiple samples of the same cardinality/size as your original data. We can't expect to improve the models' predictive power by synthetically increasing the size of the training set; however, we may decrease the variance by narrowly tuning the prediction to the expected outcome.
- *Boosting* is a two-step approach that aims to *reduce bias* in parameter estimation. First, we use subsets of the original data to produce a series of moderately performing models and then "boost" their performance by combining them together using a particular cost function (e.g., Accuracy). Unlike bagging, in classical boosting, the subset creation is not random and depends upon the performance of the previous models: every new subset contains the elements that were (likely to be) misclassified by previous models. Usually, when using boosting, we prefer weaker classifiers. For example, a prevalent choice is to use a stump (level-one decision tree) in AdaBoost (Adaptive Boosting).

6.4.1 Bagging

One of the most well-known meta-learning methods is bootstrap aggregating or *bagging*. It builds multiple models with bootstrap samples using a single algorithm. The models' predictions are combined with voting (for classification) or averaging (for numeric prediction). Voting means the bagging model's prediction is based on the majority of learners' prediction for a class. Bagging is especially good with unstable learners like decision trees or SVM models. To illustrate the bagging method, we will again use the quality of life and chronic disease dataset we saw earlier in Chap. 5. Just like we did in the second practice problem in this chapter, we will use CHARLSONSCORE as the class label, which has 11 different levels.

```
qol <-
    read.csv("https://umich.instructure.com/files/481332/download?download_frd=1")
qol <- qol[!qol$CHARLSONSCORE==-9 , -c(1, 2)]
qol$CHARLSONSCORE <- as.factor(qol$CHARLSONSCORE)
```

To apply bagging(), we can download and install the ipred package first. After loading the package, we build a bagging model with CHARLSONSCORE as class label and all other variables in the dataset as predictors. We can specify the number of voters (decision tree models we want to have), which defaults to 25.

```
# install.packages("ipred")
library(ipred)
## Warning: package 'ipred' was built under R version 4.1.1
set.seed(123)
mybag<-bagging(CHARLSONSCORE ~ ., data=qol, nbagg=25)
```

The result, mybag, is a complex class object that includes y (vector of responses), X (data frame of predictors), mtrees (multiple trees as a list of length *nbagg* containing the trees for each bootstrap sample, OOB (logical indicating whether the out-of-bag estimate should be computed), err error (if OOB = TRUE, the out-of-bag estimate of misclassification or root mean squared error or the Brier score for censored data), and comb (Boolean indicating whether a combination of models was requested). Now we will use the predict() function to apply this forecasting model. For evaluation purposes, we create a table to inspect the re-substitution error.

```
bt_pred <- predict(mybag, qol)
agreement <- bt_pred==qol$CHARLSONSCORE
prop.table(table(agreement))
## agreement
##      FALSE        TRUE
## 0.00128866 0.99871134
```

This model works very well with its training data. It labeled 99.8% of the cases correctly. To evaluate its performance on testing data, we apply the caret train () function again with 10 repeated CVs as a re-sampling method. In caret, the bagged trees method is called treebag.

```
library(caret)
set.seed(123)
ctrl <- trainControl(method="repeatedcv", number = 10, repeats = 10)
train(CHARLSONSCORE ~ ., data=as.data.frame(qol),
      method="treebag", trControl=ctrl)
##   Accuracy   Kappa
##   0.5199428  0.2120838
```

The results indicate a marginal accuracy of 52% and a fair Kappa statistic. This result is better than the one we got earlier using the ksvm() function alone (~50%). Here, we combined the prediction results of 38 decision trees to get this accuracy. It seems that we can't forecast CHARLSONSCORE too well; however, other QoL outcomes may have higher prediction accuracy. For instance, we may predict QOL_Q_01 with *accuracy* = 0.6 and κ = 0.42.

```
set.seed(123)
ctrl <- trainControl(method="repeatedcv", number = 10, repeats = 10)
train(as.factor(QOL_Q_01) ~ . , data=as.data.frame(qol),
      method="treebag", trControl=ctrl)
```

In addition to decision tree classification, caret allows us to explore alternative bag() functions. For instance, instead of bagging based on decision trees, we can bag using a SVM model. caret provides a nice setting for SVM training, making predictions, and counting votes in a list object svmBag. We can examine these objects by using the str() function.

```
str(svmBag)
```

Clearly, fit provides the training functionality, pred the prediction and forecasting on new data, and aggregate is a way to combine many models and achieve voting-based consensus. Using the member operator, the $ sign, we can explore these three types of elements of the svmBag object. For instance, the fit element may be extracted from the SVM object by

```
svmBag$fit
```

The SVM bag fit relies on the kernlab::ksvm() function. The other two methods, pred and aggregate, may be explored in a similar way. They follow the SVM model building and testing process we saw earlier. This svmBag object could be used as an optional setting in the train() function. However, this option requires that all features are linearly independent, which may be rare in real-world data.

6.4.2 Boosting

Bagging uses equal weights for all learners we include in the model. *Boosting* is different as it employs nonuniform weights. Suppose we have the first learner correctly classifying 60% of the observations. This 60% of data may be less likely to be included in the training dataset for the next learner. So, we have more learners working on the remaining "hard-to-classify" observations.

Mathematically, the boosting technique uses a weighted sum of functions to predict the outcome class labels. We can try to fit the true model using weighted additive modeling. We start with a random learner that can classify some of the observations mostly correctly, possibly with some errors.

$$\widehat{y}_1 = l_1.$$

This l_1 is our first learner and $\widehat{y}_1$ denotes its predictions (this equation is in matrix form). Then, we can calculate the residuals of our first learner.

$$\varepsilon_1 = y - v_1 \times \widehat{y}_1,$$

where v_1 is a shrinkage parameter to avoid overfitting. Next, we fit the residual with another learner. This learner minimizes the following objective function $\sum_{i=1}^{N} \|y_i - l_{k-1} - l_k\|$. Here k $= 2$. Then we obtain a second model l_2 with:

$$\widehat{y}_2 = l_2.$$

After that, we can update the residuals:

$$\varepsilon_2 = \varepsilon_1 - v_2 \times \widehat{y}_2.$$

We repeat this residual fitting until adding another learner l_k results in updated residual ε_k that is smaller than a small predefined threshold. In the end, we will have an additive model like:

$$L = v_1 \times l_1 + v_2 \times l_2 + \ldots + v_k \times l_k,$$

where we ensemble k weak learners to generate a stronger meta model.

Schapire and Freund[5] found that although individual learners trained on the pilot observations might be very weak in predicting in isolation, boosting the collective power of all of them is expected to generate a model *no worse than the best of all individual constituent models* included in the boosting ensemble. Usually, the boosting results are quite better than the top individual model. Although boosting can be used for almost all models, it's most commonly applied to decision trees.

6.4.3   *Random Forests*

Random forests, or decision tree forests, represent a class of boosting methods focusing on decision tree learners. Random forests (RF) represent ensembles of a large number of (typically weaker) classifiers such as individual decision trees that provide independent class predictions. Then, for any testing set, the RF aggregates the predictions of all individual trees to pool the most likely class label which becomes the RF prediction. If and when a large number of relatively independent

---

[5]https://doi.org/10.1006/jcss.1997.1504

tree models reach a consensus, i.e., majority vote, this forecasting outcome is expected to outperform any specific individual decision tree model. Whereas many of the trees in the forest may yield vastly incorrect and wild predictions, any consistent pattern emerging from other trees would suggest strong candidate predictions that pull the consensus in a uniform (correct) direction. The main assumptions of the random forest ensemble method include (1) existence of an actual signal encoded in the data features that may guide the individual tree into a nonrandom guessing pattern, and (2) the individual trees in the forest should be fairly independently trained to output predictions with low correlations.

6.4.4 Random Forest Algorithm (Pseudo Code)

As RF relies on bagging to generate a meta-ensemble regression or classification, it uses averaging of a large number of weak (noisy), mostly independent, and approximately unbiased models. This average pooling naturally reduces the performance variance. RF can be applied to any family of classifiers, and is particularly useful with decision trees, which tend to capture complex high-dimensional interactions. When grown sufficiently deep, the RFs have relatively low bias in their predictions. Individual trees are commonly expected to generate noisy predictions. Therefore, the expectation of the subsequent RF average pooling of the identically distributed B trees is the same as the expectation of each of the constituent trees. Hence, the bias of bagged trees in the RF will be the same as the bias of any one of the individual trees. However, the RF improvement over each individual decision tree prediction rapidly decreases the forecasting variance. In boosting methods, the decision trees are not necessarily independent, but are grown adaptively to reduce the bias.

Recall that by the central limit theorem (CLT),[6] the average of B independent random variables from a distribution with a variance σ^2, has a much lower variance $\frac{\sigma^2}{B}$, which goes to zero as the sample size $B \to \infty$. However, when the random and identically distributed variables are not independent, then the variance of arithmetic mean could be much larger. For instance, if pairwise correlations of the variables is nontrivial, $\rho > 0$, the variance of the sampling distribution of the average would be on the order of $O(\sigma^2)$. More specifically, in this case, the variance would be

$$\left(\rho + \frac{1-\rho}{B}\right)\sigma^2 \underset{B \to \infty}{\longrightarrow} \rho\sigma^2.$$

In other words, bagging-dependent tree has less benefit on reducing prediction variability in the *average* pooled predictor. In RF, the improvement of prediction is based on the variance reduction of bagging, which is achieved by reducing tree

---

[6] https://doi.org/10.1080/10691898.2008.11889560

correlations using tree-growing process based on *random selection of the input variables*.

Below is a pseudo code illustrating the core parts of a random forest approach for regression or classification:

- Given a number of trees B, iterate over each tree index ($1 \le b \le B$):

  - Draw a bootstrap sample Z^* of size N from the training data
  - Grow a random forest tree T_b to the bootstrapped data, by recursively repeating these steps for each terminal node of the current tree, until the minimum node size n_{min} is reached

    - Choose a random set of $m \gg p$ variables
    - Decide on an optimal variable split among the m features
    - Split the node into two children nodes based on the features

- Compile an output by ensembling the trees, $\{T_b\}_1^B$.

The *RF prediction* given a new testing case x is given by:

- For *regression problems*, pool across all random forest trees, $\widehat{f}_B^{RF}(x) = \frac{1}{B} \times \sum_{b=1}^{B} T_b(x)$, and

- For *classification problems*: Suppose the b-th tree in the RF generates a class prediction $\widehat{C}_b(x)$. Then, the RF output (prediction) is

$$\widehat{C}_B^{RF}(x) = \left(\begin{matrix} \text{majority} \\ \text{vote} \end{matrix} \right) \{\widehat{C}_b(x)\}.$$

At each iteration, the bootstrapped sample dataset affects the growth of each tree. Prior to deciding whether and how to split a leaf node, we *randomly* choose $m \le p$ features as candidate splitting variables. In general, $1 \le m \sim \sqrt{p} \gg p$. Suppose the parameter vector Ω_b characterizes the b-th random forest tree in terms of splitting variables, node cut-points, and terminal-node values. In the RF regression setting, growing B trees $\{T(x|\Omega_b)\}_1^B$ yields the following random forest regression predictor

$$\widehat{f}_B^{RF}(x) = \frac{1}{B} \sum_{b=1}^{B} T(x|\Omega_b).$$

6.4.4.1   Training Random Forests

One approach to train and build random forests uses the `randomForest::`
`randomForest()` method, which has the following invocation:

```
model <- randomForest(expression, data, ntree=500, mtry=sqrt(p))
```

- *expression*: the class variable and features we want to include in the model.
- *data*: training data containing class and features.
- *ntree*: number of voting decision trees
- *mtry*: optional integer specifying the number of features to randomly select at
  each split. The parameter p stands for the number of features in the data.

Let's build a random forest using the quality of life dataset.

```
# install.packages("randomForest")
library(randomForest)
set.seed(123)
rf <- randomForest(as.factor(QOL_Q_01) ~ . , data=qol); rf
##            OOB estimate of  error rate: 38.4%
## Confusion matrix:
##      1  2    3    4   5  6 class.error
## 1 14 10   14    5   0  0   0.6744186
## 2  3 73  120   14   0  1   0.6540284
## 3  1 23  558  205   3  1   0.2945638
## 4  0  2  164  686  36  4   0.2309417
## 5  0  0    7  100  92  0   0.6447076
## 6  0  1   34   81   5 11   0.9166667
```

By default the model contains 500 voter trees and tries six variables at each split.
Its OOB (out-of-bag) error rate is about 38%, which corresponds with a moderate
accuracy (62%). Note that the OOB error rate is not a re-substitution error. Next to
the confusion matrix, we see the reported OOB error rate for all specific classes. All
of these error rates are reasonable estimates of future performances with unseen data.
We can see that this model is so far the best of all models, although it is still not
highly predictive of QOL_Q_01.

6.4.4.2   Evaluating Random Forest Performance

In addition to model building, the `caret` package also supports model evaluation. It
reports more detailed model performance evaluations. As usual, we need to specify
the re-sampling method and a parameter grid. Let's use a 10-fold CV re-sampling
method as an example. The grid for this model contains information about the `mtry`
parameter (the only tuning parameter for random forest). Previously, we tried the
default value $\sqrt{38} = 6$ (38 is the number of features). This time we could compare
multiple `mtry` parameters.

```
library(caret)
ctrl <- trainControl(method="cv", number=10)
grid_rf <- expand.grid(mtry=c(2, 4, 8, 16))
```
Next, we apply the `train()` function with our `ctrl` and `grid_rf` settings.
```
set.seed(123)
m_rf <- train(as.factor(QOL_Q_01) ~ ., data = qol, method = "rf",
                metric = "Kappa", trControl = ctrl, tuneGrid = grid_rf)
m_rf
##   mtry  Accuracy   Kappa
##    2    0.5760034  0.3465920
##    4    0.6039266  0.4004127
##    8    0.6125122  0.4197845
##   16    0.6180824  0.4372678
## Kappa was used to select the optimal model using the largest value.
## The final value used for the model was mtry = 16.
```

This call may take a while to complete. The result appears to be a good model, when `mtry=16` we reached a moderately high accuracy (0.62) and good `kappa` statistic (0.44). This is a good result for a meta-learner of 6 dispersed classes (`table (as.factor(qol$QOL_Q_01))`). More examples of using `randomForest ()` and interpreting its results are shown in Chap. 5.

6.4.5 Adaptive Boosting

We may achieve even higher accuracy using **AdaBoost**. Adaptive boosting (AdaBoost) can be used in conjunction with many other types of learning algorithms to improve their performance. The output of the other learning algorithms ('weak learners') is combined into a weighted sum that represents the final output of the boosted classifier. AdaBoost is adaptive in the sense that subsequent weak learners are tweaked in favor of those instances misclassified by the previous classifiers.

For binary cases, we could use the method `ada::ada()` and for multiple classes (multinomial/polytomous outcomes) we can use the package `adabag`. The `adabag::boosting()` function allows us to specify a method by setting `coeflearn`. The two main types of adaptive boosting methods that are commonly used include the `AdaBoost.M1` algorithm, e.g., `Breiman` and `Freund`, or the Zhu's `SAMME` algorithm.[7] The key parameter in the `adabag::boosting()` method is *coeflearn*

- *Breiman* (default), corresponding to $\alpha = \frac{1}{2} \times \ln\left(\frac{1-\text{err}}{\text{err}}\right)$, using the AdaBoost.M1 algorithm, where α is the weight updating coefficient,
- *Freund*, corresponding to $\alpha = \ln\left(\frac{1-\text{err}}{\text{err}}\right)$, or
- *Zhu*, corresponding to $\alpha = \ln\left(\frac{1-\text{err}}{\text{err}}\right) + \ln\left(n\text{classes} - 1\right)$.

The generalizations of AdaBoost for multiple classes (≥ 2) include `AdaBoost. M1` (where individual trees are required to have an error $< \frac{1}{2}$) and `SAMME` (where

---

[7]https://doi.org/10.18637/jss.v054.i02

individual trees are required to have an error $< 1 - \frac{1}{nclasses}$). Let's see some examples using these three alternative adaptive boosting methods.

```
# Prep the data
qol <-
    read.csv("https://umich.instructure.com/files/481332/download?download_frd=1")
qol <- qol[!qol$CHARLSONSCORE==-9 , -c(1, 2)]
qol$CHARLSONSCORE <- as.factor(qol$CHARLSONSCORE)
qol <- qol[!qol$CHARLSONSCORE==-9 , -c(1, 2)]
qol$cd <- qol$CHRONICDISEASESCORE>1.497
qol$cd <- factor(qol$cd, levels=c(F, T),
                    labels = c("minor_disease", "severe_disease"))
qol <- qol[!qol$CHRONICDISEASESCORE==-9, ]
# install.packages("ada"); install.packages("adabag")
library("ada"); library("adabag")
set.seed(123)
qol_boost <- boosting(cd ~ . , data=qol[, -37], mfinal = 100,
                            coeflearn = 'Breiman')
mean(qol_boost$class==qol$cd)
## [1] 0.86621
set.seed(123)
qol_boost <- boosting(cd ~ . , data=qol[, -37], mfinal = 100,
                            coeflearn = 'Breiman')
mean(qol_boost$class==qol$cd)
## [1] 0.86621
set.seed(1234)
qol_boost <- boosting(cd ~ . , data=qol[, -37], mfinal = 100,
                            coeflearn = 'Zhu')
mean(qol_boost$class==qol$cd)
## [1] 0.9378995
```

We observe that the Zhu approach achieves the best results, average *accuracy* = 0.78. Notice that the default method is M1 Breiman and mfinal is the number of boosting iterations.

6.5 Practice Problems

6.5.1 Problem 1: Google Trends and the Stock Market

Use the Google trend data. Fit a neural network model with the Google Trends data we saw earlier. This time use Investing as target and Unemployment, Rental, RealEstate, Mortgage, Jobs, DJI_Index, StdDJI as predictors. Use three hidden nodes.

Note: remember to change the columns you want to include in the test dataset when predicting. The following number is the correlation between predicted and observed values.

```
google_model3 <- neuralnet(Investing~Unemployment+Rental+RealEstate+Mortgage+
                           Jobs+DJI_Index+StdDJI, data=google_train, hidden = 3)
plot(google_model3)
google_pred3<-compute(google_model3, google_test[, c(1:5, 7:8)])
pred_results3<-google_pred3$net.result
cor(pred_results3, google_test$Investing)
```

Each run may generate slightly different results since the weights are generated randomly.

6.5.2   Problem 2: Quality of Life and Chronic Disease

Use the quality of life and chronic disease and the corresponding meta-data doc, which we used in Chap. 5. Load the data first. In this case study, we want to use the variable CHARLSONSCORE as our target variable.

```
qol <-
   read.csv("https://umich.instructure.com/files/481332/download?download_frd=1")
featureLength <- dim(qol)[2]
str(qol[, c((featureLength-3):featureLength)])
```

Delete the first two columns (we don't need ID variables) and rows that have missing values in CHARLSONSCORE(where CHARLSONSCOREequals "-9")!qol $CHARLSONSCORE==-9 means we want all the rows that have CHARLSONSCORE not equal to -9. The exclamation sign (!) indicates "exclude". Also, we need to convert our categorical variable CHARLSONSCORE into a factor.

```
qol <- qol[!qol$CHARLSONSCORE==-9 , -c(1, 2)]
qol$CHARLSONSCORE<-as.factor(qol$CHARLSONSCORE)
featureLength <- dim(qol)[2]
str(qol[, c((featureLength-3):featureLength)])
## 'data.frame':    2328 obs. of  4 variables:
## $ TOS_Q_03          : int  4 4 4 4 4 4 4 4 4 4 ...
## $ TOS_Q_04          : int  5 5 5 5 5 5 5 5 5 5 ...
## $ CHARLSONSCORE     : Factor w/ 11 levels "0","1","2","3",..: 3 3 4  ...
## $ CHRONICDISEASESCORE: num  1.6 1.6 1.54 2.97 1.28 1.28 1.31 1.67  ...
```

Separate the dataset into training and test datasets using the $75\%-25\%$ rule. Then, build an SVM model using all other variables in the dataset to be predictor variables. Try to add different costs of misclassification to the model. Rather than the default C = 1 we use C = 2 and C = 3. Assess the model performance utilizing different kernels.

```
sub <- sample(nrow(qol), floor(nrow(qol)*0.75))
qol_train <- qol[sub, ]
qol_test <- qol[-sub, ]
qol_clas2 <- ksvm(CHARLSONSCORE~., data=qol_train, kernel="rbfdot", C=2)
qol_clas2
qol.pred2 <- predict(qol_clas2, qol_test)
agreement <- qol.pred2==qol_test$CHARLSONSCORE
prop.table(table(agreement))
tab <- table(qol.pred2, qol_test$CHARLSONSCORE)
tab_df <- tidyr::spread(as.data.frame(tab), key = Var2, value = Freq)
sum(diag(table(hand_letter_predictions, hand_letters_test$letter)))
plot_ly(x = colnames(tab), y = colnames(tab), z = as.matrix(tab_df[, -1]),
        type = "heatmap")
```

Output for C = 3.

```
qol_clas3 <- ksvm(CHARLSONSCORE~., data=qol_train, kernel="rbfdot", C=3)
qol_clas3
qol.pred3 <- predict(qol_clas3, qol_test)
agreement <- qol.pred3==qol_test$CHARLSONSCORE
prop.table(table(agreement))
tab <- table(qol.pred3, qol_test$CHARLSONSCORE)
tab_df <- tidyr::spread(as.data.frame(tab), key = Var2, value = Freq)
sum(diag(table(hand_letter_predictions, hand_letters_test$letter)))
plot_ly(x = colnames(tab), y = colnames(tab), z = as.matrix(tab_df[, -1]),
        type = "heatmap")
```

Readers can practice these techniques using other data from the list of DSPA case studies.

Chapter 7
Qualitative Learning Methods—Text Mining, Natural Language Processing, and Apriori Association Rules Learning

As we have seen in the previous chapters, traditional statistical analyses and classical data modeling are applied to *relational data* where the observed information is represented by tables, vectors, arrays, tensors, or data-frames containing binary, categorical, original, or numerical values. Such representations provide incredible advantages (e.g., quick reference and dereference of elements, search, discovery, and navigation), but also limit the scope of applications. Relational data objects are quite effective for managing information that is based only on existing attributes. However, when data science inference needs to utilize attributes that are not included in the relational model, alternative nonrelational representations are necessary. For instance, imagine that our data object includes qualitative data or free text (e.g., physician/nurse clinical notes, biospecimen samples) containing information about medical condition, treatment, or outcome. It may be difficult, or sometimes even impossible, to include raw text in fully automated data analytic protocols solely using classical procedures and statistical models available for relational datasets. In this chapter, we will present ML/AI methods for qualitative and unstructured data.

7.1 Natural Language Processing (NLP) and Text Mining (TM)

Natural language processing (NLP) and text mining (TM) refer to automated machine-driven algorithms for semantic mapping, information extraction, and understanding of (natural) human language. Sometimes, this involves deriving salient information from large amounts of unstructured text. To do so, we need to build semantic and syntactic mapping algorithms for effective processing of heavy text. Recall the related NLP/TM work we did in Chap. 5 demonstrating an interesting text classifier using the naïve Bayes algorithm.

© The Author(s), under exclusive license to Springer Nature Switzerland AG 2023
I. D. Dinov, *Data Science and Predictive Analytics*, The Springer Series in Applied Machine Learning, https://doi.org/10.1007/978-3-031-17483-4_7

In this section, we will present details about various text processing strategies in R. Specifically, we will present simulated and real examples of text processing and computing document term frequency (TF), inverse document frequency (IDF), and cosine similarity transformation.

7.1.1   A Simple NLP/TM Example

Text mining and text analytics (TM/TA) involve examining large volumes of unstructured text (corpus) aiming to obtain interpretable information, discover context, identify linguistic motifs, or transform the text and derive quantitative data that can be further analyzed. Natural language processing (NLP) is one example of a TM analytical technique. Whereas TM's goal is to discover relevant contextual information, which may be unknown, hidden, or obfuscated, NLP is focused on linguistic analysis that trains a machine to interpret voluminous textual content. To decipher the semantics and ambiguities in human-interpretable language, NLP employs automatic summarization, tagging, disambiguation, extraction of entities and relations, pattern recognition, and frequency analyses. The US International Trade Commission reports an International Data Corporation (IDC) Estimate[1] of the expected total amount of information by 2025—a staggering 175 Zettabytes ($1\ ZB = 10^{21} = 2^{70}$ bytes). The amount of data we obtain and record doubles every 12–14 months (Kryder's law).[2] A small fraction of this massive information ($<0.0001\%$ or $<1\ PB = 10^{15}$ bytes) represents newly written or transcribed text, including software code. However, it is impossible (cf. efficiency, time, resources) for humans to read, synthesize, curate, interpret, and react to all this information without direct assistance of TM/NLP. The information content in text could be substantially higher than that of other information media. Remember that *"a picture may be worth a thousand words,"* yet *"a word may also be worth a thousand pictures."* As an example, the simple sentence *"The second edition of the data science and predictive analytics textbook includes 14 Chapters"* takes 93 bytes to store the text as a character array. However, a color image showing this sentence as a scale vector graphic or printed text could be much larger, e.g., 10 megabytes (MB), and a high definition video of a speaker reading the same sentence could easily surpass 50 MB. Text mining and natural language processing may be used to automatically analyze and interpret written, coded, or transcribed content to assess news, moods, emotions, sentiments, and biosocial trends related to specific topics.

---

[1] https://www.usitc.gov/publications/332/executive_briefings/ebot_data_centers_around_the_world.pdf

[2] https://doi.org/10.7243/2053-7662-4-3

In general, text analysis protocols involve:

- Construction of a document-term matrix (DTM) from the input documents, vectorizing the text, e.g., creating a map of single words or `n-grams` into a vector space. In other words, we generate a *vectorizer function mapping terms to indices*.
- Application of a model-based statistical analysis or a model-free machine learning technique for prediction, clustering, classification, similarity search, network/sentiment analysis, or forecasting using the DTM. This step also includes tuning and internally validating the performance of the method.
- Evaluation of the technique on new validation data.

Define and Load Unstructured-Text Documents
Let's create some documents we can use to demonstrate the use of the `tm` package to do text mining. The five documents below represent portions of the syllabi of five recent courses taught by the author[3]

- HS650: Data Science and Predictive Analytics (DSPA)
- Bioinformatics 501: Mathematical Foundations for Bioinformatics
- HS 853: Scientific Methods for Health Sciences: Special Topics
- HS851: Scientific Methods for Health Sciences: Applied Inference
- HS550: Scientific Methods for Health Sciences: Fundamentals

We import the syllabi into several separate segments represented as `documents`. In this example, we will use the `rvest::read_html()` method to load in the 5 course syllabi directly from the corresponding course websites.

```
doc1 <- "HS650: The Data Science and Predictive Analytics (DSPA) course (offered
as a massive open online course, MOOC, as well as a traditional University of
Michigan class) aims to build computational abilities, inferential thinking, and
practical skills for tackling core data scientific challenges. It explores
foundational concepts in data management, processing, statistical computing, and
dynamic visualization using modern programming tools and agile web-services.
Concepts, ideas, and protocols are illustrated through examples of real
observational, simulated and research-derived datasets. Some prior quantitative
experience in programming, calculus, statistics, mathematical models, or linear
algebra will be necessary. This open graduate course will provide a general
overview of the principles, concepts, techniques, tools and services for
managing, harmonizing, aggregating, preprocessing, modeling, analyzing and
interpreting large, multi-source, incomplete, incongruent, and heterogeneous data
(big data). The focus will be to expose students to common challenges related to
handling big data and present the enormous opportunities and power associated
with our ability to interrogate such complex datasets, extract useful
information, derive knowledge, and provide actionable forecasting. Biomedical,
healthcare, and social datasets will provide context for addressing specific
driving challenges. Students will learn about modern data analytic techniques and
develop skills for importing and exporting, cleaning and fusing, modeling and
visualizing, analyzing and synthesizing complex datasets. The collaborative
design, implementation, sharing and community validation of high-throughput
```

---

[3] https://www.socr.umich.edu/people/dinov/courses.html

analytic workflows will be emphasized throughout the course."
doc2 <- " Bioinformatics 501: The Mathematical Foundations for Bioinformatics
course covers some of the fundamental mathematical techniques commonly used in
bioinformatics and biomedical research. These include: 1) principles of multi-
variable calculus, and complex numbers/functions, 2) foundations of linear
algebra, such as linear spaces, eigen-values and vectors, singular value
decomposition, spectral graph theory and Markov chains, 3) differential equations
and their usage in biomedical system, which includes topic such as existence and
uniqueness of solutions, two dimensional linear systems, bifurcations in one and
two dimensional systems and cellular dynamics, and 4) optimization methods, such
as free and constrained optimization, Lagrange multipliers, data denoising using
optimization and heuristic methods. Demonstrations using MATLAB, R, and Python
are included throughout the course."
doc3 <- "HS 853: This course covers a number of modern analytical methods for
advanced healthcare research. Specific focus will be on reviewing and using
innovative modeling, computational, analytic and visualization techniques to
address concrete driving biomedical and healthcare applications. The course will
cover the 5 dimensions of big data (volume, complexity, multiple scales, multiple
sources, and incompleteness). HS853 is a 4 credit hour course (3 lectures + 1
lab/discussion). Students will learn how to conduct research, employ and report
on recent advanced health sciences analytical methods; read, comprehend and
present recent reports of innovative scientific methods; apply a broad range of
health problems; and experiment with real big data. Topics Covered include:
Foundations of R, Scientific Visualization, Review of Multivariate and Mixed
Linear Models, Causality/Causal Inference and Structural Equation Models,
Generalized Estimating Equations, PCOR/CER methods Heterogeneity of Treatment
Effects, big data, Big-Science, Internal statistical cross-validation, Missing
data, Genotype-Environment-Phenotype, associations, Variable selection
(regularized regression and controlled/knockoff filtering), medical imaging,
Databases/registries, Meta-analyses, classification methods, Longitudinal data
and time-series analysis, Geographic Information Systems (GIS), Psychometrics and
Rasch measurement model analysis, MCMC sampling for Bayesian inference, and
Network Analysis"

doc4 <- "HS 851: This course introduces students to applied inference methods in
studies involving multiple variables. Specific methods that will be discussed
include linear regression, analysis of variance, and different regression models.
This course will emphasize the scientific formulation, analytical modeling,
computational tools and applied statistical inference in diverse health-sciences
problems. Data interrogation, modeling approaches, rigorous interpretation and
inference will be emphasized throughout. HS851 is a 4 credit hour course (3
lectures + 1 lab/discussion). Students will learn how to: Understand the
commonly used statistical methods of published scientific papers , Conduct
statistical calculations/analyses on available data , Use software tools to
analyze specific case-studies data , Communicate advanced statistical
concepts/techniques , Determine, explain and interpret assumptions and
limitations. Topics Covered include   Epidemiology , Correlation/SLR , and slope
inference, 1-2 samples , ROC Curve , ANOVA , Non-parametric inference ,
Cronbach's α, Measurement Reliability/Validity , Survival Analysis ,
Decision theory , CLT/LLNs - limiting results and misconceptions , Association
Tests , Bayesian Inference , PCA/ICA/Factor Analysis , Point/Interval Estimation
(CI) - MoM, MLE , Instrument performance Evaluation , Study/Research Critiques ,
Common mistakes and misconceptions in using probability and statistics,
identifying potential assumption violations, and avoiding them."
doc5 <- "HS550: This course provides students with an introduction to probability
reasoning and statistical inference. Students will learn theoretical concepts and
apply analytic skills for collecting, managing, modeling, processing,
interpreting and visualizing (mostly univariate) data. Students will learn the
basic probability modeling and statistical analysis methods and acquire knowledge
to read recently published health research publications. HS550 is a 4 credit hour
course (3 lectures + 1 lab/discussion). Students will learn how to: Apply data
management strategies to sample data files , Carry out statistical tests to

answer common healthcare research questions using appropriate methods and software tools , Understand the core analytical data modeling techniques and their appropriate use Examples of Topics Covered , EDA/Charts , Ubiquitous variation , Parametric inference , Probability Theory , Odds Ratio/Relative Risk , Distributions , Exploratory data analysis , Resampling/Simulation , Design of Experiments , Intro to Epidemiology , Estimation , Hypothesis testing , Experiments vs. Observational studies , Data management (tables, streams, cloud, warehouses, DBs, arrays, binary, ASCII, handling, mechanics) , Power, sample-size, effect-size, sensitivity, specificity , Bias/Precision , Association vs. Causality , Rate-of-change , Clinical vs. Stat significance , Statistical Independence Bayesian Rule."

Create a New VCorpus Object

The `VCorpus` object includes all the text and some meta-data (e.g., indexing) about the text.

```
docs <- c(doc1, doc2, doc3, doc4, doc5)
class(docs) ## [1] "character"
```

Then let's make a `VCorpus` object using the `tm` package. To complete this task, we need to know the source type. Here `docs` is a vector with "character" class so we should use `VectorSource()`. If it is a data frame, we should use `DataframeSource()` instead. `VCorpus()` creates a *volatile corpus*, which is the data type used by the `tm` package for text mining.

```
library(tm)
doc_corpus <- VCorpus(VectorSource(docs))
doc_corpus    ## Content:  documents: 5
doc_corpus[[1]]$content
```

```
## [1] "HS650: The Data Science and Predictive Analytics (DSPA) course
(offered as a massive open online course, MOOC, as well as a traditional
University of Michigan class) aims to build computational abilities,
inferential thinking, and practical skills for tackling core data
scientific challenges. It explores foundational concepts in data
management, processing, statistical computing, and dynamic
visualization using modern programming tools and agile web-services.
Concepts, ideas, and protocols are illustrated through examples of real
observational, simulated and research-derived datasets. Some prior
quantitative experience in programming, calculus, statistics,
mathematical models, or linear algebra will be necessary. This open
graduate course will provide a general overview of the principles,
concepts, techniques, tools and services for managing, harmonizing,
aggregating, preprocessing, modeling, analyzing and interpreting
large, multi-source, incomplete, incongruent, and heterogeneous data
(big data). The focus will be to expose students to common challenges
related to handling big data and present the enormous opportunities and
power associated with our ability to interrogate such complex datasets,
```

extract useful information, derive knowledge, and provide actionable forecasting. Biomedical, healthcare, and social datasets will provide context for addressing specific driving challenges. Students will learn about modern data analytic techniques and develop skills for importing and exporting, cleaning and fusing, modeling and visualizing, analyzing and synthesizing complex datasets. The collaborative design, implementation, sharing and community validation of high-throughput analytic workflows will be emphasized throughout the course."

This is a list that contains the information for the five documents we have created. Now we can apply the tm_map() function on this object to edit the text. Similarly to human semantic language understanding, the goal here is to algorithmically process the text and output (structured) quantitative information as a signature tensor representing the original (unstructured) text.

Transform Text to Lowercase
The text itself contains upper case letters as well as lower case letters. The first thing to do is to convert everything to lowercase.

```
doc_corpus <- tm_map(doc_corpus, tolower)
doc_corpus[[1]]
```

```
## [1] "hs650: the data science and predictive analytics (dspa) course
(offered as a massive open online course, mooc, as well as a traditional
university of michigan class) aims to build computational abilities,
inferential thinking, and practical skills for tackling core data
scientific challenges. it explores foundational concepts in data
management, processing, statistical computing, and dynamic
visualization using modern programming tools and agile web-services.
concepts, ideas, and protocols are illustrated through examples of real
observational, simulated and research-derived datasets. some prior
quantitative experience in programming, calculus, statistics,
mathematical models, or linear algebra will be necessary. this open
graduate course will provide a general overview of the principles,
concepts, techniques, tools and services for managing, harmonizing,
aggregating, preprocessing, modeling, analyzing and interpreting
large, multi-source, incomplete, incongruent, and heterogeneous data
(big data). the focus will be to expose students to common challenges
related to handling big data and present the enormous opportunities and
power associated with our ability to interrogate such complex datasets,
extract useful information, derive knowledge, and provide actionable
forecasting. biomedical, healthcare, and social datasets will provide
context for addressing specific driving challenges. students will learn
about modern data analytic techniques and develop skills for importing
and exporting, cleaning and fusing, modeling and visualizing, analyzing
and synthesizing complex datasets. the collaborative design,
implementation, sharing and community validation of high-throughput
analytic workflows will be emphasized throughout the course."
```

Text Preprocessing

Removing stopwords: These documents contain a lot of "stopwords" or common words that have important semantic meaning but low analytic value. We can remove these by the following command.

```
stopwords("english")
##   [1] "i"          "me"          "my"           "myself"      "we"
##   [6] "our"        "ours"        "ourselves"    "you"         "your"
##  [11] "yours"      "yourself"    "yourselves"   "he"          "him"
##  [16] "his"        "himself"     "she"          "her"         "hers"
##  [21] "herself"    "it"          "its"          "itself"      "they"
##  [26] "them"       "their"       "theirs"       "themselves"  "what"
##  [31] "which"      "who"         "whom"         "this"        "that"
##  [36] "these"      "those"       "am"           "is"          "are"
##  [41] "was"        "were"        "be"           "been"        "being"
##  [46] "have"       "has"         "had"          "having"      "do"
##  [51] "does"       "did"         "doing"        "would"       "should"
##  [56] "could"      "ought"       "i'm"          "you're"      "he's"
##  [61] "she's"      "it's"        "we're"        "they're"     "i've"
##  [66] "you've"     "we've"       "they've"      "i'd"         "you'd"
##  [71] "he'd"       "she'd"       "we'd"         "they'd"      "i'll"
##  [76] "you'll"     "he'll"       "she'll"       "we'll"       "they'll"
##  [81] "isn't"      "aren't"      "wasn't"       "weren't"     "hasn't"
##  [86] "haven't"    "hadn't"      "doesn't"      "don't"       "didn't"
##  [91] "won't"      "wouldn't"    "shan't"       "shouldn't"   "can't"
##  [96] "cannot"     "couldn't"    "mustn't"      "let's"       "that's"
## [101] "who's"      "what's"      "here's"       "there's"     "when's"
## [106] "where's"    "why's"       "how's"        "a"           "an"
## [111] "the"        "and"         "but"          "if"          "or"
## [116] "because"    "as"          "until"        "while"       "of"
## [121] "at"         "by"          "for"          "with"        "about"
## [126] "against"    "between"     "into"         "through"     "during"
## [131] "before"     "after"       "above"        "below"       "to"
## [136] "from"       "up"          "down"         "in"          "out"
## [141] "on"         "off"         "over"         "under"       "again"
## [146] "further"    "then"        "once"         "here"        "there"
## [151] "when"       "where"       "why"          "how"         "all"
## [156] "any"        "both"        "each"         "few"         "more"
## [161] "most"       "other"       "some"         "such"        "no"
## [166] "nor"        "not"         "only"         "own"         "same"
## [171] "so"         "than"        "too"          "very"
doc_corpus <- tm_map(doc_corpus, removeWords, stopwords("english"))
doc_corpus[[1]]
```

We removed all the stopwards included in the `stopwords("english")` list. You can always make your own stop-word list and just use `doc_corpus<--tm_map(doc_corpus, removeWords, your_own_words_list)` to apply this list. From the output of `doc1`, we notice that the removal of stopwords may create extra blank spaces. Thus, the next step would be to remove them.

```
doc_corpus <- tm_map(doc_corpus, stripWhitespace)
doc_corpus[[1]]
```

Remove punctuation: Now we notice the irrelevant punctuation in the text, which can be removed by using a combination of `tm_map()` and `removePunctuation()` functions.

```
doc_corpus<-tm_map(doc_corpus, removePunctuation)
doc_corpus[[2]]
```

```
## [1] "bioinformatics 501 mathematical foundations bioinformatics
course covers fundamental mathematical techniques commonly used
bioinformatics biomedical research include 1 principles multivariable
calculus complex numbersfunctions 2 foundations linear algebra linear
spaces eigenvalues vectors singular value decomposition spectral graph
theory markov chains 3 differential equations usage biomedical system
includes topic existence uniqueness solutions two dimensional linear
systems bifurcations one two dimensional systems cellular dynamics 4
optimization methods free constrained optimization lagrange
multipliers data denoising using optimization heuristic methods
demonstrations using matlab r python included throughout course"
```

The above tm_map commands changed the structure of our doc_corpus object. We can apply the PlainTextDocument function to convert it back to the original format.

```
doc_corpus<-tm_map(doc_corpus, PlainTextDocument)
```

Stemming is the process of removal of plurals and action suffixes. Let's inspect the first three documents. We notice that there are some words ending with "ing," "es," "s."

```
doc_corpus[[1]]$content
```

```
## [1] "hs650 data science predictive analytics dspa course offered
massive open online course mooc well traditional university michigan
class aims build computational abilities inferential thinking
practical skills tackling core data scientific challenges explores
foundational concepts data management processing statistical
computing dynamic visualization using modern programming tools agile
webservices concepts ideas protocols illustrated examples real
observational simulated research derived datasets prior quantitative
experience programming calculus statistics mathematical models linear
algebra will necessary open graduate course will provide general
overview principles concepts techniques tools services managing
harmonizing aggregating preprocessing modeling analyzing interpreting
large multisource incomplete incongruent heterogeneous data big data
focus will expose students common challenges related handling big data
present enormous opportunities power associated ability interrogate
complex datasets extract useful information derive knowledge provide
actionable forecasting biomedical healthcare social datasets will
provide context addressing specific driving challenges students will
learn modern data analytic techniques develop skills importing
exporting cleaning fusing modeling visualizing analyzing synthesizing
complex datasets collaborative design implementation sharing
community validation high throughput analytic workflows will emphasized
throughout course"
```

If we have multiple terms that only differ in their endings (e.g., past, present, present perfect continuous tense), the algorithm will treat them differently because it does not understand language semantics the way a human would. To make things easier for the computer, we can delete these endings by "stemming" documents. Remember to load the package `SnowballC` before using the function `stemDocument()`. The earliest stemmer was written by Julie Beth Lovins in 1968, which had great influence on all subsequent work. Currently, one of the most popular stemming approaches was proposed by Martin Porter and is used in `stemDocument()`.[4]

```
# install.packages("SnowballC")
library(SnowballC)
doc_corpus<-tm_map(doc_corpus, stemDocument)
doc_corpus[[1]]$content
```

```
## [1] "hs650 data scienc predict analyt dspa cours offer massiv open
onlin cours mooc well tradit univers michigan class aim build comput abil
inferenti think practic skill tackl core data scientif challeng explor
foundat concept data manag process statist comput dynam visual use
modern program tool agil webservic concept idea protocol illustr exampl
real observ simul researchderiv dataset prior quantit experi program
calculus statist mathemat model linear algebra will necessari open
graduat cours will provid general overview principl concept techniqu
tool servic manag harmon aggreg preprocess model analyz interpret larg
multigsour incomplot incongru heterogen data big data focus will expos
student common challeng relat handl big data present enorm opportun
power associ abil interrog complex dataset extract use inform deriv
knowledg provid action forecast biomed healthcar social dataset will
provid context address specif drive challeng student will learn modern
data analyt techniqu develop skill import export clean fuse model visual
analyz synthes complex dataset collabor design implement share
communiti valid highthroughput analyt workflow will emphas throughout
cours"
```

This stemming process has to be done after the `PlainTextDocument` function because `stemDocument` only can be applied to plain text.

The *Bags of Words* strategy is very useful to be able to tokenize text documents into `n-grams`, sequences of words, e.g., a `2-gram` represents two-word phrases that appear together in order. This allows us to form bags of words and extract information about word ordering. The *bag of words model* is a common way to represent documents in matrix form based on their term frequencies (TFs). We can construct an $n \times t$ document-term matrix (DTM), where n is the number of documents, and t is the number of unique terms. Each column in the DTM represents a unique term, the $(i,j)^{th}$ cell represents how many of term j are present in document i.

---

[4]https://doi.org/10.1108/eb046814

The basic bag of words model is invariant to ordering of the words within a document. Once we compute the DTM, we can use machine learning techniques to interpret the derived signature information contained in the resulting matrices.

Document-Term Matrix

Now the doc_corpus object is quite clean. Next, we can make a document-term matrix to explore all the terms in 5 documents. The document-term matrix is a bunch of dummy variables that tell us if a given term appears in a specific document.

```
doc_dtm <- TermDocumentMatrix(doc_corpus)
doc_dtm
## <<TermDocumentMatrix (terms: 336, documents: 5)>>
## Non-/sparse entries: 489/1191
## Sparsity           : 71%
## Maximal term length: 27
## Weighting          : term frequency (tf)
```

The summary of the document-term matrix is informative. We have 336 different terms in the 5 documents. There are 489 nonzero and 1191 sparse entries. Thus, the sparsity is $\frac{1191}{(489+1191)} \approx 71\%$, which measures the term sparsity across documents. A high sparsity indicates that the terms are not often repeated among different documents.

Recall that we applied the PlainTextDocument function to your doc_corpus object. This removes all document metadata. To relabel the documents in the document-term matrix, we can use the following commands:

```
doc_dtm$dimnames$Docs<-as.character(1:5)
inspect(doc_dtm)
## <<TermDocumentMatrix (terms: 336, documents: 5)>>
## Non-/sparse entries: 489/1191
## Sparsity           : 71%
## Maximal term length: 27
## Weighting          : term frequency (tf)
## Sample             :
##          Docs
## Terms     1 2 3 4 5
##   analyt  3 0 3 1 2
##   cours   4 2 3 3 2
##   data    7 1 2 3 6
##   infer   0 0 2 6 2
##   method  0 2 5 3 2
##   model   3 0 4 3 3
##   statist 2 0 1 5 4
##   student 2 0 1 2 4
##   use     2 3 1 3 2
##   will    6 0 3 4 3
```

We might want to find and report the frequent terms using this document-term matrix.

```
findFreqTerms(doc_dtm, lowfreq = 2)
##   [1] "abil"        "address"     "advanc"      "algebra"     "analysi"
##   [6] "analyt"      "analyz"      "appli"       "appropri"    "associ"
##  [11] "assumpt"     "bayesian"    "big"         "bigdata"     "bioinformat"
##  [16] "biomed"      "calculus"    "challeng"    "common"      "complex"
##  [21] "comput"      "concept"     "conduct"     "core"        "cours"
##  [26] "cover"       "credit"      "data"        "dataset"     "design"
##  [31] "dimension"   "drive"       "dynam"       "emphas"      "epidemiolog"
##  [36] "equat"       "estim"       "exampl"      "experi"      "focus"
##  [41] "foundat"     "general"     "handl"       "health"      "healthcar"
##  [46] "heterogen"   "hour"        "hs550"       "includ"      "incomplet"
##  [51] "infer"       "inform"      "innov"       "interpret"   "interrog"
##  [56] "knowledg"    "labdiscuss"  "learn"       "lectur"      "limit"
##  [61] "linear"      "manag"       "mathemat"    "measur"      "method"
##  [66] "misconcept"  "model"       "modern"      "multipl"     "multivari"
##  [71] "observ"      "open"        "optim"       "power"       "present"
##  [76] "principl"    "probabl"     "problem"     "process"     "program"
##  [81] "provid"      "publish"     "read"        "real"        "recent"
##  [86] "regress"     "report"      "research"    "review"      "sampl"
##  [91] "scienc"      "scientif"    "skill"       "softwar"     "specif"
##  [96] "statist"     "student"     "studi"       "system"      "techniqu"
## [101] "test"        "theori"      "throughout"  "tool"        "topic"
## [106] "two"         "understand"  "use"         "variabl"     "visual"
## [111] "will"
```

This gives us the terms that appear in at least two documents. High-frequency terms like comput, statist, model, healthcar, and learn make perfect sense to be included in this shortlist, as these courses cover modeling, statistical, and computational methods with applications to health sciences.

The tm package provides the functionality to compute the correlations between terms. Here is a mechanism to determine the words that are highly correlated with statist, ($\rho(statist, ?) \geq 0.8$).

```
findAssocs(doc_dtm, "statist", corlimit = 0.8)
## $statist
## epidemiolog  interpret    publish    softwar     studi  understand
##        0.92       0.92       0.92       0.92      0.92        0.92
##      specif      appli
##        0.85       0.84
```

7.1.2   Case Study: Job Ranking

Next, we will mine an interesting dataset containing both quantitative and qualitative (free text) elements. The 2011 USA Jobs Ranking dataset is available in the SOCR data archive. More recent jobs description data are provided by the US Bureau of Labor Statistics (BLS)[5] and can be used to practice similar *mixed data* modeling approaches.

---

[5] https://www.bls.gov/oes/current/oes_nat.htm

```
library(rvest)
wiki_url <-
    read_html("https://wiki.socr.umich.edu/index.php/SOCR_Data_2011_US_JobsRanking")
html_nodes(wiki_url, "#content")
job <- html_table(html_nodes(wiki_url, "table")[[1]])
head(job)
## # A tibble: 6 x 10
##    Index Job_Title   Overall_Score Average_Incom Work_Environment Stress
##    <int> <chr>           <int>          <int>          <dbl>        <dbl>
## 1      1 Software          60          87140           150         10.4
## 2      2 Mathematician     73          94178           89.7        12.8
## 3      3 Actuary          123          87204           179.        16.0
## 4      4 Statistician     129          73208           89.5        14.1
## 5      5 Computer_Sci     147          77153           90.8        16.5
```

Note that low or high job indices represent more or less desirable jobs, respectively. Thus, in 2011, the most desirable job among top 200 common jobs would be Software Engineer. The aim of our study now is to explore the difference between the *top 30* desirable jobs and the *bottom 100* jobs based on their textural job descriptions (JDs). We will go through the same procedure as we did earlier in the course syllabi example. The documents we are using represent the Description column (a text vector of JDs) in the dataset.

Step 1: Make a VCorpus object

```
jobs <- as.list(job$Description)
jobCorpus <- VCorpus(VectorSource(jobs))
Step 2: clean the VCorpus object
jobCorpus <- tm_map(jobCorpus, tolower)
for(j in seq(jobCorpus)) { jobCorpus[[j]] <- gsub("_", " ", jobCorpus[[j]]) }
```

Here we used a loop to substitute "_" (underscore) with blank space. This is necessary as the underscore character connecting words will cause problems with using removePunctuation to separate terms. In this situation, global pattern matching, gsub, will find and replace the underscores with spaces.

```
jobCorpus <- tm_map(jobCorpus, removeWords, stopwords("english"))
jobCorpus <- tm_map(jobCorpus, removePunctuation)
jobCorpus <- tm_map(jobCorpus, stripWhitespace)
jobCorpus <- tm_map(jobCorpus, PlainTextDocument)
jobCorpus <- tm_map(jobCorpus, stemDocument)
```

Step 3: Build document-term matrix
Term Document Matrix (TDM) objects (tm::DocumentTermMatrix) contain a sparse term-document matrix or document-term matrix and attribute weights of the matrix. First, we should ensure that we got a clean VCorpus object.

```
jobCorpus[[1]]$content
## [1] "research design develop maintain softwar system along hardwar develop
medic scientif industri purpos"
```

Then we can start to build the DTM and reassign labels to the `Docs`.

```
dtm<-DocumentTermMatrix(jobCorpus)
dtm
## <<DocumentTermMatrix (documents: 200, terms: 846)>>
## Non-/sparse entries: 1818/167382
## Sparsity           : 99%
## Maximal term length: 15
## Weighting          : term frequency (tf)
dtm$dimnames$Docs <- as.character(1:200)
inspect(dtm[1:10, 1:10])
## <<DocumentTermMatrix (documents: 10, terms: 10)>>
## Non-/sparse entries: 2/98
## Sparsity           : 98%
## Maximal term length: 7
## Weighting          : term frequency (tf)
##      Terms
## Docs 16wheel abnorm access accid accord account accur achiev act activ
##   1        0      0      0     0      0       0     0      0   0     0
##   10       0      0      0     0      0       0     0      0   0     0
##   2        0      0      0     0      0       0     0      0   0     0
##   3        0      0      0     1      0       0     0      0   0     0
##   4        0      0      0     0      0       0     0      0   0     0
##   5        0      0      0     0      0       0     0      0   0     0
##   6        0      0      0     0      0       0     0      0   0     0
##   7        0      0      0     0      0       0     0      0   0     0
##   8        0      0      0     0      1       0     0      0   0     0
##   9        0      0      0     0      0       0     0      0   0     0
```

Let's subset the `dtm` into top 30 jobs and bottom 100 jobs.

```
dtm_top30 <- dtm[1:30, ]
dtm_bot100 <- dtm[101:200, ]
dtm_top30
## <<DocumentTermMatrix (documents: 30, terms: 846)>>
## Non-/sparse entries: 293/25087
## Sparsity           : 99%
## Maximal term length: 15
## Weighting          : term frequency (tf)
dtm_bot100
## <<DocumentTermMatrix (documents: 100, terms: 846)>>
## Non-/sparse entries: 870/83730
## Sparsity           : 99%
## Maximal term length: 15
## Weighting          : term frequency (tf)
```

In this case, since the sparsity is very high, we can try to remove some of the words that rarely appear in the job descriptions.

```
dtms_top30 <- removeSparseTerms(dtm_top30, 0.90)
dtms_top30
## <<DocumentTermMatrix (documents: 30, terms: 19)>>
## Non-/sparse entries: 70/500
## Sparsity           : 88%
## Maximal term length: 10
## Weighting          : term frequency (tf)
dtms_bot100 <- removeSparseTerms(dtm_bot100, 0.94)
dtms_bot100
## <<DocumentTermMatrix (documents: 100, terms: 14)>>
## Non-/sparse entries: 122/1278
## Sparsity           : 91%
## Maximal term length: 10
## Weighting          : term frequency (tf)
```

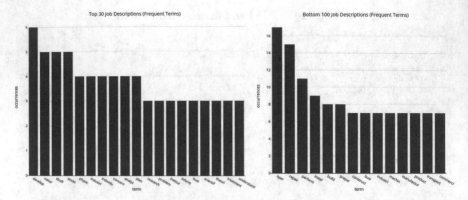

Fig. 7.1 Term frequency distributions for the job descriptions

On the top, instead of the initial 846 terms, we only have 19 terms appearing in at least 10% of the JDs. Similarly, in the bottom, instead of the initial 846 terms, we only have 14 terms appearing in at least 6% of the bottom 100 jobs.

Similar to what we did in Chap. 5, visualization of the terms-world clouds can be accomplished in R by combining functionalities from the tm and wordcloud packages. First, we can count the term frequencies in two document-term matrices (Fig. 7.1).

```
library(plotly)
# Let's calculate & sort the cumulative frequencies of words across documents
freq1 <- sort(colSums(as.matrix(dtms_top30)), decreasing=T); freq1
##    develop      assist      natur       studi      analyz     concern    individu
##          6           5          5           5           4          4           4
##   industri      physic       plan        busi      inform     institut     problem
##          4           4          4           3           3          3           3
freq2 <- sort(colSums(as.matrix(dtms_bot100)), decreasing=T); freq2
# Plot frequent words (for bottom 100 jobs)
wf2=data.frame(term=names(freq2), occurrences=freq2)
df.freq2 <- subset(wf2, freq2>2)
plot_ly(data=df.freq2, x=~term, y=~occurrences, type="bar") %>%
  layout(title="Bottom 100 Job Descriptions (Frequent Terms)")
# Plot frequent words (for top 30 jobs)
wf1=data.frame(term=names(freq1), occurrences=freq1)
df.freq1 <- subset(wf1, freq1>2)
plot_ly(data=df.freq1, x=~term, y=~occurrences, type="bar") %>%
  layout(title="Top 30 Job Descriptions (Frequent Terms)")
```

```
# what are common (frequently occurring words) in top 30 and bottom 100 jobs?
intersect(df.freq1$term, df.freq2$term)
## [1] "industri" "busi"
```

Then we apply the wordcloud() function to the freq dataset (Fig. 7.2).

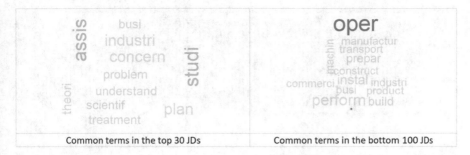

| Common terms in the top 30 JDs | Common terms in the bottom 100 JDs |

Fig. 7.2 Word clouds of frequent terms in top and bottom job descriptions

```
library(wordcloud)
set.seed(123)
# wordcloud(names(freq1), freq1)
wordcloud(names(freq1), freq1, min.freq=2, colors=brewer.pal(6,"Spectral"))
# Color code the frequencies using an appropriate color map:
wordcloud(names(freq2), freq2, min.freq=5, colors=brewer.pal(6, "Spectral"))
```

It becomes apparent that top 30 jobs tend to focus more on research or discovery and include frequent keywords like "study," "theory," and "science." The bottom 100 jobs are more focused on mechanistic operations of objects or equipment, with frequent keywords like "operation," "repair," and "perform."

7.1.3 Area Under ROC Curve

In Chap. 9, we will discuss the *receiver operating characteristic (ROC)* curve. We can use document-term matrices to build classifiers and use the *area under the ROC curve* to evaluate those classifiers. Assume we want to predict whether a job ranks top 30 in the job list. The first task would be to create an indicator of high rank (job is in the top 30 list). We can use the ifelse() function that we are already familiar with.

```
job$highrank <- ifelse(job$Index<30, 1, 0)
```

Next, we load the glmnet package to help us build, evaluate, and visualize job-ranking prediction models using the JD text.

```
# install.packages("glmnet")
library(glmnet)
```

The function we will be using is the cv.glmnet(), where cv stands for cross-validation. Since the derived job ranking variable highrank is binary, we specify the option family='binomial'. Also, we want to use a 10-fold CV method for internal statistical (resampling-based) prediction validation (Fig. 7.3).

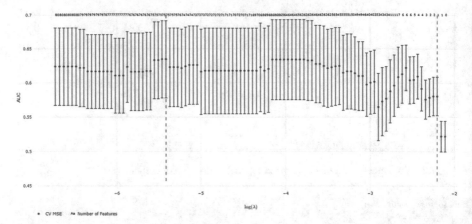

Fig. 7.3 Tracking performance of various regularized linear models (LASSO) for predicting job-ranking using the JD-derived (unweighted) document term matrix (DTM). The top and bottom horizontal axes encode the relation between the number of salient features (top) and the regularization weight (bottom, λ in logarithmic scale). The vertical axis represents the AUC performance measure. The vertical orange and green lines represent the minimal λ and one standard error (1SE) cut offs, respectively

```r
set.seed(25)
fit <- cv.glmnet(x = as.matrix(dtm), y = job[['highrank']],
                 family = 'binomial',
                 alpha = 1, # lasso penalty
                 type.measure = "auc", # use area under ROC curve metric
                 nfolds = 10, # 10-fold cross-validation
                 thresh = 1e-3, # high value yields less accurate, faster training
                 maxit = 1e3)  # lower number of iterations yields faster training
print(paste("max AUC =", round(max(fit$cvm), 4))) ## [1] "max AUC = 0.6348"
plotCV.glmnet <- function(cv.glmnet.object, name="") {
  df <- as.data.frame(cbind(x=log(cv.glmnet.object$lambda),
                      y=cv.glmnet.object$cvm, errorBar=cv.glmnet.object$cvsd),
                      nzero=cv.glmnet.object$nzero)
  featureNum <- cv.glmnet.object$nzero
  xFeature <- log(cv.glmnet.object$lambda)
  yFeature <- max(cv.glmnet.object$cvm)+max(cv.glmnet.object$cvsd)
  dataFeature <- data.frame(featureNum, xFeature, yFeature)
  plot_ly(data = df) %>%
    # add error bars for each CV-mean at log(lambda)
    add_trace(x = ~x, y = ~y, type = 'scatter', mode = 'markers',
        name = 'CV MSE', error_y = ~list(array = errorBar)) %>%
    # add the lambda-min and lambda 1SD vertical dash lines
    add_lines(data=df, x=c(log(cv.glmnet.object$lambda.min),
                  log(cv.glmnet.object$lambda.min)),
              y=c(min(cv.glmnet.object$cvm)-max(df$errorBar),
              max(cv.glmnet.object$cvm)+max(df$errorBar)),
              showlegend=F, line=list(dash="dash"), name="lambda.min",
              mode = 'lines+markers') %>%
    add_lines(data=df, x=c(log(cv.glmnet.object$lambda.1se),
                  log(cv.glmnet.object$lambda.1se)),
              y=c(min(cv.glmnet.object$cvm)-max(df$errorBar),
              max(cv.glmnet.object$cvm)+max(df$errorBar)),
              showlegend=F, line=list(dash="dash"), name="lambda.1se") %>%
    # Add Number of Features Annotations on Top
    add_trace(dataFeature, x = ~xFeature, y = ~yFeature, type = 'scatter',
```

```
              name="Number of Features",
          mode = 'text', text = ~featureNum, textposition = 'middle right',
          textfont = list(color = '#000000', size = 9)) %>%
    layout(title = paste0("Cross-Validation MSE (", name, ")"),
                        xaxis = list(title=paste0("log(",TeX("\\lambda"),")")),
          side="bottom", showgrid=TRUE), # type="Log"
          hovermode="x unified", legend=list(orientation='h'), # xaxis2=ax,
          yaxis = list(title = cv.glmnet.object$name, side="left",
          showgrid = TRUE))
  }
  plotCV.glmnet(fit, "LASSO")
```

Here x is a matrix of covariates and y is the response variable (outcome vector). The graph shows the corresponding AUC performance metrics for each model, depending on the number of features included in the model (see top horizontal axis). We also reported the optimal AUC among all models. The resulting $AUC \sim 0.63$ represents a relatively good prediction model for this small sample size.

7.1.4 TF-IDF

To enhance the utility of the DTM matrix, we introduce the *TF-IDF (term frequency-inverse document frequency)* concept. Unlike pure frequency, TF-IDF measures the relative importance of a term. If a term appears in almost every document, the term will be considered common with high information capacity. Alternatively, rare terms would be considered as less informational.

7.1.4.1 Term Frequency (TF)

The term frequency ratio is

$$TF = \frac{\text{a term's occurrences in a document}}{\text{the number of occurrences of the most frequent word within the same document}}.$$

$$TF(t, d) = \frac{f_d(t)}{\max_{w \in d} f_d(w)}.$$

7.1.4.2 Inverse Document Frequency (IDF)

The *TF* definition may allow high scores for irrelevant words that naturally show up often in a long text, even if these may have been triaged in a prior preprocessing step. The *IDF* attempts to rectify that. *IDF* represents the inverse of the share of the documents in which the regarded term can be found. The lower the number of documents containing the term, relative to the size of the corpus, the higher the term factor.

IDF involves a logarithm function because otherwise the effective scoring penalty of showing up in two documents would be too extreme. Typically, the IDF for a term found in just one document is twice the IDF for another term found in two docs. The ln() function rectifies this bias of ranking in favor of rare terms, even if the TF-factor may be high. It is rather unlikely that a term's relevance is only high in one doc and not all others,

$$IDF(t, D) = \ln \left(\frac{|D|}{|\{d \in D : t \in d\}|} \right).$$

7.1.4.3   TF-IDF

Both TF and IDF yield high scores for highly relevant terms. TF relies on local information (search over d), whereas IDF incorporates a more global perspective (search over D). The product TF $\times$ IDF, gives the classical TF-IDF formula. However, alternative expressions may be formulated to get other univariate expressions using alternative weights for TF and IDF:

$$TF\_IDF(t, d, D) = TF(t, d) \times IDF(t, D).$$

An example of an alternative TF-IDF metric can be defined by:

$$TF\_IDF'(t, d, D) = \frac{IDF(t, D)}{|D|} + TF\_IDF(t, d, D).$$

Let's make another DTM with TF-IDF weights and compare the differences between the *unweighted* and *weighted* DTM.

```
dtm.tfidf<-DocumentTermMatrix(jobCorpus, control=list(weighting=weightTfIdf))
dtm.tfidf
## <<DocumentTermMatrix (documents: 200, terms: 846)>>
## Non-/sparse entries: 1818/167382
## Sparsity           : 99%
## Maximal term length: 15
## Weighting          : (normalized) (tf-idf)
dtm.tfidf$dimnames$Docs <- as.character(1:200)
inspect(dtm.tfidf[1:9, 1:10])
## <<DocumentTermMatrix (documents: 9, terms: 10)>>
## Non-/sparse entries: 2/88
## Sparsity           : 98%
## Maximal term length: 7
## Weighting          : (normalized) (tf-idf)
inspect(dtm[1:9, 1:10])
## <<DocumentTermMatrix (documents: 9, terms: 10)>>
## Non-/sparse entries: 2/88
## Sparsity           : 98%
## Maximal term length: 7
## Weighting          : term frequency (tf)
```

Inspecting the two different DTMs we can see that TF-IDF is not only counting the frequency but also assigning different weights to each term according to the

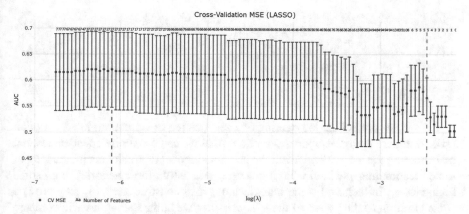

Fig. 7.4 Regularized linear model (LASSO) for predicting job-ranking using JD-derived TF-IDF-weighted document term matrix. The top and bottom horizontal axes encode the relation between the number of salient features (top) and the regularization weight (bottom). The vertical axis represents the AUC performance measure. The vertical orange and green lines represent the minimal lambda and 1SE cut offs, respectively

importance of the term. Next, we are going to fit another model with this new DTM (dtm.tfidf) (Fig. 7.4).

```
set.seed(1234)
fit1 <- cv.glmnet(x = as.matrix(dtm.tfidf), y = job[['highrank']],
            family = 'binomial',
            alpha = 1, # lasso penalty
            type.measure = "auc", # use area under ROC curve
            nfolds = 10, # 10-fold cross-validation
            thresh = 1e-3, # high value is less accurate, faster training
            maxit = 1e3) # lower number of iterations for faster training
print(paste("max AUC =", round(max(fit1$cvm), 4))) ## [1] "max AUC = 0.5738"
plotCV.glmnet(fit1, "LASSO")
```

This performance is about the same as the previous jobs ranking prediction classifier (based on the unweighted DTM). Due to random sampling, each run of the protocols may generate slightly different results. The idea behind using TF-IDF is that one would expect to get more unbiased estimates of word importance. If the document includes stopwords, like "the" or "one," the unweighted DTM may distort the results, but TF-IDF can help fix this problem.

Next, we can report a more intuitive representation of the job ranking prediction reflecting the agreement of the binary (top-30 or not) classification between the real labels and the predicted labels. Note that this specific validation uses the training data itself; however, later we will illustrate model performance assessment using independent testing data.

```
# Binarize the LASSO probability prediction, also try newx=as.matrix(dtm)
preffit1 <- predict(fit1, newx=as.matrix(dtm.tfidf),
                    s="lambda.min", type = "class")
binPredfit1 <- ifelse(preffit1 < 0.5, 0, 1)
table(binPredfit1, job[['highrank']])
## binPredfit1   0   1
##           0 171   0
##           1   0  29
```

Let's try to predict the job ranking of a new (testing or validation) job description (JD). There are many BLS job descriptions[6] that we can use for independent testing, by extracting the JD text and using the pretrained model to predict the job ranking of the corresponding positions. Trying several alternative job categories, e.g., some high-tech or fin-tech and some manufacturing and construction jobs, may provide some intuition to the power of the jobs-classifier we built. Below, we will compare the BLS JDs for the positions of *accountant*, *attorney*, and *machinist*.

```
# install.packages("text2vec"); install.packages("data.table")
library(text2vec)
library(data.table)
# Choose PUBLIC ACCOUNTANT JD 1430, https://www.bls.gov/ocs/ocsjobde.htm
xTestAccountant <- "Performs professional auditing work in a public accounting firm. Work
requires at least a bachelor's degree in accounting. Participates in or conducts audits to
ascertain the fairness of financial representations made by client companies. May also assist the
client in improving accounting procedures and operations. Examines financial reports, accounting
records, and related documents and practices of clients. Determines whether all important matters
have been disclosed and whether procedures are consistent and conform to acceptable practices.
Samples and tests transactions, internal controls, and other elements of the accounting system(s)
as needed to render the accounting firm's final written opinion. As an entry level public
accountant, serves as a junior member of an audit team. Receives classroom and on-the-job training
to provide practical experience in applying the principles, theories, and concepts of accounting
and auditing to specific situations. (Positions held by trainee public accountants with advanced
degrees, such as MBA's are excluded at this level.) Complete instructions are furnished and work
is reviewed to verify its accuracy, conformance with required procedures and instructions, and
usefulness in facilitating the accountant's professional growth. Any technical problems not
covered by instructions are brought to the attention of a superior. Carries out basic audit tests
and procedures, such as: verifying reports against source accounts and records; reconciling bank
and other accounts; and examining cash receipts and disbursements, payroll records, requisitions,
receiving reports, and other accounting documents in detail to ascertain that transactions are
properly supported and recorded. Prepares selected portions of audit working papers"

xTestAttorney <- "Performs consultation, advisory and/or trail work and carries out the legal
processes necessary to effect the rights, privileges, and obligations of the organization. The
work performed requires completion of law school with an L.L.B. degree or J.D. degree and
admission to the bar. Responsibilities or functions include one or more of the following or
comparable duties:
1. Preparing and reviewing various legal instruments and documents, such as contracts, leases,
licenses, purchases, sales, real estate, etc.;
2. Acting as agent of the organization in its transactions;
3. Examining material (e.g., advertisements, publications, etc.) for legal implications; advising
officials of proposed legislation which might affect the organization;
4. Applying for patents, copyrights, or registration of the organization's products, processes,
devices, and trademarks; advising whether to initiate or defend lawsuits;
5. Conducting pre trial preparations; defending the organization in lawsuits;
6. Prosecuting criminal cases for a local or state government or defending the general public (for
example, public defenders and attorneys rendering legal services to students); or
7. Advising officials on tax matters, government regulations, and/or legal rights.
Attorney jobs are matched at one of six levels according to two factors:
```

---

[6]https://www.bls.gov/ocs/ocsjobde.htm

1. Difficulty level of legal work; and
2. Responsibility level of job.
Attorney jobs which meet the above definitions are to be classified and coded in accordance with a chart available upon request.
Legal questions are characterized by: facts that are well-established; clearly applicable legal precedents; and matters not of substantial importance to the organization. (Usually relatively limited sums of money, e.g., a few thousand dollars, are involved.)
a. legal investigation, negotiation, and research preparatory to defending the organization in potential or actual lawsuits involving alleged negligence where the facts can be firmly established and there are precedent cases directly applicable to the situation;
b. searching case reports, legal documents, periodicals, textbooks, and other legal references, and preparing draft opinions on employee compensation or benefit questions where there is a substantial amount of clearly applicable statutory, regulatory, and case material;
c. drawing up contracts and other legal documents in connection with real property transactions requiring the development of detailed information but not involving serious questions regarding titles to property or other major factual or legal issues.
d. preparing routine criminal cases for trial when the legal or factual issues are relatively straightforward and the impact of the case is limited; and
e. advising public defendants in regard to routine criminal charges or complaints and representing such defendants in court when legal alternatives and facts are relatively clear and the impact of the outcome is limited primarily to the defendant.

Legal work is regularly difficult by reason of one or more of the following: the absence of clear and directly applicable legal precedents; the different possible interpretations that can be placed on the facts, the laws, or the precedents involved; the substantial importance of the legal matters to the organization (e.g., sums as large as $100,000 are generally directly or indirectly involved); or the matter is being strongly pressed or contested in formal proceedings or in negotiations by the individuals, corporations, or government agencies involved.
a. advising on the legal implications of advertising representations when the facts supporting the representations and the applicable precedent cases are subject to different interpretations;
b. reviewing and advising on the implications of new or revised laws affecting the organization;
c. presenting the organization's defense in court in a negligence lawsuit which is strongly pressed by counsel for an organized group;
d. providing legal counsel on tax questions complicated by the absence of precedent decisions that are directly applicable to the organization's situation;
e. preparing and prosecuting criminal cases when the facts of the cases are complex or difficult to determine or the outcome will have a significant impact within the jurisdiction; and
f. advising and representing public defendants in all phases of criminal proceedings when the facts of the case are complex or difficult to determine, complex or unsettled legal issues are involved, or the prosecutorial jurisdiction devotes substantial resources to obtaining a conviction."

xTestMachinist <- "Produces replacement parts and new parts in making repairs of metal parts of mechanical equipment. Work involves most of the following: interpreting written instructions and specifications; planning and laying out of work; using a variety of machinist's handtools and precision measuring instruments; setting up and operating standard machine tools; shaping of metal parts to close tolerances; making standard shop computations relating to dimensions of work, tooling, feeds, and speeds of machining; knowledge of the working properties of the common metals; selecting standard materials, parts, and equipment required for this work; and fitting and assembling parts into mechanical equipment. In general, the machinist's work normally requires a rounded training in machine-shop practice usually acquired through a formal apprenticeship or equivalent training and experience. Industrial machinery repairer. Repairs machinery or mechanical equipment. Work involves most of the following: examining machines and mechanical equipment to diagnose source of trouble; dismantling or partly dismantling machines and performing repairs that mainly involve the use of handtools in scraping and fitting parts; replacing broken or defective parts with items obtained from stock; ordering the production of a replacement part by a machine shop or sending the machine to a machine shop for major repairs; preparing written specifications for major repairs or for the production of parts ordered from machine shops; reassembling machines; and making all necessary adjustments for operation. In general, the work of a machinery maintenance mechanic requires rounded training and experience usually acquired through a formal apprenticeship or equivalent training and experience. Excluded from this classification are workers whose primary duties involve setting up or adjusting machines. Vehicle and mobile equipment mechanics and repairers. Repairs, rebuilds, or overhauls major assemblies of internal combustion automobiles, buses, trucks, or tractors. Work involves most of the following: Diagnosing the source of trouble and determining the extent of repairs required; replacing worn or broken parts such as piston rings, bearings, or other engine parts; grinding and adjusting valves; rebuilding carburetors; overhauling transmissions; and repairing fuel injection, lighting, and ignition systems. In general, the work of the motor vehicle mechanic requires rounded training and experience usually acquired through a formal apprenticeship or equivalent training and experience"

```
# Define testing cases (1) list, (2) Y-category (top-30 or not), (3) ID names
testJDs <- as.list(c(xTestAccountant, xTestAttorney, xTestMachinist))
testTop30 <- c(1,1,0)
testNames <- c("xTestAccountant", "xTestAttorney", "xTestMachinist")
### 1. Training Phase Labeled data
# loop to substitute "_" with blank space
for(j in seq(jobs)) {  jobs[[j]] <- gsub("_", " ", jobs[[j]]) }
prep_fun = tolower
tok_fun = word_tokenizer
trainIterator = itoken(unlist(jobs), preprocessor = prep_fun,
                tokenizer = tok_fun, ids = rownames(jobs), progressbar = FALSE)
vocab = create_vocabulary(trainIterator); vocab
vectorizer = vocab_vectorizer(vocab)
dtm_train = create_dtm(trainIterator, vectorizer)
dim(dtm_train) ## [1]  200 1113
### 2. Fit LASSO model
set.seed(1234)
fit1 <- cv.glmnet(x = dtm_train, y = job[['highrank']], family = 'binomial',
                  alpha = 1, # Lasso penalty
                  type.measure = "auc", # use the area under ROC curve measure
                  nfolds = 10, # 10-fold cross-validation
                  thresh = 1e-5, maxit = 1e4)
print(paste("max AUC =", round(max(fit1$cvm), 4))) ## [1] "max AUC = 0.6191"
#### 3. Testing Phase (new JDs)
testIterator = tok_fun(prep_fun(unlist(testJDs)))
# turn off progress bar
testIterator = itoken(testIterator, ids = testNames, progressbar = FALSE)
dtm_test = create_dtm(testIterator, vectorizer)
predictedJDs = predict(fit1, dtm_test, type = 'response')[,1]
# Type can be: "link", "response", "coefficients", "class", "nonzero"
predictedJDs
## xTestAccountant    xTestAttorney  xTestMachinist
##       0.2312489       0.1504954       0.1355345
plotCV.glmnet(fit1, "LASSO")
```

Note that at run time, the results may change somewhat. Above we assessed the JD predictive (LASSO) model using the three out of bag job descriptions—*accountant*, *attorney*, and *machinist*. The output predictions of the testing JDs show that:

- On the *training data*, the predicted probabilities rapidly decrease with the indexing of the jobs, corresponding to the *overall job ranking* (highly ranked/desired jobs are listed on the top).
- On the three *testing job description data* (accountant, attorney, and machinist), there is a clear ranking difference between the machinist and the other two professions; accountant and attorney JDs suggest that these professions are more likely to be highly desirable, i.e., high-ranked jobs.

Also see the discussion in Chap. 11 about the different *types of predictions* that can be generated as outputs of cv.glmnet regularized linear model forecasting methods.

7.1.5 Cosine Similarity

As we mentioned above, text data are often *transformed*, or weighted, by the term frequency-inverse document frequency (TF-IDF). In many text-mining applications, this preprocessing step may often yield better results compared to the raw (unweighted) term-frequencies. Alternative transformations may be based on different distance measures, such as *cosine distance*. The *cosine similarity* and distance are defined by

$$\text{Cosine Similarity} = \cos(\theta) = \frac{A \cdot B}{\|A\|_2 \|B\|_2},$$

$$\text{Cosine Distance} = 1 - \text{Cosine Similarity} = 1 - \frac{A \cdot B}{\|A\|_2 \|B\|_2},$$

where θ represents the angle between two vectors A and B in the Euclidean space spanned by the DTM matrix. Note that the cosine *similarity* of two text documents (more specifically two DTMs with or without TF-IDF weights) will always be in the range $[0, 1]$, since the term frequencies are always non-negative. In other words, the angle between two term frequency vectors cannot exceed 90°, and therefore, $0 \leq$ Cosine Distance ≤ 1. Even though it is not a proper distance metric, as in general it does not satisfy the triangle inequality, the cosine similarity is a practically useful pseudo-distance. Mind the dimensions of the corresponding matrices; dim (dtm) $= 200 \times 846$ and dim(dist $\_$ cos) $= 200 \times 200$.

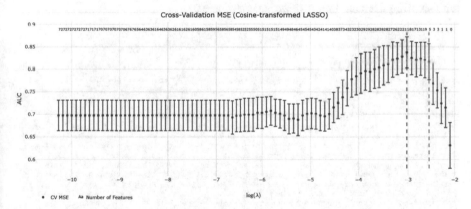

Fig. 7.5 Regularized linear model (LASSO) for predicting job-ranking following cosine-transformation. The top and bottom horizontal axes encode the relation between the number of salient features (top) and the regularization weight (bottom). The vertical axis represents the AUC performance measure. The vertical orange and green lines represent the minimal lambda and 1SE cut offs, respectively

```
cos_dist = function(mat) {  numer = tcrossprod(mat)
  denom1 = sqrt(apply(mat, 1, crossprod))
  denom2 = sqrt(apply(mat, 1, crossprod))
  1 - numer / outer(denom1,denom2)
}
# Recall fit <- cv.glmnet(x = as.matrix(dtm), y = job[['highrank']], ...)
dist_cos = cos_dist(as.matrix(dtm))   # also try with dtm_train
set.seed(1234)
fit_cos <- cv.glmnet(x = dist_cos, y=job[['highrank']], family = 'binomial',
             alpha = 1, type.measure = "auc", nfolds = 10,
             thresh = 1e-5, maxit = 1e5)
plotCV.glmnet(fit_cos, "Cosine-transformed LASSO")
print(paste("max AUC =", round(max(fit_cos$cvm), 4))) # [1] "max AUC=0.8377"
```

The AUC now is significantly higher, 0.84, which is a pretty good result, an improvement over the prior unweighted and TF-IDF-weighted DTMs, Fig. 7.5. This suggests that cosine-transforming the data improves natural language processing results and leads to a more acceptable content classifier.

7.1.6   Sentiment Analysis

In the next example, we will use the `text2vec::movie_review` dataset, which consists of 5000 movie reviews (X) paired with dichotomized `positive` or `negative` sentiments (Y). In the subsequent predictive analytics, this *sentiment* will represent the output feature (binary movie recommendation)

$$Y = \text{Sentiment} = \begin{cases} 0, & \text{negative} \\ 1, & \text{positive} \end{cases}.$$

Data Preprocessing

The `data.table` package will also be used for some data manipulation. Let's start with splitting the data into *training* and *testing* sets.

```
# install.packages("text2vec"); install.packages("data.table")
library(text2vec)
library(data.table)
data("movie_review") # Load the movie reviews data
setDT(movie_review) # coerce the movie reviews into a data.table (DT) object
setkey(movie_review, id) # create a key for the movie-reviews data table
# View(movie_review)
head(movie_review); dim(movie_review); colnames(movie_review)
## review 1: Homelessness (or Houselessness as George Carlin stated) has been an issue for years
but never a plan to help those on the street that were once considered human who did everything
from going to school, work, or vote for the matter. Most people think of the homeless as just a
lost cause while worrying about things such as racism, the war on Iraq, pressuring kids to
succeed, technology, the elections, inflation, or worrying if they'll be next to end up on the
streets.<br /><br />But what if you were given a bet to live on the streets for a month without
the luxuries you once had from a home, the entertainment sets, a bathroom, pictures on the wall, a
computer, and everything you once treasure to see what it's like to be homeless? That is Goddard
Bolt's lesson.<br /><br />Mel Brooks (who directs) who stars as Bolt plays a rich man who has
everything in the world until deciding to make a bet with a sissy rival (Jeffery Tambor) to see if
he can live in the streets for thirty days without the luxuries; if Bolt succeeds, he can do what
he wants with a future project of making more buildings. The bet's on where Bolt is thrown on the
street with a bracelet on his leg to monitor his every move where he can't step off the sidewalk.
He's given the nickname Pepto by a vagrant after it's written on his forehead where Bolt meets
other characters including a woman by the name of Molly (Lesley Ann Warren) an ex-dancer who got
divorce before losing her home, and her pals Sailor (Howard Morris) and Fumes (Teddy Wilson) who
are already used to the streets. They're survivors. Bolt isn't. He's not used to reaching mutual
agreements like he once did when being rich where it's fight or flight, kill or be killed.<br
/><br />While the love connection between Molly and Bolt wasn't necessary to plot, I found \\"Life
Stinks\\" to be one of Mel Brooks' observant films where prior to being a comedy, it shows a
tender side compared to his slapstick work such as Blazing Saddles, Young Frankenstein, or
Spaceballs for the matter, to show what it's like having something valuable before losing it the
next day or on the other hand making a stupid bet like all rich people do when they don't know
what to do with their money. Maybe they should give it to the homeless instead of using it like
Monopoly money.<br /><br />Or maybe this film will inspire you to help others.
## [1] 5000      3
## [1] "id" "sentiment" "review"
# Generate 80-20% training-testing split of the reviews
all_ids = movie_review$id
set.seed(1234)
train_ids = sample(all_ids, 5000*0.8)
test_ids = setdiff(all_ids, train_ids)
train = movie_review[train_ids, ]
test = movie_review[test_ids, ]
```

Next, we will vectorize the reviews by creating terms to *termID* mappings. Note that terms may include arbitrary *n-grams*, not just single words. The set of reviews will be represented as a sparse matrix, with rows and columns corresponding to reviews and terms, respectively. This vectorization may be accomplished in several alternative ways, e.g., by using the corpus vocabulary, feature hashing, etc.

The vocabulary-based DTM, created by the `create_vocabulary()` function, relies on all unique terms from all reviews, where each term has a unique ID. In this example, we will create the review vocabulary using an *iterator* construct abstracting the input details and enabling *in memory* processing of the (training) data by chunks.

```
# define the test preprocessing - either a simple (tolower case) function
preproc_fun = tolower
# or a more elaborate "cleaning" function
preproc_fun = function(x)                        # text data
{ require("tm")
  x  =  gsub("<.*?>", " ", x)                    # regex removing HTML tags
  x  =  iconv(x, "latin1", "ASCII", sub="")      # remove non-ASCII characters
  x  -  gsub("[^[:alnum:]]", " ", x)             # remove non-alpha-numeric values
  x  =  tolower(x)                               # convert to lowercase characters
  # x  =  removeNumbers(x)                       # removing numbers
  x  =  stripWhitespace(x)                       # removing white space
  x  =  gsub("^\\s+|\\s+$", "", x)   # remove leading and trailing white space
  return(x)
}
# define the tokenization function
token_fun = word_tokenizer
# iterator for both training and testing sets
iter_train = itoken(train$review, preprocessor = preproc_fun,
            tokenizer = token_fun, ids = train$id, progressbar = TRUE)
iter_test = itoken(test$review, preprocessor = preproc_fun,
            tokenizer = token_fun, ids = test$id, progressbar = TRUE)
reviewVocab = create_vocabulary(iter_train)
# report the head and tail of the reviewVocab
reviewVocab
## Number of docs: 4000
## 0 stopwords:  ...
## ngram_min = 1; ngram_max = 1
## Vocabulary:
##          term term_count doc_count
##      1: 00015          1          1
##      2:    03          1          1
##      3:   041          1          1
##      ---
## 35562:      a      26468       3871
## 35563:    and      26832       3864
## 35564:    the      54245       3966
```

The next step computes the *document term matrix* (DTM).

```
reviewVectorizer = vocab_vectorizer(reviewVocab)
t0 = Sys.time()
dtm_train = create_dtm(iter_train, reviewVectorizer)
dtm_test = create_dtm(iter_test, reviewVectorizer)
t1 = Sys.time()
print(difftime(t1, t0, units = 'sec')) ## Time difference of 2.434013 secs
# check the DTM dimensions
dim(dtm_train); dim(dtm_test) ## [1]  4000 35564
# confirm that the training data review DTM dimensions are consistent
# with training review IDs, i.e., #rows = number of documents, and
# #columns = number of unique terms (n-grams), dim(dtm_train)[[2]]
identical(rownames(dtm_train), train$id)  ## [1] TRUE
```

7.1.7   NLP/TM Analytics

We can now fit statistical models or derive machine learning AI predictions. Let's start by using `glmnet()` to fit a *logit model* with LASSO (L_1) regularization and 10-fold cross-validation, see Chap. 11 (Fig. 7.6).

```
library(glmnet)
nFolds = 10
t0 = Sys.time()
glmnet_classifier = cv.glmnet(x = dtm_train, y = train[['sentiment']],
        family = "binomial", alpha = 1, type.measure = "auc",
        nfolds = nFolds, thresh = 1e-2, maxit = 1e3)
lambda.best <- glmnet_classifier$lambda.min
lambda.best    ## [1] 0.009043106
t1 = Sys.time()  # report execution time
print(difftime(t1, t0, units = 'sec'))  ## Time difference of 8.660954 secs
plotCV.glmnet(glmnet_classifier)
```

Now let's look at external validation, i.e., testing the model on the independent 20% of the set aside movie reviews. The performance of the binary prediction

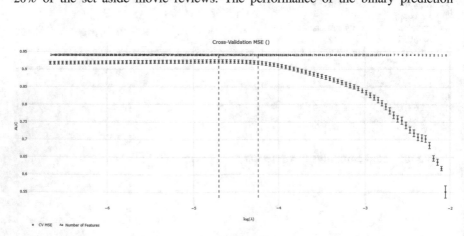

Fig. 7.6 Regularized linear model (LASSO) for predicting movie review sentiment

(binary sentiment analysis of these movie reviews) on the test data is roughly the same as we had from the internal statistical 10-fold cross-validation.

```
# report the mean internal cross-validated error
print(paste("max AUC =", round(max(glmnet_classifier$cvm), 4)))
## [1] "max AUC = 0.9221"
xTest = dtm_test    # report TESTING data prediction accuracy
yTest = test[['sentiment']]
predLASSO <- predict(glmnet_classifier,
                    s = glmnet_classifier$lambda.1se, newx = xTest)
testMSE_LASSO <- mean((predLASSO - yTest)^2); testMSE_LASSO  ## [1] 2.482202
# Binarize the LASSO probability prediction
binPredLASSO <- ifelse(predLASSO < 0.5, 0, 1)
table(binPredLASSO, yTest)
##             yTest
## binPredLASSO   0   1
##            0 449 181
##            1  38 332
glmnet:::auc(yTest, predLASSO)   # testing data AUC ## [1] 0.906773
# report top 20 negative & positive predictive terms predict==predict.cv.glmnet
sort(predict(glmnet_classifier, s=lambda.best, type="coefficients"))[1:20]
rev(sort(predict(glmnet_classifier,s=lambda.best,type="coefficients")))[1:20]
```

The (external) prediction performance, measured by AUC, on the *testing data* is about the same as the internal 10-fold stats cross-validation we reported using the *training data*.

Prediction Optimization
Earlier we saw that we can also prune the vocabulary and potentially improve prediction performance, e.g., by removing nonsalient terms like stopwords and by using *n-grams* instead of single words.

```
reviewVocab = create_vocabulary(iter_train, stopwords=tm::stopwords("english"),
    ngram = c(1L, 2L))
prunedReviewVocab = prune_vocabulary(reviewVocab, term_count_min = 10,
                    doc_proportion_max = 0.5, doc_proportion_min = 0.001)
prunedVectorizer = vocab_vectorizer(prunedReviewVocab)
t0 = Sys.time()
dtm_train = create_dtm(iter_train, prunedVectorizer)
dtm_test = create_dtm(iter_test, prunedVectorizer)
t1 = Sys.time()
print(difftime(t1, t0, units = 'sec')) ## Time difference of 2.321133 secs
```

Next, refit the model, report the performance, and examine for any improvements in the prediction accuracy (Fig. 7.7).

```
glmnet_prunedClassifier = cv.glmnet(x=dtm_train, y=train[['sentiment']],
        family = "binomial", alpha = 1, type.measure = "auc",
        nfolds = nFolds, thresh = 1e-4, maxit = 1e5)
lambda.best <- glmnet_prunedClassifier$lambda.min
lambda.best  ## [1] 0.007166507
t1 = Sys.time()  # report execution time
print(difftime(t1, t0, units = 'sec')) ## Time difference of 8.524901 secs
plotCV.glmnet(glmnet_prunedClassifier)
```

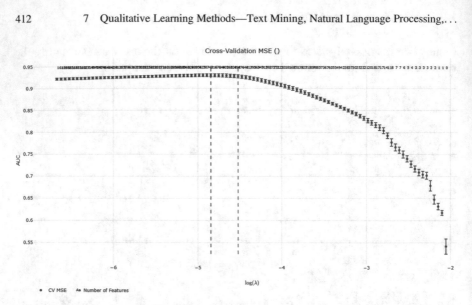

Fig. 7.7 Regularized linear model (LASSO) predicting movie review sentiment using the pruned vocabulary

```
# report the mean internal cross-validated error
print(paste("max AUC =", round(max(glmnet_prunedClassifier$cvm), 4)))
## [1] "max AUC = 0.9296"
xTest = dtm_test # report TESTING data prediction accuracy
yTest = test[['sentiment']]
predLASSO = predict(glmnet_prunedClassifier, dtm_test, type = 'response')[,1]
testMSE_LASSO <- mean((predLASSO - yTest)^2); testMSE_LASSO # 0.1232584
# Binarize the LASSO probability prediction
binPredLASSO <- ifelse(predLASSO < 0.5, 0, 1)
table(binPredLASSO, yTest)
##              yTest
## binPredLASSO   0    1
##            0  397   80
##            1   90  433
glmnet:::auc(yTest, predLASSO) # testing data AUC 0.9181407
# report the top 20 negative and positive predictive terms
summary(predLASSO)
sort(predict(glmnet_classifier, s = lambda.best, type="coefficients"))[1:20]
rev(sort(predict(glmnet_classifier, s=lambda.best, type="coefficients")))[1:20]
# Binarize the LASSO probability prediction and report the confusion matrix
binPredLASSO <- ifelse(predLASSO<0.5, 0, 1)
table(binPredLASSO, yTest)
##              yTest
## binPredLASSO   0    1
##            0  397   80
##            1   90  433
```

Using n-grams somewhat improved the sentiment prediction model.

7.2 Apriori Association Rules Learning

HTTP cookies[7] are used to track web-surfing and Internet traffic. We often notice that promotions (ads) on websites tend to match our needs, reveal our prior browsing history, or may reflect our interests. That is not an accident. Nowadays, recommendation systems[8] are highly based on machine learning methods that can learn the behavior, e.g., purchasing patterns, of individual consumers. In this section, we will uncover some of the mystery behind recommendation systems like market basket analysis. Specifically, we will (1) discuss association rules and their support and confidence, (2) present the *Apriori algorithm* for association rule learning, and (3) cover step-by-step a set of case-studies, including a toy example and studies of Head and Neck Cancer Medications, Grocery purchases, and survival of Titanic passengers.

7.2.1 Association Rules

Association rules are the result of process analytics (e.g., market basket analysis) that specify patterns of relationships among items. One specific example would be

$$\{charcoal, lighter, chicken\,wings\} \rightarrow \{barbecue\,sauce\}$$

In other words, charcoal, lighter, and chicken wings imply barbecue sauce. The curly brackets indicate that we have a set of items and the arrow suggests a direction of the association. Items in a set are called *elements*. When an item-set like $\{charcoal, lighter, chicken\,wings, barbecue\,sauce\}$ appears in our dataset with some regularity, we can mine and discover patterns of association with other item-sets. Association rules are commonly used for unsupervised discovery of knowledge rather than prediction of prespecified outcomes. In biomedical research, association rules are widely used to

- Search for interesting or frequently occurring patterns of DNA
- Discover relevant protein sequences in an analysis of cancer data
- Find patterns of medical claims that occur in combination with credit card or insurance fraud

---

[7]https://doi.org/10.1145/502152.502153
[8]https://doi.org/10.1007/978-0-387-85820-3_8

7.2.2   The Apriori Algorithm for Association Rule Learning

Association rules are mostly applied to *transactional data*, which is usually records of trade, exchange, or arrangement, e.g., medical records. These datasets are typically very large in number of transactions and features, e.g., electronic health record (EHR).[9] In such data archives, the number and complexity of transactions is high, which complicates efforts to extract patterns, conduct market analysis, or predict basket purchases.

Apriori association rules help untangle such difficult modeling problems. If we have a simple prior belief about the properties of frequent elements, we may be able to efficiently reduce the number of features or combinations that we need to look at. The Apriori algorithm is based on a simple `apriori` belief that *all subsets of a frequent item-set must also be frequent*. This is known as the **Apriori property**. In the last example, the full set {*charcoal, lighter, chicken wings, barbecue sauce*} is *frequent* if and only if itself and all of its subsets, including single elements, pairs, and triples, occur frequently. Naturally, the apriori rule is designed for finding patterns in large datasets where patterns that appear frequently are considered "interesting," "valuable," or "important."

7.2.3   Rule Support and Confidence

We can measure rule's importance by computing its **support** and **confidence** metrics. The support and confidence represent two criteria useful in deciding whether a pattern is "valuable." By setting thresholds for these two criteria, we can easily limit the number of interesting rules or item-sets reported.

For item-sets X and Y, the `support` of an item-set measures how (relatively) frequently it appears in the data

$$\text{support}(X) = \frac{\text{count}(X)}{N},$$

where N is the total number of transactions in the database and count(X) is the number of observations (transactions) containing the item-set X.

In a set-theoretic sense, the union of item-sets is an item-set itself. In other words, if $Z = \{X, Y\} = \{X \cup Y\}$, then

$$\text{support}(Z) = \text{support}(X, Y).$$

For a given rule $X \rightarrow Y$, the `rule's confidence` measures the relative accuracy of the rule

---

[9]https://doi.org/10.1109/JBHI.2017.2767063

$$\text{confidence}(X \to Y) = \frac{\text{support}(X, Y)}{\text{support}(X)} .$$

The confidence measures the joint occurrence of X and Y over the X domain. If whenever X appears Y tends to also be present, then we will have a high confidence $(X \to Y)$. This set-theoretic formulation of the confidence can also be expressed as a conditional probability, since the numerator is effectively the probability of the intersection of the events E_X and E_Y corresponding to observing the transactions X and Y, respectively. That is, the support corresponds to the conditional probability $\text{support}(X, Y) = \text{Prob}(E_X \cap E_Y)$ and

$$\text{confidence}(X \to Y) = \frac{\text{Prob}(E_X \cap E_Y)}{\text{Prob}(E_X)} \equiv \text{Prob}(E_Y | E_X).$$

Note that the ranges of the support and the confidence are $0 \le$ support, confidence ≤ 1.

One intuitive example of a strong association rule is {peanut butter} $\to$ {bread}, because it has high *support* as well as high *confidence* in grocery store transactions. Shoppers tend to purchase bread when they get peanut butter. These items tend to appear in the same baskets, which yields high confidence for the rule {peanut butter} $\to$ {bread}. Of course, there may be cases where {peanut butter} $\to$ {celery}. These recommendation systems may not be perfect and can fail in unexpected ways; see the peculiar case of how the Target store figured out a teen girl was pregnant before her parents knew.[10]

7.2.4 Building a Set of Rules with the Apriori Principle

Remember that the number of arrangements of n elements taken k at a time, i.e., the number of combinations, increases exponentially with the size of the item inventory (n). This is precisely why if a restaurant only uses 10 ingredients, there are $\binom{10}{5} = 253$ possible menu items composed of 5 ingradients for customers to order. Clearly the complexity of the number of "baskets" rapidly increases with the inventory of the available items or ingredients. For instance,

- $n = 100$ (ingredients) and $k = 50$ (menus of 50 ingredients), yields $\binom{100}{50} = 100891344545564193334812497256 > 10^{29}$ possible arrangements (combinations), and
- $n = 100$ (ingredients) and $k = 5$ (menus of only 5 ingredients), yields $\binom{100}{5} = 75287520 > 7M$ possible orders.

---

[10]https://doi.org/10.1109/BigData.Congress.2014.112

To avoid this complexity, we will introduce a two-step process of building few, simple, and informative sets of rules:

- **Step 1**: Filter all item-sets with a minimum *support* threshold. This is accomplished iteratively by increasing the size of the item-sets. In the first iteration, we compute the support of singletons, 1-item-sets. Next iteration, we compute the support of pairs of items, then triples of items, etc. Item-sets passing iteration *i* could be considered as candidates for the next iteration, *i+1*. If *{A}, {B}, {C}* are all frequent singletons, but *D* is not frequent in the first singleton-selection round, then in the second iteration we only consider the support of these pairs *{A, B}, {A, C}, {B,C}*, ignoring all pairs including *D*. This substantially reduces the cardinality of the potential item-sets and ensures the feasibility of the algorithm. At the third iteration, if *{A,C}*, and *{B,C}* are frequently occurring, but *{A, B}* is not, then the algorithm may terminate, as the support of *{A,B,C}* is trivial (does not pass the support threshold), given that *{A, B}* was not frequent enough.
- **Step 2**: Using the item-sets selected in step 1, generate new rules with *confidence* larger than a predefined minimum confidence threshold. The candidate item-sets that passed step 1 would include all frequent item-sets. For the highly supported item-set *{A, C}*, we would compute the confidence measures for *{A}* → *{C}* as well as *{C}* → *{A}* and compare these against the minimum confidence threshold. The *surviving rules are the ones with confidence levels exceeding that minimum threshold*.

7.2.5 A Toy Example

Assume that a large supermarket tracks sales data by stock-keeping unit (SKU) for each item, i.e., each item, such as "butter" or "bread," is identified by an SKU number. The supermarket has a database of transactions where each transaction is a set of SKUs that were bought together. Suppose the database of transactions consist of following item-sets, each representing a purchasing order.

```
require(knitr)
item_table = as.data.frame(t(c("{1,2,3,4}","{1,2,4}","{1,2}",
                               "{2,3,4}","{2,3}","{3,4}","{2,4}")))
colnames(item_table) <- c("choice1","choice2","choice3",
                          "choice4","choice5","choice6","choice7")
kable(item_table, caption = "Item table")
```

Item table

choice1	choice2	choice3	choice4	choice5	choice6	choice7
{1,2,3,4}	{1,2,4}	{1,2}	{2,3,4}	{2,3}	{3,4}	{2,4}

We will use *Apriori* to determine the frequent item-sets of this database. To do so, we will say that an item-set is frequent if it appears in at least 3 transactions of the database, i.e., the value 3 is the support threshold. The first step of Apriori is to count up the number of occurrences, i.e., the support, of each member item separately. By scanning the database for the first time, we obtain the following Size 1 support.

```
item_table = as.data.frame(t(c(3,6,4,5)))
colnames(item_table) <- c("items: {1}","{2}","{3}","{4}")
rownames(item_table) <- "(N=7)*support"
kable(item_table,caption = "Size 1 Support")
```

Size 1	Items: {1}	{2}	{3}	{4}
(N = 7)*support	3	6	4	5

All the singletons, item-sets of size 1, have a support of at least 3, so they are all frequent. The next step is to generate a list of all pairs of frequent items. For example, regarding the pair {1, 2}: the first table of Example 2 shows items 1 and 2 appearing together in three of the item-sets; therefore, we say that the support of the item {1, 2} is 3.

```
item_table = as.data.frame(t(c(3,1,2,3,4,3)))
colnames(item_table) <- c("{1,2}","{1,3}","{1,4}","{2,3}","{2,4}","{3,4}")
rownames(item_table) <- "N*support"
kable(item_table,caption = "Size 2 Support")
```

Size 2	{1,2}	{1,3}	{1,4}	{2,3}	{2,4}	{3,4}
N*support	3	1	2	3	4	3

The pairs {1, 2}, {2, 3}, {2, 4}, and {3, 4} all meet or exceed the minimum support of 3, so they are *frequent*. The pairs {1, 3} and {1, 4} are not and any larger set which contains {1, 3} or {1, 4} cannot be frequent. In this way, we can prune sets: we will now look for frequent triples in the database, but we can already exclude all the triples that contain one of these two pairs.

```
item_table = as.data.frame(t(c(2)))
colnames(item_table) <- c("{2,3,4}")
rownames(item_table) <- "N*support"
kable(item_table,caption = "Size 3 Support")
```

Size 3	{2,3,4}
N*support	2

In this example, there are no frequent triplets—the support of the item-set {2, 3, 4} is below the minimal threshold, and the other triplets were excluded because they were super sets of pairs that were already below the threshold. Thus, we have determined all frequent sets of items in the database and illustrated how some items were not counted because some of their subsets were already known to be below the threshold.

7.2.6   Case Study 1: Head and Neck Cancer Medications

Step 1: Data import

To demonstrate the *Apriori* algorithm in a real biomedical case study, we will use a transactional healthcare data representing a subset of the Head and Neck Cancer Medication data, which it is available in the DSPA case-studies collection as `10_medication_descriptions.csv`. It consists of inpatient medications of head and neck cancer patients.

The data are in a wide format (see Chap. 1) where each row represents a patient. During the study period, each patient had records for a maximum of five encounters. *NA* represents no medication administration records in this specific time point for the specific patient. This dataset contains a total of 528 patients.

Step 2: Exploring and Preparing the Data

Different from our data imports in the previous chapters, transactional data need to be ingested in R using the `read.transactions()` function. This function will store data as a matrix with each row representing a basket (or transaction example) and each column representing items in the transaction.

Let's load the dataset and delete the irrelevant *index* column. Using the `write.csv(R data, "path")` function, we can output our R data file into a local CSV file. To avoid generating another index column in the output CSV file, we can use the `row.names = F` option (Table 7.1).

```
med<-
 read.csv("https://umich.instructure.com/files/1678540/download?download_frd=1",
          stringsAsFactors = FALSE)
med<-med[, -1]
write.csv(med, "medication.csv", row.names=F)
library(knitr)
kable(med[1:5, ])
```

Table 7.1 Excerpt of the medication description for the first five patients

Medication description 1	Medication description 2	Medication description 3	Medication description 4	Medication description 5
acetaminophen uh	cefazolin ivpb uh	NA	NA	NA
docusate	fioricet	heparin injection	ondansetron injection uh	simvastatin
hydrocodone acet-aminophen 5 mg 325 mg	NA	NA	NA	NA
fentanyl injection uh	NA	NA	NA	NA
cefazolin ivpb uh	hydrocodone acet-aminophen 5 mg 325 mg	NA	NA	NA

Now we can use `read.transactions()` in the `arules` package to read the CSV file we just outputted.

```
# install.packages("arules")
library(arules)
Med <- read.transactions("medication.csv", sep = ",",
                         skip = 1, rm.duplicates=TRUE)
summary(med)
## transactions as itemMatrix in sparse format with
##   528 rows (elements/itemsets/transactions) and
##   88 columns (items) and a density of 0.02085486
## most frequent items:
##                 fentanyl injection uh  hydrocodone acetaminophen 5mg 325mg
##                                   211                                  165
##                    cefazolin ivpb uh                    heparin injection
##                                   108                                  105
## hydrocodone acetamin 75mg 500mg 15ml                              (Other)
##                                    60                                  320
## element (itemset/transaction) length distribution:
## sizes
##   1   2   3   4   5
## 248 166  79  23  12
```

Here we use the option `rm.duplicates` $=$ T because we may have similar medication administration records for two different patients. The option `skip` $= 1$ means we skip the heading line in the CSV file. Now we get transactional data with unique rows.

The summary of a transactional data contains rich information. The first block of information tells us that we have 528 rows and 88 different medicines in this matrix. Using the density number we can calculate how many non *NA* medication records are in the data. In total, we have $528 \times 88 = 46,464$ positions in the matrix. Thus, there are $46,464 \times 0.0209 = 971$ medicines prescribed during the study period.

The second block lists the most frequent medicines and their frequencies in the matrix. For example, "`fentanyl injection uh`" appeared 211 times, which represents a proportion of $211/528 = 0.4$ of the (treatment) transactions. Since fentanyl[11] is frequently used to help prevent pain after surgery or other medical treatments, we can see that many of these patients may have undergone some significant medical procedures that require postoperative pain management.

The summary reports statistics about the size of the transaction, e.g., 248 patients had only one medicine in the study period, while 12 of them had 5 medication records, one for each time point. On average, a random 10-tuple of patients are expected to take 18 different medications, i.e., each patient is expected to take between 1 and 2 different medicines.

---

[11] https://doi.org/10.1016/j.jpain.2014.08.010

7.2.6.1   Visualizing Item Support—Item Frequency Plots

The summary may still appear to be fairly abstract, and we can visualize some specific information.

```
inspect(med[1:5,])
##      items
## [1] {acetaminophen uh,
##        cefazolin ivpb uh}
## [2] {docusate,
##        fioricet,
##        heparin injection,
##        ondansetron injection uh,
##        simvastatin}
## [3] {hydrocodone acetaminophen 5mg 325mg}
## [4] {fentanyl injection uh}
## [5] {cefazolin ivpb uh,
##        hydrocodone acetaminophen 5mg 325mg}
```

The inspect() function can explicate the transactional dataset, e.g., we can report the medication records of each patient formatted as item-sets. We can further analyze the frequent terms using itemFrequency(). This will show all item frequencies alphabetically ordered from the first five outputs (Figs. 7.8 and 7.9).

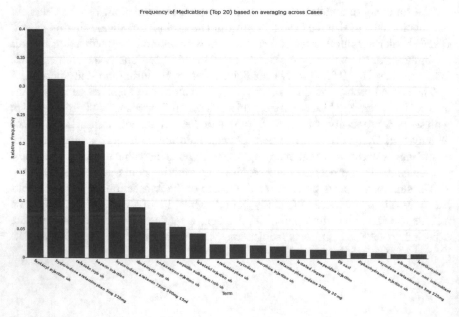

Fig. 7.8 Medication frequency distribution

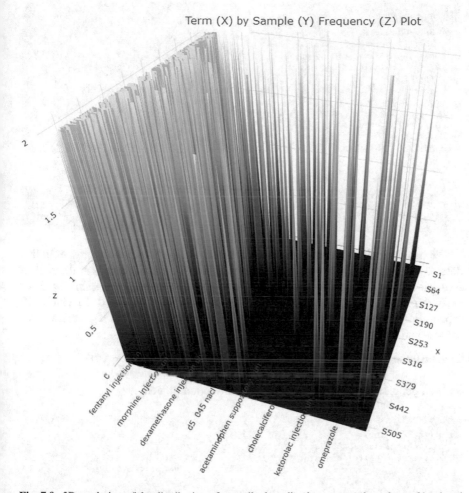

Fig. 7.9 3D rendering of the distribution of prescribed medications across the cohort of head and neck patients

```
library(plotly)
itemFrequency(med[, 1:5])
##                  09 nacl                        09 nacl bolus
##              0.013257576                          0.003787879
##    acetaminophen  multiroute      uh acetaminophen codeine 120 mg 12 mg 5 ml
##              0.001893939                          0.001893939
##        acetaminophen codeine 300mg 30 mg
##              0.020833333
mat <- as.matrix(med@data)    # View matrix as an image # image(mat)
# capture the row/column names
rowNames <- med@itemInfo$labels
colNames <- paste0("S", c(1:dim(mat)[2]))
rownames(mat) <- rowNames
colnames(mat) <- colNames
# convert matrix to DF for processing, order rows based on their average (across
subjects/cases/columns), back to matrix for display
df <- as.data.frame(1*mat)
```

```
df$avg <- rowMeans(df)
dfOrdered <- df[order(df$avg, decreasing = T), ]
matOrdered <- as.matrix(dfOrdered)
# track the ordered row names
rowNames <- rownames(dfOrdered)
colNames <- colnames(dfOrdered)
# 2D top 20 terms bar plot
# To order the meds based on "avg", instead of alphabetically (mind the "-" sign
to order Large to small!)
plot_ly(x = reorder(rowNames[c(1:20)], -dfOrdered[1:20, "avg"]),
        y=dfOrdered[1:20, "avg"], name="Top 20 Meds", type="bar") %>%
  layout(title='Frequency of Medications (Top 20) based on averaging across
Cases', xaxis = list(title="Term"), yaxis = list(title="Relative Frequency"))
```

```
# 3D surface plot
plot_ly(x = colNames, y = rowNames, z = 2*matOrdered, type = "surface") %>%
  layout(title='Term (X) by Sample (Y) Frequency (Z) Plot',
    xaxis=list(title="Term"),yaxis=list(title="Sample ID")) %>% hide_colorbar()
```

We can only display the top 20 medicines that are most frequently present in this dataset. Consistent with the prior summary() output, fentanyl is still the most frequent item. Alternatively, we can also try to plot the items with a threshold for support. Instead of topN = 20, we can use the option support = 0.1, which will report all the items that have a support greater or equal to 0.1. Let's generalize this process and define a new function,

itemFrequencyPlotly(transactionObject, numTopItemps = 10),

that can generate frequency plots for any transaction object.

```
# define a generic plot_ly ItemFrequency plotting function
itemFrequencyPlotly <-
  function(transactionObject, numTopItemps = 10, name="") {
        name <- ifelse(name=="",
                paste0('Frequency of Items (Top ', numTopItemps,
                       ' ) based on averaging across Cases'),
                paste0('Frequency of Items (Top ', numTopItemps,
                       ' ) based on averaging across Cases (Data=', name, ')'))
  mat <- as.matrix(transactionObject@data)
  rowNames <- transactionObject@itemInfo$labels
  colNames <- paste0("S", c(1:dim(mat)[2]))
  rownames(mat) <- rowNames
  colnames(mat) <- colNames
  # convert matrix to DF for processing, order rows based on their
  # average (across subjects/cases/columns), back to matrix for display
  df <- as.data.frame(1*mat)
  df$avg <- rowMeans(df)
  dfOrdered <- df[order(df$avg, decreasing = T), ]
  matOrdered <- as.matrix(dfOrdered)
  # track the ordered row names
  rowNames <- rownames(dfOrdered)
  colNames <- colnames(dfOrdered)
  plot_ly(
    x=reorder(rowNames[c(1:numTopItemps)], -dfOrdered[1:numTopItemps,"avg"]),
    y=dfOrdered[1:numTopItemps, "avg"],
    name=paste0("Top ", numTopItemps, " Meds"), type="bar")  %>%
    layout(title=name, xaxis = list(title="Terms"),
            yaxis = list(title="Relative Frequency"))
}
```

7.2.6.2 Visualizing Transaction Data—Plotting the Sparse Matrix

The sparse matrix will show what medications were prescribed for each patient. Below we only show the top 20 medications for the first 15 cases (Fig. 7.10).

```
plot_ly(x=reorder(rowNames[c(1:20)],-dfOrdered[1:20,"avg"]),y=colNames[1:15],
        z=2*matOrdered[1:15, 1:20], type="heatmap") %>%
  layout(title='Heatmap - Top-20 Medications for the first 15 Cases') %>%
  hide_colorbar()
```

This image has 15 rows (translations), as we only specified the first 15 patients, and 20 columns (top 20 medications). Although the picture may be a little hard to interpret, it gives a sense of what kind of medicine is prescribed for these head and neck cancer patients. Let's see an expanded graph including the top 30 medications for a random roster of 50 patients (Fig. 7.11).

```
subset_int <- sample(ncol(matOrdered), 50, replace = F)
# image(med[subset_int, ])

plot_ly(x=rowNames[1:30], y=colNames[subset_int],
        z=2*t(matOrdered[1:30, subset_int]), type="heatmap") %>%
  layout(title='Heatmap - Bottom-30 Medications for a Random set of 50 Patients')
%>% hide_colorbar()
```

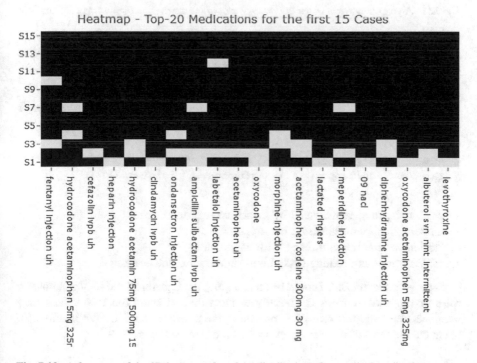

Fig. 7.10 A fragment of the 2D heatmap plot of the distribution of prescribed medications

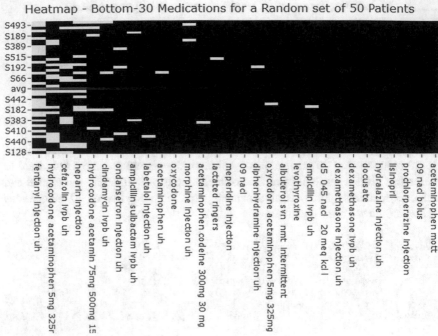

Fig. 7.11 An expanded view of the 2D heatmap plot of the distribution of prescribed medications

This graph shows clearly that some medications are more commonly prescribed than others. Next we can fit the *Apriori* model to identify transactional relations.

Step 3: Training a model on the data

With the data in place, we can build the *association rules* using the `arules::apriori()` function.

```
myrules <- apriori(data=mydata,
parameter=list(support=0.1, confidence=0.8, minlen=1))
```

- *data*: a sparse matrix crcatcd by `read.transacations()`
- *support*: minimum threshold for support
- *confidence*: minimum threshold for confidence
- *minlen*: minimum required rule items (in our case, medications)

Setting up the threshold could be challenging; too high threshold may generate no rules or common-sense and noninformative rules, whereas too low values may overlook too many relevant rules present in the transactional data. We'll start with using the default setting `support = 0.1, confidence = 0.8`.

```
apriori(med)
## Parameter specification:
## confidence minval smax arem aval originalSupport maxtime support
minlen
## 0.8 0.1 1 none FALSE TRUE 5 0.1 1
## maxlen target ext
## 10 rules TRUE
## Absolute minimum support count: 52
## set item appearances ... [0 item(s)] done [0.00s].
## set transactions ... [88 item(s), 528 transaction(s)] done [0.00s].
## sorting and recoding items ... [5 item(s)] done [0.00s].
## creating transaction tree ... done [0.00s].
## checking subsets of size 1 2 done [0.00s].
## writing ... [0 rule(s)] done [0.00s].
## creating S4 object ... done [0.00s].
## set of 0 rules
```

Not surprisingly, we obtained 0 rules, as the default confidence setting is too high. In practice, we might need some time to fine-tune these thresholds, which may require certain familiarity with the underlying process or embedding human clinical knowledge into the AI decision support. Let's try setting support = 0.01 and confidence = 0.25. This requires rules that have appeared in at least 1% of the head and neck cancer patients in the study. Also, the rules have to have at least 25% accuracy. Moreover, minlen = 2 would be a very helpful option because it removes all rules that have fewer than two items.

```
med_rule <-apriori(med,parameter=list(support=0.01,confidence=0.25,minlen=2))
##   maxlen target  ext
##       10  rules TRUE
## Algorithmic control:
##  filter tree heap memopt load sort verbose
##     0.1 TRUE TRUE  FALSE TRUE    2    TRUE
## Absolute minimum support count: 5
med_rule
## set of 29 rules
```

The result suggests we have a new med_rule object consisting of 29 rules.

Step 4: Evaluating model performance
First, we can obtain the overall summary of this set of rules.

```
summary(med_rule)
## set of 29 rules
## rule length distribution (lhs + rhs):sizes
## 2 3 4
## 13 12 4
## summary of quality measures:
## support confidence coverage lift
## Min.   :0.01136 Min.   :0.2500 Min.   :0.01894 Min.   :0.7583
## 1st Qu.:0.01705 1st Qu.:0.3390 1st Qu.:0.03788 1st Qu.:1.3333
## Median :0.01894 Median :0.4444 Median :0.06250 Median :1.7481
```

```
## Mean :0.03448 Mean :0.4491 Mean :0.08392 Mean :1.8636
## 3rd Qu.:0.03788 3rd Qu.:0.5000 3rd Qu.:0.08902 3rd Qu.:2.2564
## Max. :0.11174 Max. :0.8000 Max. :0.31250 Max. :3.9111
## mining info:
## data ntransactions support confidence
## med 528 0.01 0.25
```

We have 13 rules that contain 2 items; 12 rules containing 3 items; and the remaining 4 rules contain 4 items. The `lift` column shows how much more likely one medicine is to be prescribed to a patient given another medicine is prescribed. It is obtained by the following formula

$$\text{lift}(X \to Y) = \frac{\text{confidence}(X \to Y)}{\text{support}(Y)}.$$

Note that $\text{lift}(X \to Y)$ is the same as $\text{lift}(Y \to X)$. The range of lift is $[0, \infty)$ and higher lift is better. We don't need to worry about the support, since we already set a threshold that the support must exceed. Using the `arulesViz` package we can visualize the confidence and support scatter plots for all the rules (Fig. 7.12).

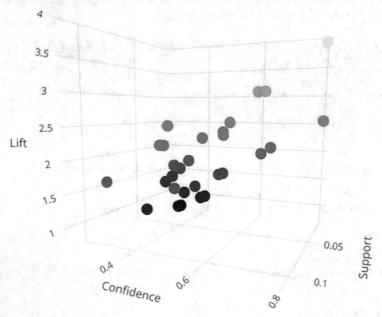

Fig. 7.12 3D Scatterplot of *confidence, support,* and *lift* for all 29 apriori-derived rules

```
# install.packages("arulesViz")
library(arulesViz)
sortedRule <- sort(med_rule)
x1   <- sortedRule@quality$support
y1   <- sortedRule@quality$confidence
z1   <- sortedRule@quality$lift
col1 <- sortedRule@quality$count
ruleNames <- paste0("Rule", c(1:length(sortedRule@quality$support)))
plot_ly(x = ~x1, y = ~y1, z = ~z1, color = ~z1, name=ruleNames) %>%
  add_markers() %>%
  layout(title=paste0("Arule Support-Confidence-Lift Plot (for all ",
                      length(sortedRule@quality$support), " rules)"),
         scene = list(xaxis = list(title = 'Support'),
                      yaxis = list(title = 'Confidence'),
                      zaxis = list(title = 'Lift'))) %>% hide_colorbar()
```

Again, we can utilize the `inspect()` function to see any of these specific rules, e.g., top three association rules.

```
inspect(med_rule[1:3])
##      lhs                                rhs                 support
confidence
## [1] {acetaminophen uh}              => {cefazolin ivpb uh} 0.01136364 0.4615385
## [2] {ampicillin sulbactam ivpb uh} => {heparin injection} 0.01893939 0.3448276
## [3] {ondansetron injection uh}     => {heparin injection} 0.01704545 0.2727273
##      coverage   lift     count
## [1] 0.02462121 2.256410  6
## [2] 0.05492424 1.733990 10
## [3] 0.06250000 1.371429  9
```

Here, `lhs` and `rhs` refer to the "left hand side" and "right hand side" of the rule, respectively. The `lhs` is the given (observed) condition and `rhs` represents the predicted association (outcome). Using the first row as an example: If a head-and-neck patient has been prescribed acetaminophen (pain reliever and fever reducer), it is likely that the same patient may also be prescribed *cefazolin* (antibiotic prescribed for treatment of resistant bacterial infections), as bacterial infections are associated with fevers and some cancers.

Step 5: Sorting the set of association rules
Sorting the resulting association rules corresponding to high **lift** values will help us identify the most useful rules.

```
inspect(sort(med_rule, by="lift")[1:3])
##      lhs                                      rhs                  support
confidence    coverage     lift count
## [1] {fentanyl injection uh,
##      heparin injection,
##      hydrocodone acetaminophen 5mg 325mg} => {cefazolin ivpb uh} 0.01515152
0.8000000 0.01893939 3.911111    8
## [2] {cefazolin ivpb uh,
##      fentanyl injection uh,
##      hydrocodone acetaminophen 5mg 325mg} => {heparin injection} 0.01515152
0.6153846 0.02462121 3.094505    8
## [3] {heparin injection,
##      hydrocodone acetaminophen 5mg 325mg} => {cefazolin ivpb uh} 0.03787879
0.6250000 0.06060606 3.055556   20
```

These rules may need to be interpreted by clinicians and experts in the specific context of the study. For instance, the first row, *{fentanyl, heparin, hydrocodone acetaminophen}* implies *{cefazolin}*. *Fentanyl* and hydrocodone acetaminophen are both pain relievers that may be prescribed after surgery to relieve moderate to severe pain based on a narcotic opioid pain reliever (*hydrocodone*) and a nonopioid pain reliever (acetaminophen).

Heparin is usually used before surgery to reduce the risk of blood clots. The third rule suggests that surgery patients that are treated with *heparin* may also need *cefazolin* to prevent post-surgical bacterial infection. *Cefazolin* is an antibiotic used for the treatment of bacterial infections and to prevent group *B streptococcal disease* around the time of delivery and before general surgery.

Step 6: Taking subsets of association rules

If we are more interested in investigating associations that are linked to a specific medicine, we can narrow the rules down by making subsets. Let us try investigating rules related to fentanyl, since it appears to be the most frequently prescribed medicine. Fentanyl is used in the management of chronic cancer pain.

```
fi_rules<-subset(med_rule, items %in% "fentanyl injection uh")
inspect(fi_rules)
##        lhs                                        rhs
support confidence    coverage        lift count
## [1]  {ondansetron injection uh}                 => {fentanyl injection uh}
0.01893939   0.3030303 0.06250000 0.7582938    10
## [2]  {fentanyl injection uh,
##       ondansetron injection uh}                 => {hydrocodone acetaminophen 5mg
325mg} 0.01136364   0.6000000 0.01893939 1.9200000    6
## [3]  {hydrocodone acetaminophen 5mg 325mg,
##       ondansetron injection uh}                 => {fentanyl injection uh}
0.01136364   0.3750000 0.03030303 0.9383886    6
...
```

Earlier, we saw that the R expression *%in%* is a simple intuitive interface to the function match(), which is used as a binary operator returning a logical vector indicating if there is a match (T) or not (F) for its left operand within the right table object. In total, there are 14 rules related to this item. Let's plot them.

7.2.7   Graphical Depiction of Association Rules

Next we will demonstrate the graphical exploratory analytics of the derived association rules (Figs. 7.13 and 7.14).

```
plot(sort(fi_rules, by="lift"), method = "graph", engine = "htmlwidget",
     control=list(main = list(title="Grouped Matrix for the 14 Fentanyl-
associated Rules")))


subrules2 <- sample(subset(fi_rules, lift > 2), 5)
plot(sort(subrules2, by="lift"), method="grouped",
     control=list(type="items"), engine = "htmlwidget")
```

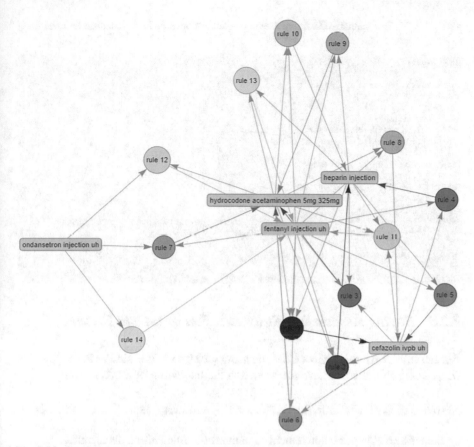

Fig. 7.13 Graphical rendering of the apriori-derived rules. At run time, this is an interactive plot that supports dynamic mouse control and exploratory analytics

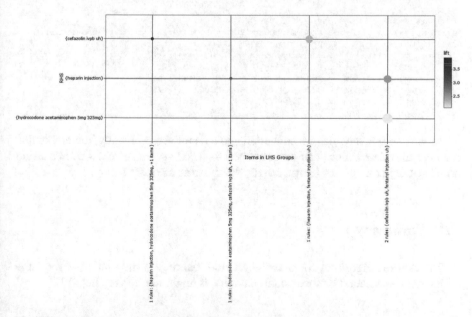

Fig. 7.14 Explicating some of the LHS→RHS association rules

```
plot(sort(fi_rules, by="lift"), method="grouped",  k = 7,
     control=list(type="items"), engine = "htmlwidget")
m <- rules2matrix(sort(fi_rules, by="lift")[1:10], measure = "lift")
plot(fi_rules[1:10], method = "matrix", engine = "htmlwidget")
## Grouped matrix
# create a matrix with LHSs grouped in k = 10 groups
m <- rules2groupedMatrix(sort(fi_rules, by="lift")[1:10], k = 10)
inspect(fi_rules[m$clustering_rules == 1])
##      lhs                         rhs
support confidence    coverage        lift count
## [1] {ondansetron injection uh} => {fentanyl injection uh}
0.01893939  0.3030303 0.06250000 0.7582938    10
## [2] {cefazolin ivpb uh,
##        fentanyl injection uh,
##       heparin injection}         => {hydrocodone acetaminophen 5mg 325mg}
0.01515152  0.8000000 0.01893939 2.5600000     8
# the corresponding plot
plot(fi_rules, method = "grouped matrix", k = 7, engine = "htmlwidget")
plot(fi_rules, method="graph", measure = "support", engine="htmlwidget",
     shading = "lift", control = list(verbose = TRUE))
```

7.2.8   Saving Association Rules to a File or a Data Frame

We can save these rules into a CSV file using `write()`. It is similar to the function `write.csv()` that we have mentioned in the beginning of this case study.

```
write(med_rule, file = "medrule.csv", sep=",", row.names=F)
```

Sometimes it is more convenient to convert the rules into a data frame.

```
med_df <- as(med_rule, "data.frame")
str(med_df)
## 'data.frame':    29 obs. of  6 variables:
## $ rules     : chr  "{acetaminophen uh} => {cefazolin ivpb uh}" "{ampicillin
sulbactam ivpb uh} => {heparin injection}" "{ondansetron injection uh} =>
{heparin injection}" "{ondansetron injection uh} => {fentanyl injection uh}" ...
## $ support   : num  0.0114 0.0189 0.017 0.0189 0.0303 ...
## $ confidence: num  0.462 0.345 0.273 0.303 0.485 ...
## $ coverage  : num  0.0246 0.0549 0.0625 0.0625 0.0625 ...
## $ lift      : num  2.256 1.734 1.371 0.758 1.552 ...
## $ count     : int  6 10 9 10 16 13 21 17 48 48 ...
```

As we can see, the rules are converted into a factor vector. Finally, remember that matrices and data-frames can be converted to `arules` *transactions* format using `arulesObject <- as(input.df, "transactions")`.

7.3   Summary

- The Apriori algorithm for association rule learning is only suitable for large transactional data. For some small datasets, it might not be very helpful.

- It is useful for discovering associations, mostly in early phases of an exploratory study.
- Some rules can be built due to chance and may need further verification.

7.4 Practice Problems

7.4.1 Groceries

In this practice problem, we will investigate the associations of frequently purchased groceries using the *grocery* dataset in the R base. First, let's load the data.

```
data("Groceries")
summary(Groceries)
## transactions as itemMatrix in sparse format with
##  9835 rows (elements/itemsets/transactions) and
##  169 columns (items) and a density of 0.02609146
## most frequent items:
##       whole milk other vegetables    rolls/buns          soda
##             2513            1903          1809          1715
##            yogurt         (Other)
##             1372           34055
```

We will try to find out the top five frequent grocery items and plot them (Fig. 7.15).

```
# itemFrequencyPlot(Groceries, topN=5)
itemFrequencyPlotly(Groceries, 10, "groceries")
```

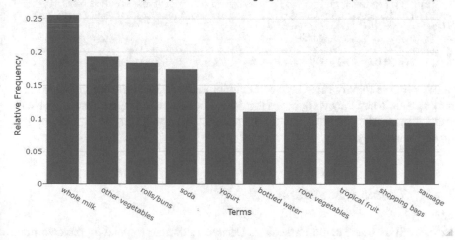

Fig. 7.15 Term frequency distribution (grocery data)

Then, try to use support = 0.006, confidence = 0.25, minlen = 2 to set up the grocery association rules. Sort the top three rules with highest lift.

```
## Apriori Parameter specification:
## confidence minval smax arem aval originalSupport maxtime support
minlen
## 0.25 0.1 1 none FALSE TRUE 5 0.006 2
## maxlen target ext
## 10 rules TRUE
## Absolute minimum support count: 59
## set of 463 rules
## lhs rhs support confidence coverage lift count
## [1] {herbs} => {root vegetables} 0.007015760 0.4312500 0.01626843
3.956477 69
## [2] {berries} => {whipped/sour cream} 0.009049314 0.2721713
0.03324860 3.796886 89
## [3] {tropical fruit,
## other vegetables,
## whole milk} => {root vegetables} 0.007015760 0.4107143 0.01708185
3.768074 69
```

The number of rules (463) appears excessive. We can try stringer parameters. In practice, it is more possible to observe underlying rules if you set a higher confidence. Here we set the confidence = 0.6.

```
groceryrules <- apriori(Groceries,
                  parameter=list(support=0.006, confidence=0.6, minlen=2))
## Absolute minimum support count: 59
groceryrules
## set of 8 rules
inspect(sort(groceryrules, by = "lift")[1:3])
##     lhs                             rhs            support     confidence
## [1] {butter, whipped/sour cream} => {whole milk} 0.006710727 0.6600000
## [2] {butter, yogurt}             => {whole milk} 0.009354347 0.6388889
## [3] {root vegetables, butter}    => {whole milk} 0.008235892 0.6377953
##      coverage    lift     count
## [1] 0.01016777 2.583008 66
## [2] 0.01464159 2.500387 92
## [3] 0.01291307 2.496107 81
```

We observe mainly rules between dairy products. It makes sense that customers pick up milk when they walk down the dairy products aisle. Experiment further with various parameter settings and try to interpret the results in the context of this grocery case study.

7.4.2 Titanic Passengers

Next, we'll use the Titanic Passengers Dataset. Let's start by loading the data first.

```r
dat <-
    read.csv("https://umich.instructure.com/files/9372716/download?download_frd=1")
# Choose only the key data features
dat <- dat[ , c("pclass", "survived", "sex", "age", "fare", "cabin")]
# Factorize categorical features
dat$pclass <- as.factor(dat$pclass)
dat$survived <- factor(dat$survived, levels = c("0", "1"))
dat$sex <- as.factor(dat$sex)
# Convert the Cabin number to a character A-F, Z=missing cabin ID
dat$cabin <- substring(dat$cabin,1,1)
for (i in 1:length(dat$cabin))
    if ((dat$cabin[i]=="")) dat$cabin[i] <- "Z"
dat$cabin <- as.factor(dat$cabin)
# Convert the Ticket Fair from numeric to categorical label
f <- as.character(dat$fare)
for (i in 1:length(dat$fare)) {
  if (is.na(dat$fare[i])) f[i] <- as.character("low")
  else if (dat$fare[i]<50) f[i] <- as.character("low")
  else if (50<=dat$fare[i] && dat$fare[i]<100) f[i] <- as.character("medium")
  else if (100<=dat$fare[i] && dat$fare[i]<200)  f[i] <- as.character("high")
  else f[i] <- as.character("extreme")   #  if (200<=dat$fare[i])
}
dat$fare <- as.factor(f)
table(as.factor(dat$fare))
## extreme    high    low  medium
##      38      46   1067     158
# Convert Age from numeric to categorical (Decade-of-life) label
f <- as.character(dat$age)
for (i in 1:length(dat$age)) {
  if (is.na(dat$age[i])) f[i] <- as.character("1")
  else {
    a = 1 + dat$age[1] %/% 10  # integer division by 10 (per decade of life)
    f[i] <- as.character(a)
  }
}
dat$age <- as.factor(f)
table(as.factor(dat$age))
##   1   2   3   4   5   6   7   8   9
## 345 143 344 232 135  70  32   7   1
str(dat)
## 'data.frame':    1309 obs. of  6 variables:
## $ pclass  : Factor w/ 3 levels "1","2","3": 1 1 1 1 1 1 1 1 1 1 ...
## $ survived: Factor w/ 2 levels "0","1": 2 2 1 1 2 2 1 2 1 ...
## $ sex     : Factor w/ 2 levels "female","male": 1 2 1 2 1 2 1 2 1 2 ...
## $ age     : Factor w/ 9 levels "1","2","3","4",..: 3 1 1 4 3 5 7 4 ...
## $ fare    : Factor w/ 4 levels "extreme","high",..: 1 2 2 2 2 3 4 3 ...
## $ cabin   : Factor w/ 9 levels "A","B","C","D",..: 2 3 3 3 3 5 4 1 ...
```

We can also mine the derived association rules and explicate patterns and motifs present in the transactional data that may have relevance in the context of the study.

```
library(arules)
rules <- apriori(dat, parameter = list(minlen=5, supp=0.02, conf=0.8))
## Absolute minimum support count: 26
inspect(rules[1:20])
##      lhs                                         rhs          support
## [1] {pclass=3, survived=0, sex=male, age=5}   => {cabin=Z}    0.02062643
## [2] {pclass=3, sex=male, age=5, cabin=Z}      => {survived=0} 0.02062643
## [3] {pclass=3, survived=0, sex=male, age=5}   => {fare=low}   0.02139037
## [4] {pclass=3, sex=male, age=5, fare=low}     => {survived=0} 0.02139037
## [5] {pclass=3, survived=0, age=5, cabin=Z}    => {fare=low}   0.02750191
## [6] {pclass=3, survived=0, age=5, fare=low}   => {cabin=Z}    0.02750191
## [7] {pclass=3, age=5, fare=low, cabin=Z}      => {survived=0} 0.02750191
...

##      confidence coverage   lift     count
## [1] 0.9642857  0.02139037 1.244822 27
## [2] 0.9310345  0.02215432 1.506458 27
## [3] 1.0000000  0.02139037 1.226804 28
## [4] 0.9333333  0.02291826 1.510177 28
## [5] 1.0000000  0.02750191 1.226804 36
## [6] 0.9729730  0.02826585 1.256037 36
## [7] 0.8780488  0.03132162 1.420724 36
...
```

We can focus on the binary *survival* outcome (Survived = 1/0).

```
# examine the rules with containing "Survived=1" in the RHS
rules <- apriori(dat, parameter = list(minlen=3, supp=0.02, conf=0.7),
   appearance=list(rhs="survived=1", default="lhs"), control=list(verbose=F))
rules.sorted <- sort(rules, by="lift")
inspect(head(rules.sorted, 30))
##      lhs              rhs                support confidence  coverage     lift
count
## [1] {sex=female,
##       cabin=B}     => {survived=1} 0.02750191  1.0000000 0.02750191 2.618000
36
## [2] {pclass=1,
##       sex=female,
##       cabin=B}     => {survived=1} 0.02750191  1.0000000 0.02750191 2.618000
36
## [3] {pclass=1,
##       sex=female,
##       fare=medium} => {survived=1} 0.05271199  1.0000000 0.05271199 2.618000
69
...
```

Prune any redundant association rules. For instance, some rules may provide no extra knowledge. Rules that are highly related with prior rules may be redundant. Pruning reduces the number of rules from *27 to 18*.

```
# search for redundant rules
rules_lift <- sort(rules, by = 'lift')
rules_pruned <- rules_lift[!is.redundant(rules_lift, measure="lift")]
inspect(head(rules_pruned, 30))
##      lhs                                      rhs          support    confidence
## [1] {sex=female, cabin=B}                 => {survived=1} 0.02750191 1.0000000
## [2] {pclass=1, sex=female, fare=medium}   => {survived=1} 0.05271199 1.0000000
## [3] {pclass=1, sex=female, age=4}         => {survived=1} 0.02826585 0.9736842
...
## [18] {pclass=1, cabin=D}                  => {survived=1} 0.02139037 0.7000000
##      coverage   lift     count
## [1] 0.02750191 2.618000 36
## [2] 0.05271199 2.618000 69
## [3] 0.02902979 2.549105 37
...
## [18] 0.03055768 1.832600 28
```

The package `arulesViz` supplies rule-visualization routines using scatter, bubble, and parallel coordinates plots. The visualization of the frequent item sets using parallel coordinates allows all items to be placed on the vertical axis with their position determined by their group and by the frequency of the item in descending order, vertical ranking based on the support of the 1-itemset containing the item.[12] To render the maximal frequent item sets, all subsets are implicitly drawn as sub-segments of one polyline. All item sets are visualized as parallel coordinate polylines. The *support* can be mapped to line color or width. This shows effectively that item sets that share common parts may have overlapping polylines (Figs. 7.16, 7.17 and 7.18).

```
library(arulesViz)
plot(rules)
```

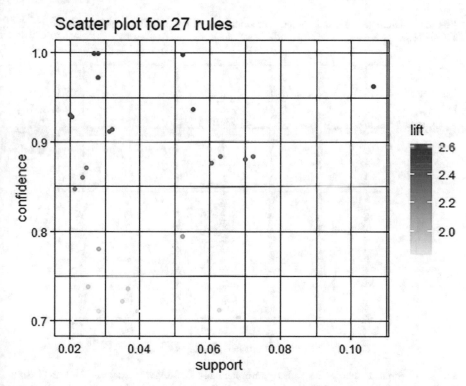

Fig. 7.16 Support, confidence, and lift correspondences (pruned Titanic passengers data association rules)

---

[12] https://doi.org/10.1007/978-3-030-04921-8_12

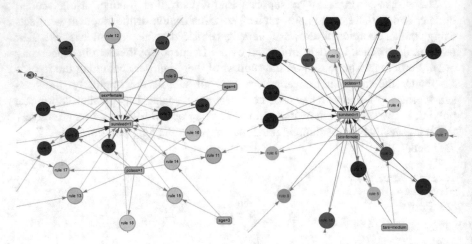

Fig. 7.17 Alternative dynamic graph representations of the pruned association rules using the Titanic passengers data

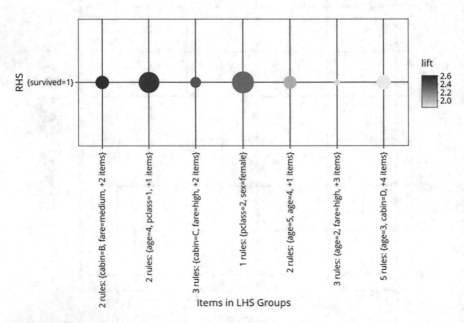

Fig. 7.18 Pruned association rules corresponding to survival outcome in the Titanic passenger's data

```
# scatter plot of association rules
plot(rules_pruned, method="graph", control=list(verbose = FALSE),
     engine="htmlwidget")
# interactive association network graph
plot(rules_pruned, method="graph", measure = "support", engine="htmlwidget",
     nodeCol=rainbow(14), shading = "lift", control = list(verbose = FALSE))
```

```
inspect(rules_pruned[m$clustering_rules == 1])
##      lhs                        rhs              support    confidence coverage
## [1] {sex=female, cabin=B} => {survived=1} 0.02750191 1.0000000  0.02750191
## [2] {pclass=1, fare=high} => {survived=1} 0.02597403 0.7391304  0.03514133
##      lift       count
## [1] 2.618000 36
## [2] 1.935043 34
# the corresponding plot
plot(rules_pruned, method = "grouped matrix", k = 7, engine = "htmlwidget")
```

Consider plotting *all rules* (not only the pruned list of association rules) and examine rules predicting passenger death (use `"survived=0"`).

Readers may also these TM/NLP techniques for other applications, e.g.,

- MIMIC-III, a freely accessible critical care database[13]
- Other data from the DSPA list of case-studies
- Other available free text documents or transactional data archives

---

[13] https://doi.org/10.1038/sdata.2016.35

Chapter 8
Unsupervised Clustering

As we learned in Chaps. 3, 4, 5 and 6, supervised regression and classification techniques facilitate explicit forecasting and prediction of specific observable outcomes. However, these approaches typically require a priori human supervised class labels or explicit predefined outcomes. In many situations, e.g., exploratory data analytics or open-ended study paradigms, such explicit outcomes may not be readily available, may not be desirable, or could require additional time and resources to define, derive, or generate.

Clustering can help us conduct complex data-driven studies where automated segregation of participants, grouping of cases, or cohort clustering may be beneficial for capturing similar traits, characterizing common behaviors, or phenotype categorization of heterogeneous phenomena. Each derived group or categorical label can be subsequently interpreted in terms of the observed data features. Complementary to various confirmatory analytic methods used in supervised strategies for predicting specific outcomes, clustering may be used for exploratory data analytics and *unsupervised learning*.

In this chapter, we will (1) present clustering as a machine learning task, (2) explain the *silhouette* plots for assessing the reliability of clustering, (3) discuss the *k-Means* clustering algorithm and how to tune it, (4) show examples of several interesting case studies, including Divorce and Consequences on Young Adults, Pediatric Trauma, and Youth Development, and (5) demonstrate hierarchical, spectral, and Gaussian mixture-model clustering approaches.

8.1 ML Clustering

As we mentioned earlier, clustering is a machine learning technique that bundles unlabeled cases and outcome-free data into distinct groups. Scatter plots we saw in previous chapters represent a simple visual illustration of the clustering process.

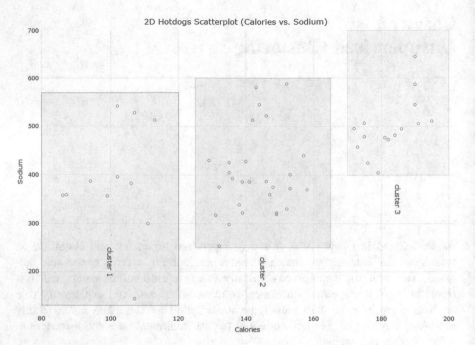

Fig. 8.1 Hotdog data scatterplot—calories vs. sodium, with geometric pseudo-clusters

Let's start with a simple hotdogs example. Assume we don't know much about the ingredients of frankfurters (hotdogs) and we look at the graph shown on Fig. 8.1.

In terms of their *calories* and *sodium* content, these hotdogs appear to be separated into three different clusters. *Cluster 1* has hotdogs of low calories and medium sodium content; *Cluster 2* has both calorie and sodium at medium levels; *Cluster 3* has both sodium and calories at high levels. We can make a bold guess about the ingredients used in the hotdogs in these three clusters. For cluster 1, it could be mostly *chicken* meat since it has low calories. The second cluster might be *beef* and the third one is likely to be *pork*, because beef hotdogs have considerably fewer calories and less salt than pork hotdogs. However, this is just heuristic guessing. Some hotdogs have a mixture of two or three types of meat. The real situation is resembling somewhat our initial guess, however with some random noise, especially in cluster 2.

Figure 8.2 shows a more nuanced scatter of the primary type of meat used for each hotdog designated by color and glyph-symbol for meat-type. In this chapter, we will demonstrate strategies to algorithmically tackle the problem of automatically deriving such groupings or clustering labels.

8.2   Silhouette Plots

Silhouette plots represent graphical depictions of the individual data points and their corresponding cluster-wide silhouette values, which are useful for interpretation of the performance and validation of the consistency of various clustering algorithms.

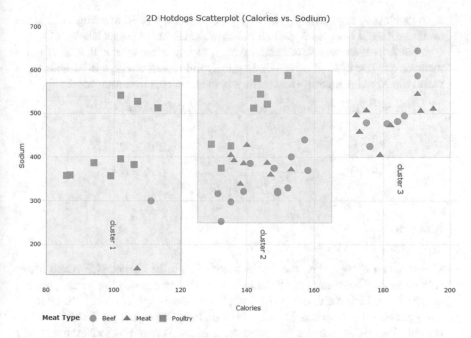

Fig. 8.2 Hotdog data scatterplot—calories (horizontal axis), sodium (vertical axis), and meat ingredients (colors and glyph-type), with geometric pseudo-clusters

The silhouette value, $sil \in [-1, 1]$, measures the similarity (cohesion) of a data point to its cluster relative to other clusters (separation). Silhouette plots rely on a distance metric, e.g., the Euclidean distance, Manhattan distance, Minkowski distance,[1] etc. The qualitative mapping between silhouette values and their interpretations is summarized below:

- A high silhouette value suggests that the data matches its own cluster well.
- A clustering algorithm performs well when most Silhouette values are high.
- A low silhouette value indicates poor matching within the neighboring cluster.
- Poor clustering may imply that the algorithm configuration may have too many or too few clusters.

Suppose a clustering method groups all data points (objects), $\{X_i\}_i$, into k clusters; in most clustering techniques, the hyperparameter k is required, but can be tuned to acheive better clustering results. For each object, we can define the following pair of similarity measures to track its within-cluster and between-cluster similarity.

- d_i as the *average dissimilarity* of X_i with all other data points within its cluster. The internal dissimilarity d_i captures the quality of the assignment of X_i to its current class label. Smaller or larger d_i values suggest better or worse overall assignment for

---

[1] https://doi.org/10.1109/ACCESS.2020.3003086

X_i to its cluster, respectively. The average dissimilarity of X_i to a cluster C is the average distance between X_i and all points in the cluster of points labeled C.

- l_i as the *lowest average dissimilarity* of X_i to any other cluster that X_i is not a member of. The cluster corresponding to l_i, the lowest average dissimilarity, is called the X_i **neighboring cluster**, as it is the next best fit cluster for X_i.

Then, the **silhouette** (value) of each object X_i is defined by

$$-1 \leq s_i = \frac{l_i - d_i}{\max\{l_i, d_i\}} \equiv \begin{cases} 1 - \dfrac{d_i}{l_i}, & \text{if } d_i < l_i \\ 0, & \text{if } d_i = l_i \leq 1. \\ \dfrac{l_i}{d_i} - 1, & \text{if } d_i > l_i \end{cases}$$

Note that:

- $-1 \leq s_i \leq 1$,
- $s_i \to 1$ when $d_i \gg l_i$, i.e., the dissimilarity of X_i to its cluster C is much lower relative to its dissimilarity to other clusters, indicating a good (cluster assignment) match. Thus, high Silhouette values imply the data is appropriately clustered.
- Conversely, $-1 \leftarrow s_i$ when $l_i \gg d_i$, d_i is large, implying a poor match of X_i with its current cluster C, relative to neighboring clusters. X_i may be more appropriately clustered in its neighboring cluster.
- $s_i \sim 0$ means that the X_i may lie on the border between two natural clusters.

Cluster-wide silhouette values represent the pooled overall averages of the corresponding point-based silhouette values for all members of each class.

8.3   The k-Means Clustering Algorithm

The *k-means* algorithm is one of the most commonly used ML clustering algorithms. It has resemblance to the familiar *k-nearest neighbors (kNN)* presented in Chap. 5. The distinction is that in clustering, we don't have a priori predetermined labels, and the k-means algorithm is trying to deduce the missing intrinsic groupings in the data.

Similar to kNN, most of the times, k-means relies on the Euclidean distance ($|\cdot|_2$ norm), however Manhattan distance ($|\cdot|_1$ norm), the more general Minkowski distance $\left(\left(\sum_{i=1}^{n} |p_i - q_i|^c\right)^{\frac{1}{c}}\right)$, Mahalanobis distance (for $x, y \in \mathbb{R}$ and a given a nonsingular covariance matrix S, $d(x, y) = \sqrt{(x-y)^t S^{-1}(x-y)}$), or other distance functions may also be used. For $c = 2$, the Minkowski distance represents the classical Euclidean distance, which is commonly used in k-means clustering

$$\text{dist}(x, y) = \sqrt{\sum_{n=1}^{n} (x_i - y_i)^2}.$$

8.3.1 Pseudocode

Given a specific distance function, we can group neighbors of observations into separate clusters according to their paired distances. Suppose we are trying to use k-means clustering to group a set of observations $\{x_1, x_2, \cdots, x_n\}$, $x_i \in \mathbb{R}^d$, into $k \leq n$ classes $S = \{S_1, S_2, \cdots, S_k\}$. Effectively, the algorithm aims to *minimize* the within-cluster sum of squares, i.e., enforce lower intraclass variance. Let μ_i be the mean of all points in the group S_i. Then the k-means optimizes the following objective function

$$\arg\min_S \sum_{i=1}^{k} \sum_{x \in S_i} |x - \mu_i|^2 = \arg\min_S \sum_{i=1}^{k} |S_i| \mathrm{Var}(S_i) \approx \arg\min_S \sum_{i=1}^{k} \frac{1}{|S_i|} \sum_{x, y \in S_i} |x - y|^2.$$

Since $|S_i| \sum_{x \in S_i} |x - \mu_i|^2 = \sum_{x \neq y \in S_i} |x - y|^2$, the left and right hand side optimization problems yield equivalent solutions. Also, as the total variance remains unchanged, this *within-group minimization* problem is equivalent to a corresponding *between clusters (dual) maximization* problem involving the sum squared deviations *between* points in different clusters.

The generic **k-means protocol** is as follows:

- *Initiation*: First, define k points as cluster centers. Often these points are k random points from the dataset. For example, if $k = 3$ we choose 3 random points in the dataset as initial cluster centers.
- *Assignment*: Second, determine the maximum extent of the cluster boundaries by computing the distances between each point and the current cluster centers. For each point, we assign the cluster label based on its shortest distance to a cluster center. Now the data are separated into k initial clusters. The assignment of each observation to a cluster is based on computing the least within-cluster sum of squares (i.e., minimize the intra-group dissimilarity) according to the chosen distance. Mathematically, this is equivalent to Voronoi tessellation[2] of the space of the observations according to their mean distances. Voronoi partitioning of the observations can be accomplished by assigning each point x_p to a single class $S^{(t)}$, where at each iteration i, $m_i^{(t)}$ denotes the group means of $S_i^{(t)}$.

$$S_i^{(t)} = \left\{ x_p : \| x_p - m_i^{(t)} \|^2 \leq \| x_p - m_j^{(t)} \|^2, \ 1 \leq j \leq k \right\}.$$

- *Update*: Third, update the centers of the current clusters to the new *means* of all points in the current cluster vicinity (based on the shortest distances from current centroid locations). This updating phase is the essence of the *k-means* algorithm. The updating step recomputes the new centroids for each cluster using

---

[2] https://doi.org/10.1137/S0036144599352836

$$m_i^{(t+1)} = \frac{1}{\left| S_i^{(t)} \right|} \sum_{x_j \in S_i^{(t)}} x_j.$$

Although there is no guarantee that the *k-means* algorithm converges to a global optimum, in practice, the algorithm tends to converge, i.e., the assignments of objects into groups stabilizes to a local minimum represented by one of only a finite number of such Voronoi partitionings. This SOCR 2D Interactive Voronoi Tessellation App[3] provides an interactive demonstration of this iterative parcellation process where we can use parameters to manually control the dynamics of the iterative process.

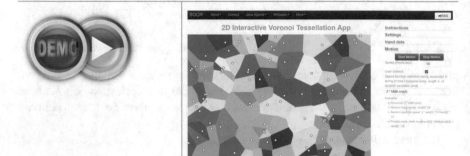

statistics@umich.edu

https://socr.umich.edu/HTML5/others/Voronoi_App/

8.3.2   Choosing the Appropriate Number of Clusters

In principle, neither a large nor a small number of clusters are desirable. If the number of clusters is too large, the induced object grouping may be too specific to be meaningfully interpreted. On the other hand, having too few groups might be overly broad or excessively general to be useful. As we mentioned in Chap. 5, $k = \sqrt{\frac{n}{2}}$ may be a good place to start. However, it might generate too many cluster groups. Again, the *elbow method* may be used to determine the relationship between the number of clusters k and the homogeneity of the observations within each cluster.

---

[3] https://socr.umich.edu/HTML5/others/Voronoi_App/

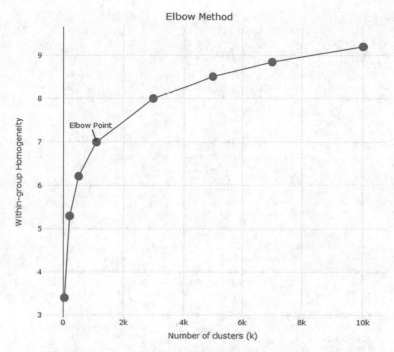

Fig. 8.3 Schematic of the elbow method for determining reasonable estimates of the hyperparameter k by plotting the within-group homogeneity against the number of clusters

Graphing the within-group homogeneity against *k* identifies if there exists a clearly defined "elbow point," suggesting a minimum number *k* corresponding to relatively large within-group homogeneity (Fig. 8.3).

Figure 8.3 shows that homogeneity barely increases above the "elbow point." There are various ways to measure homogeneity within a cluster; further details about these choices are provided here.[4]

Let's try to develop a new method `drawElbowGraph()` that automatically identifies an optimal *elbow* point and determines an appropriate value for the number of clusters *k*.

---

[4] https://doi.org/10.1023/A:1012801612483

```r
estimateElbowPoint <- function(xValues, yValues) { # Estimate Elbow point
  # Determine the extreme values to create line
  max_x_x <- max(xValues)
  max_x_y <- yValues[which.max(xValues)]
  max_y_y <- min(yValues)
  max_y_x <- xValues[which.min(yValues)]
  max_df  <- data.frame(x = c(max_y_x, max_x_x), y = c(max_y_y, max_x_y))
  # Create a straight line between the extreme values
  fit <- lm(max_df$y ~ max_df$x)
  # compute Euclidean Distance from point to line
  distances <- c()
  for(i in 1:length(xValues)) { distances <- c(distances,
                   abs(coef(fit)[2]*xValues[i] - yValues[i] + coef(fit)[1]) /
                        sqrt(coef(fit)[2]^2 + 1^2))  }
  # Determine the Max distance point
  x_max_dist <- xValues[which.max(distances)]
  y_max_dist <- yValues[which.max(distances)]
  return(c(x_max_dist, y_max_dist, max(distances)))
}
# Define elbow-drawing function
drawElbowGraph <- function(x_K_clusters, y_WGH_values) {
  nbValues = length(y_WGH_values)
  extremes_lineSlope = (y_WGH_values[nbValues] - y_WGH_values[1]) /
                        (x_K_clusters[nbValues] - x_K_clusters[1])
  extremes_orth_lineSlope = -1 / extremes_lineSlope
  elbowPoint_orth_proj = c(elbowPoint[1] + elbowPoint[3]/2,
                elbowPoint[2] + extremes_orth_lineSlope * (elbowPoint[3]/2))
  e1 = c(x_K_clusters[nbValues]-x_K_clusters[1], y_WGH_values[nbValues]-
             y_WGH_values[1])  # bottom-left (origin) point
  e2 = c(elbowPoint[1]-x_K_clusters[1], elbowPoint[2]-y_WGH_values[1])
                 # elbow point, e2
  p = ((e1 %*% e2)[1,1]/(e1 %*% e1)[1,1]) * e1 + c(x_K_clusters[1],
             y_WGH_values[1]); p  # Projection point
  distP <- e2-p
  dist <- sqrt((distP %*% distP)[1,1])
  distLabel <- (e2+p)/2 + c(100, 2)
  plot_ly(x = ~x_K_clusters, y = ~y_WGH_values, type="scatter",
               mode = "markers+lines", name="Data") %>%
    add_lines(x=c(x_K_clusters[1], x_K_clusters[nbValues]), name="reference",
               y = c(y_WGH_values[1], y_WGH_values[nbValues]),
               type = 'scatter', mode = 'lines') %>%
    add_lines(x = c(elbowPoint[1], p[1]), y = c(elbowPoint[2], p[2]),
               type = 'scatter', name="Max Distance (Elbow)", mode = 'lines') %>%
    layout(title='Within-Group Homogeneity (WGH) vs. number of clusters (k)',
           xaxis = list(title="k"), # scaleanchor="y"),
           yaxis = list(title="WGH Value"), #, scaleanchor="x"))
           legend = list(orientation = 'h'),
           annotations = list(text=paste0("MaxDist=", round(dist, 3)),
                   x=distLabel[1], y=distLabel[2], textangle=0, showarrow=T,
                   xref = "x", yref = "y", ax = 80, ay = -40))
}
# Test the function: drawElbowGraph()
x <- c(30, 200, 500, 1096.663, 3000, 5000, 7000, 10000)
y <- function(x) {   return (log(x))   }
elbowPoint = estimateElbowPoint(xValues = x, yValues = y(x))
drawElbowGraph(x_K_clusters=x, y_WGH_values=y(x))
```

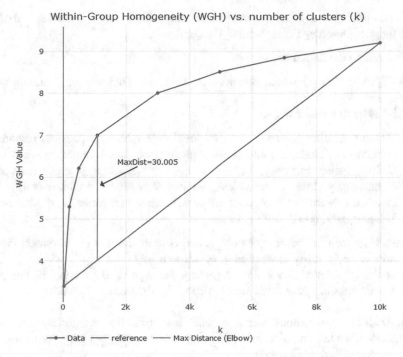

Fig. 8.4   Graphical illustration of the `drawElbowGraph()` optimization method

Note: Recall that the projection, $\vec{Q}$, of a point, $\vec{P}$, onto a line, $\vec{l}$, is defined as the vector $\vec{Q} = \dfrac{\langle \vec{P} \mid \vec{l} \rangle}{\langle \vec{l} \mid \vec{l} \rangle} \vec{l}$. In Fig. 8.4, the *max-distance* is the length $\left\| \vec{Q} \right\|$ and $\vec{Q} \perp \vec{l}$. However, since the scales of the horizontal and vertical axes in Fig. 8.4 are different, $\vec{Q}$ *appears* to be a vertical line (it's not!) and it represents the maximum distance between the blue curve to the reference orange line.

8.3.3   Case Study 1: Divorce and Consequences on Young Adults

Step 1: Collecting data
This example uses the Divorce and Consequences on Young Adults dataset. This is a longitudinal study focused on examining the consequences of recent parental divorce for young adults (initially ages 18–23) whose parents had divorced within 15 months of the study's first wave (1990–1991). The sample consisted of 257 White respondents with newly divorced parents. Here we have a subset of this dataset with

47 respondents available in the supporting case studies folder, CaseStudy01_Divorce_YoungAdults_Data.csv.

The features in the data include:

- **DIVYEAR**: Year in which parents were divorced. Dichotomous variable with 1989 and 1990
- **Child affective relations**:
  - Momint: Mother intimacy. Interval level data with four possible responses (1. extremely close, 2. quite close, 3. fairly close, and 4. not close at all)
  - Dadint: Father intimacy. Interval level data with four possible responses (1. extremely close, 2. quite close, 3. fairly close, and 4. not close at all)
  - Live with mom: Polytomous variable with three categories (1. mother only, 2. father only, and 3. both parents)

- **momclose**: measure of how close the child is to the mother (1. extremely close, 2. quite close, 3. fairly close, and 4. not close at all).
- **Depression**: Interval level data regarding feelings of depression in the past 4 weeks. Possible responses are 1. often, 2. sometimes, 3. hardly ever, and 4. never
- **Gethitched**: Polytomous variable with four possible categories indicating respondent's plan for marriage (1- marry fairly soon, 2- marry sometime, 3- never marry, 8- don't know).

Step 2: Exploring and preparing the data
Let's load the dataset and report a summary of all variables.

```
divorce<-
  read.csv("https://umich.instructure.com/files/399118/download?download_frd=1")
summary(divorce)
##      DIVYEAR          momint          dadint          momclose
##  Min.   :89.00   Min.   :1.000   Min.   :1.000   Min.   :1.000
##  1st Qu.:89.00   1st Qu.:1.000   1st Qu.:2.000   1st Qu.:1.000
##  Median :90.00   Median :1.000   Median :2.000   Median :2.000
##  Mean   :89.68   Mean   :1.809   Mean   :2.489   Mean   :1.809
##  3rd Qu.:90.00   3rd Qu.:3.000   3rd Qu.:3.000   3rd Qu.:2.000
##  Max.   :90.00   Max.   :4.000   Max.   :4.000   Max.   :4.000
##     depression       livewithmom      gethitched
##  Min.   :1.000   Min.   :1.000   Min.   :1.000
##  1st Qu.:2.000   1st Qu.:1.000   1st Qu.:2.000
##  Median :3.000   Median :1.000   Median :2.000
##  Mean   :2.851   Mean   :1.489   Mean   :2.213
##  3rd Qu.:4.000   3rd Qu.:2.000   3rd Qu.:2.000
##  Max.   :4.000   Max.   :9.000   Max.   :8.000
```

According to the summary, DIVYEAR is actually a dummy variable (either 89 or 90). We can re-code (binarize) the DIVYEAR using the `ifelse()` function (mentioned in Chap. 7). The following line of code generates a new indicator variable for *divorce year = 1990*.

```
divorce$DIVYEAR<-ifelse(divorce$DIVYEAR==89, 0, 1)
```

We also need another preprocessing step to deal with livewithmom, which has missing values, livewithmom=9. We can impute these using momint and dadint variables for each specific participant.

```
table(divorce$livewithmom)
##  1  2  9
## 31 15  1
divorce[divorce$livewithmom==9, ]
##     DIVYEAR momint dadint momclose depression livewithmom gethitched
## 45       1      3      1        3          3           9          2
```

For instance, respondents that feel much closer to their dads may be assigned divorce$livewithmom==2, suggesting they most likely live with their fathers. Of course, alternative imputation strategies are also possible.

```
divorce[45, 6]<-2
divorce[45, ]
##     DIVYEAR momint dadint momclose depression livewithmom gethitched
## 45       1      3      1        3          3           2          2
```

Step 3 - Training a model on the data

The function kmeans() provides one interface to the *k-means* clustering method using the following invocation syntax.

```
myclusters <- kmeans(mydata, k)
```

- *mydata*: dataset in a matrix form
- *k*: number of clusters we want to create

The *output* consists of

- *myclusters$cluster*: vector indicating the cluster number for every observation
- *myclusters$center*: a matrix showing the mean feature values for every center
- *mycluster$size*: a table showing how many observations are assigned to each cluster

Before we perform clustering, we need to standardize the features to avoid biasing the clustering based on features that use large-scale values. Note that distance calculations are sensitive to measuring units. The method as.data.frame() converts the dataset into a data frame allowing us subsequently to use a combination of lapply() and scale() to standardize the data.

```
di_z<- as.data.frame(lapply(divorce, scale))
str(di_z)
```

The resulting dataset, di_z, is standardized, so all features are unit less and follow approximately standardized normal distribution.

Next, we need to select a proper k hyperparameter. We have a relatively small dataset with 47 observations. Obviously, we cannot have a parameter k exceeding 10. The rule of thumb suggests $k = \sqrt{47/2} = 4.8$. This would be relatively large also because we may expect less than 10 observations for each cluster and it is likely that some clusters may only have one or no observations. A better choice for the parameter may be 3. Let's see if this value works.

```
library(stats)
set.seed(321)
diz_clussters<-kmeans(di_z, 3)
```

Step 4: Evaluating model performance
Let's look at the clusters created by the *k-means* model.

```
diz_clussters$size
## [1] 15 19 13
```

At first glance, it seems that three worked well for the number of clusters. We don't have any cluster that contains a small number of observations. The three clusters have a relatively equal number of respondents.

Silhouette plots represent the most appropriate evaluation strategy to assess the quality of the clustering. In our case, two data points correspond to negative Silhouette values, suggesting these cases may be "mis-clustered," or perhaps are ambiguous as the Silhouette value is close to 0. We observe that the average Silhouette is reasonable, about 0.2 (Fig. 8.5).

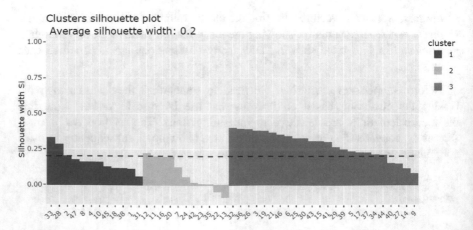

Fig. 8.5 A silhouette plot of all data points in the three clusters

```
require(cluster)
dis = dist(di_z)
sil = silhouette(diz_clussters$cluster, dis)
summary(sil)
## Silhouette of 47 units in 3 clusters from silhouette.default(x =
diz_clussters$cluster, dist = dis) :
## Cluster sizes and average silhouette widths:
##           15          19          13
## 0.1026558 0.2381074 0.1216357
## Individual silhouette widths:
##       Min.  1st Qu.   Median     Mean  3rd Qu.      Max.
## -0.04724  0.08985  0.15871  0.16266  0.23772  0.38138
plot(sil, col=c(1:length(diz_clussters$size)))
ggplotly(factoextra::fviz_silhouette(sil, label=T, palette="jco"))
```

The next step would be to interpret the clusters in the context of this social study.

```
diz_clussters$centers
# DIVYEAR momint dadint momclose depression livewithmom gethitched
# 1 0.5004720 1.1698438 -0.07631029 1.2049200 -0.1112567 0.1591755
-0.1390230
# 2 0.0985208 -0.1817299 -0.70455885 -0.2023993 -0.1362761 1.3770536
0.4549845
# 3 -0.2953914 -0.5016290 0.36107795 -0.5096937 0.1180883 -0.7107373
-0.1390230
```

These results facilitate interpretation of the underlying factors associated with the derived three-cluster labels. For instance, *cluster 1* corresponds to divyear = mostly 90, moment = very close, dadint = not close, livewithmom = mostly mother, depression = not often, (gethiched) marry = will likely not get married. Cluster 1 represents mostly adolescents that are closer to mom than dad. These young adults do not often feel depressed and they may avoid getting married. These young adults tend to not be too emotional and do not value family. We can see that these three different clusters appear to contain three complementary types of young adults. Bar plots also provide an alternative strategy to visualize the difference between clusters (Fig. 8.6).

```
df <- as.data.frame(t(diz_clussters$centers))
rowNames <- rownames(df)
colnames(df) <- paste0("Cluster",c(1:3))
plot_ly(df, x = rownames(df), y = ~Cluster1, type='bar', name='Cluster1') %>%
  add_trace(y = ~Cluster2, name = 'Cluster2') %>%
  add_trace(y = ~Cluster3, name = 'Cluster3') %>%
  layout(title="Explicating Derived Cluster Labels",
         yaxis = list(title = 'Cluster Centers'), barmode = 'group')
```

Step 5: Usage of cluster information

Clustering results could be utilized as new information augmenting the original dataset. For instance, we can add a *cluster* label in our divorce dataset.

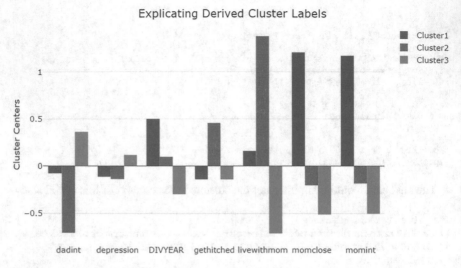

Fig. 8.6 A bar plot explicating the relations between derived clusters and observed characteristics

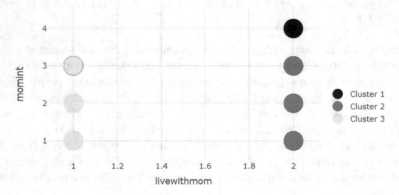

Fig. 8.7 A scatterplot explicating the relations between living with mom, feeling close to mom, and the derived cluster classes

```
divorce$clusters <- diz_clussters$cluster
divorce[1:5, ]
```

We can also examine the relationship between living with mom and feeling close to mom by displaying a scatter plot of these two variables. If we suspect that young adults' personality might affect this relationship, then we could consider the potential personality (cluster type) in the plot. The cluster labels associated with each participant are printed in different positions relative to each pair of observations, (livewithmom, momint) (Fig. 8.7).

```
clusterNames <- paste0("Cluster ", divorce$clusters)
plot_ly(data=divorce,x=~livewithmom,y=~momint, type="scatter",mode="markers",
        color = ~clusters, marker = list(size = 30), name=clusterNames) %>%
  hide_colorbar()
```

Figure 8.7 shows that living with mom does not necessarily mean young adults will feel close to mom and there are some clear cluster dependencies.

8.3.4 Model Improvement

Let's still use the divorce data to illustrate a model improvement using **k-means++**. Appropriate initialization of the **k-means** algorithm is of paramount importance. The **k-means++** extension provides a practical strategy to obtain an optimal initialization for k-means clustering using a predefined `kpp_init` method.

```
# install.packages("matrixStats")
library(matrixStats)
## Warning: package 'matrixStats' was built under R version 4.1.2
kpp_init = function(dat, K) {
  x = as.matrix(dat)
  n = nrow(x)
  # Randomly choose a first center
  centers = matrix(NA, nrow=K, ncol=ncol(x))
  # set.seed(123)
  centers[1,] = as.matrix(x[sample(1:n, 1),])
  for (k in 2:K) {
    # Calculate dist^2 to closest center for each point
    dists = matrix(NA, nrow=n, ncol=k-1)
    for (j in 1:(k-1)) {
      temp = sweep(x, 2, centers[j,], '-')
      dists[,j] = rowSums(temp^2)
    }
    dists = rowMins(dists)
    # Draw next center with probability proportional to dist^2
    cumdists = cumsum(dists)
    prop = runif(1, min=0, max=cumdists[n])
    centers[k,] = as.matrix(x[min(which(cumdists > prop)),])
  }
  return(centers)
}
set.seed(12345)
clust_kpp = kmeans(di_z, kpp_init(di_z, 3), iter.max=100, algorithm='Lloyd')
```

We can observe some differences in the results.

```
clust_kpp$centers
```

The resulting classification is not a substantial improvement—the new overall average Silhouette value remains 0.2 for **k-means++**, compared with the value of 0.2 reported for the earlier k-means clustering. However, the earlier three-group clustering is significantly distinct from the newly generated pair of clusters (Fig. 8.8).

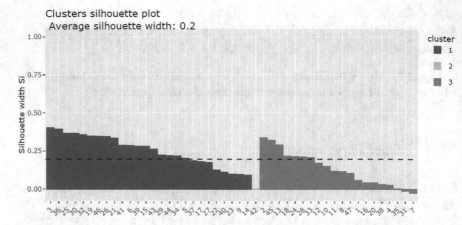

Fig. 8.8 A silhouette plot of all data points derived by the new *k-means++* approach

```
sil2 = silhouette(clust_kpp$cluster, dis)
summary(sil2)
## Silhouette of 47 units in 3 clusters from
## silhouette.default(x = clust_kpp$cluster, dist = dis) :
## Cluster sizes and average silhouette widths:
##        26          1          20
## 0.2525363 0.0000000 0.1306386
plot(sil2, col=1:length(diz_clussters$size), border=NA)
ggplotly(factoextra::fviz_silhouette(sil2, label=T, palette="jco"))
```

8.3.4.1   Tuning the Hyperparameter *k*

Similar to the approaches we used for estimating hyperparameters for the kNN and SVM methods, we can tune the **k-means** parameters, including centers initialization and the number of clusters, *k* (Fig. 8.9).

```
n_rows <- 21
mat = matrix(0,nrow = n_rows)
for (i in 2:n_rows){
  set.seed(321)
  clust_kpp = kmeans(di_z, kpp_init(di_z,i), iter.max=100, algorithm='Lloyd')
  sil = silhouette(clust_kpp$cluster, dis)
  mat[i] = mean(as.matrix(sil)[,3])
}
colnames(mat) <- c("Avg_Silhouette_Value"); mat
df <- data.frame(k=2:n_rows,sil=mat[2:n_rows])
plot_ly(df, x=~k, y=~sil, type='scatter',mode='lines', name='Silhouette') %>%
  layout(title="Average Silhouette Graph")
```

This suggests that $k = 2$ or 8 may be appropriate numbers of clusters to use in this case.

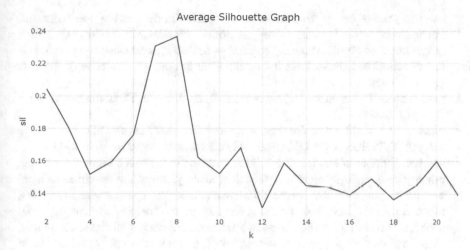

Fig. 8.9 Average silhouette plot of *k-means++* method against number of clusters

We can also experiment with other parameter settings, e.g., set the maximal iteration of the algorithm and rerun the model with optimal values of the hyperparameter $k = 2$ or $k = 8$.

8.3.5 Case Study 2: Pediatric Trauma

The next example demonstrates the use of the *k-means* clustering method on a larger dataset of trauma-exposed children.

Step 1: Collecting data
The dataset we will interrogate now includes Services Utilization by Trauma-Exposed Children in the US data, which is located in the supplementary canvas case studies folder. This case study examines associations between post-traumatic psychopathology and service utilization by trauma-exposed children. The variables in this dataset include:

- **id**: Case identification number
- **sex**: Female or male, dichotomous variable (1 = female, 0 = male)
- **age**: Age of child at time of seeking treatment services. Interval-level variable, score range = 0–18
- **race**: Race of child seeking treatment services. Polytomous variable with four categories (1 = black, 2 = white, 3 = Hispanic, 4 = other)
- **cmt**: The child was exposed to child maltreatment trauma—dichotomous variable (1 = yes, 0 = no)

- **traumatype**: Type of trauma exposure the child is seeking treatment for. Polytomous variable with five categories ("sexabuse" = sexual abuse, "physabuse" = physical abuse, "neglect" = neglect, "psychabuse" = psychological or emotional abuse, "dvexp" = exposure to domestic violence or intimate partner violence)
- **ptsd**: The child has current post-traumatic stress disorder. Dichotomous variable (1 = yes, 0 = no)
- **dissoc**: The child currently has a dissociative disorder (PTSD dissociative subtype, DESNOS, DDNOS). Interval-level variable, score range = 0–11
- **service**: Number of services the child has utilized in the past 6 months, including primary care, emergency room, outpatient therapy, outpatient psychiatrist, inpatient admission, case management, in-home counseling, group home, foster care, treatment foster care, therapeutic recreation or mentor, department of social services, residential treatment center, school counselor, special classes or school, detention center or jail, probation officer. Interval-level variable, score range = 0–19

Note: These data (`Case_04_ChildTrauma._Data.csv`) are tab delimited.

Step 2: Exploring and preparing the data
First, we need to load the dataset into R and report its summary and dimensions.

```
trauma<-
    read.csv("https://umich.instructure.com/files/399129/download?download_frd=1",
        sep = " ")
summary(trauma); dim(trauma)
## [1] 1000    9
```

In the summary, we see two factors—`traumatype` and `race`. The first one, `traumatype` codes the real classes we are interested in. If the clusters created by the model are quite similar to the trauma types, our model may have a quite reasonable interpretation. Let's also create a dummy variable for each racial category.

```
trauma$black<-ifelse(trauma$race=="black", 1, 0)
trauma$hispanic<-ifelse(trauma$race=="hispanic", 1, 0)
trauma$other<-ifelse(trauma$race=="other", 1, 0)
trauma$white<-ifelse(trauma$race=="white", 1, 0)
```

Then, we will remove the (outcome-type) class variable, `traumatype`, from the dataset to avoid biasing the clustering algorithm. Thus, we are simulating a real biomedical case study where we do not necessarily have the actual class information available, i.e., classes are latent features.

```
trauma_notype<-trauma[, -c(1, 5, 6)]
```

Step 3: Training a model on the data
Similar to the first case study, let's standardize the dataset and fit a k-means model.

```
tr_z<- as.data.frame(lapply(trauma_notype, scale))
str(tr_z)
## 'data.frame':    1000 obs. of  10 variables:
## $ sex     : num  0.988 0.988 -1.012 -1.012 0.988 ...
## $ age     : num  -0.997 1.677 -0.997 0.674 -0.662 ...
## $ ses     : num  -0.468 -0.468 -0.468 -0.468 -0.468 ...
## $ ptsd    : num  1.564 -0.639 -0.639 -0.639 1.564 ...
## $ dissoc  : num  0.819 -1.219 0.819 0.819 0.819 ...
## $ service : num  2.314 0.678 -0.303 0.351 1.66 ...
## $ black   : num  2 2 2 2 2 ...
## $ hispanic: num  -0.333 -0.333 -0.333 -0.333 -0.333 ...
## $ other   : num  -0.333 -0.333 -0.333 -0.333 -0.333 ...
## $ white   : num  -1.22 -1.22 -1.22 -1.22 -1.22 ...
set.seed(1234)
trauma_clusters<-kmeans(tr_z, 5)
```

Here we use $k = 5$ in the hope that we have five clusters corresponding to the five trauma types. In this case study, we have 1000 observations and $k = 5$ may be a reasonable option.

Step 4: Evaluating model performance
To assess the clustering model results, we can examine the resulting clusters (Fig. 8.10).

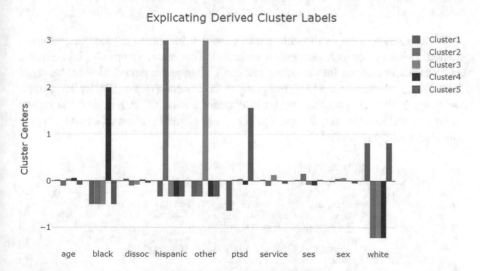

Fig. 8.10 Bar plot of clusters against observed pediatric phenotypes

```
trauma_clusters$centers
myColors <- c("darkblue", "red", "green", "brown", "pink", "purple",
              "lightblue", "orange", "gray", "yellow")
df <- as.data.frame(t(trauma_clusters$centers))
rowNames <- rownames(df)
colnames(df) <- paste0("Cluster", c(1:dim(trauma_clusters$centers)[1]))
plot_ly(df, x = rownames(df), y=~Cluster1, type='bar', name = 'Cluster1') %>%
  add_trace(y = ~Cluster2, name = 'Cluster2') %>%
  add_trace(y = ~Cluster3, name = 'Cluster3') %>%
  add_trace(y = ~Cluster4, name = 'Cluster4') %>%
  add_trace(y = ~Cluster5, name = 'Cluster5') %>%
  layout(title="Explicating Derived Cluster Labels",
         yaxis = list(title = 'Cluster Centers'), barmode = 'group')
```

On this bar plot, the bars in each cluster represents sex, age, ses, ptsd, dissoc, service, black, hispanic, other, and white, respectively. It is quite obvious that each cluster has a unique fingerprint of features.

Next, we can compare the *k-means* computed cluster labels to the *original labels*. Let's evaluate the similarities between the automated cluster labels and their real class counterparts (trauma type) using a confusion matrix table, where rows represent the k-means clusters, columns show the actual labels, and the cell values include the frequencies of the corresponding pairings.

```
trauma$clusters<-trauma_clusters$cluster
table(trauma$clusters, trauma$traumatype)
##
##     dvexp neglect physabuse psychabuse sexabuse
## 1     36     243         0        143        0
## 2    100       0         0          0        0
## 3    100       0         0          0        0
## 4      0       0       100          0      100
## 5     14     107         0         57        0
```

We can see that all of the children in cluster 4 belong to dvexp (exposure to domestic violence or intimate partner violence). The model groups all physabuse and sexabuse cases into *cluster1* but can't distinguish between them. Majority (200/250) of all dvexp children are grouped in *clusters 4 and 5*. Finally, neglect and psychabuse types are mixed in *clusters 2 and 3*. Let's review the output Silhouette value summary. It works well as only a small portion of samples appear mis-clustered (Fig. 8.11).

```
dis_tra = dist(tr_z)
sil_tra = silhouette(trauma_clusters$cluster, dis_tra)
summary(sil_tra)
## Silhouette of 1000 units in 5 clusters from silhouette.default(x =
trauma_clusters$cluster, dist = dis_tra) :
## Cluster sizes and average silhouette widths:
##      422       100       100       200       178
## 0.2166778 0.3353976 0.3373487 0.2836607 0.1898492
## Individual silhouette widths:
##    Min. 1st Qu.  Median    Mean 3rd Qu.    Max.
## 0.03672 0.19967 0.23675 0.24924 0.30100 0.41339
windows(width=7, height=7)
plot(sil_tra, col=1:length(trauma_clusters$centers[ ,1]), border=NA)
```

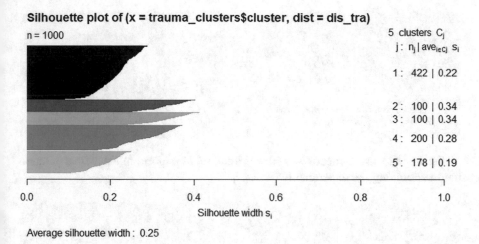

Fig. 8.11   Silhouette plot of the five k-means derived pediatric trauma clusters

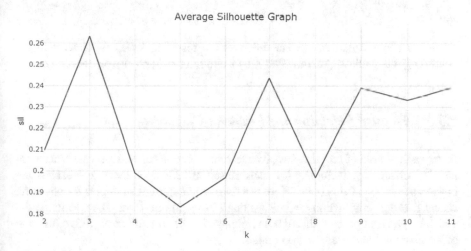

Fig. 8.12   Pediatric trauma average silhouette plot of *k-means++* method against number of clusters

```
# report the overall mean silhouette value
mean(sil_tra[,"sil_width"])
## [1] 0.249238
# The sil object colnames  are ("cluster", "neighbor", "sil_width")
```

Next, let's try to tune k with **k-means++** and see if $k = 5$ appears to be optimal
(Fig. 8.12).

```
mat = matrix(0,nrow = 11)
for (i in 2:11){
  set.seed(321)
  clust_kpp = kmeans(tr_z, kpp_init(tr_z, i), iter.max=100, algorithm='Lloyd')
  sil = silhouette(clust_kpp$cluster, dis_tra)
  mat[i] = mean(as.matrix(sil)[,3])
}
mat
df <- data.frame(data.frame(k=2:11, sil=mat[2:11]))
plot_ly(df, x=~k,y=~sil, type='scatter', mode='lines', name='Silhouette') %>%
  layout(title="Average Silhouette Graph")
```

Finally, let's use **k-means++** with $k = 3$ and set the algorithm's maximal iteration before rerunning the experiment.

```
set.seed(1234)
clust_kpp = kmeans(tr_z, kpp_init(tr_z, 3), iter.max=100, algorithm='Lloyd')
sil = silhouette(clust_kpp$cluster, dis_tra)
summary(sil)
## Cluster sizes and average silhouette widths:
##      600          100          300
##  0.3083487 0.3606939 0.1408309
mean(sil[,"sil_width"])
## [1] 0.2633279
```

As we showed earlier, we can interpret the resulting kmeans clusters in the context of this pediatric trauma study, by examining clust_kpp$centers.

8.3.6   Feature Selection for k-Means Clustering

A very active area of research involves feature selection for unsupervised machine-learning clustering, including k-means clustering. Most of these approaches are beyond the scope of this book. Here is a list of some current strategies for choosing salient features in situations where we don't have ground-truth labels to guide the variable-selection process through an optimization of an explicit objective function of the observed and predicted outcomes.

- For Gaussian model-based clustering, the *mclust* package provides the functionality to learn and report the clusters, as well as perform variable selection using the package *clustvarsel*.
- A review of possible clustering strategies for feature selection.[5]
- Unsupervised feature selection for k-means clustering provides specifics for variable selection for the k-means algorithm.[6]

---

[5]https://doi.org/10.1201/9781315373515-2

[6]https://dl.acm.org/doi/abs/10.5555/2984093.2984111

- This feature selection for clustering paper[7] presents an approach where features are ranked according to their importance on clustering and then a subset of important features is chosen.

8.4 Hierarchical Clustering

Recall from Chap. 5 that there are three large classes of unsupervised clustering methods—*Bayesian*, *partitioning-based*, and *hierarchical*. Hierarchical clustering represents a family of techniques that build hierarchies of clusters using one of two complementary strategies:

- *Generative* methods (also known as *agglomerative*) represent bottom-up approaches that are initialized with each individual observation being its own cluster, and the iterative protocol aggregates observations (i.e., merges clusters) by pairing similar clusters, which results in higher hierarchy levels.
- *Discriminative* methods (also known as *divisive*) represent reversed top-down techniques that are initialized by all observations belonging to a single cluster, which is recursively split into higher hierarchical levels.

In both situations, cluster splits and merges are determined by minimizing some objective function using a greedy algorithm (e.g., gradient descent). It's common to illustrate hierarchical clustering results as dendrograms or tree graphs. One example of genomics data hierarchical clustering using probability distributions is available here.[8]

Decisions about merging or splitting nodes in the hierarchy heavily depend on the specific distance metric used to measure the dissimilarity between sets of observations in the original cluster and the candidate children (sub)clusters. It's common to employ standard metrics (d) for measuring distances between pairs of observations (e.g., Euclidean, Manhattan, Mahalanobis) and a linkage criterion connecting cluster-dissimilarity of sets to the paired distances of observations in the cluster sets. For examples, maximum/complete linkage clustering $\max\{d(a,b) : a \in A, b \in B\}$, minimum/single linkage clustering $\min\{d(a,b) : a \in A, b \in B\}$, and mean linkage clustering $\frac{1}{|A|.|B|} \sum_{a \in A} \sum_{b \in B} d(a, b)$.

There are a number of R *hierarchical clustering* packages, including:

- `hclust` in base R
- `agnes` in the `cluster` package

Alternative distance measures (or linkages) can be used in all Hierarchical Clustering approaches, e.g., *single*, *complete*, and *ward*. We will demonstrate

---

[7] https://doi.org/10.1007/3-540-45571-X_13

[8] https://doi.org/10.1016/j.jtbi.2016.07.032

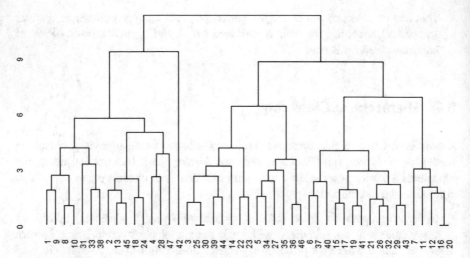

Fig. 8.13 Hierarchical dendrogram illustrating implicit graphical neighborhoods in the first case study (divorce and consequences on young adults)

hierarchical clustering using case study 1 (Divorce and Consequences on Young Adults). Let's set $k = 3$ and recall that we have to use normalized data for hierarchical clustering.

```
library(cluster)
divorce_sing = agnes(di_z, diss=FALSE, method='single')
divorce_comp = agnes(di_z, diss=FALSE, method='complete')
```

```
divorce_ward = agnes(di_z, diss=FALSE, method='ward')
sil_sing = silhouette(cutree(divorce_sing, k=3), dis)
sil_comp = silhouette(cutree(divorce_comp, k=3), dis)
# try 10 clusters, see plot above
sil_ward = silhouette(cutree(divorce_ward, k=10), dis)
```

You can generate the hierarchical plot by `ggdendrogram` in the package `ggdendro` (Figs. 8.13 and 8.14).

```
# install.packages("ggdendro")
library(ggdendro)
ggdendrogram(as.dendrogram(divorce_ward), leaf_labels=FALSE, labels=FALSE)
mean(sil_ward[,"sil_width"])  ## [1] 0.2398738
ggdendrogram(as.dendrogram(divorce_ward),leaf_labels=TRUE, labels=T, size=10)
```

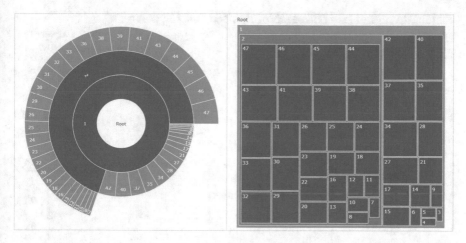

Fig. 8.14 Sunburst (left) and treemap (right) plots illustrating the derived hierarchical structure of the data in case study 1. At runtime, these dynamic plots support mouse interactions

```
library(data.tree)
DD_hcclust <- as.hclust(divorce_ward)
DD <- as.dendrogram(divorce_ward)
# Dendrogram     > Graph(Nodes)
DD_Node <- data.tree::as.Node(DD)
DD_Node$attributesAll
# Get nodes, labels, values, IDs
IDs <- DD_Node$Get("name")
labels = DD_Node$Get("name")
parents = DD_Node$Get(function(x) x$parent$name)
values = as.numeric(DD_Node$Get("name"))
## Warning: NAs introduced by coercion
df <- as.data.frame(cbind(labels=labels, parents=parents, values=values))
# remove node self-loops
df1 <- subset(df, as.character(labels) != as.character(parents))
# remove duplicates
df2 <- distinct(df1, labels, .keep_all= TRUE)
plot_ly(df2, labels=~labels, parents=~parents,values=~values,type='sunburst')
plot_ly(df2, labels=~labels, parents=~parents,values=~values, type='treemap')
```

Generally speaking, the best results are expected from using the *wald* linkage, yet, often trying *complete* and *other* linkages is valuable. We can see that the hierarchical clustering result (average silhouette value $\sim$0.24) mostly agrees with the prior *k-means* (0.2) and *k-means++* (0.2) results (Fig. 8.15).

Silhouette plot of (x = cutree(divorce_ward, k = 10), dist = dis)

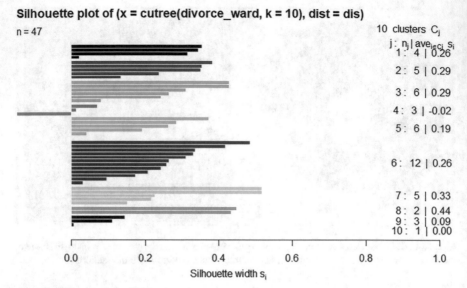

Average silhouette width : 0.24

Fig. 8.15 Silhouette plot of the 10 derived hierarchical clustering labels, case study 1 (divorce and consequences on young adults)

```
summary(sil_ward)
## Silhouette of 47 units in 10 clusters from silhouette.default(x =
cutree(divorce_ward, k = 10), dist = dis) :
##  Cluster sizes and average silhouette widths:
##          4          5          6          3          6         12
## 0.25905454 0.29195989 0.29305926 -0.02079056 0.19263836 0.26268274
##          5          2          3          1
## 0.32594365 0.44074717 0.08760990 0.00000000
## Individual silhouette widths:
##    Min. 1st Qu.  Median    Mean 3rd Qu.    Max.
## -0.1477  0.1231  0.2577  0.2399  0.3524  0.5176
plot(sil_ward, col=1:length(unique(sil_ward[,1])))
```

8.5 Spectral Clustering

Spectral clustering relies on a decomposition of the data similarity-matrix in terms of its spectrum of eigenvalues. The similarity matrix of the data is computed using the pairwise distances between all observations in the dataset. This spectral decomposition is used to reduce the data dimensionality prior to clustering. Typically, one precomputes the distance matrix first and feeds it as an input to a specified clustering method.

For a given dataset, the similarity matrix is a symmetric matrix $A = \{a_{ij} \geq 0\}_{ij}$ encoding the similarity measures between pairs of data points indexed by $1 \leq i, j \leq n$.

Most spectral clustering methods employ a traditional *cluster method* like k-means clustering applied on the eigenvectors of the *Laplacian* similarity matrix. There are alternative approaches to define a Laplacian that lead to different mathematical interpretations of the spectral clustering protocol. The *relevant eigenvectors* correspond to the few *smallest eigenvalues* of the Laplacian, excluding the smallest eigenvalue, which is typically 0. This process (finding the smallest eigenvalues) is analogous to computing the *largest* few eigenvalues of an operator representing a *function* of the original Laplacian.

The underlying philosophy of spectral clustering has roots in physics, e.g., partitioning of a mass-spring system. In particle physics, the analytical concept corresponding to physical mass is typically represented as a mass-characteristic (e.g., stiffness parameter), which can be related to weights of edges describing pairwise similarities of a particle to other related particle (in our case—data points). In spectral clustering analytics, the eigenvalue problem corresponds to physical transversal vibration modes of mass-spring systems.

Mathematically, the graph Laplacian matrix corresponding to the dataset is the matrix $L = D - A$, where $D = \{d_{i,i} = \sum_j a_{i,j}; d_{i \neq j} = 0\}$ is a diagonal matrix of vertex degrees and A is the data similarity matrix. Tightly coupled spring masses in a physical system jointly move in space around the equilibrium state in low-frequency vibration modes. Eigenvector components that correspond to the smallest eigenvalues of the Laplacian can be used to derive clustering of the masses (i.e., data points).

For instance, the *normalized cuts* spectral clustering algorithm partitions points in B into two sets B_1 and B_2 based on the eigenvector v corresponding to the *second-smallest* Laplacian eigenvalue, where the *symmetrized-and-normalized* Laplacian matrix is defined by

$$L^{\text{norm}} = I - \left(D^{-1/2} A D^{-1/2} \right).$$

Similarly, we can take the eigenvector corresponding to the *largest eigenvalue* of the adjacency matrix

$$P = D^{-1} A.$$

The key is to compute the spectrum of the Laplacian and use the corresponding eigenvectors to cluster the observations in many alternative ways. For instance, the cases can be partitioned by computing the median, m, of the components of the *second smallest eigenvector v* and then mapping all points whose component in v is greater than m in B_1 and the remaining cases in its complement, B_2. Repeated partitioning of the data into the subsets using this protocol will induce a classification scheme (*spectral clustering*) of the data.

The unnormalized spectral clustering pseudo algorithm is listed below.

- *Input*: *Similarity matrix*, $A \in \mathbb{R}^n \times \mathbb{R}^n$, $k =$ number of clusters.
- Construct a *similarity graph* modeling the local neighborhood relationships, where the similarity function encodes mainly local neighborhoods. For instance,

a Gaussian similarity function $a(x_i, x_j) = \exp\left(-\frac{\|x_i - x_j\|^2}{2\sigma^2}\right)$, where σ controls the width of the neighborhoods.

- Let W be its *weighted adjacency matrix*, corresponding to the similarity graph, $W = (w_{i,j})_{i,j}$, where $w_{i,j} = w_{j,i}$ and $w_{i,j} = 0$ implies that the vertices x_i and x_j are not connected.
- Compute the unnormalized Laplacian L.
- Compute the first k eigenvectors of L and let $V \in \mathbb{R}^{n \times k}$ be the matrix containing these k vectors as columns.
- For $1 \leq i \leq n$, let $y_i \in \mathbb{R}^k$ be the vector corresponding to the ith row of V.
- In $\mathbb{R}^k$, cluster the points $\{y_i\}_{1 \leq i \leq n}$ in k-clusters, $\{C_i\}_{i=1}^k$, using k-means clustering.
- *Output*: Clusters $\{A_i\}_{i=1}^k$, where $A_i = \{j | y_i \in C_i\}$.

8.5.1   Image Segmentation Using Spectral Clustering

Let's look at one specific implementation of spectral clustering for segmenting/classifying a region of interest (ROI) representing brain hematoma (trauma induced bleeding in the brain) in a 2D MRI image (*MRI_ImageHematoma.jpg*) (Fig. 8.16).

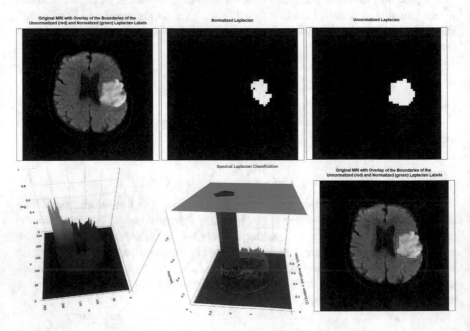

Fig. 8.16 Image segmentation using spectral clustering (brain hematoma study)

```
# Import the Brain 2D image MRI_ImageHematoma.jpg
library(jpeg)
img_url <- "https://umich.instructure.com/files/1627149/download?download_frd=1"
img_file <- tempfile(); download.file(img_url, img_file, mode="wb")
img <- readJPEG(img_file)
# install.packages("BiocManager")
# BiocManager::install("EBImage")
library("EBImage")
# take the first RGB-color channel; transpose to get it anatomically correct
# Viz - according to the width and height of the original image
img <- t(apply(img[ , , 1], 2, rev)) dim(img)[1:2]
## [1] 256 256
olddim <- c(dim(img)[1], dim(img)[2])
newdim <- c(64, 64)   # new smaller image dimensions
img1 <- resize(img, w = newdim[1], h = newdim[2])
plot_ly(z = ~img, type="surface")
# Convert image matrix to long vector (i,j, value)
imgvec <- matrix(NA, prod(dim(img1)),3)
counter <- 1
for (r in 1:nrow(img1)) {
  for (c in 1:ncol(img1)) {
    imgvec[counter,1] <- r
    imgvec[counter,2] <- c
    imgvec[counter,3] <- img1[r,c]
    counter <- counter+1
  }
}
# Compute the Similarity Matrix A
pixdiff <- 2
sigma2 <- 0.01
simmatrix <- matrix(0, counter-1, counter-1)
for(r in 1:nrow(imgvec)) {
  # Verbose
  # cat(r, "out of", nrow(imgvec), "\n")
  simmatrix[r,] <- ifelse(abs(imgvec[r,1]-imgvec[,1])<=pixdiff & abs(imgvec[r,2]-
imgvec[,2])<=pixdiff,exp(-(imgvec[r,3]-imgvec[,3])^2/sigma2),0)
}
# Compute the graph Laplacians
# U: unnormalized graph Laplacian (U=D-A)
# L: normalized graph Laplacian, which can be computed in different ways:
## L1:   Simple Laplacian: I - D^{-1} A, which can be seen as a random walk,
where D^{-1} A is the transition matrix, which yields spectral clustering with
groups of nodes such that the random walk seldom transitions from one group to
another.
## L2:   Normalized Laplacian D^{-1/2} A D^{-1/2}, or
## L3:   Generalized Laplacian: D^{-1} A.
D <- diag(rowSums(simmatrix))
Dinv <- diag(1/rowSums(simmatrix))
L <- diag(rep(1,nrow(simmatrix)))-Dinv %*% simmatrix
U <- D-simmatrix
# Compute the eigen-spectra for the normalized and unnormalized Laplacians
evL <- eigen(L, symmetric=TRUE)
evU <- eigen(U, symmetric=TRUE)
# Apply k-means clustering on the eigenspectra of both Laplacians
kmL <- kmeans(evL$vectors[,(ncol(simmatrix)-1):(ncol(simmatrix)-0)],
              centers=2,nstart=5)
segmatL <- matrix(kmL$cluster-1, newdim[1], newdim[2], byrow=T)
kmU <- kmeans(evU$vectors[,(ncol(simmatrix)-1):(ncol(simmatrix)-0)],
              centers=2,nstart=5)
segmatU <- matrix(kmU$cluster-1, newdim[1], newdim[2], byrow=T)
colorL <- rep(1, length(img))
```

```
dim(colorL) <- dim(img)
plot_ly(x=~seq(0,4, length.out=olddim[1]), y=~seq(0,4, length.out=olddim[2]),
        z=~segmatL, surfacecolor=colorL, cauto=F, cmax=1, cmin=0,
        name="L = Normalized graph Laplacian", type="surface") %>%
  add_trace(x=~seq(0, 4, length.out=olddim[1]),
        y=~seq(0, 4, length.out=olddim[2]), z=~segmatU*(1),
        colorscale = list(c(0, 1), c("tan", "red")),
        name="U = Unnormalized graph Laplacian", type="surface")  %>%
  add_trace(x = ~seq(0, 1, length.out=olddim[1]),
        y = ~seq(0, 1, length.out=olddim[2]),
        z = ~img/2, type="surface", name="Original Image", opacity=0.5) %>%
  layout(xaxis=list(name="X"), xaxis=list(name="X"),
        title="Spectral Laplacian Classification")  %>% hide_colorbar()
# Plot the pair of spectral clusters (hematoma and normal brain areas)
image(segmatL, col=grey((0:15)/15), main="Normalized Laplacian",
      xaxt = "n", yaxt = "n", asp=1)
image(segmatU, col=grey((0:15)/15), main="Unnormalized Laplacian",
      xaxt = "n", yaxt = "n", asp=1)
# Overlay the outline of the ROI-segmentation region on top of original image
image(seq(0, 1, length.out=olddim[1]), seq(0, 1, length.out=olddim[2]),
      img, col = grey((0:15)/15), xlab="",ylab="", asp=1, xaxt="n", yaxt="n",
      main="Original MRI with Overlay of the Boundaries of the \n Unnormalized
(red) and Normalized (green) Laplacian Labels")
# Compute the outline of the spectral segmentation and plot it as piecewise
polygon - line segments
segmat <- segmatU
linecol <- "red"
linew <- 3
for(r in 2:newdim[1]) {
  for (c in 2:newdim[2]) {
    if(abs(segmat[r-1,c]-segmat[r,c])>0) {
      xloc <- (r-1)/(newdim[1])
      ymin <- (c-1)/(newdim[2])
      ymax <- (c-0)/(newdim[2])
      segments(xloc, ymin, xloc, ymax, col=linecol,lwd=linew)
    }
    if(abs(segmat[r,c-1]-segmat[r,c])>0) {
      yloc <- (c-1)/(newdim[2])
      xmin <- (r-1)/(newdim[1])
      xmax <- (r-0)/(newdim[1])
      segments(xmin, yloc, xmax, yloc, col=linecol,lwd=linew)
    }
  }
}
# Add the normalized Laplacian contour
segmat <- segmatL
linecol <- "green"
linew <- 3
for(r in 2:newdim[1]) {
  for (c in 2:newdim[2]) {
    if(abs(segmat[r-1,c]-segmat[r,c])>0) {
      xloc <- (r-1)/(newdim[1])
```

```
# Add the normalized Laplacian contour
segmat <- segmatL
linecol <- "green"
linew <- 3
for(r in 2:newdim[1]) {
  for (c in 2:newdim[2]) {
    if(abs(segmat[r-1,c]-segmat[r,c])>0) {
      xloc <- (r-1)/(newdim[1])
      ymin <- (c-1)/(newdim[2])
      ymax <- (c-0)/(newdim[2])
      segments(xloc, ymin, xloc, ymax, col=linecol,lwd=linew)
    }
    if(abs(segmat[r,c-1]-segmat[r,c])>0) {
      yloc <- (c-1)/(newdim[2])
      xmin <- (r-1)/(newdim[1])
      xmax <- (r-0)/(newdim[1])
      segments(xmin, yloc, xmax, yloc, col=linecol,lwd=linew)
    }
  }
}
```

8.5.2   Point Cloud Segmentation Using Spectral Clustering

Let's try spectral clustering for segmenting point clouds using the knee pain dataset and the `kernlab::specc()` method (Fig. 8.17).

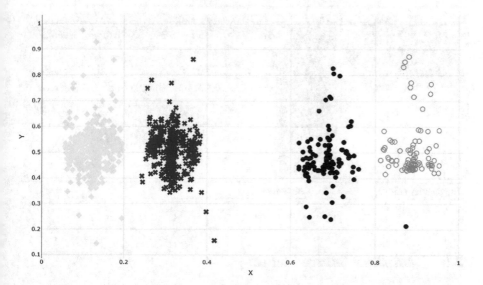

Fig. 8.17 Point cloud segmentation using spectral clustering (knee pain dataset). Colors and glyph-shapes are used to discriminate the derived class labels. The original data represents four native clusters corresponding to the front (left two scatterplots) and back (right two scatterplots) views on the left and right knee. Each point indicates the knee pain location identified by the patients

```
#Get the data first
library("XML"); library("xml2"); library("rvest")
wiki_url <- read_html("https://wiki.socr.umich.edu/index.php/SOCR_Data_KneePainData_041409")
html_nodes(wiki_url, "#content")
kneeRawData <- html_table(html_nodes(wiki_url, "table")[[2]])
normalize<-function(x) { return((x-min(x))/(max(x)-min(x))) }
kneeRawData_df <- as.data.frame(cbind(normalize(kneeRawData$x),
normalize(kneeRawData$Y), as.factor(kneeRawData$View)))
colnames(kneeRawData_df) <- c("X", "Y", "Label")
# randomize the rows of the DF as RF, RB, LF and LB labels of classes
# which are by default sequentially ordered
set.seed(1234)
kneeRawData_df <- kneeRawData_df[sample(nrow(kneeRawData_df)), ]
# summary(kneeRawData_df) # View(kneeRawData_df)
# Artificially reduce the data size from 8K to 1K to get faster results
kneeDF <- data.frame(x=kneeRawData_df[1:1000,1], y=kneeRawData_df[1:1000, 2],
                     class=as.factor(kneeRawData_df[1:1000, 3]))
head(kneeDF)
##               x          y class
## 1 0.69096672 0.4479769     1
## 2 0.88431062 0.7716763     3
# Do the spectral clustering
library(kernlab)
knee_data <- cbind(kneeDF$x, kneeDF$y); dim(knee_data)
spectral_knee <- specc(knee_data, iterations=10, centers=4)
plot_ly(x = ~knee_data[,1], y = ~knee_data[,2], type = 'scatter',
        mode = 'markers', symbol = ~unlist(spectral_knee@.Data),
        symbols = c('circle','x','o', 'diamond'),
        color = ~unlist(spectral_knee@.Data), marker = list(size = 10)) %>%
  layout("Knee-pain data (L+R & F+B) with derived Spectral Color/Symbol
        Clustering Labels", xaxis=list(title="X"), yaxis=list(title="Y")) %>%
  hide_colorbar()
```

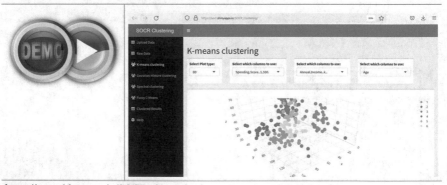

https://socr.shinyapps.io/SOCR_Clustering/

8.6   Gaussian Mixture Models

Recall the general univariate distribution mixture modeling we showed using the crystallography data in Chap. 2. Gaussian mixture modeling is a special case of distribution mixture modeling using normal distribution components (Fig. 8.18).

```r
crystallography_data <- read.csv(file =
"https://umich.instructure.com/files/11653615/download?download_frd=1", header=TRUE)
# install.packages("mixtools")
library(mixtools)
fit_Gauss <- list()
capture.output(
  for(i in 1:col_num) {    # remove all non-numeric elements (if any)
    data_no_NA <-
        crystallography_data[complete.cases(crystallography_data[, i]), i]
    length(data_no_NA)
    fit_Gauss[[i]] <- normalmixEM(data_no_NA,k=3,verb=F) # summary(fit_LN[i])
  },
  file='NUL'
)
library(plotly)
# Custom design of Normal-Mixture Model plot
normalMM.plot <- function(mix.object, dataSet, k = 3, main = "") {
  data_no_NA <- dataSet
  d3 <- function(x) { # construct the mixture using the estimated parameters
    mix.object$lambda[1]*dnorm(x, mean=mix.object$mu[1],
                               sd=mix.object$sigma[1]) +
    mix.object$lambda[2]*dnorm(x, mean=mix.object$mu[2],
                               sd=mix.object$sigma[2]) +
    mix.object$lambda[3]*dnorm(x, mean=mix.object$mu[3],
                               sd=mix.object$sigma[3])
  }
  x <- seq(min(data_no_NA), max(data_no_NA), 0.1)
  d_list <- list()
  for (i in 1:3) {
    # construct each of the Gaussian components using estimated parameters
    d_list[[i]] = mix.object$lambda[i]*dnorm(x, mean=mix.object$mu[1],
                                             sd=mix.object$sigma[i])
  }
  pl <- plot_ly() %>%
    add_trace(x=~x, y=~(10*d3(x)), type="scatter", mode="lines",
              name="Mixture of 3 Gaussian Models") %>%
    add_trace(x=~x, y=~(10*d_list[[1]]), type="scatter", mode="lines",
              name=paste0("Gaussian Mixture Component ", 1)) %>%
    add_trace(x=~x, y=~(10*d_list[[2]]), type="scatter", mode="lines",
              name=paste0("Gaussian Mixture Component ", 2)) %>%
    add_trace(x=~x, y=~(10*d_list[[3]]), type="scatter", mode="lines",
              name=paste0("Gaussian Mixture Component ", 3)) %>%
    add_trace(x = ~data_no_NA, type="histogram", histnorm = "probability",
              name = "Data histogram") %>%
    layout(title = "Gaussian Mixture Modeling (1D)",
           xaxis=list(title="data values"), yaxis=list(title="frequency"),
           legend = list(orientation='h'), bargap=0.2)
  return (pl)
}
i=1
data_no_NA <-crystallography_data[complete.cases(crystallography_data[,i]),i]
normalMM.plot(mix.object=fit_Gauss[[i]], dataSet=data_no_NA, k=3,
              main=paste0("Mixture of ", 3, " Normal Models"))
```

When modeling a process using a mixture of k Gaussian distributions, the probability of observing an outcome x_n is given by the weighted averaging (linear mixture) of the corresponding k Gaussian probabilities

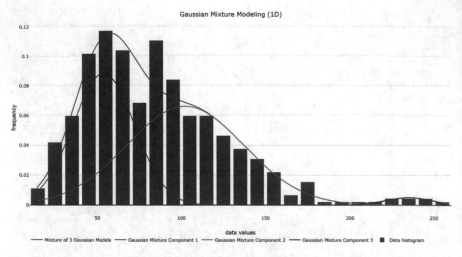

Fig. 8.18 Gaussian mixture modeling of crystallography data. This example of a mixture of three distributions illustrates the process of deriving class-labels for each data observation based on its closest match to one of the three univariate Gaussian distribution models fit to the entire dataset

$$p(x_n) = \sum_k \left(\underbrace{p(x_n | z_n = k)}_{\substack{k^{\text{th}} \text{ Gaussian} \\ \text{Probability}}} \times \underbrace{p(z_n = k)}_{\text{prior}} \right).$$

The *probability* represents the specific Gaussian mixture component, N-$(x_n | \mu_k, \Sigma_k)$, and the *prior* represents the mixture proportion. The probability $p(x_n)$ describes how each data point x_n can be generated from the prior distribution on the k model components, $\pi_k = p(z_n = k)$, choosing a cluster first, and then how to generate values of the data point from the corresponding model distribution, $N(\mu_k, \Sigma_k)$.

For a mixture of k Gaussians, the GMM distribution has $\theta = \{\mu_l, \Sigma_l, \pi_l, 1 \le l \le k\}$ parameters. We want to obtain the maximum likelihood estimate (MLE) of the unknown parameter vector θ. When all data and classes (x_i, z_i) are observed, we can maximize the data log-likelihood function for (x_i, z_i) using $p(x_i, z_i)$. However, when only a fraction of x_i's is observed, the situation is much more difficult, as we can only maximize the data log-likelihood for (x_i) based on $p(x_i)$. Using the expectation maximization (EM) algorithm,[9] we can maximize the expected data log-likelihood for (x_i, z_i) based on $p(x_i, z_i)$.

To learn the mixture models when the data and classes are fully observed, we assume that the data are independent and identically distributed (IID), which helps

---

[9]https://escholarship.org/uc/item/1rb70972

simplify the joint probability distribution. The log-likelihood decomposes into a sum of local terms. The MLE exists since the two optimization problems, for each Gaussian component (μ_k, Σ_k) and for each weight parameter π_k, are decoupled, and there exists a closed-form MLE solution

$$l_c(\theta|\text{Data}) = \sum_k \log\left(p(x_n, z_n|\theta) \equiv \underbrace{\sum_k \log\left(p(z_n|\theta)\right.}_{\text{depends on } \pi_k} + \underbrace{\sum_k \log\left(p(x_n|z_n, \theta)\right.}_{\text{depends on } (\mu_k, \Sigma_k)}$$

More explicitly,

$$l(\theta|\text{Data}) = \log\prod_n p(x_n, z_n|\theta) = \log\prod_n (p(z_n|\pi)p(x_n|z_n, \mu, \sigma))$$

$$= \sum_n \log\prod_k \pi_k^{z_n^k} + \sum_n \log\prod_k (N(x_n|\mu_k, \sigma))^{z_n^k}$$

$$= \sum_n\sum_k z_n^k \log\pi_k - \sum_n\sum_k (z_n^k \frac{1}{2\sigma^2}(x_n - \mu_k)^2) + \text{const.}$$

The corresponding MLE estimates are

- $\widehat{\pi}_k^{MLE} = \arg\max{}_\pi l(\theta|\text{Data})$,
- $\widehat{\mu}_k^{MLE} = \arg\max{}_\mu l(\theta|\text{Data}) \equiv \dfrac{\sum z_n^k x_n}{\sum z_n^k}$,
- $\widehat{\sigma}_k^{MLE} = \arg\max{}_\sigma l(\theta|\text{Data})$.

Below is a brief introduction to GMM using the `Mclust()` function in the R package `mclust`.

For multivariate mixture, there are totally 14 possible models:

- "EII" = spherical, equal volume
- "VII" = spherical, unequal volume
- "EEI" = diagonal, equal volume and shape
- "VEI" = diagonal, varying volume, equal shape
- "EVI" = diagonal, equal volume, varying shape
- "VVI" = diagonal, varying volume and shape
- "EEE" = ellipsoidal, equal volume, shape, and orientation
- "EVE" = ellipsoidal, equal volume and orientation (*)
- "VEE" = ellipsoidal, equal shape and orientation (*)
- "VVE" = ellipsoidal, equal orientation (*)
- "EEV" = ellipsoidal, equal volume and equal shape
- "VEV" = ellipsoidal, equal shape
- "EVV" = ellipsoidal, equal volume (*)
- "VVV" = ellipsoidal, varying volume, shape, and orientation

Additional practical and theoretical details about model-based clustering and discriminant analysis are available here.[10] Let's use the Divorce and Consequences on Young Adults dataset for a quick illustration where the optimal model, VEI, has three Gaussian components (Fig. 8.19).

```
library(mclust)
set.seed(1234)
gmm_clust <- Mclust(di_z)
summary(gmm_clust, parameters = TRUE)
gmm_clust$modelName
## [1] "VEI"
plot(gmm_clust$BIC, legendArgs = list(x = "bottom", ncol = 2, cex = 1))
plot(gmm_clust, what = "density")
plot(gmm_clust, what = "classification")
plot(gmm_clust, what = "uncertainty", dimens = c(6,7), main = "livewithmom vs.
gethitched")
# Mclust Dimension Reduction clustering
gmm_clustDR <- MclustDR(gmm_clust, lambda=1)
summary(gmm_clustDR)
## ----------------------------------------------------------------
## Dimension reduction for model-based clustering and classification
## ----------------------------------------------------------------
## Mixture model type: Mclust (VEI, 3)
## Clusters   n
##         1 16
##         2 11
##         3 20
## Estimated basis vectors:
##                   Dir1       Dir2
## DIVYEAR      -0.963455   0.033455
## momint        0.018017  -0.024376
## dadint       -0.020111   0.094546
## momclose     -0.018771   0.107977
## depression    0.017151   0.089764
## livewithmom   0.069653  -0.971657
## gethitched    0.255983   0.159729
##                   Dir1     Dir2
## Eigenvalues     1.9604    1.007
## Cum. %         66.0653  100.000
plot(gmm_clustDR, what = "boundaries", ngrid = 200)
plot(gmm_clustDR, what = "pairs")
plot(gmm_clustDR, what = "scatterplot")
# Plot the Silhouette plot to assess the quality of
# the clustering based on the Mixture of 3 Gaussians
silGauss = silhouette(as.numeric(gmm_clustDR$classification), dis)
plot(silGauss, col=1:length(gmm_clustDR$class2mixcomp), border=NA)
```

To assess the model, we can print the confusion matrix comparing, say, the Mclust clustering labels (3 columns) against the divorce$depression categories (4 rows).

---

[10] https://doi.org/10.1198/016214502760047131

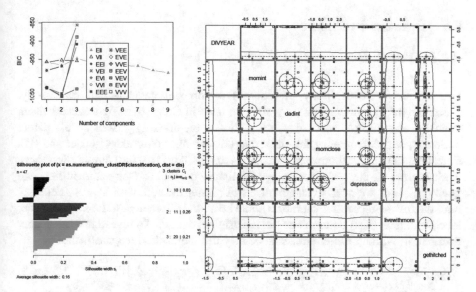

Fig. 8.19 Summary plots of multivariate Gaussian mixture modeling results (Divorce and Consequences on Young Adults dataset)

```
table(divorce$depression, qmm_clust$classification)
## 1 2 3
## 1 2 0 1
## 2 3 5 6
## 3 4 5 8
## 4 7 1 5
```

8.7 Summary

- K-means, spectral, hierarchical, and Gaussian mixture-modeling clustering may be most appropriate for exploratory data analytics but can also be used for deriving computed class labels. These techniques are highly flexible and fairly efficient in terms of tessellating data into groups.
- Clustering approaches may be used for data that has no a priori class categories (labels), i.e., for unsupervised AI/ML.
- The generated clusters may lead to phenotype stratification and/or be compared against known clinical traits.

8.8 Practice Problems

8.8.1 Youth Development

Use the Boys Town Study of Youth Development data, second case study, CaseStudy02_Boystown_Data.csv, that we used in Chap. 6, to find clusters using variables about GPA, alcohol abuse, attitudes on drinking, social status, parent closeness, and delinquency for clustering (all variables other than gender and ID). First, load the data and transfer sex, dadjob and momjob into dummy variables. Then, extract all the variables, except the first two columns (subject identifiers and genders). Next, we need to standardize and cluster the data with k = 3. You may have the following centers (numbers could be a little different). Add *k-means* cluster labels as a new (last) column back in the original dataset. To investigate the gender distribution within different clusters we may use the method aggregate().

```
boystown<-
    read.csv("https://umich.instructure.com/files/399119/download?download_frd=1",
             sep=" ")
boystown$sex<-boystown$sex-1
boystown$dadjob <- (-1)*(boystown$dadjob-2)
boystown$momjob <- (-1)*(boystown$momjob-2)
str(boystown)
boystown_sub<-boystown[, -c(1, 2)]
# Compute the averages for the variable 'sex', grouped by cluster
aggregate(data=boystown, sex~clusters, mean)
##    clusters        sex
## 1         1 0.6216216
## 2         2 0.6527778
## 3         3 0.6481481
```

Here the object clusters represents the new vector indicating the derived cluster labels. The gender distribution does not vary much between different cluster labels.

Readers may also try to apply these classification techniques to other data in the canvas archive of case studies.

Chapter 9
Model Performance Assessment, Validation, and Improvement

In previous chapters, we used several measures, such as prediction accuracy, to evaluate classification and regression models. In general, accurate predictions for one dataset do not necessarily imply that our model is perfect nor that it will reproduce when tested on external or prospective data. We need additional metrics to evaluate the model performance and ensure it is robust, reproducible, reliable, and unbiased.

In this chapter, we will (1) discuss various evaluation strategies for prediction, clustering, classification, regression, and decision-making; (2) demonstrate performance visualization, e.g., visualization of ROC curves; (3) discuss performance tradeoffs; and (4) present internal statistical cross-validation and bootstrap sampling.

9.1 Measuring the Performance of Classification Methods

Prediction accuracy represents just one evaluation aspect of classification model performance and reliability assessment of clustering methods. Different classification models and alternative clustering techniques may be appropriate for different situations. For example, when screening newborns for rare genetic defects, we may want the model to have as few true-negatives as possible. We don't want to classify anyone as "noncarriers" when they actually may have a defective gene, since early treatment might impact near- and long-term life experiences.

We can use the following three types of data to evaluate the performance of a classifier model:

- Actual class values (for supervised classification)
- Predicted class values
- Estimated probabilities of the prediction

We have already seen examples of these cases. For instance, the last type of validation relies on the predict(model, test_data) function that we used previously in the classification and regression chapters (Chaps. 3, 4, 5, and 6). Let's revisit some of the models and test data we discussed in Chap. 5—Inpatient Head and Neck Cancer Medication data. We will demonstrate prediction probability estimation using the data in CaseStudy14_HeadNeck_Cancer_Medication.csv.

```
hn_med <-
    read.csv("https://umich.instructure.com/files/1614350/download?download_frd=1",
                    stringsAsFactors = FALSE)
hn_med$seer_stage <- factor(hn_med$seer_stage)
library(tm)
hn_med_corpus <- Corpus(VectorSource(hn_med$MEDICATION_SUMMARY))
 corpus_clean <- tm_map(hn_med_corpus, tolower)
 corpus_clean <- tm_map(corpus_clean, removePunctuation)
 corpus_clean <- tm_map(corpus_clean, stripWhitespace)
 corpus_clean <- tm_map(corpus_clean, removeNumbers)
 hn_med_dtm    <- DocumentTermMatrix(corpus_clean)
 hn_med_train <- hn_med[1:562, ]
 hn_med_test  <- hn_med[563:662, ]
 hn_med_dtm_train <- hn_med_dtm[1:562, ]
 hn_med_dtm_test <- hn_med_dtm[563:662, ]
 corpus_train <- corpus_clean[1:562]
 corpus_test <- corpus_clean[563:662]
 hn_med_train$stage <- hn_med_train$seer_stage %in% c(4, 5, 7)
 hn_med_train$stage <- factor(hn_med_train$stage, levels=c(F, T),
                            labels = c("early_stage", "later_stage"))
 hn_med_test$stage <- hn_med_test$seer_stage %in% c(4, 5, 7)
 hn_med_test$stage <- factor(hn_med_test$stage, levels=c(F, T),
                            labels = c("early_stage", "later_stage"))
convert_counts <- function(x) {
  x <- ifelse(x > 0, 1, 0)
  x <- factor(x, levels = c(0, 1), labels = c("No", "Yes"))
  return(x)
}
hn_med_dict <- as.character(findFreqTerms(hn_med_dtm_train, 5))
hn_train <- DocumentTermMatrix(corpus_train, list(dictionary=hn_med_dict))
hn_test   <- DocumentTermMatrix(corpus_test, list(dictionary=hn_med_dict))
hn_train <- apply(hn_train, MARGIN = 2, convert_counts)
hn_test   <- apply(hn_test, MARGIN = 2, convert_counts)
library(e1071)
hn_classifier <- naiveBayes(hn_train, hn_med_train$stage)
pred_raw <- predict(hn_classifier, hn_test, type="raw")
head(pred_raw)
##      early_stage later_stage
## [1,]   0.8812634  0.11873664
## [2,]   0.8812634  0.11873664
## [3,]   0.8425828  0.15741724
## [4,]   0.9636007  0.03639926
## [5,]   0.8654298  0.13457022
## [6,]   0.8654298  0.13457022
```

The above output includes the prediction probabilities for the first six rows of the data. This example is based on a naïve Bayes classifier (naiveBayes); however, the same approach works for any other machine learning classification or prediction technique. The `type="raw"` indicates that the prediction call will return the *conditional a-posterior probabilities* for each class. When we set the parameter `type="class"`, the `predict()` method returns the class label corresponding to the *maximal probability*.

In addition, we can report the predicted probability with the outputs of the naïve Bayesian decision-support system

```
hn_classifier <- naiveBayes(hn_train, hn_med_train$stage)

pred_nb <- predict(hn_classifier, hn_test)
head(stats::ftable(pred_nb))
## "pred_nb" "early_stage" "later_stage"
##                        96             4
```

The general predict() method automatically subclasses to the specific predict.naiveBayes(object, newdata, type = c("class", "raw"), threshold = 0.001, ...) call, where type="raw" and type = "class" specify the output as the conditional a-posterior probabilities for each class or the class with maximal probability, respectively. Back in Chap. 5, we discussed the C5.0 and the randomForest classifiers to predict the chronic disease score in another case study, quality of life (QoL).

```
qol <-
     read.csv("https://umich.instructure.com/files/481332/download?download_frd=1")
qol <- qol[!qol$CHRONICDISEASESCORE==-9, ]
qol$cd <- qol$CHRONICDISEASESCORE>1.497
qol$cd <- factor(qol$cd, levels=c(F, T),
                 labels = c("minor_disease", "severe disease"))
qol <- qol[order(qol$ID), ]
# Remove ID (col=1) # the clinical Diagnosis (col=41) will be handled later
qol <- qol[ , -1]
set.seed(1234)          # 80-20% training-testing data split
train_index <- sample(seq_len(nrow(qol)), size = 0.8*nrow(qol))
qol_train <- qol[train_index, ]
qol_test <- qol[-train_index, ]
library(C50)
set.seed(1234)
qol_model <- C5.0(qol_train[,-c(40, 41)], qol_train$cd)
```

Below are the *probability* results of the C5.0 classification tree model prediction.

```
pred_prob <- predict(qol_model, qol_test, type="prob")
head(pred_prob)
##      minor_disease severe_disease
## 1        0.3762353      0.6237647
## 3        0.3762353      0.6237647
## 4        0.2942230      0.7057770
## 9        0.7376664      0.2623336
## 10       0.3762353      0.6237647
## 12       0.3762353      0.6237647
```

These can be contrasted against the C5.0 tree *classification* label results.

```
pred_tree <- predict(qol_model, qol_test)
head(pred_tree); head(stats::ftable(pred_tree))
## [1] severe_disease severe_disease severe_disease minor_disease  …
## Levels: minor_disease severe_disease
##  "pred_tree" "minor_disease" "severe_disease"
##                          214             229
```

Similar complementary types of outputs can be reported for most machine learning classification, regression, and prediction approaches.

9.2   Evaluation Strategies

In Chap. 5, we saw an attempt to categorize the supervised classification and unsupervised clustering methods. Similarly, the *table* below summarizes the basic types of evaluation and validation strategies for different forecasting, prediction, ensembling, and clustering techniques. (Internal) statistical cross-validation or external validation should always be applied to ensure reliability and reproducibility of the results. The SciKit clustering performance evaluation and classification metrics sections provide details about many alternative techniques and metrics for performance evaluation of clustering and classification methods.[1]

Inference	Outcome	Evaluation metrics	R functions
Classification and prediction	Binary	Accuracy, sensitivity, specificity, PPV/precision, NPV/recall, LOR	`caret:: confusionMatrix`, `gmodels::CrossTable`, `cluster::silhouette`
Classification and prediction	Categorical	Accuracy, sensitivity/specificity, PPV, NPV, LOR, Silhouette coefficient	`caret:: confusionMatrix`, `gmodels::CrossTable`, `cluster::silhouette`
Regression modeling	Real quantitative	Correlation coefficient, R^2, RMSE, mutual information, homogeneity and completeness scores	`cor`, `metrics::mse`

9.2.1   Binary Outcomes

This Table 9.1 summarizes the key measures commonly used to evaluate the performance of binary tests, classifiers, or predictions.

---

[1] https://doi.org/10.3389/fninf.2014.00014

Table 9.1 Simple performance metrics for binary outcome classifiers

Binary outcome metrics		Actual condition		Test interpret
		Absent (H_0 is true)	Present (H_1 is true)	
Test result	Negative (fail to reject H_0)	TN Condition absent + negative result = true (accurate) negative	FN Condition present + negative result = false (invalid) negative type II error (proportional to β)	NPV = $\frac{TN}{TN+FN}$
	Positive (reject H_0)	FP Condition absent + positive result = false positive type I error (α)	TP Condition present + positive result = true positive	PPV = Precision = $\frac{TP}{TP+FP}$
Test interpret	Power = $1 - \beta$ = $1 - \frac{FN}{FN+TP}$	Specificity = $\frac{TN}{TN+FP}$	Power = Recall= Sensitivity = $\frac{TP}{TP+FN}$	LOR = $\ln\left(\frac{TN \times TP}{FP \times FN}\right)$

9.2.2 Cross Tables, Contingency Tables, and Confusion-Matrices

In ML and AI, the concepts of *cross table, contingency table,* and *confusion matrix* are often used to quantify the performance of a classifier. A contingency table represents a statistical cross tabulation that summarizes the multivariate frequency distribution of two (or more) categorical variables. In the special case of cross tabulating the performance of an AI classifier relative to ground truth, this comparison is referred to as a *confusion matrix*, for supervised learning, or a *matching matrix*, for unsupervised learning. Typically, the rows and columns in these cross tables represent observed instances in predicted and actual class labels, respectively.

We already saw some confusion matrices in Chap. 8. For binary classes, these will be just 2×2 matrices where each of the cells represents the agreement, match, or discrepancy between the real and predicted class labels, indexed by the row and column indices, as illustrated below:

cross table	predict_T	predict_F
TRUE	TP	TN
FALSE	FP	FN

- **True Positive**(TP): Number of observations that are correctly classified as "yes" or "success"
- **True Negative**(TN): Number of observations that are correctly classified as "no" or "failure"
- **False Positive**(FP): Number of observations that are incorrectly classified as "yes" or "success"

- **False Negative**(FN): Number of observations that are incorrectly classified as "no" or "failure"

Using confusion matrices to measure performance: The way we calculate accuracy using these four cells is summarized by the following formula

$$\text{accuracy} = \frac{TP + TN}{TP + TN + FP + FN} = \frac{TP + TN}{\text{Total number of observations}}.$$

On the other hand, the error rate, or proportion of incorrectly classified observations is calculated using:

$$\text{error rate} = \frac{FP + FN}{TP + TN + FP + FN} \equiv \frac{FP + FN}{\text{Total number of observations}} = 1 - \text{accuracy}.$$

If we look at the numerator and denominator carefully, we can see that the error rate and accuracy add up to 1. Therefore, a 95% accuracy means 5% error rate. In R, we have multiple ways to obtain a confusion table. The simplest way would be table(). For example, in Chap. 5, to get a plain 2×2 table reporting the agreement between the real clinical cancer labels and their machine learning predicted counterparts, we saw the following example:

```
hn_test_pred <- predict(hn_classifier, hn_test)
table(hn_test_pred, hn_med_test$stage)
## hn_test_pred  early_stage later_stage
##    early_stage          73          23
##    later_stage           4           0
```

The reason we sometimes use the gmodels::CrossTable() function, e.g., see Chap. 5, is because it reports additional information about the model performance.

```
library(gmodels)
CrossTable(hn_test_pred, hn_med_test$stage)
##   Cell Contents
## |-------------------------|
## |                       N |
## |   Chi-square contribution |
## |           N / Row Total |
## |           N / Col Total |
## |         N / Table Total |
## |-------------------------|
## Total Observations in Table:  100
##              | hn_med_test$stage
## hn_test_pred | early_stage | later_stage |  Row Total |
## ------------ |------------ |------------ |----------- |
## early_stage  |          73 |          23 |         96 |
##              |       0.011 |       0.038 |            |
##              |       0.760 |       0.240 |      0.960 |
```

```
##             |     0.948 |     1.000 |           |
##             |     0.730 |     0.230 |           |
## ----------- | --------- | --------- | --------- |
## later_stage |         4 |         0 |         4 |
##             |     0.275 |     0.920 |           |
##             |     1.000 |     0.000 |     0.040 |
##             |     0.052 |     0.000 |           |
##             |     0.040 |     0.000 |           |
## ----------- | --------- | --------- | --------- |
## Column Total |        77 |        23 |       100 |
##             |     0.770 |     0.230 |           |
## ----------- | --------- | --------- | --------- |
```

The second entry in each cell of the *crossTable* table reports the Chi-square contribution. This uses the standard Chi-square formula for computing relative discrepancy between *observed* and *expected* counts. For instance, the Chi-square contribution of *cell(1,1)*, (hn_med_test$stage=early_stage and hn_test_pred=early_stage), can be computed as follows from the $\frac{(\text{Observed} - \text{Expected})^2}{\text{Expected}}$ formula. Assuming independence between the rows and columns (i.e., random classification), the *expected cell(1,1) value* is computed as the product of the corresponding row (96) and column (77) marginal counts, $\frac{96 \times 77}{100}$. Thus the Chi-square value for cell(1,1) is

$$\text{Chi} - \text{square cell}(1, 1) = \frac{(\text{Observed} - \text{Expected})^2}{\text{Expected}} = \frac{\left(73 - \frac{96 \times 77}{100}\right)^2}{\frac{96 \times 77}{100}} = 0.01145022.$$

Note, that each cell Chi-square value represents one of the four (in this case) components of the Chi-square test-statistics, which tries to answer the question if there is no association between observed and predicted class labels. That is, under the null-hypothesis there is no association between actual and observed counts for each level of the factor variable, which allows us to quantify whether the derived classification agrees with the real class annotations (labels). The aggregate sum of all Chi-square values represents the χ_o^2 statistics

$$\chi_o^2 = \sum_{\text{all categories}} \frac{(O - E)^2}{E} \sim X_{\text{df}}^2,$$

where the degrees of freedom parameter is df = (#rows − 1) × (#columns − 1).

We can calculate accuracy and error rate by hand or by using either table(), CrossTable(), or confusionMatrix().

```
accuracy <- (73+0)/100
accuracy     ## [1] 0.73
error_rate <- (23+4)/100
error_rate   ## [1] 0.27
1-accuracy   ## [1] 0.27
```

For matrices that are larger than 2 × 2, all diagonal elements count the observations that are correctly classified, and the off-diagonal elements represent incorrectly labeled cases.

9.2.3   Other Measures of Performance Beyond Accuracy

So far we discussed two performance methods—table() and CrossTable(). A third function is caret::confusionMatrix() which provides the easiest way to report model performance. Notice that the first argument is an *actual vector of the labels*, i.e., *Test _ Y* and the second argument, of the same length, represents the *vector of predicted labels*. This example was presented as the first case study in Chap. 5.

```
library(caret)
qol_pred <- predict(qol_model, qol_test)
confusionMatrix(table(qol_pred, qol_test$cd), positive="severe_disease")
```

9.2.3.1   Silhouette Coefficient

In Chap. 8, we saw the *Silhouette coefficient*, which captures the shape of the clustering boundaries. It is a function of the *intracluster distance* of a sample in the dataset (*i*). Recall that:

- d_i is the average dissimilarity of point *i* with all other data points within its cluster. Then, d_i captures the quality of the assignment of *i* to its current class label. Smaller or larger d_i values suggest better or worse overall assignment for *i* to its cluster, respectively. The average dissimilarity of *i* to a cluster *C* is the average distance between *i* and all points in the cluster of points labeled *C*.
- l_i is the lowest average dissimilarity of point *i* to any other cluster that *i* is not a member of. The cluster corresponding to l_i, the lowest average dissimilarity, is called the *i* neighboring cluster, as it is the next best fit cluster for *i*.

  Then, the *Silhouette coefficient* for a sample point *i* is:

$$-1 \leq Silhouette(i) = \frac{l_i - d_i}{\max{(l_i, d_i)}} \leq 1.$$

The *mean Silhouette value* represents the arithmetic average of all Silhouette coefficients (either within a cluster, or overall) and represents the quality of the cluster (clustering). High mean Silhouette corresponds to compact clustering (dense and separated clusters), whereas low values represent more diffused clusters. The Silhouette value is useful when the number of predicted clusters is smaller than the number of samples.

9.2.3.2   The Kappa (κ) Statistic

The Kappa statistic was originally developed to measure the reliability between two human raters.[2] It can be harnessed in machine learning applications to compare the accuracy of a classifier, where one rater represents the ground truth (for labeled data, these are the actual values of each instance) and the second rater represents the results of the automated machine learning classifier. The order of listing the **raters** is irrelevant.

Kappa statistic measures the **possibility of a correct prediction by chance alone** and answers the question of *How much better is the agreement (between the ground truth and the machine learning prediction) than would be expected by chance alone?* Its value is between 0 and 1. When $\kappa = 1$, we have a perfect agreement between a **computed** prediction (typically the result of a model-based or model-free technique forecasting an outcome of interest) and an **expected** prediction (typically random, by-chance, prediction).

A common interpretation of the Kappa statistics includes:

* *Poor* agreement: less than 0.20
* *Fair* agreement: 0.20–0.40
* *Moderate* agreement: 0.40–0.60
* *Good* agreement: 0.60–0.80
* *Very good* agreement: 0.80–1

In the above confusionMatrix output, we have a fair agreement. For different problems, we may have different interpretations of Kappa statistics. To understand Kappa statistic better, let's look at its definition.

Predicted/observed	Minor	Severe	Row sum
Minor	$A = 143$	$B = 71$	$A + B = 214$
Severe	$C = 72$	$D = 157$	$C + D = 229$
Column sum	$A + C = 215$	$B + D = 228$	$A + B + C + D = 443$

In this table, $A = 143, B = 71, C = 72, D = 157$ denote the frequencies (counts) of cases within each of the cells in the 2×2 design. Then,

$$\text{Observed Agreement} = (A + D) = 300.$$

$$\text{Expected Agreement} = \frac{(A + B) \times (A + C) + (C + D) \times (B + D)}{A + B + C + D} = 221.72.$$

$$\text{(Kappa)}\ \kappa = \frac{(\text{Observed Agreement}) - (\text{Expected Agreement})}{(A + B + C + D) - (\text{Expected Agreement})} = 0.35.$$

---

[2] https://doi.org/10.1002/sim.4780090917

In this manual calculation of kappa statistics (κ), we used the corresponding values we saw earlier in the quality of life (QoL) case study, where chronic-disease (cd) binary outcome qol$cd<-qol$CHRONICDISEASESCORE>1.497, and we also used the cd prediction (qol_pred).

```
table(qol_pred, qol_test$cd)
## qol_pred minor_disease severe_disease
## minor_disease 143 71
## severe_disease 72 157
```

According to the above table, high agreement between actual and predicted chronic-disease corresponds to the high algorithmic performance (accuracy).

```
A=143; B=71; C=72; D=157
# A+B+ C+D # 443
# ((A+B)*(A+C)+(C+D)*(B+D))/(A+B+C+D)    # 221.7201
EA=((A+B)*(A+C)+(C+D)*(B+D))/(A+B+C+D) # Expected accuracy
OA=A+D; OA    # Observed accuracy ## [1] 300
k=(OA-EA)/(A+B+C+D - EA); k # 0.3537597
# Compare against the official kappa score
confusionMatrix(table(qol_pred, qol_test$cd),
                positive="severe_disease")$overall[1] # report official Kappa
##    Kappa
## 3.537597e-01
```

The manually and automatically computed accuracies coincide ($\sim$0.35). When computing Kappa, it may be trickier to obtain the expected agreement. Probability rules tell us that the probability of the union of two *disjoint events* equals the sum of the individual (marginal) probabilities for these two events. We get a similar value in the confusionTable() output. A more straightforward way of getting the Kappa statistics is by using the Kappa() function in the vcd package.

```
# install.packages(vcd)
library(vcd)
Kappa(table(qol_pred, qol_test$cd))
##              value     ASE      z Pr(>|z|)
## Unweighted 0.3538 0.04446 7.957 1.76e-15
## Weighted   0.3538 0.04446 7.957 1.76e-15
```

The combination of Kappa() and table function yields a 2 × 4 matrix. The *Kappa statistic* is under the unweighted value. Generally speaking, predicting a severe disease outcome is a more critical problem than predicting a mild disease state. Thus, weighted Kappa is also useful. We give the severe disease a higher weight. The Kappa test result is not acceptable since the classifier may make too many mistakes for the severe disease cases. The Kappa value is 0.26374. Notice that the range of weighted Kappa may exceed [0,1].

```
Kappa(table(qol_pred, qol_test$cd),weights = matrix(c(1,10,1,10),nrow=2))
##              value      ASE        z  Pr(>|z|)
## Unweighted  0.353760 0.04446  7.95721 1.760e-15
## Weighted   -0.004386 0.04667 -0.09397 9.251e-01
```

When the predicted value is the first argument, the row and column names represent the **true labels** and the **predicted labels**, respectively.

```
table(qol_pred, qol_test$cd)
## qol_pred minor_disease severe_disease
## minor_disease 143 71
## severe_disease 72 157
```

9.2.3.3   Summary of the Kappa Score for Calculating Prediction Accuracy

Kappa compares an **Observed classification accuracy** (output of our ML classifier) with an **Expected classification accuracy** (corresponding to random chance classification). It may be used to evaluate single classifiers and/or to compare a set of different classifiers. It takes into account random chance (agreement with a random classifier). That makes **Kappa** more meaningful than simply using the **accuracy** as a single quality metric.

For instance, the interpretation of an Observed Accuracy of 80% is **relative** to the Expected Accuracy. An Observed Accuracy of 80% is more impactful for a corresponding Expected Accuracy of 50% relative to an Expected Accuracy of 75%.

9.2.3.4   Sensitivity and Specificity

Take a closer look at the confusionMatrix() output where we can find two important statistics - "sensitivity" and "specificity." Sensitivity or true positive rate measures the proportion of "success" observations that are correctly classified

$$\text{sensitivity} = \frac{TP}{TP + FN}.$$

Notice TP + FN are the total number of true "success" observations. On the other hand, specificity or true negative rate measures the proportion of "failure" observations that are correctly classified

$$\text{sensitivity} = \frac{TN}{TN + FP}.$$

Accordingly, TN + FP are the total number of true "failure" observations. In the QoL data, considering "severe_disease" as "success" and using the table() function output we can manually compute the *sensitivity* and *specificity*, as well as the corresponding *precision* and *recall* measures.

```
sens <- 131/(131+89)
sens
## [1] 0.5954545
spec <- 149/(149+74)
spec
## [1] 0.6681614
```

Another R package `caret` also provides functions to directly calculate the sensitivity and specificity.

```
library(caret)
sensitivity(qol_pred, qol_test$cd, positive="severe_disease")
## [1] 0.6885965
# specificity(qol_pred, qol_test$cd)
confusionMatrix(table(qol_pred, qol_test$cd),
positive="severe_disease")$byClass[1] # another way to report the sensitivity
## Sensitivity
##    0.6885965
# confusionMatrix(table(qol_pred, qol_test$cd),
positive="severe_disease")$byClass[2] # another way to report the specificity
```

Sensitivity and specificity both range from 0 to 1. For either measure, a value of 1 implies that the positive and negative predictions are very accurate. However, simultaneously high sensitivity and specificity may not be attainable in real world situations. There is a tradeoff between sensitivity and specificity. To compromise, some studies loosen the demands on one and focus on achieving high values on the other.

9.2.3.5   Precision and Recall

Very similar to sensitivity, *precision* measures the proportion of true "success" observations among predicted "success" observations

$$\text{precision} = \frac{\text{TP}}{\text{TP} + \text{FP}}.$$

Recall is the proportion of true "failures" among all "failures." A model with high recall captures most "interesting" cases

$$\text{recall} = \frac{\text{TP}}{\text{TP} + \text{FN}}.$$

Again, let's calculate these by hand for the QoL data and report the Area under the ROC Curve (AUC) (Fig. 9.1).

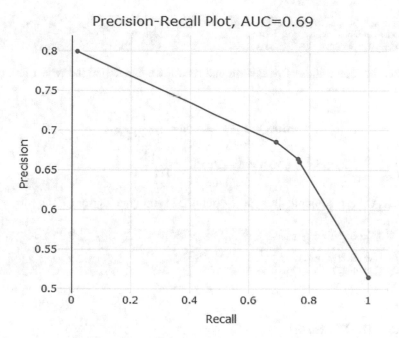

Fig. 9.1 Algorithmic performance, precision vs. recall plot

```
prec    <- 157/(157+72); prec
## [1] 0.6855895
recall <- 157/(157+71); recall
## [1] 0.6885965
library (ROCR)
library(plotly)
qol_pred <- predict(qol_model, qol_test)
qol_pred <- predict(qol_model, qol_test, type = 'prob')
pred <- prediction( qol_pred[,2], qol_test$cd)
PrecRec <- performance(pred, "prec", "rec")
PrecRecAUC <- performance(pred, "auc")
paste0("AUC=", round(as.numeric(PrecRecAUC@y.values), 2))
## [1] "AUC=0.69"
# plot(PrecRec)
plot_ly(x = ~PrecRec@x.values[[1]][2:length(PrecRec@x.values[[1]])],
        y = ~PrecRec@y.values[[1]][2:length(PrecRec@y.values[[1]])],
        name = 'Recall-Precision relation', type='scatter',
        mode='markers+lines') %>%
  layout(title=paste0("Precision-Recall Plot, AUC=",
                      round(as.numeric(PrecRecAUC@y.values[[1]]), 2)),
         xaxis=list(title="Recall"), yaxis=list(title="Precision"))
```

Another way to obtain *precision* would be posPredValue() in the caret package. Remember to specify which one is the "success" class.

```
qol_pred <- predict(qol_model, qol_test)
posPredValue(qol_pred, qol_test$cd, positive="severe_disease")
## [1] 0.6855895
```

From the definitions of **precision** and **recall**, we can derive the type 1 and type 2 errors as follows

$$\text{error}_1 = 1 - \text{Precision} = \frac{FP}{TP + FP}.$$

$$\text{error}_2 = 1 - \text{Recall} = \frac{FN}{TN + FN}.$$

Thus, we can compute the type 1 error (0.31) and type 2 error (0.31).

```
error1<-1-prec; error1
## [1] 0.3144105
error2<-1-recall; error2
## [1] 0.3114035
```

9.2.3.6   The F-Measure

The F-measure, or *F1-score*, combines precision and recall using the *harmonic mean* assuming equal weights. High F1-score means high precision and high recall. This is a convenient way of measuring model performances and comparing models

$$F1 = \frac{2 \times \text{precision} \times \text{recall}}{\text{recall} + \text{precision}} = \frac{2 \times TP}{2 \times TP + FP + FN}$$

Let's calculate the F1-score by hand using the quality of life prediction model.

```
f1 <- (2*prec*recall)/(prec+recall)
f1
## [1] 0.6870897
```

We can contrast these results against direct calculations of the F1-statistics obtained using caret.

```
precision <- posPredValue(qol_pred, qol_test$cd, positive="severe_disease")
recall <- sensitivity(qol_pred, qol_test$cd, positive="severe_disease")
F1 <- (2 * precision * recall) / (precision + recall); F1
## [1] 0.6870897
```

9.2.4   Visualizing Performance Tradeoffs (ROC Curve)

Another choice for evaluating classifiers' performance is by graphs rather than scalars, numerical vectors, or statistics. Graphs are usually more comprehensive than single statistics.

The R package ROCR provides user-friendly functions for visualizing model performance.

Here, we evaluate the model performance for the quality of life case study in Chap. 5.

```
# install.packages("ROCR")
library(ROCR)
pred <- ROCR::prediction(predictions=pred_prob[, 2], labels=qol_test$cd)
# avoid naming collision (ROCR::prediction), as
# there is another prediction function in the neuralnet package.
```

The prediction() method argument pred_prob[, 2] stores the probability of classifying each observation as "severe_disease", and we saved all model prediction information into the object pred. Receiver operating characteristic (ROC) curves[3] are often used for examining the trade-off between detecting true positives and avoiding the false positives (Fig. 9.2).

```
x <- seq(from=0, to=1.0, by=0.01) + 0.001
plot_ly(x = ~x, y = (log(100*x)+2.3)/(log(100*x[101])+2.3),
        line=list(color="lightgreen"),
        name='Test Classifier', type='scatter', mode='lines', showlegend=T) %>%
    add_lines(x=c(0,1), y=c(0,1), line=list(color="black", dash='dash'),
                name="Classifier with no predictive value") %>%
    add_segments(x=0, xend=0, y=0, yend = 1, line=list(color="blue"),
                name="Perfect Classifier") %>%
    add_segments(x=0, xend=1, y=1, yend = 1, line=list(color="blue"),
                name="Perfect Classifier 2", showlegend=F) %>%
    layout(title="ROC curve", legend = list(orientation = 'h'),
        xaxis=list(title="False Positive Rate", scaleanchor="y", range=c(0,1)),
        yaxis=list(title="True Positive Rate", scaleanchor="x"))
```

The blue line in the ROC graph represents the perfect classifier where we have 0% false positives and 100% true positives. The green line in the middle represents a test classifier. Most of our classifiers trained by real data will look like this. The black diagonal line illustrates a classifier with no predictive value. We can see that it has the same true positive rate and false positive rate. Thus, it cannot distinguish between the two states.

Classifiers with high true positive values have ROC curves near the (blue) *perfect classifier* curve. Thus, we measure the area under the ROC curve (abbreviated as AUC) as a proxy of the classifier performance. To do this, we have to change the

---

[3] https://doi.org/10.1177/0272989X8400400203

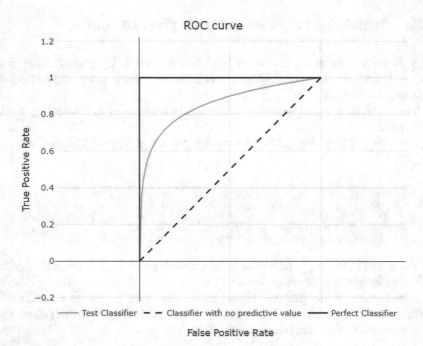

Fig. 9.2 Schematic of algorithmic performance, receiver operating characteristic (ROC) curve

scale of the graph above. Mapping 100% to 1, we have a 1×1 square. The area under perfect classifier would be 1 and area under classifier with no predictive value being 0.5. Then, 1 and 0.5 will be the upper and lower limits for our model ROC curve. For model ROC curves, the typical interpretation of the area under curve (AUC) includes

- Outstanding: 0.9–1.0
- Excellent/good: 0.8–0.9
- Acceptable/fair: 0.7–0.8
- Poor: 0.6–0.7
- No discrimination: 0.5–0.6

Note that this rating system is somewhat subjective. We can use the ROCR package to draw ROC curves.

```
roc <- performance(pred, measure="tpr", x.measure="fpr")
```

We can specify a "performance" object by providing `"tpr"` (true positive rate) and `"fpr"` (false positive rate) parameters (Fig. 9.3).

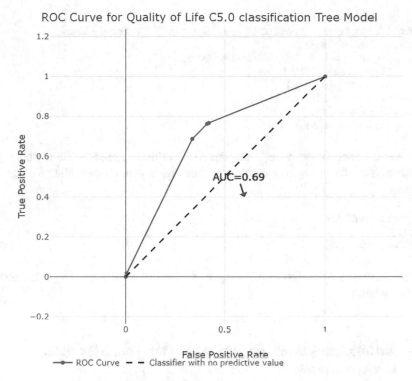

ROC Curve for Quality of Life C5.0 classification Tree Model

Fig. 9.3 Algorithmic performance, area under the ROC curve for the QoL C5.0 decision tree classification model predicting chronic disease (CD)

```
plot_ly(x = ~roc@x.values[[1]], y = ~roc@y.values[[1]],
        name = 'ROC Curve', type='scatter', mode='markers+lines') %>%
  add_lines(x=c(0,1), y=c(0,1), line=list(color="black", dash='dash'),
            name="Classifier with no predictive value") %>%
  layout(title="ROC Curve for Quality of Life C5.0 classification Tree Model",
         legend = list(orientation = 'h'),
         xaxis=list(title="False Positive Rate", scaleanchor="y", range=c(0,1)),
         yaxis=list(title="True Positive Rate", scaleanchor="x"),
         annotations = list(text=paste0("AUC=",
             round(as.numeric(performance(pred, "auc")@y.values[[1]]), 2)),
             x=0.6, y=0.4, textangle=0,
             font=list(size=15, color="blue", showarrow=FALSE)))
```

The *segments* command draws the dash line representing a classifier with no predictive value. To measure the model performance quantitatively, we need to create a new performance object with measure="auc" for the area under the curve (AUC).

```
roc_auc <- performance(pred, measure="auc")
```

Now the roc_auc is stored as a S4 object. This is quite different from data frames and matrices. First, we can use the str() function to examine its structure.

```
str(roc_auc)
## Formal class 'performance' [package "ROCR"] with 6 slots
## ..@ x.name : chr "None"
## ..@ y.name : chr "Area under the ROC curve"
## ..@ alpha.name : chr "none"
## ..@ x.values : list()
## ..@ y.values :List of 1
## .. ..$ : num 0.692
## ..@ alpha.values: list()
```

It has 6 members or "slots," and the AUC value is stored in the member y. values. To extract object members, we use the @ symbol according to str() output.

```
roc_auc@y.values
## [[1]]
## [1] 0.6915953
```

The resulting $AUC = 0.69$, which suggests a fair classifier, according to the above scoring schema.

9.3   Estimating Future Performance (Internal Statistical Cross-validation)

The evaluation methods we have talked about are all measuring re-substitution error. That involves building the model on *training data* and measuring the model performance (error/accuracy) on *testing data*. This evaluation process provides one mechanism of dealing with unseen data. Let's look at some alternative strategies.

9.3.1   The Holdout Method

The holdout method idea is to partition a dataset into two separate sets. Using the first set to create (train) the model and the other to test (validate) the model performance. In practice, we usually use a fraction (e.g., 60%, $\frac{3}{5}$) of our data for training the model, and reserve the rest (e.g., 40%, $\frac{2}{5}$) for testing. Note that the testing data may also be further split into proportions for internal repeated (e.g., cross-validation) testing and final external (independent) testing.

The partition has to be randomized. In R, the best way of doing this is to create a parameter that randomly draws numbers and use this parameter to extract random rows from the original dataset. In Chap. 6, we used this method to partition the *Google Trends* data.

Another way of partitioning is using the `caret::createDatePartition`
() method. We can subset the original dataset or any independent variable column
of the original dataset, e.g., `google_norm$RealEstate`.

```
sub <- caret::createDataPartition(google_norm$RealEstate, p=0.75, list = F)
google_train <- google_norm[sub, ]
google_test <- google_norm[-sub, ]
```

To make sure that the model can be applied to future datasets, we can partition the
original dataset into three separate subsets. In this way, we have two subsets of data
for testing and validation. The additional validation dataset can alleviate the probability that we have a good model due to chance (nonrepresentative subsets). A
common split among training, testing, and validation subsets may be 50%, 25%, and
25%, respectively.

```
sub <- sample(nrow(google_norm), floor(nrow(google_norm)*0.50))
google_train <- google_norm[sub, ]
google_test <- google_norm[-sub, ]
sub1 <- sample(nrow(google_test), floor(nrow(google_test)*0.5))
google_test1 <- google_test[sub1, ]
google_test2 <- google_test[-sub1, ]
nrow(google_norm)
## [1] 731
nrow(google_train) # training                            ## [1] 365
nrow(google_test1) # testing: internal cross validation ## [1] 183
nrow(google_test2) # testing: out of bag validation     ## [1] 183
```

However, when we only have a very small dataset, it's difficult to split off too
much data as this may excessively reduce the training sample size. There are the
following two options for evaluation of model performance with unseen data. Both
of these are implemented in the `caret` package.

9.3.2 Cross-validation

The complete details about cross-validation will be presented below. Now, we
describe the fundamentals of cross-validation as an internal statistical validation
technique. This technique is known as *k-fold cross-validation*, or *k-fold CV*, which is
a standard for estimating model performance. K-fold CV randomly partitions the
original data into k separate random subsets called folds.

A common practice is to use $k = 10$ or 10-fold CV. That is to split the data into
10 different subsets. Each time, one of the subsets is reserved for testing, and the rest
are employed for learning/building the model. This can be accomplished using the
`caret::createFolds()` method. Using `set.seed()` ensures the reproducibility of the created folds, in case you run the code multiple times. Here, we use
`1234`, a random number, to seed the fold separation. You can use any number for

set.seed(). We demonstrate the process using the normalized Google Trend dataset.

```
library("caret")
set.seed(1234)
folds <- createFolds(google_norm$RealEstate, k=10)
str(folds)
## List of 10
##  $ Fold01: int [1:73] 9 12 28 31 42 54 62 81 83 86 ...
##  $ Fold02: int [1:73] 20 23 47 61 63 72 82 88 96 100 ...
##  $ Fold03: int [1:73] 15 22 26 43 49 53 73 80 101 109 ...
##  $ Fold04: int [1:74] 5 17 38 52 55 74 91 92 141 142 ...
##  $ Fold05: int [1:73] 7 14 29 35 37 39 41 48 51 57 ...
##  $ Fold06: int [1:73] 4 18 33 36 44 59 70 77 78 112 ...
##  $ Fold07: int [1:73] 6 40 45 65 66 69 71 94 98 102 ...
##  $ Fold08: int [1:73] 19 24 27 50 60 75 76 97 99 106 ...
##  $ Fold09: int [1:74] 3 11 13 16 21 30 32 34 46 56 ...
##  $ Fold10: int [1:72] 1 2 8 10 25 67 68 105 111 126 ...
```

Another way to cross-validate is to use methods such as sparsediscrim::
cv_partition() or caret::createFolds().

```
# install.packages("sparsediscrim")
library(sparsediscrim)
folds2 = cv_partition(1:nrow(google_norm), num_folds=10)
```

And the structure of folds may be reported by

```
str(folds2)
## List of 10
## $ Fold1 :List of 2
## ..$ training: int [1:657] 1 2 3 4 5 6 7 8 9 10 ...
## ..$ test : int [1:74] 493 338 652 368 698 55 261 407 379 648 ...
...
## $ Fold10:List of 2
## ..$ training: int [1:658] 1 2 4 5 6 7 8 9 10 11 ...
## ..$ test : int [1:73] 595 57 86 83 387 666 495 715 45 96 ...
```

Now, we have 10 different subsets in the folds object. We can use lapply() to fit the model. Ninety percent of the data will be used for training so we use [-x,] to represent all observations not in a specific fold. In Chap. 6, we built a neural network model for the *Google Trends* data. We can do the same for each fold manually. Then we can train test the model and aggregate the model performance results. Finally, we can report the overall agreement (e.g., correlations between the predicted and observed RealEstate values).

```
library(neuralnet)
fold_cv <- lapply(folds, function(x){
  google_train <- google_norm[-x, ]
  google_test  <- google_norm[x, ]
  google_model <- neuralnet(RealEstate~Unemployment+Rental+Mortgage+Jobs+
                            Investing+DJI_Index+StdDJI, data=google_train)
  google_pred  <- compute(google_model, google_test[, c(1:2, 4:8)])
  pred_results <- google_pred$net.result
  pred_cor     <- cor(google_test$RealEstate, pred_results)
  return(pred_cor)
})
str(fold_cv)
## List of 10
##  $ Fold01: num [1, 1] 0.972
##  $ Fold02: num [1, 1] 0.979
##  $ Fold03: num [1, 1] 0.976
##  $ Fold04: num [1, 1] 0.975
##  $ Fold05: num [1, 1] 0.977
##  $ Fold06: num [1, 1] 0.981
##  $ Fold07: num [1, 1] 0.974
##  $ Fold08: num [1, 1] 0.973
##  $ Fold09: num [1, 1] 0.977
##  $ Fold10: num [1, 1] 0.972
```

From the output, we know that in most of the folds the model predicts very well. In a typical run, one fold may yield bad results. We can use the *mean* of these 10 correlations to represent the *overall* model performance. But first, we need to use the unlist() function to transform fold_cv into a vector.

```
mean(unlist(fold_cv)) ## [1] 0.9756676
```

This high correlation suggests a strong association between predicted and true values. Thus, the model is very good in terms of its prediction.

9.3.3   Bootstrap Sampling

The second method is called *bootstrap sampling*. In k-fold CV, each observation can only be used once for testing, i.e., sampling without replacement. Bootstrap sampling relies on a sampling *with replacement* process. Before selecting a new sample, it recycles every observation so that each observation could appear in multiple folds.

At each iteration, bootstrap sampling uses 63.2% of the original data as our training dataset and the remaining 36.8% as the test dataset. Thus, compared to k-fold CV, bootstrap sampling is less representative of the full dataset. A special case of bootstrapping is the *0.632 bootstrap* technique, which addresses this issue by changing the final performance error assessment formula to

$$\text{error} = 0.632 \times \text{error}_{\text{test}} + 0.368 \times \text{error}_{\text{train}}.$$

This synthesizes the *optimistic model performance* on training data (error$_\text{train}$) with the *pessimistic model performance* on testing data (error$_\text{test}$) by weighting the corresponding errors. This method is extremely reliable for small samples (it may be computationally intensive for large samples).

To see the (asymptotics) rationale behind the *0.632 bootstrap* technique, consider a standard training set T of cardinality n where our bootstrapping sampling generates m new training sets T_i, each of size n'. As sampling from T is uniform *with replacement*, some observations may be repeated in each sample T_i. Suppose the size of the sub-samples are of the same order as T, i.e., $n' = n$, then for large n the sample T_i is *expected* to have $\left(1 - \frac{1}{e}\right) \sim 0.632$ unique cases from the complete original collection T; the remaining proportion 0.368 are expected to be repeated duplicates. Hence the name *0.632 bootstrap* sampling. A particular training data element has a probability of $1 - \frac{1}{n}$ of not being picked for training; hence, its probability of being in the testing set is $\left(1 - \frac{1}{n}\right)^n = e^{-1} \approx 0.368$. The simulation below illustrates the *0.632* bootstrap experimentally.

```
# define the total data size
n <- 500
# define number of Bootstrap iterations
N=2000
#define resampling function, compute the proportion of uniquely selected elements
uniqueProportions <- function(myDataSet, sampleSize){
    indices <- sample(1:sampleSize,sampleSize,replace=TRUE) #sample w/ Replacement
    length(unique(indices))/sampleSize
}
# compute the N proportions of unique elements (could also use a for loop)
proportionsVector <- c(lapply(1:N, uniqueProportions, sampleSize=n),
                       recursive=TRUE)
# Expected (mean) proportion of unique elements in bootstrapping samples of n
mean(proportionsVector)
## [1] 0.632138
```

In general, for large $n \ll n'$, the sample T_i is *expected* to have $n\left(1 - e^{-n'/n}\right)$ unique cases.[4]

Having the bootstrap samples, the m models can be fitted (estimated) and aggregated, e.g., by averaging the outputs (for regression) or using voting methods (for classification). We will discuss this more in later chapters. Let's look at the implementation of the 0.632 Bootstrap technique for the *QoL* case study.

---

[4]https://doi.org/10.1177/003754979105600207

```
# Recall: qol_model <- C5.0(qol_train[,-c(40, 41)], qol_train$cd)
# predict labels of testing data
qol_pred <- predict(qol_model, qol_test)
# compute matches and mismatches of Predicted and Observed class labels
predObsEqual <- qol_pred == qol_test$cd
predObsTF <- c(table(predObsEqual)[1], table(predObsEqual)[2]); predObsTF
## FALSE   TRUE
##   143    300
# training error rate
train.err <- as.numeric(predObsTF[1]/(predObsTF[1]+predObsTF[2]))
# testing error rate, Leave-one-out Bootstrap (LOOB) Cross-Validation
B <- 10
loob.err <- NULL
N <- dim(qol_test)[1]    # size of test-dataset
for (b in 1:B) {
   bootIndices <- sample(1:N, N*0.9, replace=T)
   train <- qol_test[bootIndices, ]
   qol_modelBS <- C5.0(train[,-c(40, 41)], train$cd)
   inner.err <- NULL
   # for current iteration extract the appropriate testing cases for testing
   i <- (1:length(bootIndices))
   i <- i[is.na(match(i, bootIndices))]
   test <- qol_test[i, ]
   # predict using model at current iteration
   qol_modelBS_pred <- predict(qol_modelBS, test)
   predObsEqual <- qol_modelBS_pred == test$cd
   predObsTF <- c(table(predObsEqual)[1], table(predObsEqual)[2]); predObsTF
   # training error rate
   inner.err <- as.numeric(predObsTF[1]/(predObsTF[1]+predObsTF[2]))
   loob.err <- c(loob.err, mean(inner.err))
}
test.err <- ifelse(is.null(loob.err), NA, mean(loob.err))
# 0.632 Bootstrap error
boot.632 <- 0.368 * train.err + 0.632 * test.err; boot.632
## [1] 0.3876717
```

9.4 Improving Model Performance by Parameter Tuning

We already explored several alternative machine learning (ML) methods for prediction, classification, clustering, and outcome forecasting. In many situations, we derive models by estimating model coefficients or parameters. The main question now is: *How can we adopt crowd-sourcing advantages of social networks to aggregate different predictive analytics strategies?*

Are there reasons to believe that such **ensembles** of forecasting methods actually improve the performance or boost the prediction accuracy of the resulting consensus meta-algorithm? In this section, we are going to introduce ways to search for optimal parameters for a single ML method as well as aggregate different methods into **ensembles** to augment their collective performance, relative to any of the individual methods part of the meta-algorithm.

Recall that earlier in Chap. 6, we presented strategies for improving model performance based on *meta-learning*, *bagging*, and *boosting*. One of the methods

Table 9.2 Core parameters of several machine learning techniques

Model	Learning task	Method	Parameters
KNN	Classification	`class::knn`	`data, k`
K-means	Classification	`stats::kmeans`	`data, k`
Naive Bayes	Classification	`e1071::naiveBayes`	`train, class, laplace`
Decision trees	Classification	`C50::C5.0`	`train, class, trials, costs`
OneR rule learner	Classification	`RWeka::OneR`	`class~predictors, data`
RIPPER rule learner	Classification	`RWeka::JRip`	`formula, data, subset, na.action, control, options`
Linear regression	Regression	`stats::lm`	`formula, data, subset, weights, na.action, method`
Regression trees	Regression	`rpart::rpart`	`dep_var ~ indep_var, data`
Model trees	Regression	`RWeka::M5P`	`formula, data, subset, na.action, control`
Neural networks	Dual use	`nnet::nnet`	`x, y, weights, size, Wts, mask, linout, entropy, softmax, censored, skip, rang, decay, maxit, Hess, trace, MaxNWts, abstol, reltol`
SVM (polynomial kernel)	Dual use	`caret::train::svmLinear`	`C`
SVM (radial basis kernel)	Dual use	`caret::train::svmRadial`	`C, sigma`
SVM (general)	Dual use	`kernlab::ksvm`	`formula, data, kernel`
Random forests	Dual use	`randomForest::randomForest`	`formula, data`

for improving model performance relies on *tuning*. For a given ML technique, tuning is the process of searching through the parameter space for the optimal parameter(s). The following Table 9.2 summarizes some of the parameters used in ML techniques we covered in previous chapters.

9.4.1   Using `caret` for Automated Parameter Tuning

In Chap. 5, we used kNN and plugged in random k parameters for the number of clusters. This time we will simultaneously test multiple k values and select the parameter(s) yielding the highest prediction accuracy. Using `caret` allows us to specify an outcome class variable, covariate predictor features, and a specific ML method. In Chap. 5, we showed the Boys Town Study of Youth Development dataset, where we normalized all the features, stored them in a `boystown_n` computable object, and defined an outcome class variable (`boystown$grade`).

```
boystown <-
    read.csv("https://umich.instructure.com/files/399119/download?download_frd=1", sep=" ")
boystown$sex <- boystown$sex-1
boystown$dadjob <- -1*(boystown$dadjob-2)
boystown$momjob <- -1*(boystown$momjob-2)
boystown <- boystown[, -1]
table(boystown$gpa)
## 0  1  2  3  4  5
## 30 50 54 40 14 12
boystown$grade <- boystown$gpa %in% c(3, 4, 5)
boystown$grade <- factor(boystown$grade, levels=c(F, T),
                         labels = c("above_avg", "avg_or_below"))
normalize <- function(x) {   return((x-min(x))/(max(x)-min(x))) }
boystown_n <- as.data.frame(lapply(boystown[, -11], normalize))
str(boystown_n)
boystown_n <- cbind(boystown_n, boystown[, 11])
str(boystown_n)
colnames(boystown_n)[11] <- "grade"
```

Now that the dataset includes an explicit class variable and predictor features, we can use the KNN method to predict the outcome `grade`. Let's plug this information into the `caret::train()` function. Note that `caret` can use the complete dataset, as it will automatically do the random sampling for the internal statistical cross-validation. To make results reproducible, we may utilize the `set.seed()` function that we presented earlier.

```
library(caret)
set.seed(123)
kNN_mod <- train(grade~., data=boystown_n, method="knn")
kNN_mod; summary(kNN_mod)
## k-Nearest Neighbors
## Resampling results across tuning parameters:
##   k  Accuracy   Kappa
##   5  0.7971851  0.5216369
##   7  0.8037923  0.5282107
##   9  0.7937086  0.4973139
## Accuracy was used to select the optimal model using the largest value.
## The final value used for the model was k = 7.
```

In this case, using `str(m)` to summarize the object m may report out too much information. Instead, we can simply type the object name m to get a more concise information about it.

1. Description about the dataset: number of samples, features, and classes.
2. Re-sampling process: here it is using 25 bootstrap samples with 200 observations (same size as the observed dataset) each to train the model.
3. Candidate models with different parameters that have been evaluated: by default, `caret` uses three different choices for each parameter, but for binary parameters,

it only takes two choices TRUE and FALSE). As KNN has only one parameter k, we have three-candidate models reported in the output above.
4. Optimal model: the model with largest accuracy is the one corresponding to k = 9.

Let's see how accurate this "optimal model" is in terms of the re-substitution error. Again, we will use the predict() function specifying the object m and the dataset boystown_n. Then, we can report the contingency table showing the agreement between the predictions and real class labels.

```
set.seed(1234)
pred <- predict(kNN_mod, boystown_n)
table(pred, boystown_n$grade)
##   pred              above_avg avg_or_below
##     above_avg            132           17
##     avg_or_below           2           49
```

This model has (17 + 2)/200 = 0.09 re-substitution error (9%). This means that in the 200 observations that we used to train this model, 91% of them were correctly classified. Note that re-substitution error is different from accuracy. The accuracy of this model is 0.81, which is reported by a model summary call. As mentioned earlier, we can obtain prediction probabilities for each observation in the original boystown_n dataset.

```
head(predict(kNN_mod, boystown_n, type = "prob"))
##     above_avg avg_or_below
## 1 0.0000000    1.0000000
## 2 1.0000000    0.0000000
## 3 0.7142857    0.2857143
## 4 0.8571429    0.1428571
## 5 0.2857143    0.7142857
## 6 0.5714286    0.4285714
```

9.5   Customizing the Tuning Process

The default setting of train() might not meet the specific needs for every study. In our case, the optimal k might be smaller than 9. The caret package allows us to customize the settings for train(). Specifically, caret::trainControl() can help us to customize re-sampling methods. There are six popular re-sampling methods that we might want to use, which are summarized in this Table 9.3.

Each of these methods rely on alternative representative sampling strategies to train the model. Let's use *0.632 bootstrap* for example. Just specify method="boot632" in the trainControl() function. The number of different samples to include can be customized by the number= option. Another option in trainControl() allows specification of the model performance evaluation. We can select a preferred method of evaluation for choosing the optimal

Table 9.3 Core re-sampling methods

Resampling method	Method name	Additional options and default values
Holdout sampling	LGOCV	$p = 0.75$ (training data proportion)
k-fold cross-validation	cv	number $= 10$ (number of folds)
Repeated k-fold cross-validation	repeatedcv	number $= 10$ (number of folds), repeats $= 10$ (number of iterations)
Bootstrap sampling	boot	number $= 25$ (resampling iterations)
0.632 bootstrap	boot632	number $= 25$ (resampling iterations)
Leave-one-out cross-validation	LOOCV	None

model. For instance, the `oneSE` method chooses the simplest model within one standard error of the best performance to be the optimal model. Other strategies are also available in the `caret` package. For detailed information, type `?best` in the R console.

We can also specify a list of *k* values we want to test by creating a matrix or a grid.

```
ctrl <- trainControl(method="boot632", number=25, selectionFunction="oneSE")
grid <- expand.grid(k=c(1, 3, 5, 7, 9))
# Creates a data frame from all combinations of the supplied factors
```

Usually, to avoid ties, we prefer to choose an odd number of clusters *k*. Now the constraints are all set. We can start to select models again using `train()`.

```
set.seed(123)
kNN_mod2 <-train(grade ~ ., data=boystown_n, method="knn",
          metric="Kappa", trControl=ctrl, tuneGrid=grid)
kNN_mod2
##    k  Accuracy   Kappa
##    1  0.8748058  0.7155507
##    3  0.8389441  0.6235744
##    5  0.8411961  0.6254587
##    7  0.8384469  0.6132381
##    9  0.8341422  0.5971359
## Kappa was used to select the optimal model using  the one SE rule.
## The final value used for the model was k = 1.
```

Here we added `metric="Kappa"` to include the *Kappa statistics* as one of the criteria to select the optimal model. We can see the output accuracy for all the candidate models are better than the default bootstrap sampling. The optimal model has *k = 1*, a high accuracy of 0.861, and a high Kappa statistic, which is much better than the model we had in Chap. 5. Note that the output based on the SE rule may not necessarily choose the model with the highest accuracy or the highest Kappa statistic as the "optimal model." The tuning process is more comprehensive than only looking at one statistic.

9.6   Comparing the Performance of Several Alternative Models

Earlier in Chap. 5, we saw examples of how to choose appropriate evaluation metrics and how to contrast the performance of various AI/ML methods. Below, we illustrate model comparison based on the classification of case study 6, quality of life (QoL) dataset using bagging, boosting, random forest, SVN, k nearest neighbors, and decision trees (Figs. 9.4 and 9.5).

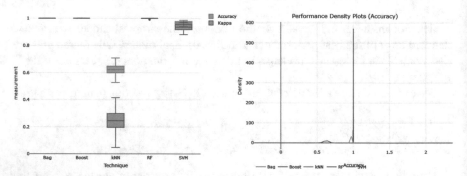

Fig. 9.4 Comparing the performance (kappa and accuracy) of several ML classifiers on the quality of life dataset

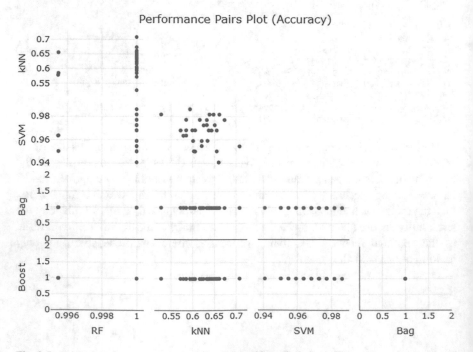

Fig. 9.5 Pairs plot of accuracy across different classifiers (QoL data)

```r
# install.packages(fastAdaboost)
library(fastAdaboost)
library(caret)    # for modeling
library(lattice)  # for plotting
control <- trainControl(method="repeatedcv", number=10, repeats=3)
## Run all subsequent models in parallel
library(doParallel)
cl <- makePSOCKcluster(5)
registerDoParallel(cl)
system.time({
  rf.fit        <- train(cd~., data=qol[, -37], method="rf", trControl=control);
  knn.fit       <- train(cd~., data=qol[, -37], method="knn", trControl=control);
  svm.fit       <- train(cd~., data=qol[, -37], method="svmRadialWeights",
                         trControl=control);
  adabag.fit    <- train(cd~., data=qol[, -37], method="AdaBag", trControl=control);
  adaboost.fit  <- train(cd~., data=qol[, -37], method="adaboost", trControl=control)
})
##    user  system elapsed
##    6.00    0.33  240.81
stopCluster(cl) # close multi-core cluster
rm(cl)
results <- resamples(list(RF=rf.fit, kNN=knn.fit, SVM=svm.fit,
                          Bag=adabag.fit, Boost=adaboost.fit))
# summary of model differences
summary(results)
## Accuracy
##              Min.   1st Qu.    Median      Mean   3rd Qu.      Max. NA's
## RF     0.9954751 1.0000000 1.0000000 0.9995489 1.0000000 1.0000000    0
## kNN    0.5270270 0.6004525 0.6238739 0.6225767 0.6475225 0.7090909    0
## SVM    0.9409091 0.9593219 0.9683971 0.9676231 0.9773499 0.9864865    0
## Bag    1.0000000 1.0000000 1.0000000 1.0000000 1.0000000 1.0000000    0
## Boost  1.0000000 1.0000000 1.0000000 1.0000000 1.0000000 1.0000000    0
## Kappa
##               Min.   1st Qu.    Median      Mean   3rd Qu.      Max. NA's
## RF     0.99092365 1.0000000 1.000000 0.9990954 1.0000000 1.0000000    0
## kNN    0.04709345 0.1967654 0.245143 0.2434337 0.2949951 0.4155251    0
## SVM    0.88132780 0.9183430 0.936674 0.9350707 0.9545693 0.9729290    0
## Bag    1.00000000 1.0000000 1.000000 1.0000000 1.0000000 1.0000000    0
## Boost  1.00000000 1.0000000 1.000000 1.0000000 1.0000000 1.0000000    0
library(tidyr)
results_long <- gather(results$values[, -1], method, measurement,
                       factor_key=TRUE) %>%
  separate(method, c("Technique", "Metric"), sep = "~")
# Compare original wide format to transformed long format
results$values[, -1]
library(plotly)
plot_ly(results_long, x=~Technique, y=~measurement, color=~Metric, type="box")
```

```
#densityplot(results, scales=scales, pch = "|") # Density plots of accuracy
densityModels <- with(results_long[which(results_long$Metric=='Accuracy'), ],
                      tapply(measurement, INDEX = Technique, density))
df <- data.frame(
  x = unlist(lapply(densityModels, "[[", "x")),
  y = unlist(lapply(densityModels, "[[", "y")),
  method = rep(names(densityModels), each = length(densityModels[[1]]$x))
)
plot_ly(df, x = ~x, y = ~y, color = ~method) %>% add_lines() %>%
  layout(title="Performance Density Plots (Accuracy)",
         legend = list(orientation='h'),
         xaxis=list(title="Accuracy"), yaxis=list(title="Density"))
densityModels <- with(results_long[which(results_long$Metric=='Kappa'), ],
                      tapply(measurement, INDEX = Technique, density))
df <- data.frame(
  x = unlist(lapply(densityModels, "[[", "x")),
  y = unlist(lapply(densityModels, "[[", "y")),
  method = rep(names(densityModels), each = length(densityModels[[1]]$x))
)
plot_ly(df, x = ~x, y = ~y, color = ~method) %>% add_lines() %>%
  layout(title="Performance Density Plots (Kappa)", legend =
list(orientation='h'),
         xaxis=list(title="Kappa"), yaxis=list(title="Density"))
# dotplot(results, scales=scales)            # Dot plots of Accuracy & Kappa
# splom(results)      # contrast pair-wise model scatterplots of prediction
accuracy (Trellis Scatterplot matrices)
# Pairs - Accuracy
results_wide <- results_long[which(results_long$Metric=='Accuracy'), -2] %>%
  pivot_wider(names_from = Technique, values_from = measurement)
df = data.frame(cbind(RF=results_wide$RF[[1]], kNN=results_wide$kNN[[1]],
                      SVM=results_wide$SVM[[1]], Bag=results_wide$Bag[[1]],
                      Boost=results_wide$Boost[[1]]))
dims <- dplyr::select_if(df, is.numeric)
dims <- purrr::map2(dims, names(dims), ~list(values=.x, label=.y))
plot_ly(type = "splom", dimensions = setNames(dims, NULL),
        showupperhalf = FALSE, diagonal = list(visible = FALSE)) %>%
  layout(title="Performance Pairs Plot (Accuracy)")
```

9.7   Forecasting Types and Assessment Approaches

Cross-validation is a strategy for validating predictive methods, classification models and clustering techniques by assessing the reliability and stability of the results of the corresponding statistical analyses (e.g., predictions, classifications, forecasts) based on independent datasets. For prediction of trend, association, clustering, and classification, a model is usually trained on one dataset (*training data*) and subsequently tested on new data (*testing or validation data*). Statistical internal cross-validation defines a test dataset to evaluate the model predictive performance as well as assess its power to avoid overfitting. *Overfitting* is the process of computing a predictive or classification model that describes random error, i.e., fits to the noise components of the observations, instead of identifying actual relationships and salient features in the data.

In this section, we will use Google Flu Trends, Autism, and Parkinson's disease case studies to illustrate (1) alternative forecasting types using linear and nonlinear predictions, (2) exhaustive and nonexhaustive internal statistical cross-validation, and (3) explore complementary predictor functions. In Chap. 5, we discussed the types of classification and prediction methods, including `supervised` and `unsupervised` learning. The former are direct and predictive (there are known outcome variables that can be predicted and the corresponding forecasts can be evaluated) and the latter are indirect and descriptive (there are no a priori labels or specific outcomes).

9.7.1 Overfitting

Before we go into the cross-validation of predictive analytics, we will present several examples of *overfitting* that illustrate why a certain amount of skepticism and mistrust may be appropriate when dealing with forecasting models based on large and complex data.

9.7.1.1 Example (US Presidential Elections)

By 2022, there were only **58 US presidential elections** and **46 presidents**. That is a small dataset and learning from it may be challenging. For instance

- If the predictor space expands to include things like *having false teeth*, it's pretty easy for the model to go from fitting the generalizable features of the data (the signal, e.g., presidential actions) to matching noise patterns (e.g., irrelevant characteristics like gender of the children of presidents, or types of dentures they may wear).
- When overfitting noise patterns takes place, the quality of the model fit assessed on the historical data may improve (e.g., better R^2, more about the Coefficient of Determination is available here). At the same time, however, the model performance may be suboptimal when used to make inferences about prospective data, e.g., future presidential elections.

9.7.1.2 Example (Google Flu Trends)

A March 14, 2014, article in Science[5] identified problems in Google Flu Trends (GFT),[6] which may be attributed in part to overfitting. The GFT was built to predict

---

[5] https://doi.org/10.1126/science.1248506

[6] https://doi.org/10.1371/journal.pone.0023610

the future Centers for Disease Control and Prevention (CDC) reports of doctor office visits for influenza-like illness (ILI). In February 2013, Nature reported that GFT was predicting more than double the proportion of doctor visits compared to the CDC forecast for the same period.

The GFT model found the best matches among 50 million web search terms to fit 1152 data points. It predicted quite high odds of finding search terms that match the propensity of the flu but are structurally unrelated and hence are not prospectively predictive. In fact, the GFT investigators reported that weeding out seasonal search terms unrelated to the flu may have been strongly correlated to the CDC data, e.g., high school basketball season. The big GFT data may have overfitted the relatively small number of cases. This false-alarm result was also paired with a false-negative finding. The GFT model also missed the nonseasonal 2009 H1N1 influenza pandemic, which provides a cautionary tale about prediction, overfitting, and prospective validation.

9.7.1.3   Example (Autism)

Autistic brains constantly overfit visual and cognitive stimuli. To an autistic person, a general conversation of several adults may seem like a cacophony due to supersensitive detail-oriented hearing and perception tuned to literally pick up all elements of the conversation and clues of the surrounding environment. At the same time, autistic brains downplay body language, sarcasm, and nonliteral cues. We can *miss the forest for the trees* when we start "overfitting," over-interpreting the noise on top of the actual salient information. Ambient noise, trivial observations, and unrelated perceptions may hide the true communication details.

Human conversations and communications involve exchanges of both critical information and random noise. Fitting a perfect model requires focus only on the "relevant" information. Overfitting occurs when attention is (excessively) consumed with peripheral noise, or worse, overwhelmed by inconsequential noise drowning the salient aspects of the communication exchange.

Any dataset is a mix of signal and noise. The main task of our brains is to sort these components and interpret the information (i.e., ignore the noise).

One person's noise is another person's treasure map!

Our predictions are most accurate if we can model as much of the signal and as little of the noise as possible. Note that in these terms, R^2 is a poor metric to identify predictive power - it measures how much of the signal **and** the noise is explained by our model. In practice, it's hard to always identify what is signal and what is noise. This is why practical applications tend to favor simpler models, since the more complicated a model is, the easier it is to overfit the noise component of the observed information.

9.8 Internal Statistical Cross-validation

Internal statistical cross-validation assesses the expected performance of a prediction method in cases (subject, units, regions, etc.) drawn from a similar population as the original training data sample. Internal validation is distinct from external validation, as the latter potentially allows for the existence of differences between the populations (training data, used to develop or train the technique, and testing data, used to independently quantify the performance of the technique). Each step in the internal statistical cross-validation protocol involves:

- Randomly partitioning a sample of data into two complementary subsets (training + testing).
- Performing the analysis, fitting or estimating the model using the training set.
- Validating the analysis or evaluating the performance of the model using a separate testing set.
- Increasing the iteration index and repeating the process. Various termination criteria can involve a fixed number, a desired mean variability, or an upper bound on the error-rate.

Here is one example of internal statistical cross-validation predictive diagnostic modeling in Parkinson's disease. To reduce the noise and variability at each iteration, the final validation results may include the averaged performance results of each iteration. In cases when new observations are hard to obtain (due to costs, reliability, time, or other constraints), cross-validation guards against testing hypotheses suggested by the data themselves (also known as Type III error or False-Suggestion).

Cross-validation is different from *conventional-validation* (e.g., 80–20% partitioning the dataset into training and testing subsets) where the prediction error (e.g., root mean square error, RMSE) evaluated on the training data is not a useful estimator of model performance, as it does not generalize across multiple samples.

In general, the errors of the conventional-valuation are based on the results of a specific test dataset and may not accurately represent the model performance. A more appropriate strategy to properly estimate model prediction performance is to use cross-validation (CV), which combines (averages) prediction errors to measure the model performance. CV corrects for the expected stochastic nature of partitioning the training and testing sets and generates a more accurate and robust estimate of the expected model performance.

Relative to a simpler model, a more complex model may *overfit the data* if it has a short foresight, i.e., it generates accurate fitting results for known data but less accurate results when predicting based on new data. Knowledge from past experiences may include either *relevant* or *irrelevant* (noise) information. In challenging data-driven prediction models when uncertainty (entropy) is high, more noise is present in past information that needs to be accounted for in prospective forecasting. However, it is generally hard to discriminate patterns from noise in complex systems (i.e., deciding which part to model and which to ignore). Models that reduce the chance of fitting noise are called *robust*.

9.8.1 Example (Linear Regression)

Let's demonstrate a simple model assessment using linear regression. Suppose we observe the response values $\{y_1, \cdots, y_n\}$, and the corresponding k predictors represented as a kD vector of covariates $\{x_1, \cdots, x_n\}$, where subjects/cases are indexed by $1 \leq i \leq n$, and the data-elements (variables) are indexed by $1 \leq j \leq k$

$$
\begin{pmatrix} x_{1,1} & \cdots & x_{1,k} \\ \vdots & \ddots & \vdots \\ x_{n,1} & \cdots & x_{n,k} \end{pmatrix}.
$$

Using least squares to estimate the linear function parameters (effect-sizes), $\beta_1, \cdots, \beta_k$, allows us to compute a hyperplane $y = a + x\beta$ that best fits the observed data $(x_i, y_i)_{1 \leq i \leq n}$. This is expressed as a matrix by

$$
\begin{pmatrix} y_1 \\ \vdots \\ y_n \end{pmatrix} = \begin{pmatrix} a_1 \\ \vdots \\ a_n \end{pmatrix} + \begin{pmatrix} x_{1,1} & \cdots & x_{1,k} \\ \vdots & \ddots & \vdots \\ x_{n,1} & \cdots & x_{n,k} \end{pmatrix} \begin{pmatrix} \beta_1 \\ \vdots \\ \beta_k \end{pmatrix}.
$$

Corresponding to the system of linear hyperplanes

$$
\begin{cases} y_1 = a_1 + x_{1,1}\beta_1 + x_{1,2}\beta_2 + \cdots + x_{1,k}\beta_k \\ y_2 = a_2 + x_{2,1}\beta_1 + x_{2,2}\beta_2 + \cdots + x_{2,k}\beta_k \\ \vdots \\ y_n = a_n + x_{n,1}\beta_1 + x_{n,2}\beta_2 + \cdots + x_{n,k}\beta_k \end{cases}.
$$

One measure to evaluate the model fit may be the mean squared error (MSE). The MSE for a given value of the parameters α and β on the observed training data $(x_i, y_i)_{1 \leq i \leq n}$ is expressed as

$$
\mathrm{MSE} = \frac{1}{n} \sum_{i=1}^{n} \left(y_i - \underbrace{(a_1 + x_{i,1}\beta_1 + x_{i,2}\beta_2 + \cdots + x_{i,k}\beta_k)}_{\text{predicted value } \hat{y}_i, \text{ at } x_{i,1}, \cdots, x_{i,k}} \right)^2.
$$

And the corresponding root mean square error (RMSE) is

$$\text{RMSE} = \sqrt{\frac{1}{n} \sum_{i=1}^{n} \left(y_1 - \underbrace{(a_1 + x_{i,1}\beta_1 + x_{i,2}\beta_2 + \cdots + x_{i,k}\beta_k)}_{\text{predicted value } \widehat{y_i}, \text{ at } x_{i,1}, \cdots, x_{i,k}} \right)^2}.$$

In the linear model case, the expected value of the MSE (over the distribution of training sets) for the *training set* is $\frac{n-k-1}{n+k+1}E$, where E is the expected value of the MSE for the *testing/validation data*. Therefore, fitting a model and computing the MSE on the training set, we may produce an over optimistic evaluation assessment (smaller RMSE) of how well the model may fit another dataset. This bias represents *in-sample* estimate of the fit, whereas we are interested in the cross-validation estimate as an *out-of-sample* estimate.

In the linear regression model, cross-validation may not be as useful, since we can compute the *exact* correction factor $\frac{n-k-1}{n+k+1}$ to obtain an estimate of the exact expected *out-of-sample* fit using the *in-sample* MSE (under)estimate. However, even in this situation, cross-validation remains useful as it can be used to select an optimal regularized cost function. In most other modeling procedures (e.g., logistic regression), there are no simple general closed-form expressions (formulas) to adjust the cross-validation error estimate from the in-sample fit estimate. Cross-validation is a generally applicable way to predict the performance of a model on a validation set using stochastic computation instead of obtaining experimental, theoretical, mathematical, or analytic error estimates.

9.8.2 Cross-validation Methods

There are two classes of cross-validation approaches: *exhaustive* and *nonexhaustive*.

9.8.2.1 Exhaustive Cross-validation

Exhaustive cross-validation methods are based on determining all possible ways to divide the original sample into training and testing data. For instance, the *Leave-m-out cross-validation* involves using m observations for testing and the remaining $(n - m)$ observations as training. The case when $m = 1$, i.e., leave-1-out method, is only applicable when n is small, due to its huge computational cost. This process is repeated on all partitions of the original sample. This method requires model fitting and validating C_m^n times (n is the total number of observations in the original sample and m is the number of observations left out for validation). This requires a very large number of *steps*.

9.8.2.2   Nonexhaustive Cross-validation

Nonexhaustive cross-validation methods avoid computing estimates/errors using all possible partitionings of the original sample, and rather use approximations. For example, in the *k-fold cross-validation*, the original sample is randomly partitioned into k equal sized subsamples, or *folds*. Of the k subsamples, a single subsample is kept as final testing data for validation of the model. The other $k - 1$ subsamples are used as training data. The cross-validation process is then repeated k times, corresponding to the k folds. Each of the k subsamples is used once as the validation data. There are corresponding k results that are averaged (or otherwise aggregated) to generate a final pooled model-quality estimation. In k-fold validation, all observations are used for both training and validation, and each observation is used for validation exactly once. In general, k is a parameter that needs to be selected by an investigator (common values may be 5 or 10).

A general case of the k-fold validation is $k = n$ (the total number of observations), when it coincides with the *leave-one-out cross-validation*. A variation of the k-fold validation is *stratified k-fold cross-validation*, where each fold has the same (approximately) mean response value. For instance, if the model represents a binary classification of cases (e.g., controls vs. patients), this implies that each fold contains roughly the same proportion of the two class labels.

Repeated random subsampling validation randomly splits the entire dataset into a training set, where the model is fit, and a testing set, where the predictive accuracy is assessed. Again, the results are averaged over all iterative splits. This method has an advantage over k-fold cross-validation, as the proportion of the training/testing split is not dependent on the number of iterations (folds). However, its drawback is that some observations may never be selected whereas others may be selected multiple times in the testing/validation subsample. As validation subsets may overlap, the results may vary each time we repeat the validation protocol, unless we set a seed point in the algorithm. Asymptotically, as the number of random splits increases, the *repeated random sub-sampling* validation approaches the *leave-k-out cross-validation*.

9.8.3   Case Studies

In the examples below, we have intentionally suppressed some of the R output to save space. This is accomplished using the Rmarkdown command, {r eval=TRUE, results='hide'}; however, the reader is encouraged to try all the protocols hands-on, make modifications, inspect, and interpret the outputs.

9.8.3.1 Example 1: Prediction of Parkinson's Disease Using `Adaptive Boosting` (AdaBoost)

This Parkinson's diseases study involves heterogeneous neuroimaging, genetics, clinical, and phenotypic data of over 600 volunteers. The multivariate data include three cohorts (HC=Healthy Controls, PD=Parkinson's, SWEDD = subjects without evidence for dopaminergic deficit). First, let's load the PPMI data, 06_PPMI_ClassificationValidationData_Short.csv, and binarize the Dx (clinical diagnoses) classes.

```
ppmi_data <-
    read.csv("https://umich.instructure.com/files/330400/download?download_frd=1",
            header=TRUE)
# binarize the Dx classes
ppmi_data$ResearchGroup <- ifelse(ppmi_data$ResearchGroup == "Control",
                            "Control", "Patient")
attach(ppmi_data); head(ppmi_data) # View (ppmi_data)
```

Next, we can try model-free predictive analytics, e.g., AdaBoost classification, and report the results.

```
# Model-free analysis, classification
# install.packages("crossval")
# install.packages("ada")
# library("crossval")
library(crossval)
library(ada)
# set up adaboosting prediction function
# Define a new AdaBoost classification result-reporting function
my.ada <- function (train.x, train.y, test.x, test.y, negative, formula){
  ada.fit <- ada(train.x, train.y)
  predict.y <- predict(ada.fit, test.x)
  #count TP, FP, TN, FN, Accuracy, etc.
  out <- confusionMatrix(test.y, predict.y, negative = negative)
 # negative  is the label of a negative "null" sample (default: "control").
  return (out)
}
```

Recall from Chap. 2 that when group sizes are imbalanced, we may need to rebalance them to avoid potential biases of dominant cohorts. In this case, we will re-balance the groups using the package SMOTE Synthetic Minority Oversampling Technique.[7] SMOTE may be used to handle class imbalance in binary or multinomial (multiclass) classification.

---

[7]https://doi.org/10.1016/j.patcog.2017.07.024

```
# balance cases
# SMOTE: Synthetic Minority Oversampling Technique to handle class imbalance in
binary classification.
set.seed(1000)
# install.packages("unbalanced") to deal with unbalanced group data
library(unbalanced)
ppmi_data$PD <- ifelse(ppmi_data$ResearchGroup=="Control", 1, 0)
uniqueID <- unique(ppmi_data$FID_IID)
ppmi_data <- ppmi_data[ppmi_data$VisitID==1, ]
ppmi_data$PD <- factor(ppmi_data$PD)
colnames(ppmi_data)
# ppmi_data.1<-ppmi_data[, c(3:281, 284, 287, 336:340, 341)]
n <- ncol(ppmi_data)
output.1 <- ppmi_data$PD
input <- ppmi_data[ , -which(names(ppmi_data) %in% c("ResearchGroup",
                    "PD", "X", "FID_IID"))]
output <- as.factor(ppmi_data$PD)
c(dim(input), dim(output))
#balance the dataset
set.seed(123)
data.1<-ubBalance(X= input, Y=output, type="ubSMOTE", percOver=300,
                  percUnder=150, verbose=TRUE)
balancedData<-cbind(data.1$X, data.1$Y)
table(data.1$Y)
nrow(data.1$X); ncol(data.1$X)
nrow(balancedData); ncol(balancedData)
nrow(input); ncol(input)
colnames(balancedData) <- c(colnames(input), "PD")
```

Next, we'll check the re-balanced cohort sizes (Fig. 9.6).

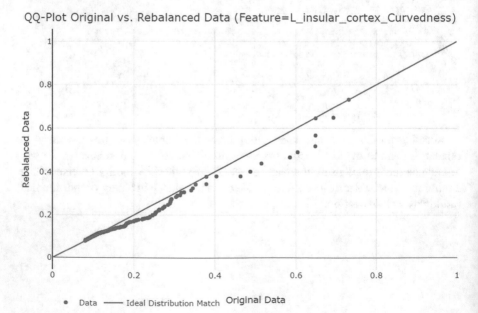

Fig. 9.6 Quantile–quantile plot of the original and rebalanced cases for the variable *L_insular_cortex_Curvedness* (Parkinson's disease data)

```
library(plotly)
###Check balance using T test
alpha.0.05 <- 0.05
test.results.bin <- NULL        # binarized/dichotomized p-values
test.results.raw <- NULL        # raw p-values
# get a better error-handling t.test function that gracefully handles NA's and
trivial variances
my.t.test.p.value <- function(input1, input2) {
    obj <- try(t.test(input1, input2), silent=TRUE)
    if (is(obj, "try-error"))  return(NA)
    else   return(obj$p.value)
}
for (i in 1:ncol(balancedData)) {
    test.results.raw[i] <- my.t.test.p.value(input[, i], balancedData [, i])
    test.results.bin[i] <- ifelse(test.results.raw[i]  > alpha.0.05, 1, 0)
    # binarize the p-value (0=significant, 1=otherwise)
    print(c("i=", i, "var=", colnames(balancedData[i]),
            "t-test_raw_p_value=", test.results.raw[i]))
}
QQ <- qqplot(input[, 5], balancedData [, 5], plot=F)
# check visually for differences between the distributions of the raw (input) and
rebalanced data (for only one variable, in this case)
plot_ly(x=~QQ$x, y=~QQ$y, type="scatter", mode="markers", name="Data") %>%
  add_trace(x=c(0,1), y=c(0,1), name="Ideal Distribution Match",
            type="scatter", mode="lines") %>%
  layout(title=paste0("QQ-Plot Original vs. Rebalanced Data (Feature=",
                      colnames(input)[5], ")"),
      xaxis=list(title="Original Data"), yaxis=list(title="Rebalanced Data"),
      hovermode = "x unified", legend = list(orientation='h'))



# Now, check visually for differences between the distributions of the raw
(input) and rebalanced data.
length(input[, 5]); length(balancedData [, 5]) # the sample-sizes changed
for (i in 1:(ncol(balancedData)-1)) {
    test.results.raw [i] <- wilcox.test(input[,i], balancedData[, i])$p.value
    test.results.bin [i] <- ifelse(test.results.raw [i] > alpha.0.05, 1, 0)
    print(c("i=", i, "Wilcoxon-test=", test.results.raw [i]))
}
print(c("Wilcoxon test results: ", test.results.bin))
```

The next step will be the actual `cross validation`.

```
X <- as.data.frame(input); Y <- output
neg <- "1"    # "Control" == "1"
X <- as.data.frame(data.1$X); Y <- data.1$Y # using Rebalanced data
set.seed(115)
cv.out <- crossval::crossval(my.ada, X, Y, K = 5, B = 1, negative = neg)
                # the label of a negative "null" sample (default: "control")
out <- diagnosticErrors(cv.out$stat)
print(cv.out$stat)
##    FP     TP    TN    FN
##   0.2 109.8  97.4   0.0
print(out)
##        acc      sens      spec       ppv       npv       lor
## 0.9990357 1.0000000 0.9979508 0.9981818 1.0000000       Inf
```

As we can see from the reported metrics, the overall averaged AdaBoost-based diagnostic predictions are quite good.

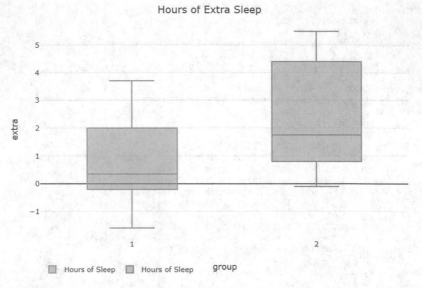

Fig. 9.7 Box plots of extra hours of sleep for the pair of groups, drug treatments (Parkinson's disease data)

9.8.3.2   Example 2: Sleep Dataset

These data contain the effect of two soporific drugs (group variable) to increase hours of sleep (treatment-compared design) on 10 patients. The data are available by default (sleep {datasets})

First, we will load the data and examine the group distributions (Fig. 9.7).

```
data(sleep); str(sleep)
X = as.matrix(sleep[, 1, drop=FALSE]) # increase in hours of sleep,
    # when drop=TRUE the result is coerced to the lowest possible dimension
Y = sleep[, 2] # drug given
plot_ly(data=sleep, x=~group, y=~extra, color=~group, type="box",
        name="Hours of Sleep") %>%
  layout(title="Hours of Extra Sleep", legend = list(orientation='h'))
levels(Y) # "1" "2"
dim(X) # 20  1
```

Next, we will define a new LDA (linear discriminant analysis) predicting function and perform the cross-validation (CV) on the resulting predictor.

```
library("MASS") # for lda function
predfun.lda = function(train.x, train.y, test.x, test.y, negative) {
    lda.fit = lda(train.x, grouping=train.y)
    ynew = predict(lda.fit, test.x)$class                    # count TP, FP etc.
    out = confusionMatrix(test.y, ynew, negative=negative)
    return( out )
}
library("crossval")    # install.packages("crossval")
set.seed(123456)
cv.out <- crossval::crossval(predfun.lda, X, Y, K=5, B=20, negative="1")
cv.out$stat
diagnosticErrors(cv.out$stat)
```

Interpreting the diagnostic results and the performance of the LDA prediction indicates the model is not particularly effective (FP = 0.6, TP = 1.13, TN = 1.4, FN = 0.87).

9.8.3.3 Example 3: Model-Based (Linear Regression) Prediction Using the Attitude Dataset

This data represents the average survey responses from about 35 employees from 30 (randomly selected) departments in a large organization. The data capture the proportion of favorable responses to seven questions in each department. Let's load and summarize the data, which is available by default in the R object attitude {datasets}.

```
data("attitude")
y = attitude[, 1]       # rating variable
x = attitude[, -1]      # date frame with the remaining variables
is.factor(y)
summary(lm(y ~ . , data=x)) # R-squared: 0.7326,  lm prediction function
```

We will demonstrate model-based analytics using lm() and lda() and will validate the forecasting using CV.

```
predfun.lm = function(train.x, train.y, test.x, test.y) {
  lm.fit = lm(train.y ~ . , data=train.x)
  ynew = predict(lm.fit, test.x )
  # compute squared error risk (MSE)
  out = mean( (ynew - test.y)^2)
  # when fitting linear model to continuous outcome variable (Y),
  # we can't use the out<-confusionMatrix(test.y, ynew, negative=negative),
  # instead, use MSE to estimate the discrepancy between observed & predicted
  return(out)
}
# prediction MSE using all variables
set.seed(123456)
cv.out.lm = crossval::crossval(predfun.lm, x, y, K=5, B=20, verbose=FALSE)
c(cv.out.lm$stat, cv.out.lm$stat.se)          # 72.581198  3.736784
# reducing to using only two variables
cv.out.lm = crossval::crossval(predfun.lm, x[, c(1, 3)], y, K=5, B=20,
                               verbose=FALSE)
c(cv.out.lm$stat, cv.out.lm$stat.se)      # 52.563957  2.015109
```

9.8.3.4   Example 4: Parkinson's Data (PPMI data)

Let's go back to the more elaborate Parkinson's disease (PD/PPMI) case, load, and preprocess the derived-PPMI data (Fig. 9.8).

```
output <- as.factor(ppmi_data$PD)
input <- ppmi_data[, -which(names(ppmi_data) %in% c("ResearchGroup", "PD",
                                                "X", "FID_IID", "VisitID"))]

X = as.matrix(input)     # Predictor variables
Y = as.matrix(output)    # Actual PD clinical assessment
dim(X); dim(Y)
fit <- lm(Y ~ X)
xResid <- scale(fit$residuals)
QQ <- qqplot(xResid, rnorm(1000), plot=F) # check visually for differences
between the distributions of the raw (input) and rebalanced data (for only one
variable, in this case)
plot_ly(x=~QQ$x, y=~QQ$y, type="scatter", mode="markers", name="Data") %>%
  add_trace(x=c(-4,4), y=c(-4,4), name="Ideal Distribution Match",
            type="scatter", mode="lines") %>%
  layout(title="QQ Normal Plot of Model Residuals",
         xaxis=list(title="Model Residuals"),
         yaxis=list(title="Normal Residuals"),
         hovermode = "x unified", legend = list(orientation='h'))
```

```
levels(as.factor(Y))          # "0" "1"
c(dim(X), dim(Y))             # 422 100 422   1
```

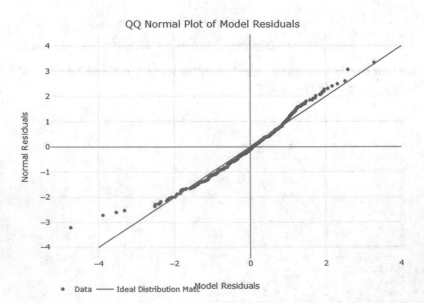

Fig. 9.8 Linear model inspection, quantile–quantile plot of model residuals vs. normal distribution (Parkinson's disease data)

Apply `cross-validation` to assess the performance of the linear model.

```
set.seed(12345)
cv.out.lda = crossval::crossval(predfun.lda, X, Y, K=5, B=20, negative="1")
diagnosticErrors(cv.out.lda$stat)
##       acc      sens      spec       ppv       npv       lor
## 0.9606635 0.9515000 0.9831967 0.9928696 0.8918216 7.0457111
```

9.8.4   Summary of CV Output

The cross-validation (CV) output object includes the following components:

- `stat.cv`: Vector of statistics returned by *predfun* for each cross-validation run
- `stat`: statistic returned by *predfun* averaged over all cross-validation runs
- `stat.se`: variability capturing the corresponding standard error across cv-iterations.

9.8.5   Alternative Predictor Functions

In Chap. 3, we have already discussed a number of `predict()` functions. Below, we will add to the collection of predictive analytics and forecasting functions using the PPMI dataset (06_PPMI_ClassificationValidationData_Short.csv).

9.8.5.1   Logistic Regression

We will learn more about the *logit* model in Chap. 11. Now, we will demonstrate the use of a logit-predictor function to forecast a binary diagnostic outcome (patient or control) using the Parkinson's disease study, 06_PPMI_ClassificationValidationData_Short.csv.

```
output <- as.factor(ppmi_data$PD)
input <- ppmi_data[, -which(names(ppmi_data) %in% c("ResearchGroup", "PD",
                                            "X", "FID_IID", "VisitID"))]
X = as.matrix(input)      # Predictor variables
Y = as.matrix(output)
```

Note that the predicted values are in *log* terms, so they need to be *exponentiated* to interpret them correctly.

```
lm.logit <- glm(as.numeric(Y) ~ ., data=as.data.frame(X), family="binomial")
ynew <- predict(lm.logit, as.data.frame(X)); #plot(ynew)
ynew2 <- ifelse(exp(ynew)<0.5, 0, 1); # plot(ynew2)
predfun.logit = function(train.x, train.y, test.x, test.y, neg)  {
    lm.logit <- glm(train.y ~ ., data = train.x, family = "binomial")
    ynew = predict(lm.logit, test.x )
    # compute TP, FP, TN, FN
    ynew2 <- ifelse(exp(ynew) < 0.5, 0, 1)    # mind exponentiation!
    out = confusionMatrix(test.y, ynew2, negative=neg)  # Binary outcome
    return( out )
}
# Reduce the bag of explanatory variables, purely to simplify the interpretation
of the analytics in this example!
input.short <- input[, which(names(input) %in% c("R_fusiform_gyrus_Volume",
    "R_fusiform_gyrus_ShapeIndex", "R_fusiform_gyrus_Curvedness",
    "Sex",   "Weight", "Age", "chr12_rs34637584_GT", "chr17_rs11868035_GT",
    "UPDRS_Part_I_Summary_Score_Baseline",
    "UPDRS_Part_I_Summary_Score_Month_03",
    "UPDRS_Part_II_Patient_Questionnaire_Summary_Score_Baseline",
    "UPDRS_Part_III_Summary_Score_Baseline",
    "X_Assessment_Non.Motor_Epworth_Sleepiness_Scale_Summary_Score_Baseline"
  ))]
X = as.matrix(input.short)
cv.out.logit = crossval::crossval(predfun.logit, as.data.frame(X), as.numeric(Y),
    K=5, B=2, neg="1", verbose=FALSE)
cv.out.logit$stat.cv
##         FP TP TN FN
## B1.F1   2 55 26  1
## B1.F2   0 61 21  3
…
## B2.F4   3 50 29  2
## B2.F5   3 58 18  5
diagnosticErrors(cv.out.logit$stat)
##       acc      sens      spec       ppv       npv       lor
## 0.9478673 0.9533333 0.9344262 0.9727891 0.8906250 5.6736914
##         FP TP TN FN
## B1.F1   2 55 26  1
## B1.F2   0 61 21  3
…
## B2.F4   3 50 29  2
## B2.F5   3 58 18  5
diagnosticErrors(cv.out.logit$stat)
##       acc      sens      spec       ppv       npv       lor
## 0.9478673 0.9533333 0.9344262 0.9727891 0.8906250 5.6736914
```

Caution Note that if you forget to exponentiate the predicted logistic model values (see *ynew2* in predict.logit), you will get nonsense results, e.g., all cases may be predicted to be in one class, or you can expect to get trivial sensitivity or negative predictive power (NPP).

9.8.5.2 Quadratic Discriminant Analysis (QDA)

In Chap. 5, we discussed the *linear* and *quadratic* discriminant analysis models. Let's now introduce a predfun.qda() function.

```
predfun.qda = function(train.x, train.y, test.x, test.y, negative) {
  library("MASS") # for lda function
  qda.fit = qda(train.x, grouping=train.y)
  ynew = predict(qda.fit, test.x)$class
  out.qda = confusionMatrix(test.y, ynew, negative=negative)
  return( out.qda )
}
cv.out.qda = crossval::crossval(predfun.qda, as.data.frame(input.short),
as.factor(Y), K=5, B=20, neg="1")
## Error in qda.default(x, grouping, ...): rank deficiency in group 1
diagnosticErrors(cv.out.lda$stat); diagnosticErrors(cv.out.qda$stat);
## Error in diagnosticErrors(cv.out.qda$stat): object 'cv.out.qda' not found
```

This error message: "**Error in qda.default(x, grouping, …): rank deficiency in group 1**" indicates that there is a rank deficiency, i.e., some variables are collinear and one or more covariance matrices cannot be inverted to obtain the estimates in group 1 (Controls)! *Removing the strongly correlated data elements ("R_fusiform_gyrus_Volume", "R_fusiform_gyrus_ShapeIndex", and "R_fusiform_gyrus_Curvedness"), resolves the rank-deficiency problem!*

```
input.short2 <- input[, which(names(input) %in% c("R_fusiform_gyrus_Volume",
  "Sex", "Weight", "Age" , "chr17_rs11868035_GT",
  "UPDRS_Part_I_Summary_Score_Baseline",
  "UPDRS_Part_II_Patient_Questionnaire_Summary_Score_Baseline",
  "UPDRS_Part_III_Summary_Score_Baseline",
  "X_Assessment_Non.Motor_Epworth_Sleepiness_Scale_Summary_Score_Baseline"))]
X = as.matrix(input.short2)
cv.out.qda = crossval::crossval(predfun.qda, as.data.frame(X), as.numeric(Y),
                    K=5, B=2, neg="1")
```

It makes sense to contrast the QDA and GLM/Logit predictions.

```
diagnosticErrors(cv.out.qda$stat);
diagnosticErrors(cv.out.logit$stat)
##        acc       sens       spec        ppv        npv        lor
## 0.9395735  0.9550000  0.9016393  0.9597990 0.8906883   5.2706226
##        acc       sens       spec        ppv        npv        lor
## 0.9478673  0.9533333  0.9344262  0.9727891 0.8906250   5.6736914
```

Clearly, both the QDA and Logit model predictions are quite similar and reliable.

9.8.6   Foundation of LDA and QDA for Prediction, Dimensionality Reduction, or Forecasting

Previously, in Chap. 5, we saw some examples of LDA/QDA methods. Now, we'll talk more about the details. Both LDA (Linear Discriminant Analysis) and QDA (Quadratic Discriminant Analysis) use probabilistic models of the class conditional distribution of the data $P(X \mid Y = k)$ for each class k. Their predictions are obtained by using Bayesian theorem (see DSPA2 Appendix):

$$P(Y = k \mid X) = \frac{P(X \mid Y = k)P(Y = k)}{P(X)} = \frac{P(X \mid Y = k)P(Y = k)}{\sum\limits_{l=0}^{\infty} P(X \mid Y = l)P(Y = l)},$$

and we select the class k, which *maximizes* this conditional probability (maximum likelihood estimation). In linear and quadratic discriminant analysis, $P(X \mid Y)$ is modeled as a multivariate Gaussian distribution with density

$$P(X \mid Y = k) = \frac{1}{(2\pi)^{\frac{n}{2}}|\Sigma_k|^{\frac{1}{2}}} \times e^{\left(-\frac{1}{2}(X - \mu_k)^T \Sigma_k^{-1}(X - \mu_k)\right)}.$$

This model can be used to classify data by using the training data to *estimate*:

- The class prior probabilities $P(Y = k)$ by counting the proportion of observed instances of class k.
- The class means μ_k by computing the empirical sample class means.
- The covariance matrices by computing either the empirical sample class covariance matrices, or by using a regularized estimator, e.g., LASSO (see Chap. 11).

In the *linear case* (LDA), the Gaussian components for each class are assumed to share the same covariance matrix $\Sigma_k = \Sigma$ for each class k. This leads to linear decision surfaces between classes. This is clear from comparing the log-probability ratios of 2 classes (k and l):

$$\text{LOR} = \log\left(\frac{P(Y = k \mid X)}{P(Y = l \mid X)}\right), \text{LOR} = 0 \Leftrightarrow$$

the two probabilities are identical, i.e., yield same class label, and

$$\text{LOR} = \log\left(\frac{P(Y = k \mid X)}{P(Y = l \mid X)}\right) = 0 \Leftrightarrow$$

$$(\mu_k - \mu_l)^T \Sigma^{-1}(\mu_k - \mu_l) = \frac{1}{2}\left(\mu_k^T \Sigma^{-1}\mu_k - \mu_l^T \Sigma^{-1}\mu_l\right).$$

However, in the more general *quadratic case* (QDA), these assumptions about the covariance matrices Σ_k of the Gaussian components are relaxed, leading to quadratic decision surfaces.

9.8.6.1 LDA (Linear Discriminant Analysis)

LDA is similar to the generalized linear model (GLM) used in ANOVA and regression analyses. LDA also attempts to express one dependent variable as a linear combination of other features or data elements. However, ANOVA uses categorical independent variables and a continuous dependent variable, whereas LDA has continuous independent variables and a categorical dependent variable (i.e., Dx/ class label). Logistic regression `logit` and `probit` regression are more similar to LDA than ANOVA, as they also explain a categorical variable by the values of continuous independent variables.

```
predfun.lda = function(train.x, train.y, test.x, test.y, neg) {
  library("MASS")
  lda.fit = lda(train.x, grouping=train.y)
  ynew = predict(lda.fit, test.x)$class
  out.lda = confusionMatrix(test.y, ynew, negative=neg)
  return( out.lda )
}
```

9.8.6.2 QDA (Quadratic Discriminant Analysis)

Similarly to LDA, the QDA prediction function can be defined by

```
predfun.qda = function(train.x, train.y, test.x, test.y, neg) {
  library("MASS") # for lda function
  qda.fit = qda(train.x, grouping-train.y)
  ynew = predict(qda.fit, test.x)$class
  out.qda = confusionMatrix(test.y, ynew, negative=neg)
  return( out.qda )
}
```

9.8.6.3 Neural Network

We introduced neural networks (NNs) in Chap. 6. Applying NNs is not straightforward. We have to create a design matrix with an indicator column for the response feature. In addition, we need to write a *predict function* to translate the output of `neuralnet()` into analytical forecasts.

```
library("neuralnet")
pred = function(nn, dat) {    # predict nn
  yhat = compute(nn, dat)$net.result
  yhat = apply(yhat, 1, which.max)-1
  return(yhat)
}
my.neural <- function (train.x,train.y, test.x, test.y,method,layer=c(5,5)) {
  train.x <- as.data.frame(train.x)
  train.y <- as.data.frame(train.y)
  colnames(train.x) <- paste0('V', 1:ncol(X))
  colnames(train.y) <- "V1"
  train_y_ind = model.matrix(~factor(train.y$V1)-1)
  colnames(train_y_ind) = paste0('out', 0:1)
  train = cbind(train.x, train_y_ind)
  y_names = paste0('out', 0:1)
  x_names = paste0('V', 1:ncol(train.x))
  nn = neuralnet(
    paste(paste(y_names, collapse='+'), '~', paste(x_names, collapse='+')),
    train, hidden=layer, linear.output=FALSE,
    lifesign='full', lifesign.step=1000)
  #predict
  predict.y <- pred(nn, test.x)
  out <- crossval::confusionMatrix(test.y, predict.y,negative = 0)
  return (out)
}
set.seed(1234)
cv.out.nn <- crossval::crossval(my.neural, scale(X), Y, K = 5,
        B = 1,layer=c(20,20),verbose = F) # scaled predictors are necessary
crossval::diagnosticErrors(cv.out.nn$stat)
##       acc      sens      spec       ppv       npv       lor
## 0.9407583 0.9016393 0.9566667 0.8943089 0.9598662 5.3101066
```

9.8.6.4   SVM

We also saw SVM in Chap. 6. Let's try cross-validation on Linear and Gaussian (radial) kernel SVM. We can expect that linear SVM should achieve a close result to Gaussian or even better than Gaussian since this dataset has a large k (# features) compared with n (# cases), which we have studied in detail in Chap. 6.

```
library("e1071")
my.svm <- function (train.x, train.y, test.x,
            test.y,method,cost=1,gamma=1/ncol(dx_norm),coef0=0,degree=3) {
  svm_l.fit <- svm(x = train.x, y=as.factor(train.y), kernel = method)
  predict.y <- predict(svm_l.fit, test.x)
  out <- crossval::confusionMatrix(test.y, predict.y, negative = 0)
  return (out)
}
set.seed(123)    # Linear kernel
cv.out.svml <- crossval::crossval(my.svm, as.data.frame(X), Y, K = 5, B = 1,
        method = "linear",cost=tune_svm$best.parameters$cost,verbose = F)
diagnosticErrors(cv.out.svml$stat)
##       acc      sens      spec       ppv       npv       lor
## 0.9573460 0.9344262 0.9666667 0.9193548 0.9731544 6.0240527
set.seed(123)    # Gaussian kernel
cv.out.svmg <- crossval::crossval(my.svm, as.data.frame(X), Y, K = 5, B = 1,
        method = "radial",cost=tune_svmg$best.parameters$cost,
        gamma=tune_svmg$best.parameters$gamma,verbose = F)
diagnosticErrors(cv.out.svmg$stat)
##       acc      sens      spec       ppv       npv       lor
## 0.9478673 0.9262295 0.9566667 0.8968254 0.9695946 5.6246961
```

Indeed, both types of kernels yield good quality predictors according to the assessment metrics reported by the `diagnosticErrors()` method.

9.8.6.5   k-Nearest Neighbors Algorithm (k-NN)

As we saw in Chap. 5, *k-NN* is a nonparametric method for either classification or regression, where the *input* consists of the k closest *training examples* in the feature space, but the *output* depends on whether k-NN is used for classification or regression:

- In *k-NN classification*, the output is a class membership (labels). Objects in the testing data are classified by a majority vote of their neighbors. Each object is assigned to a class that is most common among its k nearest neighbors (k is always a small positive integer). When $k = 1$, then an object is assigned to the class of its single nearest neighbor.
- In *k-NN regression*, the output is the property value for the object representing the average of the values of its k nearest neighbors.

Let's now build the corresponding `predfun.knn()` method.

```
#  X - as.matrix(input)  # Predictor variables X = as.matrix(input.short2)
#  Y = as.matrix(output)    # Outcome
# KNN (k-neurest neighbors)
library("class")
# knn.fit.test <- knn(X, X, cl = Y, k=3, prob=F);
# predict(as.matrix(knn.fit.test), X)$class
# table(knn.fit.test, Y); confusionMatrix(Y, knn.fit.test, negative="1")
# This can be used for polytomous variable (multiple classes)
predfun.knn = function(train.x, train.y, test.x, test.y, neg) {
  library("class")
  knn.fit = knn(train.x, test.x, cl = train.y, prob=T)
  # knn is already a prediction function!!!
  # ynew = predict(knn.fit, test.x)$class
  # no need of another prediction, in this case
  out.knn = confusionMatrix(test.y, knn.fit, negative=neg)
  return( out.knn )
}
cv.out.knn = crossval::crossval(predfun.knn, X, Y, K=5, B=2, neg="1")
#Compare all 3 classifiers (lda, qda, knn, and logit)
diagnosticErrors(cv.out.lda$stat); diagnosticErrors(cv.out.qda$stat);
diagnosticErrors(cv.out.qda$stat); diagnosticErrors(cv.out.logit$stat);
```

We can also examine the performance of k-NN prediction on the PPMI (Parkinson's disease) data. Start by partitioning the data into `training` and `testing` sets.

```
# TRAINING: 75% of the sample size
sample_size <- floor(0.75 * nrow(input))
set.seed(1234)    ## set the seed to make your partition reproducible
input.train.ind <- sample(seq_len(nrow(input)), size = sample_size)
input.train <- input[input.train.ind, ]
output.train <- as.matrix(output)[input.train.ind, ]
# TESTING DATA
input.test <- input[-input.train.ind, ]
output.test <- as.matrix(output)[-input.train.ind, ]
```

Then fit the k-NN model and report the results.

```
library("class")
knn_model <- knn(train=input.train,input.test,cl=as.factor(output.train),k=2)
summary(knn_model)
attributes(knn_model)
# cross-validation
knn_model.cv <- knn.cv(train= input.train, cl=as.factor(output.train), k=2)
summary(knn_model.cv)
```

9.8.6.6   k-Means Clustering (k-MC)

In Chap. 8, we showed that k-MC aims to partition n observations into k clusters where each observation belongs to the cluster with the nearest mean, which acts as a prototype of a cluster. The k-MC partitions the data space into Voronoi cells. In general, there is no computationally tractable solution for this, i.e., the problem is NP-hard.[8] However, there are efficient algorithms that converge quickly to local optima, e.g., the *expectation-maximization* algorithm for Gaussian mixture distribution modeling that we saw in Chap. 8. Figure 9.9 shows the results of the binary k-means clustering of the PPMI data.

```
kmeans_model <- kmeans(input.train, 2)
table (output.train, kmeans_model$cluster-1)
## output.train    0    1
##              0 173   50
##              1  65   28
layout(matrix(1, 1))
fpc::plotcluster(input.train, output.train, col = kmeans_model$cluster)
legend("topright", legend=c("0(trueLabel)+0(kmeansLabel)",
       "1(trueLabel)+0(kmeansLabel)", "0(trueLabel)+1(kmeansLabel)",
       "1(trueLabel)+1(kmeansLabel)"), col=c("red", "black", "black", "red"),
       text.col=c("red", "black", "black", "red"),
       pch = 15 , y.intersp=0.6, x.intersp=0.7, text.width = 5, cex=1)
input.train <- input.train[ , apply(input.train, 2, var, na.rm=TRUE) != 0] #
remove constant columns

cluster::clusplot(input.train, kmeans_model$cluster, color=TRUE, shade=TRUE,
labels=2, lines=0)
```

---

[8]https://doi.org/10.1007/BF00365407

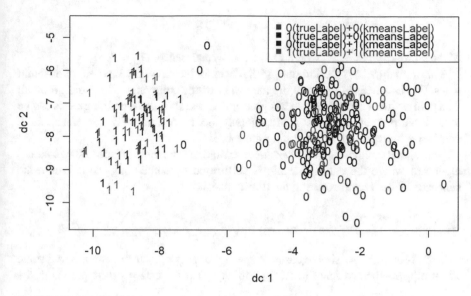

Fig. 9.9 2D projection of the k-means clustering results illustrating the performance of the binary diagnostic classifier using the Parkinson's disease data. Colors (red and black) and symbols (0 and 1) indicate the true and predicted diagnostic labels, respectively

This model can be evaluated using the method `silhouette()` in the package `cluster`. Recall from Chap. 8 that the *silhouette value* is in the range $[-1, 1]$ with negative and positive values corresponding to (mostly) "mis-labeled" and "correctly-labeled" cases, respectively.

9.8.6.7 Spectral Clustering

Expanding on the *spectral clustering* approach we covered in Chap. 8, suppose the multivariate dataset is represented as a set of data points A. We can define a similarity matrix $S = s_{(i,j)}$, where $s_{(i,j)}$ represents a measure of the similarity between points $i, j \in A$. Spectral clustering uses the spectrum of the similarity matrix of the high-dimensional data and performs dimensionality reduction for clustering into fewer dimensions. The spectrum of a matrix is the set of its eigenvalues. In general, if $T : \Omega \xrightarrow{\text{linear operator}} \Omega$ maps a vector space Ω into itself, its spectrum is the vector of scalars $\lambda = \{\lambda_i\}$ such that $(T - \lambda I)v = 0$, where I is the identity matrix and v are the eigen-vectors (or eigen-functions) for the operator T. The **determinant** of the matrix equals the product of its eigenvalues, i.e., $det(T) = \Pi_i \lambda_i$, the **trace** of the matrix $tr(T) = \Sigma_i \lambda_i$, and the **pseudo-determinant** for a singular matrix is the product of its nonzero eigenvalues, $\text{pseudo}_{det}(T) = \Pi_{\lambda_i \neq 0} \lambda_i$.

To partition the data points into two sets (S_1, S_2), suppose v is the second-smallest eigenvector of the Laplacian matrix

$$L = I - D^{-\frac{1}{2}} S D^{\frac{1}{2}}$$

of the similarity matrix S, where D is the diagonal matrix $D_{i,i} = \Sigma_j S_{i,j}$.

This actual (S_1, S_2) partitioning of the cases in the data may be done in different ways. For instance, S_1 may use the median m of the components in v and group all data points whose component in v is greater than m. Then the remaining cases can be labeled as part of S_2. This approach may be used iteratively for *hierarchical clustering* by repeatedly partitioning the subsets.

The *specc* method in the *kernlab* package implements a spectral clustering algorithm where the data-clustering is performed by embedding the data into the subspace of the eigenvectors of an affinity matrix.

```
library("kernlab")    # install.packages("kernlab")
data()  # review and choose a dataset (for example the Iris data)
```

Let's look at a few simple cases of spectral clustering. We are suppressing some of the outputs to save space (e.g., #plot(my_data, col= data_sc)).

9.8.6.8   Iris Petal Data

Let's look at the *iris* dataset we saw in Chap. 2. Figure 9.10 shows a 2D cross-section of the results of the spectral clustering of the iris data.

```
library(dplyr)
library(plotly)
my_data <- as.data.frame(iris); dim(my_data)
my_data <- as.matrix(mutate_all(my_data[, -5], function(x)
as.numeric(as.character(x))))
library(kernlab)
num_clusters <- 3
data_sc <- specc(my_data, centers= num_clusters)
data_sc
centers(data_sc)
withinss(data_sc)
plot_ly(x=~iris[,1], y=~iris[,2], type="scatter", mode="markers",
        color=~as.factor(data_sc@.Data),
        marker=list(size=15), symbol=~as.numeric(iris$Species)) %>%
  layout(title="Spectral Clustering (Iris Data)",
         xaxis=list(title=colnames(iris)[1]),
         yaxis=list(title=colnames(iris)[2]))
```

9.8.6.9   Spirals Data

Let's look at another spectral crustering example using the kernlab::spirals dataset (Fig. 9.11).

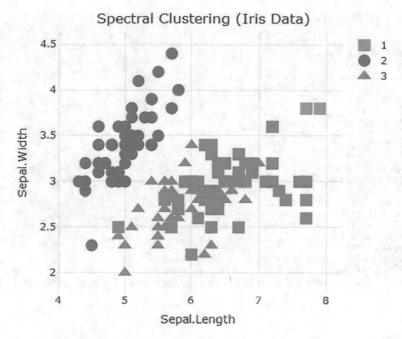

Fig. 9.10 A 2D projection of the spectral clustering results of the iris flower data. Glyph shapes (square, rectangle, and circle) indicate the actual species taxa, whereas the colors indicate the derived spectral class labels

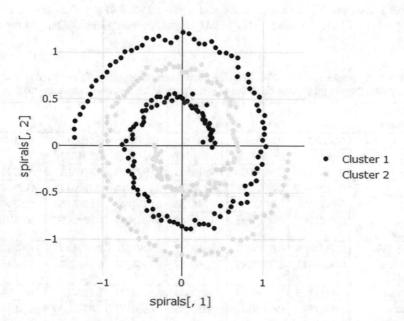

Fig. 9.11 Spectral clustering results of the 2D spirals data. The two colors indicate the derived class-labels associated with each of the two spiral arcs

```
# library("kernlab")
data(spirals)
num_clusters <- 2
data_sc <- specc(spirals, centers= num_clusters)
data_sc
## Gaussian Radial Basis kernel function.
##  Hyperparameter : sigma =  342.590151048389
## Centers:
##            [,1]         [,2]
## [1,] -0.01770984  0.1775137
## [2,]  0.01997201 -0.1761483
## Cluster size:
## [1] 150 150
## Within-cluster sum of squares:
## [1] 118.1182 117.3429
centers(data_sc)
##            [,1]         [,2]
## [1,] -0.01770984  0.1775137
## [2,]  0.01997201 -0.1761483
withinss(data_sc)
## [1] 118.1182 117.3429
clusterNames <- paste0("Cluster ", data_sc@.Data)
plot_ly(x=~spirals[,1], y=~spirals[,2], type="scatter", mode="markers",
        color = ~data_sc@.Data, name=clusterNames) %>% hide_colorbar()
```

9.8.7   Comparing Multiple Classifiers

Now let's compare all eight classifiers (AdaBoost, LDA, QDA, knn, logit, Neural Network, linear SVM and Gaussian SVM) we presented above using the PPMI dataset (06_PPMI_ClassificationValidationData_Short.csv) (Table 9.4).

Table 9.4 Aggregate results and performance metrics contrasting the performance of 10 complementary classifiers to predict the diagnosis of participants in the Parkinson's disease study

Methods/ measures	acc	sens	spec	ppv	npv	lor
AdaBoost	0.9668246	0.9866667	0.9180328	0.9673203	0.9655172	6.7199789
LDA	0.9606635	0.9515000	0.9831967	0.9928696	0.8918216	7.0457111
QDA	0.9395735	0.9550000	0.9016393	0.9597990	0.8906883	5.2706226
knn	0.6125592	0.7266667	0.3319672	0.7278798	0.3306122	0.2784748
logit	0.9478673	0.9533333	0.9344262	0.9727891	0.8906250	5.6736914
Neural network	0.9407583	0.9016393	0.9566667	0.8943089	0.9598662	5.3101066
linear SVM	0.9573460	0.9344262	0.9666667	0.9193548	0.9731544	6.0240527
Gaussian SVM	0.9478673	0.9262295	0.9566667	0.8968254	0.9695946	5.6246961
k-Means	0.4241706	0.3866667	0.5163934	0.6628571	0.2550607	−0.3957483
Spectral clustering	0.4727488	0.4683333	0.4836066	0.6904177	0.2700229	−0.1924337

```
set.seed(123)
cv.out.ada <- crossval::crossval(my.ada, as.data.frame(X), Y, K = 5, B = 1,
                                 negative = neg)
## Number of folds: 5
## Total number of CV fits: 5
## Round # 1 of 1
## CV Fit # 1 of 5
## CV Fit # 2 of 5
## CV Fit # 3 of 5
## CV Fit # 4 of 5
## CV Fit # 5 of 5
# get k-Means CV results
my.kmeans <- function (train.x, train.y, test.x, test.y, negative, formula) {
  kmeans.fit <- kmeans(scale(test.x), kpp_init(scale(test.x), 2),
                       iter.max=100, algorithm='Lloyd')
  predict.y <- kmeans.fit$cluster
  #count TP, FP, TN, FN, Accuracy, etc.
  out <- confusionMatrix(test.y, predict.y, negative = negative)
  # negative  is the label of a negative "null" sample (default: "control").
  return (out)
}
set.seed(123)
cv.out.kmeans <- crossval::crossval(my.kmeans, as.data.frame(X), Y, K = 5,
                                    B = 2, negative = neg)
# get spectral clustering CV results
my.sc <- function (train.x, train.y, test.x, test.y, negative, formula){
  sc.fit <- specc(scale(test.x), centers= 2)
  predict.y <- sc.fit@.Data
  #count TP, FP, TN, FN, Accuracy, etc.
  out <- confusionMatrix(test.y, predict.y, negative = negative)
 # negative  is the label of a negative "null" sample (default: "control").
  return (out)
}
set.seed(123)
cv.out.sc <- crossval::crossval(my.sc, as.data.frame(X), Y, K = 5,
                                B = 2, negative = neg)
library(knitr)
res_tab=rbind(diagnosticErrors(cv.out.ada$stat),
    diagnosticErrors(cv.out.lda$stat),diagnosticErrors(cv.out.qda$stat),
    diagnosticErrors(cv.out.knn$stat),diagnosticErrors(cv.out.logit$stat),
    diagnosticErrors(cv.out.nn$stat),diagnosticErrors(cv.out.svml$stat),
    diagnosticErrors(cv.out.svmg$stat),diagnosticErrors(cv.out.kmeans$stat),
    diagnosticErrors(cv.out.sc$stat))
rownames(res_tab) <- c("AdaBoost", "LDA", "QDA", "knn", "logit",
       "Neural Network", "linear SVM", "Gaussian SVM", "k-Means",
       "Spectral Clustering")
kable(res_tab, caption = "Compare Result")
```

Leaving knn, kmeans, and specc aside, the other methods achieve pretty good results. With these data, the reason for the suboptimal performance of some clustering methods (e.g., specc and kmeans) may be rooted in lack of sufficient training data or the curse of (high) dimensionality, which we saw in Chap. 4. As the data are super sparse, predicting from the nearest neighbors may not be too reliable.

Chapter 10
Specialized Machine Learning Topics

In this chapter, we will discuss some technical details about data formats, streaming, optimization of computation, and distributed deployment of optimized learning algorithms. Chapter 13 includes a deep dive into the mathematical and computational aspects of function optimization.

The Internet of Things (IoT) leads to a paradigm shift of scientific inference—from static data interrogated in a batch or distributed environment to an on-demand service-based Cloud computing. Here, we will demonstrate how to work with specialized datasets, data streams, and SQL databases, as well as develop and assess on-the-fly data modeling, classification, prediction, and forecasting methods. Important examples to keep in mind throughout this chapter include high-frequency data delivered real time in hospital ICUs (e.g., microsecond electroencephalography signals, EEGs), dynamically changing stock market data (e.g., Dow Jones Industrial Average Index, DJI), and weather patterns.

In this chapter, we will present (1) format conversion and working with XML, SQL, JSON, CSV, SAS, SQL, noSQL, Google BigQuery service, and other data objects; (2) visualization of bioinformatics and network data; (3) protocols for managing, classifying, and predicting outcomes from data streams; (4) strategies for optimization, improvement of computational performance, parallel (MPI) and graphics (GPU) computing; (5) processing of very large datasets; and (6) electronic R-markdown notebook facilitating R integration with Python, C/C++, Java, and other languages.

To make use of some complex R–Python–C++ integration libraries, we will need to start with installing and loading the R *reticulate* package. Then, we will set the environment to be able to pass objects between these three (and other) languages within the same electronic Rmarkdown notebook. This functionality makes the statistical computing environment R uniquely portable, highly interoperable, reliable, efficient, and scalable. Depending on the specific operating system and other client settings, this initialization process may need to be adjusted accordingly (follow the instructions of the *reticulate* R package).

```
# install.packages("reticulate")
library(reticulate)
library(plotly)
# specify the path of the Python version that you want to use
# py_path = "C:/Users/UserName/Anaconda3/"  # manual
py_path = Sys.which("python3")              # automated
# use_python(py_path, required = T)
Sys.setenv(RETICULATE_PYTHON = "C:/Users/UserName/Anaconda3/")
sys <- import("sys", convert = TRUE)
```

10.1   Working with Specialized Data and Databases

Unlike the case studies we saw in the previous chapters, some real-world data may not always be nicely formatted, e.g., as CSV files. Often, we collect, arrange, wrangle, and harmonize scattered information to generate computable data objects that can be further processed by various techniques. Data wrangling and preprocessing may take over 80% of the time researchers spend interrogating complex multisource data archives. The following procedures will enhance your skills collecting and handling heterogeneous real-world data. Multiple examples of handling long-and-wide data, messy and tidy data, and data cleaning strategies can be found in this JSS Tidy Data article by Hadley Wickham.[1]

10.1.1   Data Format Conversion

The R package rio imports and exports various types of file formats, e.g., tab-separated (.tsv), comma-separated (.csv), JSON (.json), Stata (.dta), SPSS (.sav and .por), Microsoft Excel (.xls and .xlsx), Weka (.arff), and SAS (.sas7bdat and .xpt) file types.

There are three core functions in the rio package: import(), convert(), and export(). They are intuitive, easy to understand, and efficient to execute. Take Stata (.dta) files as an example. Let's first download a dataset, 02_Nof1_Data. dta, from our data archive folder.

---

[1]https://doi.org/10.18637/jss.v059.i10

```
# install.packages("rio")
library(rio)
# Download the SAS .DTA file first locally. Local data can be loaded by:
# nof1<-import("02_Nof1_Data.dta")
# Or directly from canvas
# nof1<- import("https://umich.instructure.com/files/1760330/download?download_frd=1a")
# the data can also be loaded from the server remotely as well:
nof1 <- read.csv("https://umich.instructure.com/files/330385/download?download_frd=1")
str(nof1)
## 'data.frame':    900 obs. of  10 variables:
## $ ID       : int  1 1 1 1 1 1 1 1 1 1 ...
## $ Day      : int  1 2 3 4 5 6 7 8 9 10 ...
## $ Tx       : int  1 1 0 0 1 1 0 0 1 1 ...
## $ SelfEff  : int  33 33 33 33 33 33 33 33 33 33 ...
## $ SelfEff25: int  8 8 8 8 8 8 8 8 8 8 ...
## $ WPSS     : num  0.97 -0.17 0.81 -0.41 0.59 -1.16 0.3 -0.34 -0.74 ...
## $ SocSuppt : num  5 3.87 4.84 3.62 4.62 2.87 4.33 3.69 3.29 3.66 ...
## $ PMss     : num  4.03 4.03 4.03 4.03 4.03 4.03 4.03 4.03 4.03 4.03 ...
## $ PMss3    : num  1.03 1.03 1.03 1.03 1.03 1.03 1.03 1.03 1.03 1.03 ...
## $ PhyAct   : int  53 73 23 36 21 0 21 0 73 114 ...
```

The data are automatically stored as a data frame. Note that by default, the package `rio` uses `stingAsFactors=FALSE`. The package `rio` can help us export files into any other format we choose. To do this, we have to use the `export ()` function.

```
export(nof1, "C:/Users/UserName/Desktop/02_Nof1.xlsx")
```

This command exports the *Nof1* data in `xlsx` format located in the R working directory or in a user-provided directory. Mac users may have a problem exporting `*.xlsx` files using `rio` because of a lack of a zip tool, but still can output other formats such as ".csv". An alternative strategy to save an `xlsx` file is to use package `xlsx` with default `row.name=TRUE`. The package `rio` also provides a one-step process to convert-and-save data into alternative formats. The following simple code allows us to convert and save the `02_Nof1_Data.dta` file we just downloaded into a CSV file.

```
# convert("02_Nof1_Data.dta", "02_Nof1_Data.csv")
convert("C:/Users/UserName/Desktop/02_Nof1.xlsx",
        "C:/Users/UserName/Desktop/02_Nof1_Data.csv")
```

The result is a new CSV file created in the working directory. Similar transformations are available for many other file formats and data types.

10.1.2   Querying Data in SQL Databases

Look at the 2013–2015 CDC Behavioral Risk Factor Surveillance System (BRFSS) Data.[2] This file (BRFSS_2013_2014_2015.zip) includes the combined landline and

---

[2]https://doi.org/10.7326/M17-3440

cell phone dataset exported from SAS V9.3 using the XPT transport format. This dataset contains 330 variables. The data can be imported into SPSS or STATA; however, some of the variable labels may get truncated in the process of converting to the XPT format.

Caution The size of this compressed (ZIP) file is over 315*MB*! Let's start by ingesting the data for a couple of years and explore some of the information.

```
# install.packages("Hmisc")
library(Hmisc)
memory.size(max=T)
pathToZip <- tempfile()
download.file("https://www.socr.umich.edu/data/DSPA/BRFSS_2013_2014_2015.zip",
              pathToZip)
# let's just pull two of the 3 years of data (2013 and 2015)
brfss_2013 <- sasxport.get(unzip(pathToZip)[1])
brfss_2015 <- sasxport.get(unzip(pathToZip)[3])
dim(brfss_2013); object.size(brfss_2013)
## [1] 491773    336
## 685687656 bytes
# summary(brfss_2013[1:1000, 1:10])  # subsample the data
# report some summaries
brfss_2013$x.race <- as.factor(brfss_2013$x.race)
summary(brfss_2013$x.race)
unlink(pathToZip)     # clean up
```

Next, we can try to use logistic regression to find out if self-reported race/ethnicity predicts the binary outcome of having a health care plan.

```
brfss_2013$has_plan <- brfss_2013$hlthpln1 == 1
system.time(gml1 <- glm(has_plan ~ as.factor(x.race), data=brfss_2013,
              family=binomial))    # report execution time
summary(gml1)
## Coefficients:
##                      Estimate Std. Error  z value Pr(>|z|)
## (Intercept)          2.293549   0.005649  406.044  <2e-16 ***
## as.factor(x.race)2  -0.721676   0.014536  -49.647  <2e-16 ***
## as.factor(x.race)3  -0.511776   0.032974  -15.520  <2e-16 ***
## as.factor(x.race)4  -0.329489   0.031726  -10.386  <2e-16 ***
## as.factor(x.race)5  -1.119329   0.060153  -18.608  <2e-16 ***
## as.factor(x.race)6  -0.544458   0.054535   -9.984  <2e-16 ***
## as.factor(x.race)7  -0.510452   0.030346  -16.821  <2e-16 ***
## as.factor(x.race)8  -1.332005   0.012915 -103.138  <2e-16 ***
## as.factor(x.race)9  -0.582204   0.030604  -19.024  <2e-16 ***
```

We can also examine the odds (rather the log odds ratio, LOR) of having a health care plan (HCP) by race (R). The LORs are calculated for two-dimensional arrays, separately for each *race* level (presence of *health care plan* (HCP) is binary, whereas *race* (R) has 9 levels, $R_1, R_2, \ldots, R_9$). For example, the odds ratio of having a HCP for $R1 : R2$ is:

$$OR(R_1 : R_2) = \frac{\frac{P(\text{HCP}|R_1)}{1 - P(\text{HCP}|R_1)}}{\frac{P(\text{HCP}|R_2)}{1 - P(\text{HCP}|R_2)}}.$$

```
# install.packages("vcd"), the vcd package computes the LOR
library("vcd")
# *Loddsratio* computes the Log odds ratio (LOR). The raw OR=exp(Loddsratio)
lor_HCP_by_R <- loddsratio(has_plan ~ as.factor(x.race), data = brfss_2013)
lor_HCP_by_R
## log odds ratios for has_plan and as.factor(x.race)
##          1:2         2:3         3:4         4:5         5:6         6:7
## -0.72167619  0.20990061  0.18228646 -0.78984000  0.57487142  0.03400611
##          7:8         8:9
## -0.82155382  0.74980101
```

Next, let's see an example of querying a database containing structured relational records. A *query* is a machine instruction (typically represented as text) sent by a user to a remote database requesting a specific database operation (e.g., search or summary). One database communication protocol relies on SQL (Structured query language). MySQL is an instance of a database management system that supports SQL communication that many web applications utilize, e.g., *YouTube, Flickr, Wikipedia*, biological databases like *GO, ensembl*, etc. Below is an example of an SQL query using the package RMySQL. An alternative way to interface an SQL database is by using the package RODBC. Let's look at a couple of DB query examples. The first one uses the UCSC Genomics SQL server (genome-mysql.cse. ucsc.edu) and the second one uses a local client-side database service.

```
# install.packages("DBI", "RMySQL")
# install.packages("RODBC"); library(RODBC)
library(DBI); library(RMySQL)
library("stringr"); library("dplyr"); library("readr")
library(magrittr)
ucscGenomeConn <- dbConnect(MySQL(), user='genome', dbname='hg19',
                    host='genome-mysql.cse.ucsc.edu')
# dbGetInfo(ucscGenomeConn); dbListResults(ucscGenomeConn)
result <- dbGetQuery(ucscGenomeConn,"show databases;");
# List the DB tables
allTables <- dbListTables(ucscGenomeConn); length(allTables) ## [1] 12571
# Get dimensions of a table, read and report the head
dbListFields(ucscGenomeConn, "affyU133Plus2")
##  [1] "bin"        "matches"    "misMatches" "repMatches" "nCount"
##  [6] "qNumInsert" "qBaseInsert" "tNumInsert" "tBaseInsert" "strand"
## [11] "qName"      "qSize"      "qStart"     "qEnd"       "tName"
## [16] "tSize"      "tStart"     "tEnd"       "blockCount" "blockSizes"
## [21] "qStarts"    "tStarts"
affyData <- dbReadTable(ucscGenomeConn, "affyU133Plus2"); head(affyData)
## bin matches misMatches repMatches nCount qNumInsert qBaseInsert tNumInsert
## 1 585     530          4          0     23          3          41          3
## 2 585    3355         17          0    109          9          67          9
## 3 585    4156         14          0     83         16          18          2
## 4 585    4667          9          0     68         21          42          3
## 5 585    5180         14          0    167         10          38          1
## 6 585     468          5          0     14          0           0          0
...
# Select a subset, fetch the data, and report the quantiles
subsetQuery <- dbSendQuery(ucscGenomeConn,
            "select * from affyU133Plus2 where misMatches between 1 and 3")
```

```
affySmall <- fetch(subsetQuery); dim(affySmall)    ## [1] 500  22
quantile(affySmall$misMatches)
##   0% 25% 50%  75% 100%
##    1   1   2    2    3
dbClearResult(subsetQuery)
# Another query
bedFile      <- "C:/Users/UserName/Desktop/repUCSC.bed"
subsetQuery1 <- dbSendQuery(ucscGenomeConn,
                 'select genoName,genoStart,genoEnd,repName,swScore, strand,
                  repClass, repFamily from rmsk')
subsetQuery1_df <- dbFetch(subsetQuery1 , n=100) %>%
        dplyr::mutate(genoName=stringr::str_replace(genoName,'chr','')) %>%
        readr::write_tsv(bedFile, col_names=T)
message('saved: ', bedFile)
dbClearResult(subsetQuery1)
# Another DB query: Select a specific DB subset
subsetQuery2 <- dbSendQuery(ucscGenomeConn,
            "select * from affyU133Plus2 where misMatches between 1 and 4")
affyU133Plus2MisMatch <- fetch(subsetQuery2)
quantile(affyU133Plus2MisMatch$misMatches)
##   0% 25% 50%  75% 100%
##    1   1   2    3    4
affyU133Plus2MisMatchTiny_100x22 <- fetch(subsetQuery2, n=100)
dbClearResult(subsetQuery2)
dim(affyU133Plus2MisMatchTiny_100x22)  ## [1] 100  22
summary(affyU133Plus2MisMatchTiny_100x22)
...
# Once done, clear and close the connections
# dbClearResult(dbListResults(ucscGenomeConn)[[1]])
dbDisconnect(ucscGenomeConn)
```

Depending upon the DB server, to complete the above database SQL commands, it may require access and/or specific user credentials. The example below can be done by all users, as it relies only on local DB services.

```
# install.packages("RSQLite")
library("RSQLite")
# generate an empty DB stored RAM
myConnection <- dbConnect(RSQLite::SQLite(), ":memory:"); myConnection
dbListTables(myConnection)
# Add tables to the local SQL DB
data(USArrests); dbWriteTable(myConnection, "USArrests", USArrests)
dbWriteTable(myConnection, "brfss_2013", brfss_2013)
dbWriteTable(myConnection, "brfss_2015", brfss_2015)
# Check again the DB content
# allTables <- dbListTables(myConnection); length(allTables); allTables
head(dbListFields(myConnection, "brfss_2013"))
## [1] "x.state" "fmonth"  "idate"   "imonth"  "iday"    "iyear"
tail(dbListFields(myConnection, "brfss_2013"))
## [1] "rcsrace1" "rchisla1" "rcsbirth" "typeinds" "typework" "has_plan"
dbListTables(myConnection);
## [1] "USArrests" "brfss_2013" "brfss_2015"
# Retrieve the entire DB table (for the smaller USArrests table)
head(dbGetQuery(myConnection, "SELECT * FROM USArrests"))
# Retrieve just the average of one feature
myQuery <- dbGetQuery(myConnection, "SELECT avg(Assault) FROM USArrests")
head(myQuery)
```

```
##   avg(Assault)  ## 1        170.76
myQuery <- dbGetQuery(myConnection,
            "SELECT avg(Assault) FROM USArrests GROUP BY UrbanPop"); myQuery

…
# Or do it in batches (for the much larger brfss_2013 and brfss_2015 tables)
myQuery <- dbGetQuery(myConnection, "SELECT * FROM brfss_2013")
# compute the average (poorhlth) grouping by Insurance (hlthpln1)
# Try some alternatives: numadult nummen numwomen genhlth physhlth menthlth
poorhlth hlthpln1
myQuery1_13 <- dbGetQuery(myConnection,
            "SELECT avg(poorhlth) FROM brfss_2013 GROUP BY hlthpln1"); myQuery1_13
##   avg(poorhlth)
## 1     56.25466
## 2     53.99962
## 3     58.85072
## 4     66.26757
# Compare 2013 vs. 2015: Health grouping by Insurance
myQuery1_15 <- dbGetQuery(myConnection,
            "SELECT avg(poorhlth) FROM brfss_2015 GROUP BY hlthpln1"); myQuery1_15
##   avg(poorhlth)
## 1     55.75539
## 2     55.49487
## 3     61.35445
## 4     67.62125
myQuery1_13 - myQuery1_15
##   avg(poorhlth)
## 1     0.4992652
## 2    -1.4952515
## 3    -2.5037326
## 4    -1.3536797
# reset the DB query
# dbClearResult(myQuery)
dbDisconnect(myConnection) # clean up
```

10.1.3   SparQL Queries

The *SparQL Protocol and RDF Query Language* (SparQL) is a semantic database query language for RDF (Resource Description Framework) data objects. SparQL queries consist of (1) triple patterns, (2) conjunctions, and (3) disjunctions. The following example uses SparQL to query the prevalence of tuberculosis from the WikiData SparQL server and plot it on a World geographic map (Fig. 10.1).

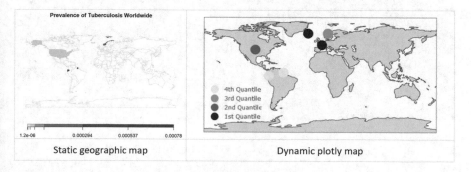

Fig. 10.1 Geographic maps showing partial SparQL results of global tuberculosis prevalence

```r
# install.packages("SPARQL"); install.packages("rworldmap")
library(SPARQL)
library(ggplot2)
library(rworldmap)
library(plotly)
# SparQL Format https://www.w3.org/2009/Talks/0615-qbe/
# W3C Turtle - Terse RDF Triple Language:
# https://www.w3.org/TeamSubmission/turtle/#sec-examples
# RDF (Resource Description Framework) is a graphical data model of (subject,
predicate, object) triples representing:
# "subject-node to predicate arc to object arc"
# Resources are represented by URIs that can be abbreviated as prefixed names
# Objects are literals: strings, integers, booleans, etc.
# Syntax
#    URIs: <http://example.com/resource> or prefix:name
#    Literals:
#              "plain string" "13.4""
#              xsd:float, or
#              "string with language" @en
#    Triple: pref:subject other:predicate "object".
wdqs <- "https://query.wikidata.org/bigdata/namespace/wdq/sparql"
query = "PREFIX wd: <http://www.wikidata.org/entity/>
    # prefix declarations
    PREFIX wdt: <http://www.wikidata.org/prop/direct/>
    PREFIX rdfs: <http://www.w3.org/2000/01/rdf-schema#>
    PREFIX p: <http://www.wikidata.org/prop/>
    PREFIX v: <http://www.wikidata.org/prop/statement/>
    PREFIX qualifier: <http://www.wikidata.org/prop/qualifier/>
    PREFIX statement: <http://www.wikidata.org/prop/statement/>
    # result clause
    SELECT DISTINCT ?countryLabel ?ISO3Code ?latlon ?prevalence ?doid ?year
    # query pattern against RDF data
    # Q36956 Hansen's disease, Leprosy https://www.wikidata.org/wiki/Q36956
    # Q15750965 - Alzheimer's disease:
                                    https://www.wikidata.org/wiki/Q15750965
    # Influenza - Q2840: https://www.wikidata.org/wiki/Q2840
    # Q12204 - tuberculosis  https://www.wikidata.org/wiki/Q12204
    # P699 Alzheimer's Disease ontology ID
    # P1193 prevalence: https://www.wikidata.org/wiki/Property:P1193
    # P17 country: https://www.wikidata.org/wiki/Property:P17
    # Country ISO-3 code: https://www.wikidata.org/wiki/Property:P298
    # Location: https://www.wikidata.org/wiki/Property:P625
    # Wikidata docs:
            https://www.mediawiki.org/wiki/Wikidata_query_service/User_Manual
    WHERE {
       wd:Q12204 wdt:P699 ?doid ; # tuberculosis P699 Disease ontology ID
       p:P1193 ?prevalencewithProvenance .
       ?prevalencewithProvenance qualifier:P17 ?country ;
       qualifier:P585 ?year ;
       statement:P1193 ?prevalence .
       ?country wdt:P625 ?latlon ;
       rdfs:label ?countryLabel ;
       wdt:P298 ?ISO3Code ;
       wdt:P297 ?ISOCode .
    FILTER (lang(?countryLabel) = \"en\")
    # FILTER constraints use boolean conditions to filter out unwanted query
results.
    #    Shortcut: a semicolon (;) can be used to separate two triple patterns
that share the same disease (?country is the shared subject above.)
```

```
   #     rdfs:label is a common predicate for giving a human-friendly label to a
resource.
   }
   # query modifiers
   ORDER BY DESC(?population)
"

# install.packages("WikidataQueryServiceR")
library(WikidataQueryServiceR)
library(mapproj)
results <- query_wikidata(sparql_query=query); head(results)
## # A tibble: 6 x 6
##     countryLabel                ISO3Code latlon  prevalence doid   year
##     <chr>                       <chr>    <chr>        <dbl> <chr>  <dttm>
## 1 Norway                        NOR      Point(~   0.0001   DOID~ 2014-01-01
## 2 United States of America USA      Point(~   0.000029 DOID~ 2014-01-01
## 3 France                        FRA      Point(~   0.0000012 DOID~ 2014-01-01
## 4 Iceland                       ISL      Point(~   0.0000043 DOID~ 2014-01-01
## 5 Ecuador                       ECU      Point(~   0.00078  DOID~ 2014-01-01
## 6 Suriname                      SUR      Point(~   0.00044  DOID~ 2014-01-01
# join the data to the geo map
sPDF <- joinCountryData2Map(results, joinCode = "ISO3",
                            nameJoinColumn = "ISO3Code")
# map the data with no legend
mapParams <- mapCountryData( sPDF, nameColumnToPlot="prevalence",
         # Alternatively , nameColumnToPlot="doid"
         addLegend='FALSE', mapTitle="Prevalence of Tuberculosis Worldwide")
#  add a modified legend using the same initial parameters as mapCountryData
do.call( addMapLegend, c( mapParams, legendLabels="all", legendWidth=0.5))
text(1, -120, "Partial view of Tuberculosis Prevalence in the World", cex=1)
View(getMap()) # write.csv(file = "C:/Users/Map.csv", getMap())
# Alternative Plot_ly Geo-map
df_cities <- results
df_cities$popm <- paste(df_cities$countryLabel, df_cities$ISO3Code,
                        "prevalence=", df_cities$prevalence)
df_cities$quart <- with(df_cities, cut(prevalence, quantile(prevalence),
                        include.lowest = T))
levels(df_cities$quart) <- paste(c("1st", "2nd", "3rd", "4th"), "Quantile")
df_cities$quart <- as.ordered(df_cities$quart)
df_cities <- tidyr::separate(df_cities, latlon, into=c("long","lat"),sep=" ")
df_cities$long <- gsub("Point\\(", "", df_cities$long)
df_cities$lat  <- gsub("\\)", "", df_cities$lat)
head(df_cities)
ge <- list(scope = 'world', showland = TRUE, landcolor = toRGB("lightgray"),
           subunitwidth = 1, countrywidth = 1, subunitcolor = toRGB("white"),
           countrycolor = toRGB("white"))
plot_geo(df_cities, lon = ~long, lat = ~lat, text = ~popm, mode="markers",
         marker = ~list(size = 20, line = list(width = 0.1)),
         color = ~quart, locationmode = 'country names') %>%
    layout(geo = ge, title = 'Prevalence of Tuberculosis Worldwide')
```

Similar geographic maps may be displayed for other processes, e.g., malaria. Note that such data are sparse as they are pulled dynamically from wikidata. Some data pulls may generate lots of data, some may be small, and still others may result in empty queries. Below is an example of a geo-map showing the global locations and population-size of various cities in millions (Fig. 10.2).

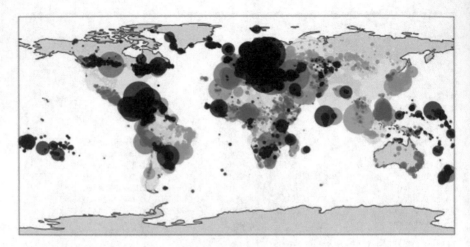

Fig. 10.2 A geographic map showing partial SparQL results of several city populations

```
library(plotly)
df_cities <- world.cities
df_cities$popm <- paste(df_cities$country.etc, df_cities$name, "Pop",
                        round(df_cities$pop/1e6,2), " million")
df_cities$quart <- with(df_cities, cut(pop, quantile(pop), include.lowest=T))
levels(df_cities$quart) <- paste(c("1st", "2nd", "3rd", "4th"), "Quantile")
df_cities$quart <- as.ordered(df_cities$quart)
ge <- list(scope = 'world', showland = TRUE, landcolor = toRGB("lightgray"),
           subunitwidth = 1, countrywidth = 1, subunitcolor =-toRGB("white"),
           countrycolor = toRGB("white"))
plot_geo(df_cities, lon = ~long, lat = ~lat, text = ~popm, mode="markers",
         marker = ~list(size = sqrt(pop/10000) + 1, line=list(width = 0.1)),
         color = ~quart, locationmode = 'country names') %>%
    layout(geo = ge, title = 'City Populations (Worldwide)')
```

10.1.4   Real Random Number Generation

We are already familiar with (pseudo) random number generation (e.g., rnorm
(100, 10, 4) or runif(100, 10,20)), which *algorithmically* generate random values subject to specified distributions. There are also web-services, e.g.,
https://random.org, that can provide *truly random* numbers based on atmospheric
noise, rather than using a pseudo random number generation protocol. Below is one
example of generating a total of 300 numbers arranged in 3 columns, each of
100 rows of random integers (in decimal format in the range [100, 200].

```
siteURL <- "https://random.org/integers/"   #    base URL
shortQuery <-"num=300&min=100&max=200&col=3&base=10&format=plain&rnd=new"
completeQuery <- paste(siteURL,shortQuery,sep="?") #concat url & query string
rngNumbers <- read.table(file=completeQuery)        # and read the data
head(rngNumbers); tail(rngNumbers)
##    V1  V2  V3
## 1 124 131 139
## 2 189 124 153
…
## 6 103 178 143
##       V1  V2  V3
## 95  197 160 142
## 96  125 175 141
…
## 100 125 189 161
```

10.1.5   Downloading the Complete Text of Web Pages

The package RCurl provides functionality for extracting and scraping information
from websites. Let's use it to demonstrate extracting information from a SOCR
website.

```
# install.packages("RCurl")
library(RCurl)
web<-getURI("https://wiki.socr.umich.edu/index.php/SOCR_Data",
            followlocation = TRUE)
str(web, nchar.max = 200)
##   chr "<!DOCTYPE html>\n<html class=\"client-nojs\" lang=\"en\"
dir=\"ltr\">\n<head>\n<meta charset=\"UTF-8\"/>\n<title>SOCR Data -
SOCR</title>\n<script>document.documentElement.className ="| …
```

The retrieved web object looks incomprehensible. This is because most websites
are wrapped in XML/HTML hypertext or include JSON formatted meta-data.
RCurl understands special HTML tags and website meta-data. To deal solely
with the web pages, the httr package provides another alternative to RCurl. It
returns a list that makes much more sense.

```
# install.packages("httr")
library(httr)
web <- GET("https://wiki.socr.umich.edu/index.php/SOCR_Data")
str(web[1:3])
## List of 3
##  $ url         : chr "https://wiki.socr.umich.edu/index.php/SOCR_Data"
##  $ status_code : int 200
##  $ headers     :List of 15
##  ..$ date                    : chr "Sun, 12 Jun 2022 20:51:17 GMT"
…
```

10.1.6   Reading and Writing XML with the XML Package

A combination of the RCurl and the XML packages could help us extract only the plain text from the specified webpages. This would be very helpful to get information from text heavy webpages.

```
Web <- getURL("https://wiki.socr.umich.edu/index.php/SOCR_Data",
              followlocation = TRUE)
library(XML)
web.parsed <- htmlParse(web, asText = T, encoding="UTF-8")
plain.text <- xpathSApply(web.parsed, "//p", xmlValue)
substr(paste(plain.text, collapse = "\n"), start=1, stop=256)
## [1] "The links below contain a number of datasets that may be used for
demonstration purposes in probability and statistics education. There are two
types of data - simulated (computer-generated using random sampling) and … "
```

Here we extracted all plain text between the starting and ending *paragraph* HTML tags, <p> and </p>. More information about extracting text from XML/HTML to text via XPath is available here.[3]

10.1.7   Web Page Data Scraping

The process of extracting data from complete web pages and storing it in structured data format is called scraping. However, before starting a data scrape from a website, we need to understand the underlying HTML structure for that specific website. Also, we have to check the terms of that website to make sure that scraping from this site is allowed.

The R package rvest is a very good place to start "harvesting" data from websites. To start with, we use read_html() to ingest the SOCR website hypertext metadata into a xmlnode object.

```
library(rvest)
SOCR <- read_html("https://wiki.socr.umich.edu/index.php/SOCR_Data"); SOCR
```

From the summary structure of SOCR, we can discover that there are two important hypertext section markups <head> and <body>. Also, notice that the SOCR data website uses <title> and </title> tags to extract the title in the <head> section. Let's use html_node() to extract title information based on this knowledge.

```
SOCR %>% html_node("head title") %>% html_text()
## [1] "SOCR Data - SOCR"
```

---

[3] https://doi.org/10.1007/978-1-4614-7900-0_4

Here we used %>% operator, or pipe, to connect two functions, see magrittr package, which creates a chain of functions to operate on the SOCR object. The first function in the chain html_node() extracts the title from the head section. Then, html_text() translates HTML formatted hypertext into English.

Another function, rvest::html_nodes() is also very helpful in scraping. Similar to html_node(), html_nodes() can help us extract multiple nodes in an xmlnode object. Assume that we want to obtain the meta elements (usually page description, keywords, author of the document, last modified, and other metadata) from the SOCR data website. We apply html_nodes() to the SOCR object for lines starting with <meta in the <head> section. It is optional to use html_attrs() (extracts attributes, text and tag name from html) to make texts prettier.

```
meta <- SOCR %>% html_nodes("head meta") %>% html_attrs(); meta
...
```

10.1.8 Parsing JSON From Web APIs

Application Programming Interfaces (APIs) allow web-accessible functions to communicate with each other. Today most API is stored in JSON (JavaScript Object Notation) format.

JSON represents a plain text format used for web applications, data structures or objects. Online JSON objects could be retrieved by packages like RCurl and httr. Let's see a JSON formatted dataset first. We can use 02_Nof1_Data.json in the class file as an example.

```
library(httr)
nof1 <- GET("https://umich.instructure.com/files/1760327/download?download_frd=1")
nof1
...
```

We can see that JSON objects tend to be simple hierarchical structures. The data structure is organized using hierarchies marked by square brackets. Each piece of information is formatted as a {key:value} pair.

The package jsonlite is a very useful tool to import online JSON formatted datasets into data frames directly. Its syntax is very straight forward.

```
# install.packages("jsonlite")
library(jsonlite)
nof1_lite <-
    fromJSON("https://umich.instructure.com/files/1760327/download?download_frd=1")
class(nof1_lite)
```

10.1.9   Reading and Writing Microsoft Excel Spreadsheets Using XLSX

We can transfer *xlsx* datasets into CSV files, save them, and use read.csv() to load the data back into R. However, R also provides an alternative read.xlsx() function in the package xlsx to simplify this process. Let's take the 02_Nof1_Data.xls data as an example.

```
# install.packages("xlsx")
library(xlsx)
nof1 <- read.xlsx("C:/Users/UserName/Desktop/02_Nof1.xlsx", 1)
str(nof1)
## 'data.frame':    900 obs. of  10 variables:
## $ ID        : num  1 1 1 1 1 1 1 1 1 1 ...
## $ Day       : num  1 2 3 4 5 6 7 8 9 10 ...
## $ Tx        : num  1 1 0 0 1 1 0 0 1 1 ...
## $ SelfEff   : num  33 33 33 33 33 33 33 33 33 33 ...
## $ SelfEff25 : num  8 8 8 8 8 8 8 8 8 8 ...
## $ WPSS      : num  0.97 -0.17 0.81 -0.41 0.59 -1.16 0.3 -0.34 -0.74 -0.38 ...
## $ SocSuppt  : num  5 3.87 4.84 3.62 4.62 2.87 4.33 3.69 3.29 3.66 ...
## $ PMss      : num  4.03 4.03 4.03 4.03 4.03 4.03 4.03 4.03 4.03 4.03 ...
## $ PMss3     : num  1.03 1.03 1.03 1.03 1.03 1.03 1.03 1.03 1.03 1.03 ...
## $ PhyAct    : num  53 73 23 36 21 0 21 0 73 114 ...
```

The last argument in the function call, 1, indicates extracting the first excel sheet, as any excel file may include a large number of tables in it. Also, we can download the xls or xlsx file into our R working directory so that it is easier to find file paths.

Sometimes more complex protocols may be necessary to ingest data from complex XLSX documents, e.g., when the XLSX doc is large, if it includes many tables, or if it is only accessible via HTTP protocol from a remote webserver. Below is an example downloading the second table, ABIDE_Aggregated_Data, from the multi-table Autism/ABIDE XLSX dataset.

```
# install.packages("openxlsx"); library(openxlsx)
tmp = tempfile(fileext = ".xlsx")
download.file(
        url = "https://umich.instructure.com/files/3225493/download?download_frd=1",
        destfile = tmp, mode="wb")
df_Autism <- openxlsx::read.xlsx(xlsxFile = tmp,
                    sheet = "ABIDE_Aggregated_Data", skipEmptyRows = TRUE)
dim(df_Autism)
## [1] 1098 2145
```

10.2 Working with Domain-Specific Data

Many powerful Machine Learning methods are applicable in a broad range of disciplines. However, each domain has specific requirements and specialized data formats that often demand customized interfaces to employ existing tools to research-specific data-driven challenges. The important field of biomedical informatics and data science (BIDS) represents one such example.

10.2.1 Working with Bioinformatics Data

Genetic data are stored in widely varying formats and usually have more feature variables than observations. They could have 1000 columns and only 200 rows. One of the commonly used preprocessing steps for such datasets is *variable selection*. We will talk about this in Chap. 11. The Bioconductor project provides powerful R functionality (packages and tools) for analyzing genomic data.[4]

10.2.2 Visualizing Network Data

Social network data and graph datasets describe the relations between nodes (vertices) using connections (links or edges) joining the node objects. Assume we have N objects, we can have $N \times (N - 1)$ directed links establishing paired associations between the nodes. Let's use an example with $N = 4$ to demonstrate a simple graph potentially modeling the following linkage table

objects	1	2	3	4
1	...	$1 \rightarrow 2$	$1 \rightarrow 3$	$1 \rightarrow 4$
2	$2 \rightarrow 1$	...	$2 \rightarrow 3$	$2 \rightarrow 4$
3	$3 \rightarrow 1$	$3 \rightarrow 2$	...	$3 \rightarrow 4$
4	$4 \rightarrow 1$	$4 \rightarrow 2$	$4 \rightarrow 3$	...

If we change the assignment mapping $a \rightarrow b$ to an indicator variable (0 or 1) capturing whether we have an edge connecting a pair of nodes, then we get the graph *adjacency matrix*. Edge lists provide an alternative way to represent network connections. Every line in the list contains a connection between two nodes (objects)

---

[4] https://www.bioconductor.org

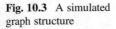 **Fig. 10.3** A simulated graph structure

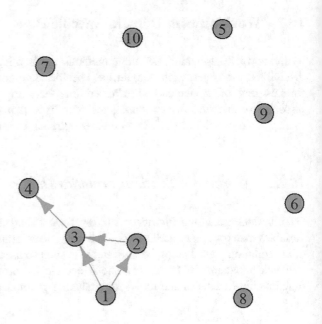

Vertex	Vertex
1	2
1	3
2	3

The above edge list is listing three network connections: object 1 is linked to object 2; object 1 is linked to object 3; and object 2 is linked to object 3. Note that edge lists can represent both *directed* and *undirected* networks or graphs.

We can imagine that if N is very large, e.g., representing large social networks, the data representation and analysis may be resource intense (memory or computation). In R, we have multiple packages that can deal with social network data. One user-friendly example is provided using the igraph package. First, let's build a toy example and visualize it using this package (Fig. 10.3).

```
# install.packages("igraph")
library(igraph)
g <- graph(c(1, 2, 1, 3, 2, 3, 3, 4), n=10)
plot(g)
```

Here c(1, 2, 1, 3, 2, 3, 3, 4) is an *edge* list with 4 pairs of node connections and n = 10 *nodes* (objects) in total. The small arrows in the graph show us directed network connections. We might notice that 5–10 nodes are scattered and disconnected from the rest of the graph. This is because they are not included in the edge list, so there are no network connections between them and the rest of the network.

Now let's explore an example of the co-appearance network of Facebook circles. The data contains anonymized `circles` (friends lists) from Facebook collected from survey participants using a Facebook app. The dataset only includes edges (88,234 circles) connecting pairs of nodes (4039 users) in a network.

The values on the connections represent the number of links/edges within a circle. We have a huge edge-list made of scrambled Facebook user IDs. Let's load this dataset into R first. The data is stored in a text file. Unlike CSV files, text files in table format need to be imported using `read.table()`. We are using the `header=F` option to let R know that we don't have a header in the text file that contains only tab-separated node pairs (indicating the social connections, edges, between Facebook users).

```
soc.net.data<-
   read.table("https://umich.instructure.com/files/2854431/download?download_frd=1",
              sep=" ", header=F)
head(soc.net.data)
##     V1 V2
## 1  0  1
## 2  0  2
...
```

The data are stored in a data frame and to make it ready for `igraph` processing and visualization, we need to convert `soc.net.data` into a matrix object.

```
soc.net.data.mat <- as.matrix(soc.net.data, ncol=2)
```

By using `ncol=2`, we create a matrix with two columns which is ready for applying the method `graph.edgelist()`.

```
# remove the first 347 edges (to wipe out the degenerate "0" node)
graph_m<-graph.edgelist(soc.net.data.mat[-c(0:347), ], directed = F)
```

Before we display the social network graph, we may want to examine our model first.

```
summary(graph_m) ## IGRAPH 80e350b U--- 4038 87887 --
```

This is an extremely brief yet informative summary. The first line `U--- 4038 87887` includes potentially four letters and two numbers. The first letter could be `U` or `D` indicating *undirected* or *directed* edges. The second letter `N` would mean that the object set has a "name" attribute, and the third letter is for weighted (`W`) graphs. Since we didn't add weight in our analysis the third letter is empty ("`-`"). The final, fourth character, also "`-`", is an indicator for bipartite graphs whose vertices can be divided into `two disjoint sets`, i.e., independent sets where each vertex from one set connects to one vertex in the other set. The two numbers following the four letters represent the `number of nodes` (4038) and the `number of edges` (87887), respectively. Now let's render the graph.

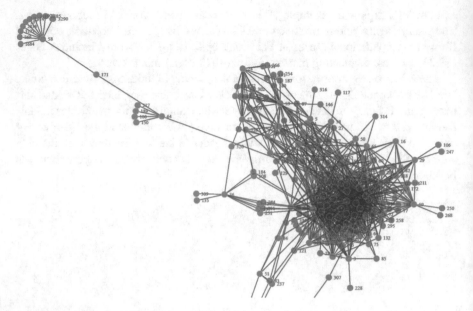

Fig. 10.4 A portion of a large Facebook friends' graph network

```
# Choose an algorithm to find network communities.
# FastGreedy algorithm is great for large undirected networks
comm_graph_m <- fastgreedy.community(graph_m)
# sizes(comm_graph_m); membership(comm_graph_m)
# Collapse the graph by communities
reduced_comm_graph_m <- simplify(contract(graph_m, membership(comm_graph_m)))
plot(graph_m, vertex.size=3, vertex.color=adjustcolor("SkyBlue2",
    alpha.f=0.7), vertex.label=NA, margin=-0.2, layout=layout.reingold.tilford)
```

We can also use D3 to display a dynamic graph (Fig. 10.4).

```
# install.packages('networkD3')
library(networkD3)
df <- as_data_frame(graph_m, what = "edges")
# JS note indexing starts at 0, not 1, make an artificial index 0 root
df1 <- rbind(c(0,1), df)
# Use D3 to display graph
simpleNetwork(df1[1:1000,], fontSize = 12, zoom = T)
```

This graph is very complicated, yet we can still see that some nodes (influencers) are surrounded by more nodes than other network members. To quantify such information we can use the degree() function which lists the number of edges for each node in the graph.

```
degree(graph_m)[100:110]
##  [1]    8   18    5   15   31   13    7 1044   12   36    4
```

Skimming the table, we can find that the 107-th user has as many as 1044 connections, which makes the user a *highly connected hub*. Likely, this node may have higher social relevance or influence.

Similarly, some edges might be more important than other edges because they serve as a bridge between different clouds or clusters of nodes. To compare their importance, we can use the betweenness centrality measurement. *Betweenness centrality* measures the centrality in a network. High centrality for a specific node indicates high importance and potential influence. The method betweenness() can help us to calculate the betweenness centrality of a given fixed network node v_o

$$g(v_0) = \sum_{s \neq v_o \neq t} \frac{\sigma_{st}(v_o)}{\sigma_{st}},$$

where σ_{st} is the total number of shortest paths from node s to node t and $\sigma_{st}(v_o)$ is the number of those paths that pass through the fixed network node v_o, which is not a leaf node on the graph.

```
betweenness(graph_m)[100:110]
```

Again, the 107-th node has the highest betweenness centrality $(3.556221e + 06)$.

We can try another example using SOCR hierarchical data, which is also available for dynamic exploration as a tree graph. Let's read its JSON data source using the jsonlite package.

```
tree.json <- fromJSON("http://socr.ucla.edu/SOCR_HyperTree.json",
                      simplifyDataFrame = FALSE)
```

This generates a list object representing the hierarchical structure of the network. Note that this is quite different from edge list. There is one root node, its sub nodes are called *children nodes*, and the terminal nodes are call *leaf nodes*. Instead of presenting the relationship between nodes in pairs, this hierarchical structure captures the level for each node. To draw the social network graph, we need to convert it as a Node object. We can utilize the as.Node() function in the data.tree package to do so.

```
# install.packages("data.tree")
library(data.tree)
tree.graph <- as.Node(tree.json, mode = "explicit")
```

Here we use the mode="explicit" option to allow "children" nodes to have their own "children" nodes. Now, the tree.json object has been separated into four different node structures - "About SOCR", "SOCR Resources", "Get Started", and "SOCR Wiki". Let's plot the first one using the igraph package.

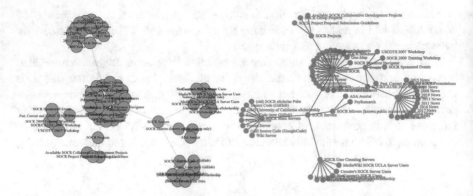

Fig. 10.5 Static (left) and dynamic (right) graph displays of the SOCR meta-data

In the example below, we are demonstrating a slightly complicated scenario where the graphs source data (in this case JSON file) includes nodes with the same *name*. In principle, this causes a problem with the graph traversal that may lead to infinite loops of node traversal. Thus, we will search for nodes with duplicated names and modify their names to make the algorithm more robust (Fig. 10.5).

```
AreNamesUnique <- function(node) {
  mynames <- node$Get("name")
  all(duplicated(mynames) == FALSE)
}
## extract Graph Nodes with Unique Names (remove duplicate nodes)
getUniqueNodes <- function(node) {
  AreNamesUnique(node)
  mynames <- node$Get("name")
  (names_unique <- ifelse (duplicated(mynames),
                      sprintf("%s_%d", mynames, sample(1:1000,1)), mynames))
  node$Set(name = names_unique)
  AreNamesUnique(node)
  return(node)
}
# Do this duplicate node renaming until there are no duplicated names
while (length(tree.graph$Get("name"))!=length(unique(tree.graph$Get("name"))))
     { getUniqueNodes(tree.graph); AreNamesUnique(tree.graph)  }
length(tree.graph$Get("name"))  ## [1] 587
length(unique(tree.graph$Get("name")))
plot(as.igraph(tree.graph$`About SOCR`), edge.arrow.size=5,  # static graph
                 edge.label.font=0.05)
## D3 dynamic plot
df <- as_data_frame(as.igraph(tree.graph$`About SOCR`), what = "edges")
df1 <- rbind(c("SOCR", "About SOCR"), df)
simpleNetwork(df1, fontSize = 12, zoom = T) # Use D3 to display graph
```

In these network graphs, the node "About SOCR", located at the center of the graph, represents the root of the tree network. Of course, we can repeat this process starting with the root of the complete hierarchical structure, SOCR.

10.3   Data Streaming

The proliferation of Cloud services and the emergence of modern technology in all aspects of human experiences leads to a tsunami of data, much of which is streamed real time. The interrogation of such voluminous data is an increasingly important area of research. *Data streams* are ordered, often unbounded, sequences of data points created continuously by a data generator. All the data mining, interrogation, and forecasting methods we discussed for traditional datasets are also applicable to data streams.

10.3.1   Definition

Mathematically, a *data stream* in an ordered sequence of data points

$$Y = \{y_1, y_2, y_3, \cdots, y_t, \cdots\},$$

where the (time) index, t, reflects the order of the observation/record, which may be single numbers, simple vectors in multidimensional space, or objects, e.g., structured Ann Arbor Weather (JSON) and its corresponding structured form. Some streaming data are *streamed* because it's too large to be downloaded shotgun style and some is *streamed* because it's continually generated and serviced. This presents the potential problem of dealing with data streams that may be unlimited.

Notes
- *Data sources*: Real or synthetic stream data can be used. Random simulation streams may be created by `rstream`. Real stream data may be piped from financial data providers, the WHO, World Bank, NCAR, and other sources.
- *Inference Techniques*: Many of the data interrogation techniques we have seen can be employed for dynamic stream data, e.g., `factas`, for PCA, `rEMM` and `birch` for clustering, etc. Clustering and classification methods capable of processing data streams have been developed, e.g., *Very Fast Decision Trees* (VFDT), *time window-based Online Information Network* (OLIN), *On-demand Classification*, and the *APRIORI* streaming algorithm.
- *Cloud distributed computing*: Hadoop2/HadoopStreaming, SPARK, Storm3/RStorm and other services provide environments to expand batch/script-based R tools to the Cloud.

10.3.2   The stream Package

The R *stream* package provides data stream mining algorithms using fpc, clue, cluster, clusterGeneration, MASS, and proxy packages. In addition, the package streamMOA provides an rJava interface to the Java-based data stream clustering algorithms available in the *Massive Online Analysis* (MOA) framework for stream classification, regression, and clustering. A deeper exposure to data streaming in R is provided in the stream package vignettes.

10.3.3   Synthetic Example—Random Gaussian Stream

This example shows the creation and loading of a *mixture of five random 2D Gaussians*, centers at (*x_coords*, *y_coords*) with paired correlations *rho_corr*, representing a simulated data stream.

10.3.4   Generate the Stream

```
# install.packages("stream")
library("stream")
## Warning: package 'stream' was built under R version 4.1.2
x_coords <- c(0.2,0.3, 0.5, 0.8, 0.9)
y_coords <- c(0.8,0.3, 0.7, 0.1, 0.5)
p_weight <- c(0.1, 0.9, 0.5, 0.4, 0.3) # A vector of probabilities that
determines the likelihood of generated a data point from a particular cluster
set.seed(12345)
stream_5G <- DSD_Gaussians(k=5, d=2, mu=cbind(x_coords,y_coords), p=p_weight)
```

10.3.4.1   K-Means Clustering

We will now try k-means (Chap. 8) and a density-based data stream clustering algorithm, D-Stream,[5] where microclusters are formed by grid cells of size *gridsize* with the density of a grid cell (Cm) being at least 1.2 times the average cell density. The model is updated with the next 500 data points from the stream.

```
dstream <- DSC_DStream(gridsize = 0.1, Cm = 1.2)
update(dstream,  stream_5G,  n=500)
```

First, let's run the k-means clustering with $k = 5$ clusters and plot the resulting micro- and macroclusters (Fig. 10.6).

---

[5]https://doi.org/10.1007/s11390-014-1416-y

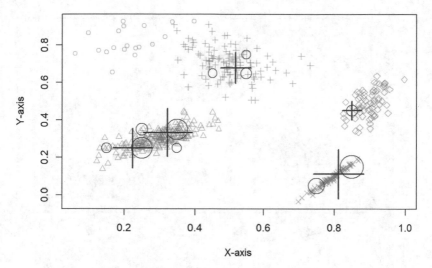

Fig. 10.6 Results of the (online) k-means stream clustering ($k = 5$) showing the resulting micro (red circles)- and macro (blue crosshairs)-clusters

```
kmc <- DSC_Kmeans(k = 5)
recluster(kmc,    dstream)
plot(kmc, stream_5G, type = "both", xlab="X-axis", ylab="Y-axis")
```

In this clustering plot, *microclusters are shown as circles* and *macroclusters are shown as crosshairs* whose sizes represent the corresponding cluster weight estimates. Prior to updating the model with the next 1000 data points from the stream, we specify the grid cells as micro-clusters, grid cell size (gridsize = 0.1), and a microcluster (Cm = 1.2) that specifies the density of a grid cell as a multiple of the average cell density.

```
dstream <- DSC_DStream(gridsize = 0.1, Cm = 1.2)
update(dstream,   stream_5G,   n=1000)
```

We can re-cluster the data using k-means with five clusters and plot the resulting *micro-* and *macro*clusters (Fig. 10.7).

```
km_G5 <- DSC_Kmeans(k = 5)
recluster(km_G5,    dstream)
plot(km_G5, stream_5G, type = "both")
```

Note the subtle changes in the clustering results after updating with the new batch of data.

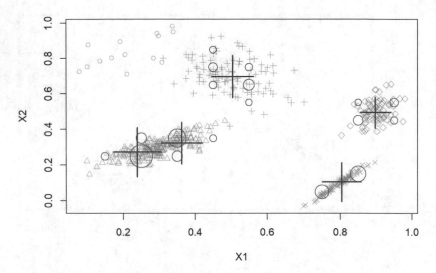

Fig. 10.7 Results of the (online) k-means stream clustering ($k = 5$) showing the resulting micro (red circles)- and macro (blue crosshairs)-clusters

10.3.5   Sources of Data Streams

10.3.5.1   Static Structure Streams

- *DSD_BarsAndGaussians* generates two uniformly filled rectangles and two Gaussian clusters with different density.
- *DSD_Gaussians* generates randomly placed static clusters with random multi-variate Gaussian distributions.
- *DSD_mlbenchData* provides streaming access to machine learning benchmark datasets found in the mlbench package.
- *DSD_mlbenchGenerator* interfaces the generators for artificial data sets defined in the mlbench package.
- *DSD_Target* generates a ball in a circle data set.
- *DSD_UniformNoise* generates uniform noise in a d-dimensional (hyper) cube.

10.3.5.2   Concept Drift Streams

- *DSD_Benchmark* provides a collection of simple benchmark problems including splitting and joining clusters, and changes in density or size, which can be used as a comprehensive benchmark set for algorithm comparison.
- *DSD_MG* is a generator to specify complex data streams with concept drift. The shape as well as the behavior of each cluster over time can be specified using keyframes.

- *DSD_RandomRBFGeneratorEvents* generates streams using radial base functions with noise. Clusters move, merge and split.

10.3.5.3 Real Data Streams

- *DSD_Memory* provides a streaming interface to static, matrix-like data (e.g., a data frame, a matrix) in memory which represents a fixed portion of a data stream. Matrix-like objects also include large objects potentially stored on disk like ff::ffdf.
- *DSD_ReadCSV* reads data line by line in text format from a file or an open connection and makes it available in a streaming fashion. This way data that is larger than the available main memory can be processed.
- *DSD_ReadDB* provides an interface to an open result set from a SQL query to a relational database.

10.3.6 Printing, Plotting, and Saving Streams

For DSD objects, some basic stream functions include print(), plot() and write_stream(). These can save part of a data stream to disk. DSD_Memory and DSD_ReadCSV objects also include member functions like reset_stream() to reset the position in the stream to its beginning.

To request a new batch of data points from the stream, we use the method get_points(). A *random cluster* (based on the probability weights in p_weight) is chosen along with a point drawn from the multivariate Gaussian distribution (*mean = mu, covariance matrix = Σ*) of that cluster. Below, we pull $n = 10$ new data points from the stream (Fig. 10.8).

```
new_p <- get_points(stream_5G, n = 100, class = TRUE)
head(new_p, n = 20)
##              X1           X2 class
## 1   0.2881355 0.2563178134     2
## 2   0.3562591 0.3547617080     2
## 3   0.5630757 0.6237138823     3
...
## 20 0.9034460 0.4165642707     5
plot(stream_5G, n = 700, method = "pc")
```

Note that if you add *noise* to your stream, e.g.,

```
stream_Noise <- DSD_Gaussians(k=5, d=4, noise=0.1, p=c
(0.1,0.5,0.3,0.9,0.1)),
```

then some noise points may not be part of any clusters and may have an NA class label.

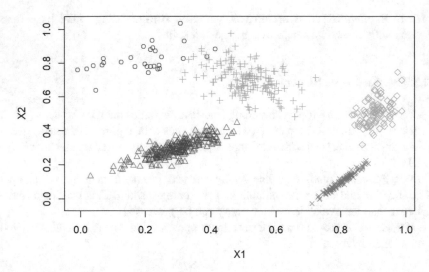

Fig. 10.8 Plotting 700 points from the 5D Gaussian mixture-model stream (DSD_Gaussians)

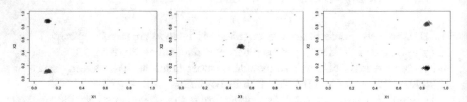

Fig. 10.9 Demonstration of online stream clustering (Benchmark(1)) of a pair of clusters moving diagonally from left to right, meeting through the center with 5% noise. At runtime, this represents a time evolution of the (online) stream data classification

10.3.7 Stream Animation

Clusters can be animated over time by `animate_data()`. Use `reset_stream ()` to start the animation at the beginning of the stream and note that this method is *not implemented* for streams of class `DSD_Gaussians`, `DSD_R`, `DSD_data. frame`, and `DSD`. We'll demonstrate this with a new `DSD_Benchmark` data stream (Fig. 10.9).

```
set.seed(12345)
stream_Bench <- DSD_Benchmark(1)
stream_Bench
## Benchmark 1: Two clusters moving diagonally from left to right,
## meeting in the center (5% noise).
## Class: DSD_MG, DSD_R, DSD_data.frame, DSD
## With 2 clusters in 2 dimensions. Time is 1
library("animation")
reset_stream(stream_Bench)
animate_data(stream_Bench, n=10000, horizon=100, xlim = c(0, 1), ylim=c(0,1))
```

This benchmark generator creates two 2D clusters moving in the plane. One moves from *top-left* to *bottom-right*, the other from *bottom-left* to *top-right*. When the pair of clusters meet at the center of the domain, they briefly overlap and then split again.

Concept drift in the stream can be depicted by requesting (10) times 300 data points from the stream and animating the plot. Fast-forwarding the stream can be accomplished by requesting, but ignoring, (2000) points in between the (10) plots.

```
for(i in 1:10) {
    plot(stream_Bench, 300, xlim = c(0, 1), ylim = c(0, 1))
    tmp <- get_points(stream_Bench, n = 2000)
}
reset_stream(stream_Bench)
# Uncomment this to see the animation
# animate_data(stream_Bench, n=8000, horizon = 120, xlim=c(0,1), ylim=c(0,1))
# Animations can be saved as HTML or GIF
# saveHTML(ani.replay(), htmlfile = "stream_Bench_Animation.html")
# saveGIF(ani.replay())
```

Streams can also be saved locally by

```
write_stream(stream_Bench, "dataStreamSaved.csv", n = 100, sep=",")
```

and loaded back in R by DSD_ReadCSV().

10.3.8 Case Study: SOCR Knee Pain Data

These data represent the X and Y spatial knee pain locations for over 8000 patients, along with *labels* about the knee *Front*, *Back*, *Left*, and *Right*. Let's try to read the SOCR Knee Pain Datasest as a stream.

```
library("XML"); library("xml2"); library("rvest")
wiki_url <- read_html("https://wiki.socr.umich.edu/index.php/SOCR_Data_KneePainData_041409")
html_nodes(wiki_url, "#content")
kneeRawData <- html_table(html_nodes(wiki_url, "table")[[2]])
normalize<-function(x)  {     return((x-min(x))/(max(x)-min(x)))  }
kneeRawData_df <- as.data.frame(cbind(normalize(kneeRawData$x),
                    normalize(kneeRawData$Y), as.factor(kneeRawData$View)))
colnames(kneeRawData_df) <- c("X", "Y", "Label")
# randomize rows of DF; cols RF, RB, LF and LB class labels are sequential
set.seed(1234)
kneeRawData_df <- kneeRawData_df[sample(nrow(kneeRawData_df)), ]
summary(kneeRawData_df)
# View(kneeRawData_df)
```

We can use the DSD::DSD_Memory class to get a stream interface for matrix or data frame objects, like the Knee pain location dataset. The number of true clusters $k = 4$ in this dataset.

```
# use data.frame to create a stream (3rd column contains label assignment)
kneeDF <- data.frame(x=kneeRawData_df[,1], y=kneeRawData_df[,2],
                    class=as.factor(kneeRawData_df[,3]))
head(kneeDF)
##                 x         y class
## 1 0.69096672 0.4479769     1
## 2 0.88431062 0.7716763     3
...
streamKnee <- DSD_Memory(kneeDF[,c("x", "y")], class=kneeDF[,"class"],
                    loop=T)
streamKnee
# Each time we get a point from *streamKnee*, the stream pointer moves to the
next position (row) in the data.
get_points(streamKnee, n=10)
##                 x         y
## 1  0.69096672 0.4479769
## 2  0.88431062 0.7716763
...
## 10 0.16323296 0.5780347
streamKnee
## Contains 8666 data points - currently at position 11 - loop is TRUE
# Stream pointer is in position 11 now
# We can redirect the current position of the stream pointer by:
reset_stream(streamKnee, pos = 200)
get_points(streamKnee, n=10)
##                 x         y
## 200 0.26465927 0.4161850
## 201 0.09033281 0.2543353
...
streamKnee
## Contains 8666 data points - currently at position 210 - loop is TRUE
```

10.3.9 *Data Stream Clustering and Classification (DSC)*

Let's demonstrate clustering using `DSC_DStream`, which assigns points to cells in a grid. First, initialize the clustering, as an empty cluster and then use the `update()` function to implicitly alter the mutable DSC object.

```
dsc_streamKnee <- DSC_DStream(gridsize = 0.1, Cm = 0.4, attraction=T)
dsc_streamKnee
# stream::update
reset_stream(streamKnee,  pos  =  1)
update(dsc_streamKnee, streamKnee,  n  =  500)
dsc_streamKnee
## Number of micro-clusters: 14
## Number of macro-clusters: 8
head(get_centers(dsc_streamKnee))
plot(dsc_streamKnee,  streamKnee, xlim=c(0,1), ylim=c(0,1))
# plot(dsc_streamKnee,  streamKnee, grid = TRUE)
# Micro-clusters are plotted in red on top of gray stream data points
# The size of the micro-clusters indicates their weight - it's proportional to
the number of data points represented by each micro-cluster.
```

The purity metric represents an external evaluation criterion of cluster quality, which is the proportion of the total number of points that were correctly classified

$$0 \leq \mathrm{Purity} = \frac{1}{N} \sum_{i=1}^{k} \max{}_j a \left| c_l \cap t_j \right| \leq 1,$$

where N = number of observed data points, k = number of clusters, c_i is the i-th cluster, and t_j is the classification that has the maximum number of points with c_i class labels. High purity suggests that we correctly label points. Next, we can use K-means clustering (Figs. 10.10 and 10.11).

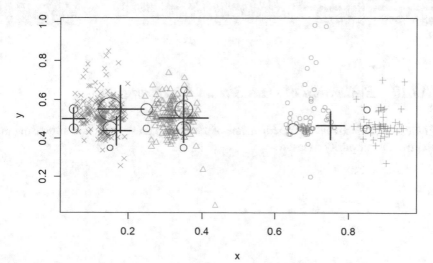

Fig. 10.10 Knee pain data stream clustering

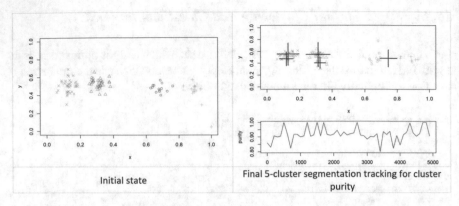

Fig. 10.11 Online stream clustering (knee pain data)

```
kMeans_Knee <- DSC_Kmeans(k = 5) #choose 4-5 clusters, as we have 4 knee labels
recluster(kMeans_Knee, dsc_streamKnee)
plot(kMeans_Knee, streamKnee, type = "both")
```

```
animate_data(streamKnee, n=1000, horizon=100, xlim = c(0, 1), ylim = c(0, 1))
```

```
# purity <- animate_cluster(kMeans_Knee, streamKnee, n=2500, type="both",
#           xlim=c(0,1), ylim=c(-,1), evaluationMeasure="purity", horizon=10)
animate_cluster(kMeans_Knee, streamKnee, horizon = 100,  n = 5000,
                measure="purity", plot.args=list(xlim = c(0,1), ylim=c(0,1)))
##    points    purity
## 1       1 0.8595152
## 2     101 0.8304348
...
## 49   4801 1.0000000
## 50   4901 0.9078947
```

10.3.10   Evaluation of Data Stream Clustering

Figure 10.12 illustrates the performance of the knee pain stream clustering using the average cluster purity measure.

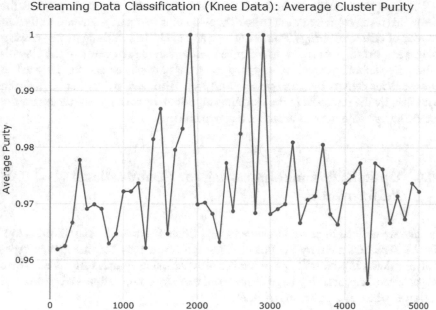

Fig. 10.12 Knee pain stream clustering performance (metric = average cluster purity measure)

```
evaluate(dsc_streamKnee, streamKnee,
         measure = c("crand", "SSQ", "silhouette"), n = 100,
         type = c("auto", "micro", "macro"), assign = "micro",
         assignmentMethod=c("auto","model","nn"), noise=c("class","exclude"))
## Evaluation results for micro-clusters.
## Points were assigned to micro-clusters.
##        cRand          SSQ  silhouette
##   0.28474810   0.53860025 -0.03565456
clusterEval <- evaluate_cluster(dsc_streamKnee, streamKnee,
             measure = c("numMicroClusters", "purity"), n=5000, horizon-100)
head(clusterEval)
library(plotly)
plot_ly(x=~clusterEval[ , "points"], y=~clusterEval[ , "purity"],
        type="scatter", mode="markers+lines") %>%
  layout(
       title="Streaming Data Classification (Knee Data): Average Cluster Purity",
       xaxis=list(title="Streaming Points"), yaxis=list(title="Average Purity"))
```

```
animate_cluster(dsc_streamKnee, streamKnee,  horizon  =  100,  n  =  5000,
                measure="purity", plot.args=list(xlim = c(0,1), ylim=c(0,1)))
##     points    purity
## 1        1 0.9736842
## 2      101 0.9764706
...
## 49    4801 0.9800000
## 50    4901 0.9750000
```

The `dsc_streamKnee` includes the clustering results, where n represents the data points taken from `streamKnee`. The evaluation `measure` can be specified as a vector of character strings. Points are assigned to clusters in `dsc_streamKnee` using `get_assignment()` and can be used to assess the quality of the classification. By default, points are assigned to *micro-clusters*, or can be assigned to *macro-cluster* centers by `assign = "macro"`. Also, new points can be assigned to clusters by the rule used in the clustering algorithm by `assignmentMethod = "model"` or using nearest-neighbor assignment (nn).

10.4   Optimization and Improving the Computational Performance

Just like we noticed in previous chapters, e.g., Chap. 9, streaming classification in R may be slow and memory-inefficient. These problems may become severe, especially for datasets with millions of records or when using complex functions. There are packages for processing large datasets and memory optimization – `bigmemory`, `biganalytics`, `bigtabulate`, etc.

10.4.1   Generalizing Tabular Data Structures with `dplyr`

We have also seen long execution times when running processes that ingest, store, or manipulate huge `data.frame` objects. The `dplyr` package, created by Hadley Wickham and Romain Francoi, provides a faster route to manage such large datasets in R. It creates an object called `tbl`, similar to `data.frame`, which has an in-memory column-like structure. R reads these objects a lot faster than data frames.

To make a `tbl` object we can either convert an existing data frame to `tbl` or connect to an external database. Converting from data frame to `tbl` is quite easy. All we need to do is call the function `as.tbl()`.

```
#install.packages("dplyr")
library(dplyr)
nof1_tbl <- as.tbl(nof1)
nof1_tbl
## # A tibble: 900 x 10
##       ID   Day   Tx SelfEff SelfEff25  WPSS SocSuppt  PMss PMss3 PhyAct
##    <dbl> <dbl> <dbl>   <dbl>     <dbl> <dbl>    <dbl> <dbl> <dbl>  <dbl>
## 1      1     1     1      33         8  0.97        5  4.03  1.03     53
## 2      1     2     1      33         8 -0.17     3.87  4.03  1.03     73
## 3      1     3     0      33         8  0.81     4.84  4.03  1.03     23
## 4      1     4     0      33         8 -0.41     3.62  4.03  1.03     36
## 5      1     5     1      33         8  0.59     4.62  4.03  1.03     21
## 6      1     6     1      33         8 -1.16     2.87  4.03  1.03      0
## 7      1     7     0      33         8   0.3     4.33  4.03  1.03     21
## 8      1     8     0      33         8 -0.34     3.69  4.03  1.03      0
## 9      1     9     1      33         8 -0.74     3.29  4.03  1.03     73
## 10     1    10     1      33         8 -0.38     3.66  4.03  1.03    114
## # ... with 890 more rows
```

This looks like a normal data frame. If you are using R Studio by viewing the `nof1_tbl` you can see the same output as `nof1`.

10.4.2   Making Data Frames Faster with data.table

Similar to `tbl`, the `data.table` package provides another alternative to data frame object representation. `data.table` objects are processed in R much faster compared to standard data frames. Also, all of the functions that can accept data frames could be applied to `data.table` objects as well. The function `fread()` is able to read a local CSV file directly into a `data.table`.

```
# install.packages("data.table")
library(data.table)
nof1 <- fread("C:/Users/UserName/Desktop/02_Nof1_Data.csv")
```

Another amazing property of `data.table` is that we can use subscripts to access a specific location in the dataset just like `dataset[row, column]`. It also allows the selection of rows with Boolean expression and direct application of functions to those selected rows. Note that column names can be used to call the specific column in `data.table`, whereas with data frames, we have to use the `dataset$columnName` syntax).

```
nof1[ID==1, mean(PhyAct)]
## [1] 52.66667
```

This useful functionality can also help us run complex operations with only a few lines of code. One of the drawbacks of using `data.table` objects is that they are still limited by the available system memory.

10.4.3   Creating Disk-Based Data Frames with ff

The `ff` (fast-files) package allows us to overcome the RAM limitations of finite system memory. For example, it helps with operating datasets with billion rows. `ff` creates objects in `ffdf` formats, which is like a map that points to a location of the data on a disk. However, this makes `ffdf` objects inapplicable for most R functions. The only way to address this problem is to break the huge dataset into small chunks. After processing a batch of these small chunks, we have to combine the results to reconstruct the complete output. This strategy is relevant in parallel computing, which will be discussed in detail in the next section. First, let's download one of the large datasets in our datasets archive, UQ_VitalSignsData_Case04.csv.

```
# install.packages("ff")
library(ff)
# vitalsigns<-read.csv.ffdf(file="UQ_VitalSignsData_Case04.csv", header=T)
vitalsigns <-
 read.csv.ffdf(file="https://umich.instructure.com/files/366335/download?download_frd=1",
                 header=T)
```

As mentioned earlier, we cannot apply functions directly on this `ff` object, e.g.,

```
mean(vitalsigns$Pulse)
## Warning in mean.default(vitalsigns$Pulse): argument is not numeric
or logical:
## returning NA
## [1] NA
```

For basic data calculations, we can download another package `ffbase`. This allows operations on `ffdf` objects using simple tasks, such as mathematical operations, query functions, summary statistics, and bigger regression models using packages like `biglm`, which will be mentioned later in this chapter.

```
library(ffbase)
mean(vitalsigns$Pulse)
```

10.4.4   Using Massive Matrices with *bigmemory*

The previously introduced packages include alternatives to `data.frames`. For instance, the `bigmemory` package creates alternative objects to 2D matrices (second-order tensors). It can store huge datasets and can be divided into small chunks that can be converted to data frames. However, we cannot directly apply machine learning methods on these types of objects. More detailed information about the `bigmemory` package is available online.[6]

10.5   Parallel Computing

In previous chapters, we saw various machine learning techniques applied as serial computing tasks. The traditional protocol involves the following steps. First, applying *function 1* to our raw data. Then, using the output from *function 1* as an input to *function 2*. This process is iterated for a series of functions. Finally, we have the terminal output generated by the last function. This serial or linear computing method is straightforward but time consuming and perhaps sub-optimal.

---

[6]https://www.bigmemory.org

Now we introduce a more efficient way of computing - *parallel computing*, which provides a mechanism to deal with different tasks at the same time and combine the outputs for all of the processes to get the final answer faster. However, parallel algorithms may require special conditions and cannot be applied to all problems. If two tasks have to be run in a specific order, this problem cannot be parallelized.

10.5.1   Measuring Execution Time

To measure how much time can be saved for different methods, we can use the function system.time().

```
system.time(mean(vitalsigns$Pulse))
```

This means calculating the mean of the Pulse column in the vitalsigns dataset takes 0.001 seconds. These values will vary between computers, operating systems, and states of operations.

10.5.2   Parallel Processing with Multiple Cores

We will introduce two packages for parallel computing multicore and snow (their core components are included in the package parallel). They both have a different way of multitasking. However, to run these packages, you need to have a relatively modern multicore computer. Let's check how many cores your computer has. This function parallel::detectCores() provides this functionality. parallel is a base package, so there is no need to install it prior to using it.

```
library(parallel)
detectCores()
## [1] 8
```

This reports that there are eight (8) cores on the computer used to compile and knit the Rmarkdown source of the DSPA book content. In this case, we can run up to 6–7 parallel jobs on this computer, never use all cores for computing as this will overwhelm the core state of the machine. The multicore package simply uses the multitasking capabilities of the *kernel*, the computer's operating system, to "fork" additional R sessions that share the same memory. Imagine that we open several R sessions in parallel and let each of them do part of the work. Now, let's examine how this can save time when running complex protocols or dealing with large datasets. To start with, we can use the mclapply() function, which is similar to lapply(), which applies functions to a vector and returns a vector of lists. Instead of applying functions to vectors mcapply() divides the complete computational task and delegates portions of it to each available core. We will apply a simple, yet time consuming, task - generating random numbers - for demonstrating this procedure. Also, we can use the `system.time()` to track the time differences.

```
set.seed(123)
system.time(c1 <- rnorm(10000000))
##    user  system elapsed
##    1.64    0.03    1.70
# Note the multi core calls require use of the package parallel
library(parallel)
numWorkers <- 4 # number of cores to use, check available cores: detectCores()
cl <-makeCluster(numWorkers, type="PSOCK")
system.time(c2 <- unlist(parLapply(cl,1:10, function(x) { rnorm(10000000) })))
stopCluster(cl)
##    user  system elapsed
##    0.98    0.35    2.36
```

The `unlist()` is used at the end to combine results from different cores into a single vector. Each line of code creates 10,000,000 random numbers. The generation of the `c1` output uses the default R single core invocation, which uses the most CPU time. The `c2` output uses four cores to complete the task (each core handles the same, 10,000,000, random number generations, and uses less time than the first (nonparallelized) test. Clearly, using additional cores significantly shrinks the overall execution time.

The `snow` package also allows parallel computing on multicore multiprocessor machines or a network of multiple machines. It might be more difficult to use, but it is also certainly more flexible. First we can set how many cores we want to use via the `makeCluster()` function.

```
# install.packages("snow")
library(snow)
cl <- makeCluster(2)
```

This call might cause a pop-up message warning about access through the firewall. To do the same task, we can use the `parLapply()` function in the `snow` package. Note that we have to call the object we created with the previous `makeCluster()` function.

```
system.time(c2 <- unlist(parLapply(cl, c(5000000, 5000000),
                            function(x) {rnorm(x)})))
##    user  system elapsed
##    0.25    0.18    0.91
```

While using `parLapply()`, we have to specify the matrix and the function that will be applied to this matrix. Remember to stop the cluster we made after completing the task, to release back the system resources.

```
stopCluster(cl)
```

10.5.3   Parallelization Using `foreach` and `doParallel`

The `foreach` package provides another option of parallel computing. It relies on a
loop-like process basically applying a specified function for each item in the set,
which again is somewhat similar to `apply()`, `lapply()` and other regular
functions. The interesting thing is that these loops can be computed in parallel
saving substantial amounts of time. The `foreach` package alone cannot provide
parallel computing. We have to combine it with other packages like `doParallel`.
Let's reexamine the task of creating a vector of 10,000,000 random numbers. First,
register the four compute cores using `registerDoParallel()`.

```
# install.packages("doParallel")
library(doParallel)
cl<-makeCluster(4)
registerDoParallel(cl)
```

Then we can examine the time saving `foreach` command.

```
#install.packages("foreach")
library(foreach)
system.time(c4 <- foreach(i=1:4, .combine = 'c') %dopar% rnorm(2500000) )
##     user  system elapsed
###    0.24    0.16    0.66
```

Here we used four items (each item runs on a separate core), `.combine—c`
allows `foreach` to combine the results with the parameter `c()` generating the
aggregate result vector.

Also, don't forget to close the `doParallel` by registering the sequential
backend.

```
unregister <- registerDoSEQ()
```

10.5.4   GPU Computing

Modern computers have graphics cards, GPU (graphics processing unit), that consist
of thousands of cores; however, they are very specialized, unlike the standard CPU
chip. If we can use this feature for parallel computing, we may reach amazing
performance improvements, at the cost of complicating the processing algorithms
and increasing the constraints on the data format. Specific disadvantages of GPU
computing include relying on a proprietary manufacturer (e.g., NVidia) frameworks
and Complete Unified Device Architecture (CUDA) programming language. CUDA

allows programming of GPU instructions into a common computing language. This paper[7] provides one example of using GPU computation to significantly improve the performance of advanced neuroimaging and brain mapping processing of multidimensional data. The specialized R package gputools is created for parallel computing using NVidia CUDA.

10.6   Deploying Optimized Learning Algorithms

As we mentioned earlier, some tasks can be parallelized easier than others. In real world situations, we can pick the algorithms that lend themselves well to parallelization. Some of the R packages that allow parallel computing using ML algorithms are listed below.

10.6.1   Building Bigger Regression Models with biglm

The R biglm package allows training regression models with data from SQL databases or large data chunks obtained from the ff package. The output is similar to the standard lm() function that builds linear models. However, biglm operates efficiently on massive datasets.

10.6.2   Growing Bigger and Faster Random Forests with bigrf

The bigrf package can be used to train random forests combining the foreach and doParallel packages. In Chap. 9, we presented random forests as machine learners ensembling multiple tree learners. With parallel computing, we can split the task of creating thousands of trees into smaller tasks that can be outsourced to each available CPU core. We only need to combine the results at the end. Then, we will obtain the exact same output in a relatively shorter amount of time.

---

[7] https://doi.org/10.1016/j.cmpb.2010.10.013

10.6.3   *Training and Evaluation Models in Parallel with* `caret`

Combining the `caret` package with `foreach`, we can obtain a powerful method to deal with time-consuming tasks like building a random forest learner. Utilizing the same example we presented in Chap. 9, we can see the time difference of utilizing the `foreach` package.

```
# library(caret)
system.time(m_rf <- train(CHARLSONSCORE ~ ., data=qol, method="rf",
                          metric="Kappa", trControl=ctrl, tuneGrid=grid_rf))
##    user  system elapsed
## 273.09    2.29  282.00
```

It took several minutes to finish this task in the standard (single core) execution model, relying purely on the regular `caret` function. Below, this same model training completes much faster using parallelization; about 1/4 of the time compared to the standard call above.

```
set.seed(123)
cl <- makeCluster(4)
registerDoParallel(cl)
getDoParWorkers() ## [1] 4
system.time(m_rf <- train(CHARLSONSCORE ~ ., data = qol, method = "rf",
                          metric="Kappa", trControl=ctrl, tuneGrid=grid_rf))
##    user  system elapsed
##    4.91    0.06   56.72
unregister<-registerDoSEQ()
stopCluster(cl)
```

Note that the call to `train` remains the same, no need to specify parallelization in the call. It automatically utilizes all available resources, in this case 4 cores. The execution time is significantly reduced from about 280 seconds (in the standard single core environment) down to 50 seconds (in the cluster setting).

10.7   R Notebook Support for Other Programming Languages

```
library(tidyverse)
library(kableExtra)
library(gridExtra)
library(viridis)
```

The R markdown notebook allows the user to execute jobs in a number of different kinds of software platforms. In addition to R, one can define Python,

C/C++, and many other languages. Below is the current complete list of `knitr`
package supported scripting and compiled languages included in R.

```
names(knitr::knit_engines$get())
## [1] "awk" "bash" "coffee" "gawk" "groovy" "haskell"
## [7] "lein" "mysql" "node" "octave" "perl" "psql"
## [13] "Rscript" "ruby" "sas" "scala" "sed" "sh"
## [19] "stata" "zsh" "asis" "asy" "block" "block2"
## [25] "bslib" "c" "cat" "cc" "comment" "css"
## [31] "ditaa" "dot" "embed" "exec" "fortran" "fortran95"
## [37] "go" "highlight" "js" "julia" "python" "R"
## [43] "Rcpp" "sass" "scss" "sql" "stan" "targets"
## [49] "tikz" "verbatim" "glue" "glue_sql" "gluesql"
```

In this section, we will demonstrate the use of Python within R and the seamless
integration between R, Python, and C/C++ libraries. This functionality substantially enriches the already comprehensive collection of thousands of existent R
libraries, as well as provides a mechanism to improve significantly the performance
of any R protocol by outsourcing some of the heavy-duty calculations to external
(compiled) C/C++ executables.

10.7.1   R-Python Integration

RStudio provides a quick demo of the *reticulate* package, which provides access to
tools and enables the interoperability between Python and R. We will demonstrate
this interoperability by fitting some models using Python's *scikit-learn* library.[8]

10.7.2   Installing Python

Users need to first install Python on their local machines by downloading the
software for the appropriate operating system.

- Windows: For *Windows OS*, depending on the system's processor (CPU chipset),
  it's recommended to download the appropriate *Windows x86-64 executable
  installer*, for 64-bit systems, or *Windows x86 executable installer*, for 32-bit
  systems. In general, installing the more powerful 64-bit version is recommended
  to improve performance.
- Mac OS: For *OS system*, please make sure to download the proper version of the
  macOS 64-bit/32-bit installer.

---

[8]https://scikit-learn.org/

Under the download heading "*Stable Releases*", select any Python 3 version. Note that certain configurations may require downloading and installing an earlier Python version ≤3.8.

Note There may be a temporary incompatibility issue between the reticulate package and the latest Python version (e.g., ≥3.9). It may be safer to download and install a slightly older Python 3 version. If downloading the LATEST Python 3 release fails the testing below, try to reinstall an earlier Python version and try the tests below again.

Once downloaded, run the installer following the prompts.

10.7.3   Install the reticulate Package

We need to load the (preinstalled) *reticulate* package and point to the specific directory of the local Python installation on your local machine. You can either manually type in the PATH to Python or use Sys.which("python3") to find it automatically, which may not work well if you don't have the system environmental variables correctly set.

10.7.4   Installing and Importing Python Modules

Additional Python modules can be installed either using a *shell/terminal* window for Mac OS system or *cmd* window for Windows OS. In the command shell window, type in pip install and append it by the names of the modules you want to install (e.g., pip install pandas) and press *Enter*. The module should be automatically downloaded and installed on the local machine. Please make sure to install all the required modules (e.g., pandas, sklearn) before you move onto the next stage. Some of these additional packages may be automatically installed by a conda python installation.

Following a successful installation of the add-on packages, we can import python and any additional modules into the R environment. Note the new notebook specification {python}, instead of {r}, in the chunk of executable code.

Note RStudio version must be ≥1.2 to allow passing objects between R, Python, and any other of the languages that can be invoked in the R markdown notebook.

```
# import the necessary python packages (pandas) and sub-packages
# (sklearn.tree.DecisionTreeClassifier)
import pandas
from sklearn.model_selection import train_test_split
from sklearn.tree import DecisionTreeClassifier
```

10.7.5   Python-Based Data Modeling

Let's load the iris data in R, pass it onto Python, and split it into training and testing sets using the sklearn.tree.train_test_split() method.

```
# Define the data in R but make it available in the Python env context (py$)
iris[1:6,]
##   Sepal.Length Sepal.Width Petal.Length Petal.Width Species
## 1          5.1         3.5          1.4         0.2  setosa
## 2          4.9         3.0          1.4         0.2  setosa
## 3          4.7         3.2          1.3         0.2  setosa
## 4          4.6         3.1          1.5         0.2  setosa
## 5          5.0         3.6          1.4         0.2  setosa
## 6          5.4         3.9          1.7         0.4  setosa
# repl_python()
py$iris_data <- iris
```

Note that some of the *code in this section* in the Rmarkdown notebook, delimited between ```` ```{python} ... ``` ````, is python, not R, e.g., train_test_split(), DecisionTreeClassifier().

```
# Python block of code in Rmd notebook
# report the first 5 cases of the data within Python
print(r.iris[1:6])
# Split the data in Python (use random seed for reproducibility)
##   Sepal.Length Sepal.Width Petal.Length Petal.Width Species
## 1          4.9         3.0          1.4         0.2  setosa
## 2          4.7         3.2          1.3         0.2  setosa
## 3          4.6         3.1          1.5         0.2  setosa
## 4          5.0         3.6          1.4         0.2  setosa
## 5          5.4         3.9          1.7         0.4  setosa
train, test = train_test_split(r.iris, test_size = 0.4, random_state = 4321)
X = train.drop('Species', axis = 1)
y = train.loc[:, 'Species'].values
X_test = test.drop('Species', axis = 1)
y_test = test.loc[:, 'Species'].values
```

Let's pull back into R the first 5 training observations (X) from the Python object. Note that X is a *Python object* generated in the Python chunk that we are now processing within the R chunk. Mind the use of the py$ prefix to the object (py$X). As the train_test_split() method does random selection of rows (cases) into the training and testing sets, the top five cases reported in the initial ordering of the cases by R may be different from the top five cases reported after the Python block processing.

```
# R block of code in Rmd
py$X %>% head(6)
##     Sepal.Length Sepal.Width Petal.Length Petal.Width
## 41          4.5         2.3          1.3         0.3
## 16          5.4         3.9          1.3         0.4
## 26          5.0         3.4          1.6         0.4
## 99          5.7         2.8          4.1         1.3
## 5           5.4         3.9          1.7         0.4
## 85          6.0         3.4          4.5         1.6
```

Next, we will fit a *simple decision tree* model within `Python` using `sklearn` on the training data and evaluate its performance on the independent testing set and visualize the results in R.

```
# Python block; Model fitting in Python
tree = DecisionTreeClassifier(random_state=4321)
clf = tree.fit(X, y)
pred = clf.predict(X_test)
pred[1:6]
## array(['setosa', 'virginica', 'virginica', 'setosa', 'virginica'],
##       dtype=object)
```

10.7.6   Visualization of the Results in R

To begin with, we will pull the `Python` pandas dataset into an R object.

```
# R block; Store python pandas object as R tibble and identify correctly and
# incorrectly predicted labels
library(kableExtra)
library(tibble)
foo <- py$test %>% as_tibble() %>% rename(truth = Species) %>%
  mutate(predicted = as.factor(py$pred), correct = (truth == predicted))
foo %>% head(5) %>% select(-Petal.Length, -Petal.Width) %>%
  kable() %>% kable_styling()
```

Sepal.Length	Sepal.Width	truth	predicted	correct
5.4	3.4	setosa	setosa	TRUE
5.1	3.3	setosa	setosa	TRUE
5.9	3.2	versicolor	virginica	FALSE
6.3	3.3	virginica	virginica	TRUE
5.1	3.8	setosa	setosa	TRUE

Finally, we can plot in R the testing-data results and compare the *real* iris flower taxa labels (colors) and their *predicted-label* counterparts (shapes) (Fig. 10.13).

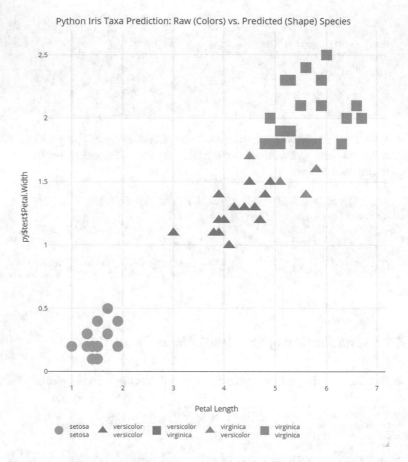

Fig. 10.13 Iris data R-python interface, data transfer, clustering, and result visualization

```
# R block of code
library(plotly)
plot_ly(py$test, x=~py$test$Petal.Length, y=~py$test$Petal.Width,
        color = ~py$test$Species, symbol = ~as.factor(py$pred),
        type="scatter", marker = list(size = 20), mode="markers") %>%
  layout(title="Python Iris Taxa Prediction: Raw (Colors) vs. Predicted (Shape)
Species",
        xaxis=list(title="Petal Length"), xaxis=list(title="Petal Width"),
        legend = list(orientation='h'))
```

10.7.7   R Integration with C/C++

There are many alternative ways to blend R and C/C++/Cpp code. The simplest
approach may be to use inline C++ functional directly in R via the cppFunction().

Alternatively, we can keep C++ source files completely independent and sourceCpp() them into R for indirect use. Here is an example of a stand-alone C++ program meanCPP() computing the mean and standard deviation of a vector input. To try this, save the C++ code below in a text file: meanCPP.cpp and invoke it within R. Note that the C++ code can also include R method calls, e.g., *sdR()*!

Note: This R/C++ integration requires the Rtools package and the *make* function, as well as proper PATH environment variable setting, which can be checked and set as indicated below.

```
writeLines(strsplit(Sys.getenv("PATH"), ";")[[1]])
### <Start_CPP_Code>
# #include <Rcpp.h>
# using namespace Rcpp;  // this is a required name-space declaration in the C++
code
#
# /*** functions that will be used within R are prefixed with: `//
[[Rcpp::export]]`.
#    We can compile the C++ code within R by *sourceCpp("/path_to/meanCPP.cpp")*.
#    These compiled functions can be used in R, but can't be saved in a `.Rdata`
files
#    and need to always be reloaded prior to reuse after `R` restart.
# */
#
# // [[Rcpp::export]]
# double meanCPP(NumericVector vec) {
#    int n = vec.size();
#    double total = 0;
#
#    for(int i = 0, i < n; ++i) { // mind the C++ indexing starts at zero, not 1,
as in R
#      total += vec[i];
#    }
#    return total/n;
# }
# /*** R
# # This is R code embedded in C++ to compute the SD of a vector
# sdR <- function (vec) {
#    return(sd(vec))
# }
# */
### <End_CPP_Code>
```

Next, we will demonstrate the R and C++ integration.

```r
### R code
# First source C++ code: for local C++ files: sourceCpp("/path/meanCPP.cpp")
library(devtools)
library(Rcpp)
sourceURL <-
        "https://www.socr.umich.edu/people/UserName/courses/DSPA_notes/meanCPP.cpp"
localSource <- "meanCPP.cpp"
download.file(url=sourceURL, destfile=localSource)
sourceCpp("meanCPP.cpp")
## > sdR <- function(vec) {
## +     return(sd(vec))
## + }
# Call outside C++ meanCPP() method
r_vec <- rnorm(10^8) # generate 100M random values & compare computational
complexity
system.time(m1 <- mean(r_vec))      # R solution
##    user  system elapsed
##    0.27    0.00    0.27
system.time(m2 <- meanCPP(r_vec)) # C++ solution
##    user  system elapsed
##    0.14    0.00    0.14
round(m1-m2, 5)  # Difference of mean calculations?
# Compare the sdR() function defined within C++ using R methods to base::sd()
s1 <- sdR(r_vec); round(s1, 3) # remember the data is N(mean=0, sd=1)
s2 <- sd(r_vec)
round(s1-s2, 5)
```

Notice that the C++ method *meanCPP()* is faster in computing the *mean* compared to the native R *base::mean()*.

10.8   Practice Problem

Try to analyze the co-appearance network in the novel "*Les Miserables*". The data contains the weighted network of co-appearances of characters in Victor Hugo's novel "Les Miserables". Nodes represent characters as indicated by the labels and edges connect any pair of characters that appear in the same chapter of the book. The values on the edges are the number of such co-appearances.

```r
miserablese <-
    read.table("https://umich.instructure.com/files/330389/download?download_frd=1",
               sep="", header=F)
head(miserablese)
##                V1             V2
## 1          Myriel       Napoleon
## 2          Myriel MlleBaptistine
## 3          Myriel    MmeMagloire
## 4 MlleBaptistine    MmeMagloire
## 5          Myriel   CountessDeLo
## 6          Myriel       Geborand
```

Also, try to interrogate other larger datasets we have using alternative parallel computing and big data analytics.

Chapter 11
Variable Importance and Feature Selection

As we mentioned earlier in Chap. 4, variable selection is very important when dealing with bioinformatics, healthcare, and biomedical data where we may have more features than observations. Instead of trying to interrogate the complete data in its native high-dimensional state, we can apply variable selection, or feature selection, to focus on the most salient information contained in the observations. Due to the presence of intrinsic and extrinsic noise, the volume and complexity of big health data, as well as different methodological and technological challenges, the process of identifying the salient features may resemble finding a needle in a haystack. We will illustrate alternative strategies for feature selection using filtering (e.g., correlation-based feature selection), wrapping (e.g., recursive feature elimination), and embedding (e.g., variable importance via random forest classification) techniques.

The process of variable selection relates to *dimensionality reduction*, which we saw in Chap. 4; however, there are also differences between these techniques. Relative to the lower variance estimates in *continuous dimensionality reduction*, the intrinsic characteristics of the *discrete feature selection* process yields higher variance in bootstrap estimation and cross-validation. Table 11.1 summarizes the synergies between feature selection and dimenssionality reduction strategies.

In this Chapter, we will present alternative methods for quantifying variable importance and selection of salient features. Examples of these include filtering, wrapper, and embedding techniques, including random forest feature importance and variable selection using *decoy features* (knockoffs) with control for the false discovery rate of selecting inconsequential features as salient.

11.1 Feature Selection Methods

There are three major classes of variable or feature selection techniques—filtering-based, wrapper-based, and embedded methods.

© The Author(s), under exclusive license to Springer Nature Switzerland AG 2023   579
I. D. Dinov, *Data Science and Predictive Analytics*, The Springer Series in Applied
Machine Learning, https://doi.org/10.1007/978-3-031-17483-4_11

Table 11.1 Similarities and differences between dimensionality reduction and variable selection

Method	Process type	Goals	Approach
Variable selection	Discrete process	To select unique representative features from each group of *similar* features	To identify highly correlated variables and choose a representative feature by postprocessing the data
Dimension reduction	Continuous process	To denoise the data, enable simpler prediction, or group features so that low impact features have smaller weights	Find the *essential*, $k \gg n$, components, factors, or clusters representing linear, or nonlinear, functions of the n variables which maximize an objective function like the proportion of explained variance

11.1.1   Filtering Techniques

Univariate   Univariate filtering methods focus on selecting single features with high scores based on some statistics like χ^2 or Information Gain Ratio. Each feature is viewed as independent of the others, effectively ignoring interactions between features. Examples include χ^2, Euclidean distance, i-test, and information gain.[1]

Multivariate   Multivariate filtering methods rely on various (multivariate) statistics to select the principal features. They typically account for between-feature interactions by using higher-order statistics like correlation. The basic idea is that we iteratively triage variables that have high correlations with other covariates. Examples of such methods include correlation-based feature selection, Markov blanket filter, and fast correlation-based feature selection.[2]

11.1.2   Wrapper

Deterministic   Deterministic wrapper feature selection methods either start with no features (forward-selection) or with all features included in the model (backward-selection) and iteratively refine the set of chosen features according to some model quality measures. The iterative process of adding or removing features may rely on statistics like the Jaccard similarity coefficient. Examples of these include sequential forward selection, recursive feature elimination, and beam search.

Randomized   Stochastic wrapper feature selection procedures utilize a binary feature-indexing vector indicating whether or not each variable should be included in the list of salient features. At each iteration, we *randomly* perturb the vector of

---

[1] https://doi.org/10.1093/bioinformatics/btm344

[2] https://doi.org/10.1109/DMIA.2015.17

binary indicators and compare the combinations of features before and after the random inclusion-exclusion indexing change. Finally, we pick the indexing vector corresponding with the optimal performance based on some metric like acceptance probability measures. The iterative process continues until no improvement of the objective function is observed. Examples include simulated annealing, genetic algorithms, and estimation of distribution algorithms.

11.1.3 Embedded Techniques

Embedded feature selection techniques are based on various classifiers, predictors, or clustering procedures. For instance, we can accomplish feature selection by using decision trees where the separation of the training data relies on features associated with the highest information gain. Further tree branching separating the data deeper may utilize *weaker* features. This process of choosing the vital features based on their separability characteristics continues until the classifier generates group labels that are mostly homogeneous within clusters/classes and largely heterogeneous across groups, and when the information gain of further tree branching is marginal. The entire process may be iterated multiple times and select the features that appear most frequently. Common examples of these include decision trees, random forests, weighted naive Bayes, and feature selection using weighted-SVM.

The different types of feature selection methods have their own pros and cons. In this chapter, we are going to introduce the randomized wrapper method using the Boruta package, which utilizes a random forest classification method to output *variable importance measures* (VIMs). Then, we will compare its results with recursive feature elimination, a classical deterministic wrapper method.

11.1.4 Random Forest Feature Selection

Let's start by examining random forest based feature selection, as an embedded technique. The good performance of random forest as a classification, regression, and clustering method is coupled with its ease-of-use, accurate, and robust results. Having a random forest, or more broadly a decision tree, prediction naturally leads to feature selection by using the mean decrease impurity or the mean accuracy decrease criteria.

The many decision trees captured in a random forest include explicit conditions at each branching node, which are based on single features. The intrinsic bifurcation conditions splitting the data may be based on cost function optimization using the *impurity*, see Chap. 5. For classification problems, we can also use alternative metrics, such as information gain or entropy. These measures capture the importance of variables by computing its impact (how much is the feature-based splitting decision decreasing the weighted impurity in a tree). In random forests, the ranking of feature importance, which is based on the average impurity decrease due to each variable, leads to effective feature selection.

11.1.5   Case Study—ALS

Step 1: Collecting Data
Let's use case study 15, amyotrophic lateral sclerosis (ALS), to examine the patterns, symmetries, associations, and causality in a rare but devastating disease, amyotrophic lateral sclerosis, also known as *Lou Gehrig disease*.[3] This ALS case study reflects a large clinical trial including big, multisource, and heterogeneous data elements. It would be interesting to interrogate the data and attempt to derive potential biomarkers that can be used for detecting, prognosticating, and forecasting the progression of this neurodegenerative disorder. Overcoming many scientific, technical, and infrastructure barriers is required to establish complete, efficient, and reproducible protocols for such complex data. These pipeline workflows start with ingesting the raw data, preprocessing, aggregating, harmonizing, analyzing, visualizing, and interpreting the findings.

In this case study, the training dataset consists of 2223 observations and 131 numeric variables. We select the functional rating scale slope, ALSFRS slope, as our outcome variable, as it captures the patients' clinical decline over a year. Although we have more observations than features, this is one of the examples where multiple features are highly correlated. Therefore, we need to preprocess the variables before commencing with feature selection.

Step 2: Exploring and Preparing the Data
The dataset is located in the DSPA case studies archive. We can use read.csv() to directly import the CSV dataset into R using the URL reference.

```
ALS.train <-
    read.csv("https://umich.instructure.com/files/1789624/download?download_frd=1")
summary(ALS.train)
```

There are 131 features and some of the variables represent statistics, e.g., *max, min,* and *median* values, of the corresponding clinical measurements.

---

[3] https://doi.org/10.1056/NEJM200105313442207

Step 3: Training a Model on the Data

Now let's explore the `Boruta()` function in the `Boruta` package to perform variable selection, based on random forest classification. `Boruta()` includes the following components:

```
vs <- Boruta(class~features, data=Mydata, pValue = 0.01, mcAdj = TRUE,
 maxRuns = 100, doTrace=0, getImp = getImpRfZ, ...)
```

- `class`: variable for class labels
- `features`: potential features to select from
- `data`: dataset containing classes and features
- `pValue`: confidence level. Default value is 0.01 (for applying multiple variable selection)
- `mcAdj`: Default TRUE to apply a multiple comparisons adjustment using the Bonferroni method
- `maxRuns`: maximal number of importance source runs. You may increase it to resolve attributes left Tentative
- `doTrace`: verbosity level. Default 0 means no tracing, 1 means reporting decision about each attribute as soon as it is justified, 2 means same as 1, plus at each importance source run reporting the number of attributes. The default is 0 where we don't do the reporting
- `getImp`: function used to obtain attribute importance. The default is *getImpRfZ*, which runs random forest from the ranger package and gathers Z-scores of mean decrease accuracy measure.

The resulting `vs` object is of class `Boruta` and contains two important components

- `finalDecision`: a factor of three values: `Confirmed`, `Rejected`, or `Tentative`, containing the final results of the feature selection process
- `ImpHistory`: a data frame of importance of attributes gathered in each importance source run. Besides the predictors' importance, it contains maximal, mean, and minimal importance of shadow attributes for each run. Rejected attributes get `-Inf` importance. This output is set to NULL if we specify `holdHistory=FALSE` in the Boruta call.

Caution Running the code below will take several minutes.

```r
# install.packages("Boruta")
library(Boruta)
set.seed(123)
als <- Boruta(ALSFRS_slope ~ . -ID, data=ALS.train, doTrace=0)
print(als)
## Boruta performed 99 iterations in 3.764011 mins.
##  27 attributes confirmed important: ALSFRS_Total_max,
als$ImpHistory[1:6, 1:10]
```

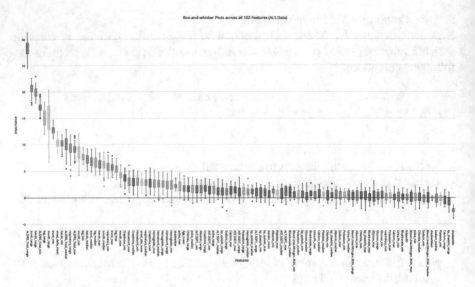

Fig. 11.1 A box and whisker plot of the Boruta-derived variable importance (ALS data)

This is a fairly time-consuming computation. Boruta determines the *important* attributes from *unimportant* and *tentative* features. Here the importance is measured by the out-of-bag (OOB) error. The OOB estimates the prediction error of machine learning methods (e.g., random forests and boosted decision trees) that utilize bootstrap aggregation to subsample training data. OOB represents the mean prediction error on each training sample x_i, using only the trees that did not include x_i in their bootstrap samples. Out-of-bag estimates provide *internal* assessment of the learning accuracy and avoid the need for an independent *external* validation dataset.

The importance scores for all features at every iteration are stored in the data frame als$ImpHistory. Let's plot a graph depicting the essential features (Fig. 11.1). Again, running this code will take several minutes to complete.

```
library(plotly)
df_long <- tidyr::gather(as.data.frame(als$ImpHistory), feature, measurement)
plot_ly(df_long, y = ~measurement, color = ~feature, type = "box") %>%
   layout(title="Box-and-whisker Plots across all 102 Features (ALS Data)",
        xaxis=list(title="Features", categoryorder ="total descending"),
        yaxis=list(title="Importance"),showlegend=F)
```

We have already seen similar groups of boxplots back in Chap. 2. In Fig. 11.1, variables to the left correspond to higher importance, relative to their less-important counterparts to the right.

It may be desirable to get rid of tentative features. Notice that this function should be used only when strict decision is highly desired because this test is much weaker than Boruta and can lower the confidence of the final result.

```
final.als <- TentativeRoughFix(als)
print(final.als)
## Boruta performed 99 iterations in 3.764011 mins.
## Tentatives roughfixed over the last 99 iterations.
##  28 attributes confirmed important: ALSFRS_Total_max,
## ALSFRS_Total_median, ALSFRS_Total_min, ALSFRS_Total_range,
## Creatinine_max and 23 more;
##  71 attributes confirmed unimportant: Age_mean, Albumin_max,
## Albumin_median, Albumin_min, Albumin_range and 66 more;
final.als$finalDecision
##                         Age_mean                   Albumin_max
##                         Rejected                      Rejected
…
##                        trunk_min                   trunk_range
##                        Confirmed                     Confirmed
##                    Urine.Ph_max              Urine.Ph_median
##                         Rejected                      Rejected
##                    Urine.Ph_min
##                         Rejected
## Levels: Tentative Confirmed Rejected
getConfirmedFormula(final.als)
## ALSFRS_slope ~ ALSFRS_Total_max + ALSFRS_Total_median + ALSFRS_Total_min +
##     ALSFRS_Total_range + Creatinine_max + Creatinine_median +
##     Creatinine_min + hands_max + hands_median + hands_min + hands_range +
##     Hemoglobin_median + leg_max + leg_median + leg_min + leg_range +
##     mouth_max + mouth_median + mouth_min + mouth_range + onset_delta_mean+
##     respiratory_median + respiratory_min + respiratory_range +
##     trunk_max + trunk_median + trunk_min + trunk_range
# report the Boruta "Confirmed" & "Tentative" features, removing "Rejected"
print(final.als$finalDecision[final.als$finalDecision %in%
    c("Confirmed", "Tentative")])
# how many are actually "confirmed" as important/salient?
impBoruta <- final.als$finalDecision[final.als$finalDecision %in%
    c("Confirmed")]; length(impBoruta)
## [1] 28
```

This shows 28 final features selected as salient in predicting ALSFRS slope changes.

Step 4: Evaluating Model Performance
Let's compare the `Boruta` results against a classical variable selection method: *recursive feature elimination (RFE)*. First, we need to load two packages `caret` and `randomForest`. Similar to the examples in Chap. 9, we must specify a resampling method. Here, we use *10-fold CV* to do the resampling.

```
library(caret)
library(randomForest)
set.seed(123)
control <- rfeControl(functions = rfFuncs, method = "cv", number=10)
```

After these preparations we can perform RFE variable selection.

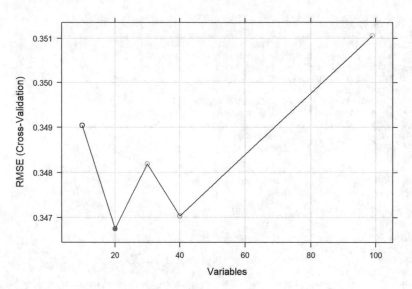

Fig. 11.2 Relation between number of variables and CV-RMSE of the recursive feature elimination variable selection model

```
rf.train <- rfe(ALS.train[, -c(1, 7)], ALS.train[, 7],
                sizes=c(10, 20, 30, 40), rfeControl=control)
rf.train
## Recursive feature selection
## Outer resampling method: Cross-Validated (10 fold)
##  Variables   RMSE Rsquared    MAE  RMSESD RsquaredSD  MAESD Selected
##         10 0.3490   0.6831 0.2479 0.03305    0.05288 0.01580
##         20 0.3468   0.6876 0.2463 0.03110    0.04798 0.01396        *
##         30 0.3482   0.6852 0.2479 0.03253    0.04827 0.01474
##         40 0.3470   0.6876 0.2473 0.03411    0.04927 0.01494
##         99 0.3511   0.6807 0.2499 0.03300    0.04967 0.01472
## The top 5 variables (out of 20):
##    ALSFRS_Total_range, hands_range, trunk_range, ALSFRS_Total_min, mouth_range
```

This calculation may take a long time to complete. The RFE invocation is different from Boruta. Here, we have to specify the feature data frame and the class labels separately. Also, the sizes= option allows us to specify the number of features we want to include in the model. Let's try sizes=c(10, 20, 30, 40) to compare the model performance for alternative numbers of features.

To visualize the results, we can plot the five different feature size combinations listed in the summary. The one with 20 features has the lowest RMSE measure. This result is similar to the Boruta output, which selected around 30 features (Fig. 11.2).

```
plot(rf.train, type=c("g", "o"), cex=1, col=1:5)
```

Using the functions predictors() and getSelectedAttributes(), we can compare the final results of the two alternative feature selection methods.

```
predRFE <- predictors(rf.train)
predBoruta <- getSelectedAttributes(final.als, withTentative = F)
```

The results are almost identical.

```
intersect(predBoruta, predRFE)
## [1] "ALSFRS_Total_max" "ALSFRS_Total_median" "ALSFRS_Total_min"
## [4] "ALSFRS_Total_range""Creatinine_max" "hands_max"
## [7] "hands_median" "hands_min" "hands_range"
## [10] "leg_median" "leg_min" "leg_range"
## [13] "mouth_median" "mouth_min" "mouth_range"
## [16] "onset_delta_mean" "respiratory_range" "trunk_median"
## [19] "trunk_min" "trunk_range"
```

There are 20 common variables chosen by the two techniques. This agreement suggests that both the Boruta and RFE methods are consistent and robust. Also, notice that the Boruta method can give similar results without utilizing the *size* option. If we want to consider 10 or more different sizes, the procedure will be quite time consuming. Thus, Boruta method is effective when dealing with complex real-world problems.

Next, we can contrast the Boruta feature selection results against another classical variable selection method—*stepwise model selection*. Let's start with fitting a bidirectional stepwise linear model-based feature selection.

```
data2 <- ALS.train[, -1]
# Define a base model - intercept only
base.mod <- lm(ALSFRS_slope ~ 1 , data= data2)
# Define the full model - including all predictors
all.mod <- lm(ALSFRS_slope ~ . , data= data2)
# ols_step <- lm(ALSFRS_slope ~ ., data=data2)
ols_step <- step(base.mod, scope = list(lower = base.mod, upper = all.mod),
direction = 'both', k=2, trace = F)
summary(ols_step); # ols_step
## Residuals:
##      Min      1Q   Median      3Q      Max
## -2.22558 -0.17875 -0.02024  0.17098  1.95100
## Coefficients:
##                        Estimate Std. Error t value Pr(>|t|)
## (Intercept)           4.176e-01  6.064e-01   0.689 0.491091
## ALSFRS_Total_range   -2.260e+01  1.359e+00 -16.631  < 2e-16 ***
## ALSFRS_Total_median  -3.388e-02  2.868e-03 -11.812  < 2e-16 ***
## ...
## Gender_mean          -3.360e-02  1.751e-02  -1.919 0.055066 .
## Creatinine_min        7.643e-04  4.977e-04   1.536 0.124771
## Signif. codes:  0 '***' 0.001 '**' 0.01 '*' 0.05 '.' 0.1 ' ' 1
## Residual standard error: 0.3355 on 2191 degrees of freedom
## Multiple R-squared:  0.7135, Adjusted R-squared:  0.7094
## F-statistic:   176 on 31 and 2191 DF,  p-value: < 2.2e-16
```

We can report the stepwise "Confirmed" (important) features.

```
# get the shortlisted variable
stepwiseConfirmedVars <- names(unlist(ols_step[[1]]))
# remove the intercept
stepwiseConfirmedVars <-
              stepwiseConfirmedVars[!stepwiseConfirmedVars %in% "(Intercept)"]
print(stepwiseConfirmedVars)
##  [1] "ALSFRS_Total_range"  "ALSFRS_Total_median" "ALSFRS_Total_min"
##  [4] "Calcium_range"       "Calcium_max"         "bp_diastolic_min"
##  [7] "onset_delta_mean"    "Calcium_min"         "Albumin_range"
## [10] "Glucose_range"       "ALT.SGPT._median"    "AST.SGOT._median"
## [13] "Glucose_max"         "Glucose_min"         "Creatinine_range"
## [16] "Potassium_range"     "Chloride_range"      "Chloride_min"
## [19] "Sodium_median"       "respiratory_min"     "respiratory_range"
## [22] "respiratory_max"     "trunk_range"         "pulse_range"
## [25] "Bicarbonate_max"     "Bicarbonate_range"   "Chloride_max"
## [28] "onset_site_mean"     "trunk_max"           "Gender_mean"
## [31] "Creatinine_min"
```

Comparing the overlap between the feature selection results of `Boruta` and `step-wise` feature selection.

```
library(mlbench)
library(caret)
# estimate variable importance
predStepwise <- varImp(ols_step, scale=FALSE)
# summarize importance
print(predStepwise)
##                         Overall
## ALSFRS_Total_range    16.630592
## ALSFRS_Total_median   11.812263
…
## Creatinine_min         1.535642
# Boruta vs. Stepwise feature selection
intersect(predBoruta, stepwiseConfirmedVars)
## [1] "ALSFRS_Total_median" "ALSFRS_Total_min"    "ALSFRS_Total_range"
## [4] "Creatinine_min"      "onset_delta_mean"    "respiratory_min"
## [7] "respiratory_range"   "trunk_max"           "trunk_range"
```

There are about nine common variables chosen by the Boruta and step-wise feature selection methods. There is another more elaborate stepwise feature selection technique that is implemented in the function `MASS::stepAIC()` that is useful for a wider range of object classes.

11.2   Regularized Linear Modeling and Controlled Variable Selection

Many biomedical and biosocial studies involve large amounts of complex data, including cases where the number of features (k) is large and may exceed the number of cases (n). In such situations, parameter estimates are difficult to compute or may be unreliable as the system is underdetermined. Regularization provides one approach to improve model reliability, prediction accuracy, and result interpretability. It is based on augmenting the fidelity term of the objective function used in the model fitting process with a regularization term that provides restrictions on the parameter space.

Classical techniques for choosing *important* covariates to include in a model of complex multivariate data rely on various types of stepwise variable selection processes. These tend to improve prediction accuracy in certain situations, e.g., when a small number of features are strongly predictive, or heavily associated, with the clinical outcome or the specific biosocial trait. However, the prediction error may be large when the model relies purely on a fidelity term. Including an additional regularization term in the optimization of the cost function improves the prediction accuracy. For example, below we show that by shrinking large regression coefficients, ridge regularization reduces overfitting and improves prediction error. Similarly, the *least absolute shrinkage and selection operator (LASSO)* employs regularization to perform simultaneous parameter estimation and variable selection. LASSO enhances the prediction accuracy and provides a natural interpretation of the resulting model. *Regularization* refers to forcing certain characteristics on the model, or the corresponding scientific inference. Examples include discouraging complex models or extreme explanations, even if they fit the data, enforcing model generalizability to prospective data, or restricting model overfitting of accidental samples.

Next, we will extend the mathematical foundation we presented in Chap. 3 and discuss computational protocols for handling complex high-dimensional data. In addition, we will illustrate model estimation by controlling the false-positive rate of selection of salient features and demonstrate fitting effective forecasting models.

11.2.1 General Questions

Applications of regularized linear modeling techniques will help us address problems like these:

- How to deal with extremely high-dimensional data (hundreds or thousands of features)?
- Why mix fidelity (model fit) and regularization (model interpretability) terms in objective function optimization?
- How to reduce the false-positive rate, increase scientific validation, and improve result reproducibility (e.g., Knockoff filtering)?

11.2.2 Model Regularization

In data-driven sciences, *regularization* is the process of introducing constraints, adding information to, or smoothing a model aiming to generate a realistic solution to an ill-posed (or under-determined) problem, to prevent overfitting, or to improve the model interpretability.

Regularization of objective functions is a commonly used strategy to solve ill-posed optimization problems (Chap. 13). This involves introducing another regularization term penalizing the model for not complying with the additional constraints or increasing the magnitude of the cost function to enforce convergence of the model to an "optimal" or a "unique" solution. The example below illustrates a schematic of regularization.

Suppose we fit several different (polynomial) models that have near perfect model-fidelity, i.e., all models go very close to the set of anchor points we specified. In that sense, all models represent near-perfect solutions to this unconstrained, not-regularized, optimization problem. They all fit the data well. Now, we can introduce an additional constraint that we want a simple model, e.g., smooth, low order, differentiable, integrable. We are looking for models that are easy to interpret and use in practice. This demand can be satisfied by adding a *regularization term* to the objective function. In addition to requiring that the model passes through (or near-by) each of the anchor points, we can require that the model is "simple." In the example below, which of the different models appear simpler? The *fidelity* of the model is captured by how closely it fits the set of anchor points (see RMSE error). The model *regularizer* enforces simple model representation, i.e., higher interpretability is associated with lower polynomial order.

The following example demonstrates the heuristics of fitting a regularized model where the objective function is a mixture of a fidelity term (polynomial fit to data) and a penalty term (enforcing conditions restricting the model flexibility to specific points) (Fig. 11.3).

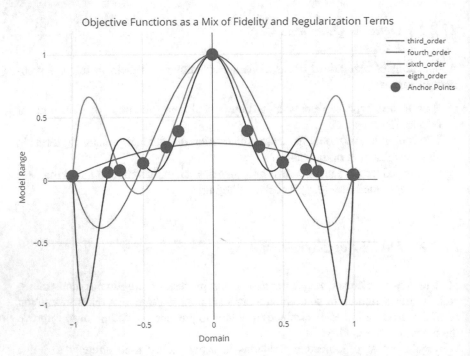

Fig. 11.3 A simple example of a regularized model where the objective function is a mixture of a fidelity term (polynomial fit) and a penalty term (enforcing anchoring points)

```r
# define a function of interest e.g., Runge's function
runge <- function(x) {  runge <- 1/(1+25*x^2)    }
# define the anchor (knot) points
knots <- seq(-1, 1, 0.01)
# library(rSymPy)
library(polynom)
library(tidyverse)
library(ModelMetrics)
lag_poly <- function(order) {
  X_nodes <- seq(-1, 1, 2/order)
  Y_coor <- runge(X_nodes)
  f <- as.function(poly.calc(X_nodes,Y_coor))
  RMSE = rmse(f(knots), runge(knots))
  print(paste("The ", order,
              " order polynomial interpolation has this RMS Error:", RMSE))
  X <- data.frame(X_nodes)
  Y <- data.frame(Y_coor)
  lag_poly <- c(f, X, Y)
}
#Adding OTHER order functions here
third_order <- lag_poly(3)
## [1] "The  3  order polynomial interpolation has this RMS Error: 0.243252"
forth_order <- lag_poly(4)
## [1] "The  4  order polynomial interpolation has this RMS Error: 0.278492"
sixth_order <- lag_poly(6)
## [1] "The  6  order polynomial interpolation has this RMS Error: 0.273265"
eigth_order <- lag_poly(8)
## [1] "The  8  order polynomial interpolation has this RMS Error: 0.367531"
# twentyth_order <- lag_poly(20)
# unlist other created polynomials
X_dat <- c(unlist(flatten(third_order[2])), unlist(flatten(forth_order[2])),
  unlist(flatten(sixth_order[2])), unlist(flatten(eigth_order[2])) )
Y_dat <-c(unlist(flatten(third_order[3])), unlist(flatten(forth_order[3])),
  unlist(flatten(sixth_order[3])), unlist(flatten(eigth_order[3])) )
Labels <- c(rep("third_order",4), rep("forth_order",5),
  rep("sixth_order",7), rep("eigth_order",9) )
dat <- data.frame(X=X_dat,Y=Y_dat,label=Labels) # print(second_order[[2]])
ord=8
X_nodes <- seq(-1, 1, 2/ord)
Y_coor <- runge(X_nodes)
# fit8 <  lm(Y_coor ~ poly(X_nodes, 8, raw-TRUE))
library(plotly)
xSample <- seq(-1, 1, length.out = 1000)
plot_ly(x=~xSample, y=~third_order[[1]](xSample), type="scatter",
        mode="lines", name="third_order") %>%
  add_trace(x=~xSample, y=~forth_order[[1]](xSample), mode="lines",
            name="forth_order") %>%
  add_trace(x=~xSample, y=~sixth_order[[1]](xSample), mode="lines",
            name="sixth_order") %>%
  add_trace(x=~xSample, y=~eigth_order[[1]](xSample), mode="lines",
            name="eigth_order") %>%
  add_markers(x=~dat$X, y=~dat$Y, mode="markers", name="Anchor Points",
              marker=list(size=20)) %>%
  layout(title="Objective Functions as a Mix of Fidelity and Regularization Terms",
         xaxis=list(title="Domain"), yaxis=list(title="Model Range"))
```

11.2.3   Matrix Notation

Let's recall the basics of matrix notation, linear algebra, and matrix computing we covered in Chap. 3. At the core of matrix, manipulations are scalars, vectors, and matrices.

- y_i: output or response variable, $i = 1, \ldots, n$ (cases, subjects, units, etc.)
- x_{ij}: input, predictor, or feature variable, $1 \leq j \leq k$, $1 \leq i \leq n$.

- $y = \begin{pmatrix} y_1 \\ y_2 \\ \vdots \\ y_n \end{pmatrix}$, and $X = \begin{pmatrix} x_{1,1} & x_{1,2} & \cdots & x_{1,k} \\ x_{2,1} & x_{2,2} & \cdots & x_{2,k} \\ \vdots & \vdots & \ddots & \vdots \\ x_{n,1} & x_{n,2} & \cdots & x_{n,k} \end{pmatrix}_{\text{cases} \times \text{features}}$

11.2.4   Regularized Linear Modeling

If we assume that the covariates are orthonormal, i.e., we have a special kind of a *design matrix* $X^{\mathrm{T}}X = I$, then the *ordinary least squares (OLS) estimates* minimize the following objective function

$$\min_{\beta \in \mathbb{R}^k} \left\{ \frac{1}{N} \parallel y - X\beta \parallel_2^2 \right\}.$$

The closed-form mathematical expression for OLS estimates is

$$\widehat{\beta}^{\mathrm{OLS}} = \left(X^{\mathrm{T}}X\right)^{-1} X^{\mathrm{T}}y.$$

Regularized *LASSO estimates* minimize a modified cost function

$$\min_{\beta \in \mathbb{R}^k} \left\{ \frac{1}{N} \parallel y - X\beta \parallel_2^2 + \lambda \parallel \beta \parallel_1 \right\}.$$

These LASSO estimates may be expressed as a soft-thresholding function of the OLS estimates

$$\widehat{\beta}_j = S_{N\lambda}\left(\widehat{\beta}_j^{\mathrm{OLS}}\right) = \widehat{\beta}_j^{\mathrm{OLS}} \max\left(0, 1 - \frac{N\lambda}{\left|\widehat{\beta}_j^{\mathrm{OLS}}\right|}\right),$$

where $S_{N\lambda}$ is a soft thresholding operator translating values *towards* zero. This is different from the hard thresholding operator, which *sets* smaller values to zero and leaves larger ones unchanged.

Similarly, the regularized *Ridge regression* minimizes a similar objective function (using a different norm)

$$\min_{\beta \in \mathbb{R}^k} \left\{ \frac{1}{N} \parallel y - X\beta \parallel_2^2 + \lambda \parallel \beta \parallel_2^2 \right\}.$$

This yields the ridge estimates $\widehat{\beta}_j = (1 + N\lambda)^{-1} \widehat{\beta}_j^{OLS}$. Thus, ridge regression shrinks all coefficients by a uniform factor, $(1 + N\lambda)^{-1}$, and does not set any coefficients to zero.

Best subset selection regression, also known as orthogonal matching pursuit (OMP), minimizes the same cost function with respect to the zero-norm:

$$\min_{\beta \in \mathbb{R}^k} \left\{ \frac{1}{N} \parallel y - X\beta \parallel_2^2 + \lambda \parallel \beta \parallel_0 \right\},$$

where $\parallel . \parallel_0$ is the "ℓ^0 norm", defined for $z \in R^d$ as $\parallel z \parallel_o = m$, where exactly m components of z are nonzero. In this case, a closed form of the parameter estimates is

$$\widehat{\beta}_j = H_{\sqrt{N\lambda}} \left(\widehat{\beta}_j^{OLS} \right) = \widehat{\beta}_j^{OLS} I \left(\left| \widehat{\beta}_j^{OLS} \right| \geq \sqrt{N\lambda} \right),$$

where H_α is a hard-thresholding function and I is an indicator function (it is 1 if its argument is true, and 0 otherwise).

The LASSO estimates may share similar features selection/estimates with both Ridge and Best (OMP). This is because they both shrink the magnitude of all the coefficients, like ridge regression, but also set some of them to zero, as in the best subset selection case. Ridge regression scales all the coefficients by a constant factor, whereas LASSO translates the coefficients towards zero by a constant value and then sets the small values to zero.

11.2.4.1 Ridge Regression

Ridge regression[4] relies on L^2 regularization to improve the model prediction accuracy. It improves prediction error by shrinking large regression coefficients and reducing overfitting. By itself, ridge regularization does not perform variable selection and does not really help with model interpretation.

Let's show an example using the MLB dataset 01a_data.txt, which includes player's Name, Team, Position, Height, Weight, and Age (Fig. 11.4). We may fit in any regularized linear mode, e.g., Weight $\sim$ Age + Height.

---

[4] https://doi.org/10.1002/wics.14

```
# install.packages("doParallel")
library("doParallel")
library(plotly)
library(tidyr)
# https://umich.instructure.com/courses/38100/files/folder/data    (01a_data.txt)
data <-
    read.table('https://umich.instructure.com/files/330381/download?download_frd=1',
              as.is=T, header=T)
attach(data); str(data)
## 'data.frame':    1034 obs. of  6 variables:
## $ Name    : chr  "Adam_Donachie" "Paul_Bako" "Ramon_Hernandez" "Kevin_Millar"
...
## $ Team    : chr  "BAL" "BAL" "BAL" "BAL" ...
## $ Position: chr  "Catcher" "Catcher" "Catcher" "First_Baseman" ...
## $ Height  : int  74 74 72 72 73 69 69 71 76 71 ...
## $ Weight  : int  180 215 210 210 188 176 209 200 231 180 ...
## $ Age     : num  23 34.7 30.8 35.4 35.7 ...
# Training Data
# Full Model: x <- model.matrix(Weight ~ ., data = data[1:900, ])
# Reduced Model
x <- model.matrix(Weight ~ Age + Height, data = data[1:900, ])
# creates a design (model) matrix, and adds 1 column for outcome
y <- data[1:900, ]$Weight
# Testing Data
x.test <- model.matrix(Weight ~ Age + Height, data = data[901:1034, ])
y.test <- data[901:1034, ]$Weight
# install.packages("glmnet")
library("glmnet")
library(doParallel)
cl <- makePSOCKcluster(6)
registerDoParallel(cl); getDoParWorkers()
# getDoParName(); getDoParVersion()
cv.ridge <-  cv.glmnet(x, y, type.measure="mse", alpha=0, parallel=T)
## alpha=1 for Lasso, alpha=0 for Ridge, and 0<alpha<1 to blend ridge & lasso
plotCV.glmnet <- function(cv.glmnet.object, name="") {
  df <- as.data.frame(cbind(x=log(cv.glmnet.object$lambda),
         y=cv.glmnet.object$cvm,
         errorBar=cv.glmnet.object$cvsd), nzero=cv.glmnet.object$nzero)
  featureNum <- cv.glmnet.object$nzero
  xFeature <- log(cv.glmnet.object$lambda)
  yFeature <- max(cv.glmnet.object$cvm)+max(cv.glmnet.object$cvsd)
  dataFeature <- data.frame(featureNum, xFeature, yFeature)
  plot_ly(data = df) %>%
    # add error bars for each CV-mean at Log(lambda)
    add_trace(x = ~x, y = ~y, type = 'scatter', mode = 'markers',
        name = 'CV MSE', error_y = ~list(array = errorBar)) %>%
    # add the lambda-min and lambda 1SD vertical dash lines
    add_lines(data=df, x=c(log(cv.glmnet.object$lambda.min),
              log(cv.glmnet.object$lambda.min)),
              y=c(min(cv.glmnet.object$cvm)-max(df$errorBar),
              max(cv.glmnet.object$cvm)+max(df$errorBar)),
              showlegend=F, line=list(dash="dash"), name="lambda.min",
              mode = 'lines+markers') %>%
    add_lines(data=df, x=c(log(cv.glmnet.object$lambda.1se),
              log(cv.glmnet.object$lambda.1se)),
              y=c(min(cv.glmnet.object$cvm)-max(df$errorBar),
              max(cv.glmnet.object$cvm)+max(df$errorBar)),
              showlegend=F, line=list(dash="dash"), name="lambda.1se") %>%
```

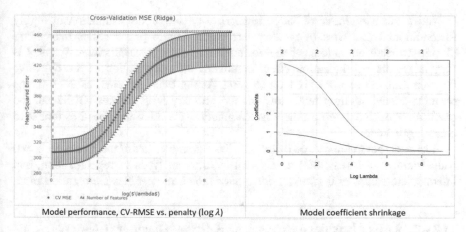

Fig. 11.4 Regularized linear model, `Weight ~ Age + Height`, with Ridge penalty term

```
# Add Number of Features Annotations on Top
add_trace(dataFeature, x = ~xFeature, y = ~yFeature, type = 'scatter',
    name="Number of Features",
    mode = 'text', text = ~featureNum, textposition = 'middle right',
    textfont = list(color = '#000000', size = 9)) %>%
layout(title = paste0("Cross-Validation MSE (", name, ")"),
            xaxis = list(title=paste0("log(",TeX("\\lambda"),")"),
            side="bottom", showgrid=TRUE), # type="Log"
            hovermode = "x unified", legend = list(orientation='h'),
            yaxis = list(title = cv.glmnet.object$name, side="left",
            showgrid = TRUE))
}
plotCV.glmnet(cv.ridge, "Ridge")
coef(cv.ridge)
## 4 x 1 sparse Matrix of class "dgCMatrix"
##                    s1
## (Intercept) -47.6548795
## (Intercept)    .
## Age           0.6050286
## Height        3.1470597
sqrt(cv.ridge$cvm[cv.ridge$lambda == cv.ridge$lambda.1se])
## [1] 18.01748
#plot variable feature coefficients against the shrinkage parameter lambda.
glmmod <-glmnet(x, y, alpha = 0)
plot(glmmod, xvar="lambda")
grid()

# for plot_glmnet with ridge/lasso coefficient path labels
# install.packages("plotmo")
library(plotmo)
plot_glmnet(glmmod, lwd=4)          #default colors
```

In Fig. 11.4, different colors represent the vector of features, and the corresponding coefficients, displayed as a function of the regularization parameter, λ. The top horizontal axis indicates the number of nonzero coefficients at the current value of λ. For LASSO regularization, this top-axis corresponds to the effective degrees of freedom (df) for the model.

Notice the usefulness of Ridge regularization for model estimation in highly ill-conditioned problems $(n \gg k)$ where slight feature perturbations may cause disproportionate alterations of the corresponding weight calculations. When λ is very large, the regularization effect dominates the optimization of the objective function and the coefficients tend to zero. At the other extreme, as $\lambda \to 0$, the resulting model solution tends towards the ordinary least squares (OLS) and the coefficients exhibit large oscillations. In practice, we often may need to tune λ to balance this tradeoff.

Also note that in the `cv.glmnet` call, the extreme values of the parameter $\alpha = 0$ (ridge) and $\alpha = 1$ (LASSO) correspond to different types of regularization, and intermediate values of $0 < \alpha < 1$ corresponds to *elastic net* blended regularization.

11.2.4.2 Least Absolute Shrinkage and Selection Operator (LASSO) Regression

Estimating the linear regression coefficients in a linear regression model using LASSO involves minimizing an objective function that includes an L^1 regularization term which tends to shrink the number of features. A descriptive representation of the fidelity (left) and regularization (right) terms of the objective function are shown below

$$\underbrace{\sum_{i=1}^{n}\left[y_i - \beta_0 - \overbrace{\sum_{j=1}^{k}\beta_j x_{ij}}^{\text{linear model}}\right]^2}_{\text{fidelity term}} + \lambda \underbrace{\sum_{j=1}^{k}|\beta_j|}_{\text{regularization term}} .$$

LASSO jointly achieves model quality, reliability, and variable selection by penalizing the sum of the absolute values of the regression coefficients. This forces the shrinkage of certain coefficients effectively acting as a variable selection process. This is similar to ridge regression's penalty on the sum of the squares of the regression coefficients, although ridge regression only shrinks the magnitude of the coefficients without truncating them to 0.

Let's show how to select the regularization weight parameter λ using `training` data and report the error using `testing` data.

```
mod.lasso <-  cv.glmnet(x, y, alpha = 1, thresh = 1e-12, parallel = T)
## alpha =1 for Lasso, alpha = 0 for ridge, 0<alpha<1 for elastic net blend
lambda.best <- mod.lasso$lambda.min
lambda.best
## [1] 0.05406379
lasso.pred <- predict(mod.lasso, newx = x.test, s = lambda.best)
LASSO.RMS <- mean((y.test - lasso.pred)^2); LASSO.RMS
## [1] 261.8045
```

Retrieve and report the model coefficient estimates.

```
mod.lasso <-  glmnet(x, y, alpha = 1)
predict(mod.lasso, s = lambda.best, type = "coefficients")
## 4 x 1 sparse Matrix of class "dgCMatrix"
##                        s1
## (Intercept) -182.1429000
## (Intercept)            .
## Age            0.9667182
## Height         4.8309312
lasso.test.r2 <-  1 - mean((y.test - lasso.pred)^2)/mean((y.test -
mean(y.test))^2)
```

Perhaps obtain a classical OLS linear model and contrast the parameter estimates.

```
lm.fit <-  lm(Weight ~ Age + Height, data = data[1:900, ])
summary(lm.fit)
## Coefficients:
##               Estimate Std. Error t value Pr(>|t|)
## (Intercept) -184.3736    19.4232  -9.492  < 2e-16 ***
## Age            0.9799     0.1335   7.341 4.74e-13 ***
## Height         4.8561     0.2551  19.037  < 2e-16 ***
## Residual standard error: 17.5 on 897 degrees of freedom
## Multiple R-squared:  0.3088, Adjusted R-squared:  0.3072
## F-statistic: 200.3 on 2 and 897 DF,  p-value: < 2.2e-16
```

The OLS linear (unregularized) model has slightly larger coefficients and greater MSE than LASSO, which attests to the shrinkage of LASSO (Fig. 11.5).

```
lm.pred <-  predict(lm.fit, newx = x.test)
LM.RMS <- mean((y - lm.pred)^2); LM.RMS
## [1] 305.1995
lm.test.r2 <-  1 - mean((y - lm.pred)^2) / mean((y.test - mean(y.test))^2)
plot_ly(x = c("OLS", "LASSO", "Ridge"),
        y = c(lm.test.r2, lasso.test.r2, ridge.test.r2),
        name = paste0("Model ", TeX("R^2") ," Performance"), type="bar") %>%
  layout(title=paste0("Model ", TeX("R^2") ," Performance"))
```

Compare the results of the three alternative models (LM, LASSO, and Ridge) for these data and contrast the derived RMS results.

```
library(knitr) # kable function to convert tabular R-results into Rmd tables
# create table as data frame
RMS_Table = data.frame(LM=LM.RMS, LASSO=LASSO.RMS, Ridge=ridge.RMS)

# convert to markdown
kable(RMS_Table, format="pandoc", caption="Test Dataset RSS Results",
align=c("c", "c", "c"))
stopCluster(cl)
```

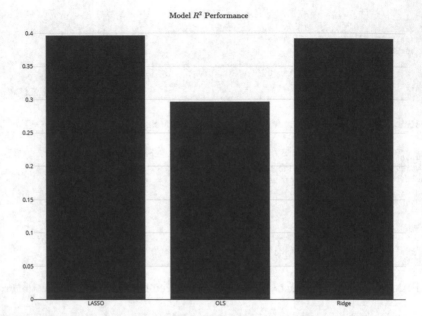

Fig. 11.5 Performance comparison (R^2 measure) of three linear models, Weight ~ Age + Height, using OLS, Ridge, and LASSO parameter estimation strategies

LM	LASSO	Ridge
305.1995	261.8045	263.8461

As both the *inputs* (features or predictors) and the *output* (response) are observed for the testing data, we can build a learner examining the relationship between the two types of features (controlled covariates and observable responses). Most often, we are interested in forecasting or predicting responses based on prospective (new, testing, or validation) data.

11.2.5 Predictor Standardization

Prior to fitting regularized linear modeling and estimating the effects, covariates may be standardized. Scaling the features ensures the measuring units of the features do not bias the distance measures or norm estimates. Standardization can be accomplished by using the classic "z-score" formula. This puts each predictor on the same scale (unitless quantities)—the mean is 0 and the variance is 1. We use $\widehat{\beta}_o = \overline{y}$, for the mean intercept parameter, and estimate the coefficients of the remaining predictors. To facilitate interpretation of the results, after the model is estimated, in the context of the specific case study, we can transform the results back to the original scale/ units.

11.2.6 Estimation Goals

The basic model-based inference problem is this: given a set of predictors X, find a function, $f(X)$, to model or predict the outcome Y. Let's denote the objective (loss or cost) function by $L(y, f(X))$. It determines adequacy of the fit and allows us to estimate the *squared error loss*

$$L(y, f(X)) = (y - f(X))^2.$$

We are looking to find f that minimizes the *expected loss*

$$E\left[(Y - f(X))^2\right] \Rightarrow f = E[Y|X = x].$$

11.2.7 Linear Regression

For a linear model:

$$Y_i = \beta_0 + x_{i,1}\beta_1 + x_{i,2}\beta_2 + \ldots + x_{i,k}\beta_k + \epsilon,$$

let's assume that

- The model shorthand matrix notation is $Y = X\beta + \epsilon$.
- And the expectation of the observed outcome given the data, $E[Y|X = x]$, is a linear function, which in certain situations can be expressed as

$$\arg\min_{\beta} \sum_{i=1}^{n} \left(y_i - \sum_{j=1}^{k} x_{ij}\beta_j \right)^2 = \arg\min_{\beta} \sum_{i=1}^{n} (y_i - x_i^T \beta)^2.$$

Multiplying both hand-sides on the left by $X^T = X'$, which is the transpose of the design matrix X (recall that matrix multiplication is not always commutative) yields

$$X^T Y = X^T (X\beta) = (X^T X)\beta.$$

To solve for the effect-size coefficients, β, we can multiply both sides of the equation by the inverse of its (right hand side) multiplier

$$(X^T X)^{-1}(X^T Y) = (X^T X)^{-1}(X^T X)\beta = \beta.$$

The *ordinary least squares (OLS)* estimate of β is given by

$$\widehat{\beta} = \arg \min_{\beta} \sum_{i=1}^{n} \left(y_i - \sum_{j=1}^{k} x_{ij}\beta_j \right)^2 = \arg \min_{\beta} \ \| y - X\beta \|_2^2 \Rightarrow$$

$$\widehat{\beta}^{\text{OLS}} = (X'X)^{-1}X'y \Rightarrow \widehat{f}(x_i) = x_i'\widehat{\beta}.$$

11.2.8 Drawbacks of Linear Regression

Despite its wide use and elegant theory, linear regression has some shortcomings, e.g.,

- Prediction accuracy—Often can be improved upon.
- Model interpretability—Linear model does not automatically do variable selection.

11.2.8.1 Assessing Prediction Accuracy

Given a new input, x_0, how do we assess our prediction $\widehat{f}(x_0)$? We can use the *Expected Prediction Error (EPE)*

$$\begin{aligned} \text{EPE}(x_0) &= E\left[\left(Y_0 - \widehat{f}(x_0)^2\right)\right] \\ &= \text{Var}(\varepsilon) + \text{Var}\left(\widehat{f}(x_0)\right) + \text{Bias}\left(\widehat{f}(x_0)^2\right) \\ &= \text{Var}(\varepsilon) + \text{MSE}\left(\widehat{f}(x_0)\right) \end{aligned}$$

where

- $\text{Var}(\varepsilon)$: irreducible error variance
- $\text{Var}\left(\widehat{f}(x_0)\right)$: sample-to-sample variability of $\widehat{f}(x_0)$ and
- $\text{Bias}\left(\widehat{f}(x_0)\right)$: average difference of $\widehat{f}(x_0)$ and $f(x_0)$

11.2.8.2 Estimating the Prediction Error

One common approach to estimating prediction error include

- Randomly splitting the data into "training" and "testing" sets, where the testing data has m observations that will be used to independently validate the model quality. We estimate/calculate $\widehat{f}$ using training data;
- Estimating prediction error using the *testing set MSE*

$$\widehat{\text{MSE}}\left(\widehat{f}\right) = \frac{1}{m} \sum_{i=1}^{m} \left(y_i - \widehat{f}(x_i)\right)^2.$$

Ideally, we want our model/predictions to perform well with new or prospective data.

11.2.8.3   Improving the Prediction Accuracy

If $f(x) \approx$ linear, $\widehat{f}$ will have low bias but possibly high variance, e.g., in high-dimensional setting due to correlated predictors, when k features $\gg n$ cases, or under-determination, when $k > n$. The goal is to minimize total error by trading off bias and precision.

$$\text{MSE}\left(\widehat{f}(x)\right) = \text{Var}\left(\widehat{f}(x)\right) + \text{Bias}\left(\widehat{f}(x)\right)^2.$$

We can sacrifice bias to reduce variance, which may lead to decrease in MSE. So, regularization allows us to tune this tradeoff. We aim to predict the outcome variable, $Y_{n \times 1}$, in terms of other features $X_{n,k}$. Assume a first-order relationship relating Y and X is of the form $Y = f(X) + \epsilon$, where the error term is $\epsilon \sim N(0, \sigma)$. An estimate model $\widehat{f}(X)$ can be computed in many different ways (e.g., using least squares calculations for linear regressions, Newton-Raphson, steepest descent, stochastic gradient descent, or other methods). Then, we can decompose the expected squared prediction error at x as

$$E(x) = E\left[\left(Y - \widehat{f}(x)\right)^2\right] = \underbrace{\left(E\left[\widehat{f}(x)\right] - f(x)\right)^2}_{\text{Bias}^2} + \underbrace{E\left[\left(\widehat{f}(x) - E\left[\widehat{f}(x)\right]\right)^2\right]}_{\text{precision (variance)}}$$

$$+ \underbrace{\sigma^2}_{\text{irreducible error (noise)}}.$$

When the true Y vs. X relation is not known, infinite data may be necessary to calibrate the model $\widehat{f}$ and it may be impractical to jointly reduce both the model *bias* and *variance*. In general, minimizing the *bias* at the same time as minimizing the *variance* may not be possible. Figure 11.6 illustrates diagrammatically the tradeoffs between *bias* (centrality) and *precision* (variance).

Fig. 11.6 A schematic of
the *bias* and *precision*
tradeoffs

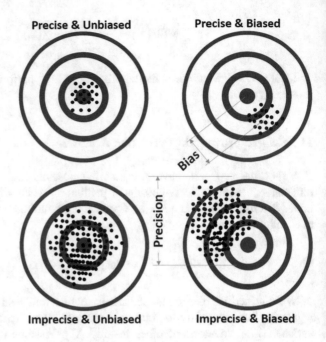

Precise & Unbiased   **Precise & Biased**

Imprecise & Unbiased   **Imprecise & Biased**

11.2.9   Variable Selection

Oftentimes, we are only interested in using a subset of the original features as model predictors. Thus, we need to identify the most relevant predictors, which usually capture the big picture of the process. This helps us avoid overly complex models that may be difficult to interpret. Typically, when considering several models that achieve similar results, it's natural to select the simplest of them.

Linear regression does not directly determine the importance of features to predict a specific outcome. The problem of selecting critical predictors is therefore very important.

Automatic feature subset selection methods should directly determine an optimal subset of variables. Forward or backward stepwise variable selection and forward stagewise are examples of classical methods for choosing the best subset by assessing various metrics like MSE, C_p (convergence probability), AIC (Akaike information criterion), or BIC (Bayesian information criterion).[5]

---

[5]https://doi.org/10.1080/03610918.2012.737491

11.2.10   Simple Regularization Framework

As before, we start with a given X and look for a (linear) function, $f(X) = \sum_{j=1}^{p} x_j \beta_j$, to model or predict y subject to certain objective cost function, e.g., squared error loss. Adding a second term to the cost function minimization process yields (model parameter) estimates expressed as

$$\widehat{\beta}(\lambda) = \arg\min_{\beta} \left\{ \sum_{i=1}^{n} \left(y_i - \sum_{j=1}^{k} x_{ij}\beta_j \right)^2 + \lambda J(\beta) \right\}.$$

In the above expression, $\lambda \geq 0$ is the regularization (tuning or penalty) parameter, $J(\beta)$ is a user-defined penalty function—typically, the intercept is not penalized.

11.2.10.1   Role of the Penalty Term

Consider $\arg\min J(\beta) = \sum_{j=1}^{k} \beta_j^2 = \| \beta \|_2^2$ (Ridge Regression, RR). Then, the formulation of the regularization framework is

$$\widehat{\beta}(\lambda)^{RR} = \arg\min_{\beta} \left\{ \sum_{i=1}^{n} \left(y_i - \sum_{j=1}^{k} x_{ij}\beta_j \right)^2 + \lambda \sum_{j=1}^{k} \beta_j^2 \right\}.$$

Alternatively, the optimization problem is

$$\widehat{\beta}(t)^{RR} = \arg\min_{\beta} \sum_{i=1}^{n} \left(y_i - \sum_{j=1}^{k} x_{ij}\beta_j \right)^2,$$

subject to

$$\sum_{j=1}^{k} \beta_j^2 \leq t.$$

11.2.10.2   Role of the Regularization Parameter

The regularization parameter $\lambda \geq 0$ directly controls the bias-variance trade-off

- $\lambda = 0$ corresponds to OLS, and
- $\lambda \to \infty$ puts more weight on the penalty function and results in more shrinkage of the coefficients, i.e., we introduce bias at the sake of reducing the variance.

The choice of λ is crucial and will be discussed below as each λ results in a different solution $\widehat{\beta}(\lambda)$.

11.2.10.3   LASSO

The LASSO (Least Absolute Shrinkage and Selection Operator) regularization relies on:

$$\operatorname{argmin}J(\beta) = \sum_{j=1}^{k} |\beta_j| = \| \beta \|_1,$$

which leads to the following objective function

$$\widehat{\beta}(\lambda)^L = \arg\min_{\beta} \left\{ \sum_{i=1}^{n} \left(y_i - \sum_{j=1}^{k} x_{ij}\beta_j \right)^2 + \lambda \sum_{j=1}^{k} |\beta_j| \right\}.$$

In practice, subtle changes in the penalty terms frequently lead to big differences in the results. Not only does the regularization term shrink coefficients towards zero, but it sets some of them to be exactly zero. Thus, it performs continuous variable selection, hence the name, least absolute shrinkage and selection operator (LASSO).

11.2.11   General Regularization Framework

The general regularization framework involves optimization of a more general objective function

$$\min_{f \in \mathcal{H}} \sum_{i=1}^{n} \{L(y_i, f(x_i)) + \lambda J(f)\},$$

where $\mathcal{H}$ is a space of possible functions, L is the *fidelity term*, e.g., squared error, absolute error, zero-one, negative log-likelihood (GLM), hinge loss (support vector machines), and J is the *regularizer*, e.g., ridge regression, LASSO, adaptive LASSO, group LASSO, fused LASSO, thresholded LASSO, generalized LASSO, constrained LASSO, elastic-net, Dantzig selector, SCAD, MCP, and smoothing splines.[6]

This represents a very general and flexible framework that allows us to incorporate prior knowledge (sparsity, structure, etc.) into the model estimation.

11.2.12 Likelihood Ratio Test (LRT), False Discovery Rate (FDR), and Logistic Transform

These concepts will be important in theoretical model development as well as in the applications we show below.

11.2.12.1 Likelihood Ratio Test (LRT)

The likelihood ratio test (LRT) compares the data fit of two models. For instance, removing predictor variables from a model may reduce the model quality (i.e., a model will have a lower log likelihood). To statistically assess whether the observed difference in model fit is significant, the LRT compares the difference of the log likelihoods of the two models. When this difference is statistically significant, the full model (the one with more variables) represents a better fit to the data, compared to the reduced model. LRT is computed using the log likelihoods (ll) of the two models

$$\mathrm{LRT} = -2\ln\left(\frac{L(m_1)}{L(m_2)}\right) = 2(ll(m_2) - ll(m_1)),$$

where

- m_1 and m_2 are the reduced and the full models, respectively.
- $L(m_1)$ and $L(m_2)$ denote the likelihoods of the two models.
- $ll(m_1)$ and $ll(m_2)$ represent the *log likelihood* (natural log of the model likelihood function).

As $n \to \infty$, the distribution of the LRT is asymptotically chi-squared with degrees of freedom equal to the number of parameters that are reduced (i.e., the number of variables removed from the model). In our case, $LRT \sim \chi^2_{df=2}$, as we have an intercept and one predictor (SE), and the null model is empty (no parameters).

[6]https://doi.org/10.1214/11-AOS878

11.2.12.2   False Discovery Rate (FDR)

The FDR rate measures the performance of a test:

$$\underbrace{\text{FDR}}_{\text{False Discovery Rate}} = \underbrace{E}_{\text{expectation}} \underbrace{\left(\frac{\text{\#False Positives}}{\text{total number of selected features}} \right)}_{\text{False Discovery Proportion}}.$$

The Benjamini–Hochberg (BH) FDR procedure[7] involves ordering the p-values, specifying a target FDR, calculating, and applying the threshold. Below we show how this is accomplished in R.

```
# List the p-values (these are typically computed by some statistical
# analysis, later these will be ordered from smallest to largest)
pvals <- c(0.9, 0.35, 0.01, 0.013, 0.014, 0.19, 0.35, 0.5, 0.63, 0.67,
           0.75, 0.81, 0.01, 0.051)
length(pvals)     # [1] 14
alpha.star <- 0.05     # enter the target FDR
pvals <- sort(pvals); pvals  # order the p-values small to large
#calculate the threshold for each p-value
# threshold[i] = alpha*(i/n), where i is the index of the ordered p-value
threshold <- alpha.star*(1:length(pvals))/length(pvals)
# for each index, compare the p-value against its threshold
cbind(pvals, threshold, pvals<=threshold)
##         pvals    threshold
##  [1,] 0.010 0.003571429 0
##  [2,] 0.010 0.007142857 0
##  [3,] 0.013 0.010714286 0
##  [4,] 0.014 0.014285714 1
##  [5,] 0.051 0.017857143 0
...
## [13,] 0.810 0.046428571 0
## [14,] 0.900 0.050000000 0
```

Starting with the smallest p-value and moving up, we find that the largest k for which the corresponding p-value is less than its threshold, α^*, which yields an index $\widehat{k} = 4$.

Next, the algorithm rejects the null hypotheses for the tests that correspond to p-values with indices $k \leq \widehat{k} = 4$, i.e., we determine that $p_{(1)}$, $p_{(2)}$, $p_{(3)}$, $p_{(4)}$ survive FDR correction for multiple testing.

Note: Since we controlled the FDR at $\alpha^* = 0.05$, we expect that on average only 5% of the tests that we rejected are spurious. In other words, of the FDR-corrected p-values, only about $\alpha^* = 0.05$ are expected to represent false-positives, e.g., features chosen to be salient, when in fact they are not really important.

As a comparison, the *Bonferroni corrected* α-value for these data is $\frac{0.05}{14} = 0.0036$. Note that Bonferroni coincides with the 1-st threshold value corresponding to the

---

[7]https://doi.org/10.1214/193940307000000158

smallest p-value. If we had used this correction for multiple testing, then we would have concluded that *none* of our 14 results were significant!

11.2.12.3   Graphical Interpretation of the Benjamini–Hochberg (BH) Method

There's an intuitive graphical interpretation of the BH calculations.

- Sort the p-values from largest to smallest
- Plot the ordered p-values $p_{(k)}$ on the y-axis versus their indices on the x-axis
- Superimpose on this plot a line that passes through the origin and has slope α^*

Any p-value that falls on or below this line corresponds to a significant result (Fig. 11.7).

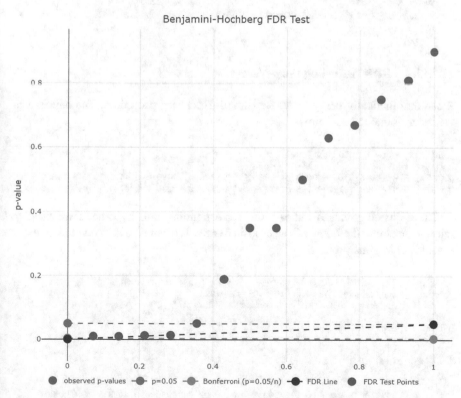

Fig. 11.7 Empirical demonstration of the Benjamini–Hochberg false discovery rate correction for multiple testing

```r
# generate the "relative-indices" (i/n) that will be plotted on the x-axis
x.values<-(1:length(pvals))/length(pvals)
# select observations that are less than threshold
for.test <- cbind(1:length(pvals), pvals)
pass.test <- for.test[pvals <= 0.05*x.values, ]
pass.test
##        pvals
## 4.000 0.014
# use largest k to color points that meet Benjamini-Hochberg FDR test
last<-ifelse(is.vector(pass.test), pass.test[1],pass.test[nrow(pass.test),1])
par(mar=c(4.1, 4.1, 1.1, 4.1))  # widen right margin to make room for labels
plot_ly(x=~x.values, y=~pvals, type="scatter", mode="markers",
        marker=list(size=15), name="observed p-values", symbols='o') %>%
  # add bounding horizontal lines | add naive threshold line
  add_lines(x=~c(0,1), y=~c(0.05, 0.05), mode="lines",
            line=list(dash='dash'), name="p=0.05") %>%
  # add conservative Bonferroni line
  add_lines(x=~c(0,1), y=~c(0.05/length(pvals), 0.05/length(pvals)),
    mode="lines", line=list(dash='dash'), name="Bonferroni (p=0.05/n)") %>%
  # add FDR line
  add_lines(x=~c(0,1), y=~c(0, 0.05), mode="lines", line=list(dash='dash'),
            name="FDR Line") %>%
  # highlight largest k to color points meeting Benjamini-Hochberg FDR test
  add_trace(x=~x.values[1:last], y=~pvals[1:last],
            mode="markers",symbols='0', name="FDR Test Points") %>%
  layout (title="Benjamini-Hochberg FDR Test", legend=list(orientation='h'),
          xaxis=list(title=expression(i/n)), yaxis=list(title="p-value"))
```

11.2.12.4   FDR Adjusting the *p*-Values

R can automatically perform the Benjamini–Hochberg procedure. The adjusted *p*-values are obtained as follows.

```r
pvals.adjusted <- p.adjust(pvals, "BH")
pvals.adjusted
## [1] 0.0490000 0.0490000 0.0490000 0.0490000 0.1428000 0.4433333 0.6125000
## [8] 0.6125000 0.7777778 0.8527273 0.8527273 0.8723077 0.8723077 0.9000000
```

The adjusted *p*-values indicate the corresponding null hypothesis we need to reject to preserve the initial α^* false-positive rate. We can also compute the adjusted *p*-values using this protocol.

```r
# manually calculate the thresholds for the ordered p-values list
test.p <- length(pvals)/(1:length(pvals))*pvals    # test.p
# loop through each p-value and carry out the manual FDR adjustment for multiple
testing
adj.p <- numeric(14)
for(i in 1:14) {
    adj.p[i]<-min(test.p[i:length(test.p)])
    ifelse(adj.p[i]>1, 1, adj.p[i])
}
adj.p
## [1] 0.0490000 0.0490000 0.0490000 0.0490000 0.1428000 0.4433333 0.6125000
## [8] 0.6125000 0.7777778 0.8527273 0.8527273 0.8723077 0.8723077 0.9000000
```

Note that the manually computed (`adj.p`) and the automatically computed (`pvals.adjusted`) adjusted-p-values are the same.

11.2.13   Logistic Transformation

For *binary outcome variables*, or *ordinal categorical variables*, we may need to employ the `logistic curve` to transform the polytomous outcomes into real values.

The Logistic curve is $y=f(x)=\frac{1}{1+e^{-x}}$, where y and x represent probability and quantitative-predictor values, respectively. A slightly more general form is: $y=f(x)=\frac{K}{1+e^{-x}}$, where the covariate $x \in (-\infty, \infty)$ and the response $y \in [0, K]$. A logistic model example is shown on Fig. 11.8.

```
library("ggplot2")
k=7
x <- seq(-10, 10, 0.1)
plot_ly(x=~x, y=~k/(1+exp(-x)), type="scatter", mode="line",
        name="Logistic model") %>%
  layout (title="Logistic Model Y=k/(1+exp(-x)), k=7",
          xaxis=list(title="x"), yaxis=list(title="Y=k/(1+exp(-x))"))
```

The point of this logistic transformation is that

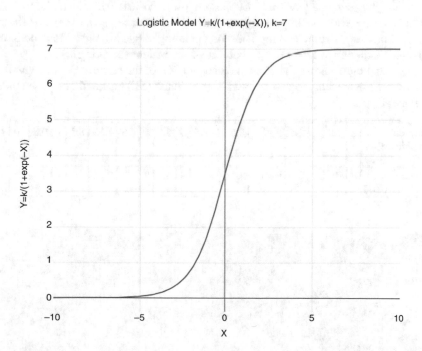

Fig. 11.8 For a given probability value p, the corresponding odds are the fraction $\frac{p}{1-p}$ and the *logit* function model is the logarithm of the odds logit $(y) = \log\left(\frac{y}{1-y}\right)$. Then, the inverse of the logit function is the plotted *sigmoid* function

$$y = \frac{1}{1 + e^{-x}} \Leftrightarrow x = \ln \frac{y}{1-y},$$

which represents the log-odds (when y is the probability of an event of interest)!!!

We use the logistic regression equation model to estimate the probability of specific outcomes

$$(\text{Estimate of}) \ P(Y = 1 | x_1, x_2, \cdots, x_l) = \frac{1}{1 + e^{-\left(a_o + \sum\limits_{k=1}^{l} a_k x_k\right)}},$$

where the coefficients a_o (intercept) and effects a_k, $k = 1, 2, \cdots, l$, are estimated using GLM according to a maximum likelihood approach. Using this model allows us to estimate the probability of the dependent (outcome) variable $Y = 1$, e.g., surviving surgery, given the observed values of the predictors X_k, $k = 1, 2, \cdots, l$.

11.2.13.1   Example: Heart Transplant Surgery

Let's look at an example of estimating the *probability of surviving a heart transplant based on surgeon's experience*. Suppose a group of 20 patients undergo heart transplantation with different surgeons having experience in the range {0(least), 2, ..., 10(most)}, representing 100s of operating/surgery hours. How does the surgeon's experience affect the probability of the patient surviving?

The data below shows the clinical outcome (CO) of the surgery (1 = survival) or (0 = death) according to the surgeon's experience (SE) in hundreds of hours of practice (Fig. 11.9).

Surgeon's Experience (SE)	1	1.5	2	2.5	3	3.5	3.5	4	4.5	5	5.5	6	6.5	7	8	8.5	9	9.5	10	10
Clinical Outcome (CO)	0	0	0	0	0	0	1	0	1	0	1	0	1	0	1	1	1	1	1	1

```
mydata <-          # 01_HeartSurgerySurvivalData.csv
    read.csv("https://umich.instructure.com/files/405273/download?download_frd=1")
# estimates a logistic regression model for the clinical outcome (CO), survival,
using the glm
mylogit <- glm(CO ~ SE, data=mydata, family = "binomial")
plot_ly(data=mydata, x=~SE, y=~CO, type="scatter", mode="markers",
        name="Data", marker=list(size=15)) %>%
  add_trace(x=~SE, y=~mylogit$fitted.values, type="scatter", mode="lines",
        name="Logit Model") %>%
  layout (title="Logistic Model Clinical Outcome ~ Surgeon's Experience",
        xaxis=list(title="SE"), yaxis=list(title="CO"), hovermode = "x unified")
```

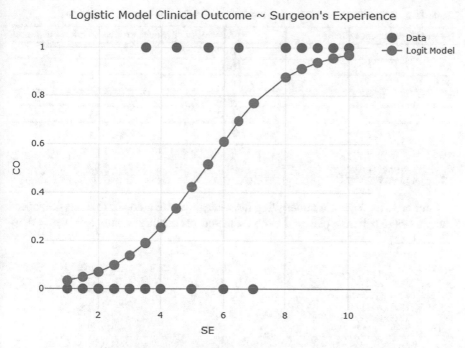

Fig. 11.9 Logistic model of binary clinical outcomes based on surgeon's experience

Figure 11.9 depicts the graph of a logistic regression curve showing the probability of surviving the surgery versus surgeon's experience. The graph shows the probability of the clinical outcome, survival (*y*-axis) versus the surgeon's experience (*x*-axis), with the logistic regression curve fitted to the data.

```
mylogit <- glm(CO ~ SE, data = mydata, family = "binomial")
summary(mylogit)
## Coefficients:
##              Estimate Std. Error z value Pr(>|z|)
## (Intercept)  -4.1030     1.7629   -2.327   0.0199 *
## SE            0.7583     0.3139    2.416   0.0157 *
```

The output indicates that a surgeon's experience (SE) is significantly associated with the probability of surviving the surgery (0.0157, Wald test). The output also provides the coefficient estimates, Intercept = −4.1030 and SE = 0.7583.

These coefficients can then be used in the logistic regression equation model to estimate the probability of surviving the heart surgery:

$$\text{Probability of surviving heart surgery } CO = \frac{1}{(1 + \exp(-(-4.1030 + 0.7583 \times SE)))} .$$

For example, for a patient who is operated on by a surgeon with 200 hours of operating experience (SE = 2), we plug in the value 2 in the equation to get the corresponding estimated probability of survival, $p = 0.07$.

Table 11.2 Probability of surviving surgery for several values of surgeons' experience

Surgeon's experience (SE)	Probability of patient survival (clinical outcome)
1	0.034
2	0.07
3	0.14
4	0.26
5	0.423

```
SE=2
CO = 1/(1+exp(-(-4.1030+0.7583*SE)))
CO  ## [1] 0.07001884
```

Similarly, for a patient undergoing heart surgery with a doctor that has 400 operating hours experience (SE = 4), the estimated probability of survival is $p = 0.26$
(Table 11.2).

```
SE=4; CO =1/(1+exp(-(-4.1030+0.7583*SE))); CO
## [1] 0.2554411
CO  ## [1] 0.2554411
for (SE in c(1:5)) {
  CO <- 1/(1+exp(-(-4.1030+0.7583*SE)));
  print(c(SE, CO))
}
## [1] 1.00000000 0.03406915
## [1] 2.00000000 0.07001884
## [1] 3.0000000 0.1384648
## [1] 4.0000000 0.2554411
## [1] 5.0000000 0.4227486
```

The output from the logistic regression analysis yields an SE effect of $\beta = 0.0157$,
which is based on the Wald z-score. In addition to the Wald method, we can calculate
the p-value for logistic regression using the likelihood ratio test (LRT), which for
these data yields 0.0006476922.

```
mylogit <- glm(CO ~ SE, data = mydata, family = "binomial")
summary(mylogit)
## Coefficients:
##              Estimate Std. Error z value Pr(>|z|)
## (Intercept)  -4.1030     1.7629  -2.327   0.0199 *
## SE            0.7583     0.3139   2.416   0.0157 *
```

Covariate	Estimate	Std. error	z value	Pr(>lzl) Wald
SE	0.7583	0.3139	2.416	0.0157 *

The *logit* of a number $0 \le p \le 1$ is given by the formula: $\text{logit}(p) = \log \frac{p}{1-p}$, and represents the log-odds ratio (of survival in this case).

```
confint(mylogit)
##               2.5 %     97.5 %
## (Intercept) -8.6083535 -1.282692
## SE           0.2687893  1.576912
```

So, why exponentiating the coefficients? Because,

$$\text{logit}(p) = \log \frac{p}{1-p} \to e^{\text{logit}(p)} = e^{\log \frac{p}{1-p}} \Rightarrow RHS = \frac{p}{1-p}, (\text{odds} - \text{ratio, OR}).$$

```
exp(coef(mylogit))    # exponentiated logit model coefficients
## (Intercept)          SE
## 0.01652254    2.13474149
```

By exponentiating the coefficient estimates, exp(coef(mylogit)), we obtain

(Intercept)	Exp(SE)
0.01652254	2.13474149 = exp(0.7583456)

which is derived from the raw estimates, coef(mylogit),

(Intercept)	SE
−4.1030298	0.7583456

```
exp(cbind(OR = coef(mylogit), confint(mylogit)))
## Waiting for profiling to be done...
##                    OR        2.5 %    97.5 %
## (Intercept) 0.01652254 0.0001825743 0.277290
## SE          2.13474149 1.3083794719 4.839986
```

	OR	2.5%	97.5%
(Intercept)	0.01652254	0.0001825743	0.277290
SE	2.13474149	1.3083794719	4.839986

We can compute the LRT and report its *p*-value by using the with() function

```
with(mylogit, df.null - df.residual)
with(mylogit, pchisq(null.deviance-deviance, df.null-df.residual,
                lower.tail = FALSE))
## [1] 0.0006476922
```

LRT p-value < 0.001 tells us that our model as a whole fits significantly better than an empty model. The deviance residual `mylogit$deviance` is $-2*log$ `likelihood`, and we can report the model's log likelihood as follows.

```
mylogit$deviance    # model residual deviance
## [1] 16.09223
-2*logLik(mylogit) # -2 * model_LL
## 'log Lik.' 16.09223 (df=2)
```

11.2.14   Implementation of Regularization

Before we dive into the theoretical formulation of model regularization, let's start with a specific application that will ground the subsequent analytics.

Example: Neuroimaging-Genetics Study of Parkinson's Disease Dataset
More information about this specific Parkinson's disease study (05_PPMI_top_UPDRS_Integrated_LongFormat1.csv) is available online.[8] The data elements include: FID_IID, L_insular_cortex_ComputeArea, L_insular_ cortex_Volume, R_insular_cortex_ComputeArea, R_insular_cortex_Volume, L_cingulate_gyrus_ComputeArea, L_cingulate_gyrus_Volume, R_cingulate_ gyrus_ComputeArea, R_cingulate_gyrus_Volume, L_caudate_ComputeArea, L_caudate_Volume, R_caudate_ComputeArea, R_caudate_Volume, L_putamen_ ComputeArea, L_putamen_Volume, R_putamen_ComputeArea, R_putamen_Volume, Sex, Weight, ResearchGroup, Age, chr12_rs34637584_GT, chr17_rs11868035_GT, chr17_rs11012_GT, chr17_rs393152_GT, chr17_rs12185268_GT, chr17_rs199533_ GT, UPDRS_part_I, UPDRS_part_II, UPDRS_part_III, and time_visit.

Note that the dataset includes missing values and repeated measures. The *goal* of this demonstration is to use OLS, `ridge regression`, and LASSO to *find the best predictive model for the clinical outcomes*—UPDRS score (vector) and Research Group (factor variable), in terms of demographic, genetics, and neuro-imaging biomarkers. We can utilize the `glmnet` package in R for most calculations.

---

[8]https://wiki.socr.umich.edu/index.php/SOCR_Data_PD_BiomedBigMetadata

```
#### Initial Stuff ####
rm(list=ls())    # clean up
# load required packages # install.packages("arm")
library(glmnet)
library(arm)
library(knitr) # kable function to convert tabular R-results into Rmd tables
# pick a random seed, but set.seed(seed) only affects the next block of code!
seed = 1234
#### Organize Data ####
# load dataset
# Data: https://umich.instructure.com/courses/38100/files/folder/data
# (05_PPMI_top_UPDRS_Integrated_LongFormat1.csv)
data1 <-
    read.table('https://umich.instructure.com/files/330397/download?download_frd=1',
               sep=",", header=T)
# For now, ignore incomplete cases, later we can use imputation, Chapter 2
data1.completeRowIndexes <- complete.cases(data1);
table(data1.completeRowIndexes)
## data1.completeRowIndexes
## FALSE   TRUE
##   609   1155
prop.table(table(data1.completeRowIndexes))
## data1.completeRowIndexes
##      FALSE       TRUE
## 0.3452381 0.6547619
attach(data1)  # View(data1[data1.completeRowIndexes, ])
# define response and predictors
y <- data1$UPDRS_part_I + data1$UPDRS_part_II + data1$UPDRS_part_III
table(y)   # Show Clinically relevant classification
y <- y[data1.completeRowIndexes]
# X-scale(data1[,]) # Scaling not needed, glmnet auto standardizes predictors
drop_features <- c("FID_IID", "ResearchGroup", "UPDRS_part_I",
                   "UPDRS_part_II", "UPDRS_part_III", "time_visit")
X <- data1[ , !(names(data1) %in% drop_features)]
X = as.matrix(X)    # remove columns: index, ResearchGroup, and y=(PDRS_part_I +
UPDRS_part_II + UPDRS_part_III)
X <- X[data1.completeRowIndexes, ]
summary(X)
…
# randomly split data into training (80%) and test (20%) sets
set.seed(seed)
train = sample(1 : nrow(X), round((4/5) * nrow(X)))
test = -train
# subset training data
yTrain = y[train]
XTrain = X[train, ]
XTrainOLS = cbind(rep(1, nrow(XTrain)), XTrain)
# subset test data
yTest = y[test]
XTest = X[test, ]
#### Model Estimation & Selection ####
# Estimate models
fitOLS = lm(yTrain ~ XTrain)  # Ordinary Least Squares
# glmnet automatically standardizes the predictors
fitRidge = glmnet(XTrain, yTrain, alpha = 0)  # Ridge Regression
fitLASSO = glmnet(XTrain, yTrain, alpha = 1)  # The LASSO
```

All readers are encouraged to fit these models, compare, and contrast the resulting *ridge* and *LASSO* model estimates.

11.2.15   *Computational Complexity*

Recall that the regularized regression estimates depend on the regularization parameter λ. Fortunately, efficient algorithms for choosing optimal λ parameters do exist. Examples of solution path algorithms include:

- LARS Algorithm for the LASSO[9]
- Piecewise linearity[10]
- Generic path algorithm[11]
- Pathwise coordinate descent[12] and
- Alternating Direction Method of Multipliers (ADMM)[13]

We will show how to visualize the relations between the regularization parameter $(\ln(\lambda))$ and the number and magnitude of the corresponding coefficients for each specific regularized regression method.

11.2.16   *LASSO and Ridge Solution Paths*

The plot for the *LASSO* results can be obtained as follows (Fig. 11.10).

```
library(RColorBrewer)
### Plot Solution Path - LASSO
plot.glmnet <- function(glmnet.object, name="") {
  df <- as.data.frame(t(as.matrix(glmnet.object$beta)))
  df$loglambda <- log(glmnet.object$lambda)
  df <- as.data.frame(df)
  data_long <- gather(df, Variable, coefficient, 1:(dim(df)[2]-1),
                      factor_key=TRUE)
  plot_ly(data = data_long) %>%
    # add error bars for each CV-mean at log(Lambda)
    add_trace(x = ~loglambda, y = ~coefficient, color=~Variable,
              colors=colorRampPalette(brewer.pal(10,"Spectral"))(dim(df)[2]),
              type = 'scatter', mode = 'lines', name = ~Variable) %>%
    layout(title = paste0(name, " Model Coefficient Values"),
           xaxis = list(title = paste0("log(",TeX("\\lambda"),")"),
           side="bottom",  showgrid = TRUE), hovermode = "x unified",
           legend = list(orientation='h'),
           yaxis = list(title = ' Model Coefficient Values', side="left",
           showgrid = TRUE))
}
plot.glmnet(fitLASSO, name="LASSO")
```

---

[9] https://doi.org/10.1214/009053604000000067

[10] https://doi.org/10.1214/009053606000001370

[11] https://doi.org/10.1080/01621459.2013.864166

[12] https://doi.org/10.1214/07-AOAS131

[13] https://doi.org/10.1561/2200000016

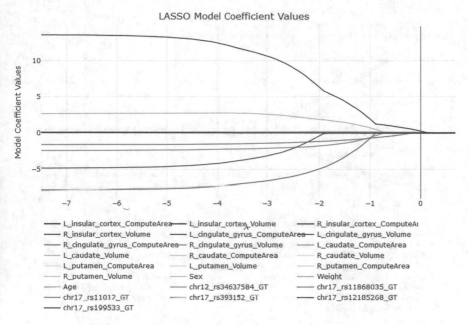

Fig. 11.10 LASSO model coefficient paths

Similarly, we can display the coefficient paths corresponding to *Ridge* regulari-zation (Fig. 11.11).

```
### Plot Solution Path - Ridge
plot.glmnet(fitRidge, name="Ridge")
```

11.2.17   *Regression Solution Paths—Ridge vs. LASSO*

Let's try to compare the paths of the *LASSO* and *Ridge* regression solutions. Below, you will see that the curves of LASSO are steeper and nondifferentiable at some points, which is the result of using the L_1 norm. On the other hand, the Ridge path is smoother and asymptotically tends to 0 as λ increases.

Let's start by examining the joint objective function (including LASSO and Ridge terms):

$$\min_{\beta} \left(\sum_i (y_i - x_i\beta)^2 + \frac{1-\alpha}{2}\|\beta\|_2^2 + \alpha\|\beta\|_1 \right),$$

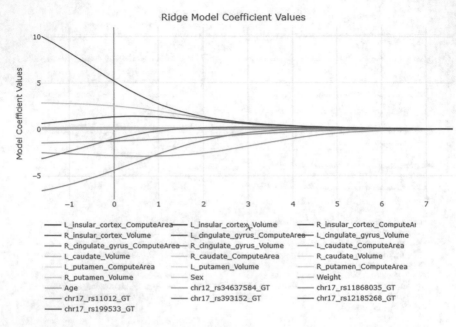

Fig. 11.11   Ridge model coefficient paths

where $\|\beta\|_1 = \sum_{j=1}^{p} |\beta_j|$ and $\|\beta\|_2 = \sqrt{\sum_{j=1}^{p} |\beta_j|^2}$ are the norms of β corresponding to

the L_1 and L_2 distance measures, respectively. The parameters $\alpha = 0$ and $\alpha = 1$ correspond to *Ridge* and *LASSO* regularization. The following two questions raise naturally.

- What if $0 < \alpha < 1$?
- How does the regularization penalty term affect the optimal solution?

In Chap. 3, we explored the minimal SSE (Sum of Square Error) for the OLS (without penalty) where the feasible parameter (β) spans the entire real solution space. In penalized optimization problems, the best solution may actually be unachievable. Therefore, we look for solutions that are "closest," within the feasible region, to the enigmatic best solution.

The effect of the penalty term on the objective function is separate from the *fidelity term* (OLS solution). Thus, the effect of $0 \leq \alpha \leq 1$ is limited to the *size and shape of the penalty region*. Let's try to visualize the feasible region as

- Centrosymmetric (disk, Euclidean distance) topology, when $\alpha = 0$
- Super diamond topology, when $\alpha = 1$

Below is a hands-on demonstration of that process using the following simple quadratic equation solver.

```
library(needs)
# Constructing Quadratic Formula
quadraticEquSolver <- function(a,b,c){
  if(delta(a,b,c) > 0){ # first case D>0
    x_1 = (-b+sqrt(delta(a,b,c)))/(2*a)
    x_2 = (-b-sqrt(delta(a,b,c)))/(2*a)
    result = c(x_1,x_2)
    # print(result)
  }
  else if(delta(a,b,c) == 0){ # second case D=0
    result = -b/(2*a)
    # print(result)
  }
  else {"There are no real roots."} # third case D<0
}
# Constructing delta
delta <- function(a,b,c) {   b^2-4*a*c  }
```

To make this realistic, we will use the MLB dataset to first fit an OLS model. The dataset contains 1034 records of *heights and weights* for some current and recent Major League Baseball (MLB) Players.

- *Height*: Player height in inch
- *Weight*: Player weight in pounds
- *Age*: Player age at time of record

Then, we can obtain the SSE for any $\|\beta\|$:

$$\text{SSE} = \left\| Y - \widehat{Y} \right\|^2 = \left(Y - \widehat{Y} \right)^{\mathrm{T}} \left(Y - \widehat{Y} \right) = Y^{\mathrm{T}}Y - 2\beta^{\mathrm{T}}X^{\mathrm{T}}Y + \beta^{\mathrm{T}}X^{\mathrm{T}}X\beta.$$

Next, we will compute the contours for SSE in several situations.

```r
library("ggplot2")
# load data
mlb <-
  read.table('https://umich.instructure.com/files/330381/download?download_frd=1',
             as.is=T, header=T)
str(mlb)
…
fit <- lm(Height ~ Weight + Age -1, data = as.data.frame(scale(mlb[,4:6])))
points = data.frame(x=c(0,fit$coefficients[1]), y=c(0,fit$coefficients[2]),
                    z=c("(0,0)","OLS Coef"))
Y=scale(mlb$Height)
X = scale(mlb[,c(5,6)])
beta1 = seq(-0.556, 1.556, length.out = 100)
beta2 = seq(-0.661, 0.3386, length.out = 100)
df <- expand.grid(beta1 = beta1, beta2 = beta2)
b = as.matrix(df)
df$sse <- rep(t(Y)%*%Y,100*100) - 2*b%*%t(X)%*%Y + diag(b%*%t(X)%*%X%*%t(b))
base <- ggplot(df) +
  stat_contour(aes(beta1, beta2, z = sse),
               breaks = round(quantile(df$sse, seq(0, 0.2, 0.03)), 0),
               size = 0.5,color="darkorchid2",alpha=0.8)+
  scale_x_continuous(limits = c(-0.4,1))+
  scale_y_continuous(limits = c(-0.55,0.4))+
  coord_fixed(ratio=1)+
  geom_point(data = points,aes(x,y))+
  geom_text(data = points,aes(x,y,label=z),vjust = 2,size=3.5)+
  geom_segment(aes(x = -0.4, y = 0, xend = 1, yend = 0),colour = "grey46",
               arrow = arrow(length=unit(0.30,"cm")),size=0.5,alpha=0.8)+
  geom_segment(aes(x = 0, y = -0.55, xend = 0, yend = 0.4),colour = "grey46",
               arrow = arrow(length=unit(0.30,"cm")),size=0.5,alpha=0.8)
plot_alpha = function(alpha=0,restrict=0.2,beta1_range=0.2,
                      annot=c(0.15,-0.25,0.205,-0.05)) {
  a=alpha; t=restrict; k=beta1_range; pos=data.frame(V1=annot[1:4])
  text=paste("(",as.character(annot[3]),",", as.character(annot[4]),")",
             sep = "")
  K = seq(0,k,length.out = 50)
  y = unlist(lapply((1-a)*K^2/2+a*K-t, quadraticEquSolver,
             a=(1-a)/2,b=a))[seq(1,99,by=2)]
  fills = data.frame(x=c(rev(-K),K), y1=c(rev(y),y), y2=c(-rev(y),-y))
  p<-base+geom_line(data=fills,aes(x = x,y = y1),
                    colour = "salmon1",alpha=0.6,size=0.7)+
    geom_line(data=fills,aes(x=x,y=y2), colour="salmon1",alpha=0.6,size=0.7)+
    geom_polygon(data = fills, aes(x, y1),fill = "red", alpha = 0.2)+
    geom_polygon(data = fills, aes(x, y2), fill = "red", alpha = 0.2)+
    geom_segment(data=pos,aes(x = V1[1] , y=V1[2], xend=V1[3], yend=V1[4]),
                 arrow = arrow(length=unit(0.30,"cm")), alpha=0.8,colour="magenta")+
    ggplot2::annotate("text", x = pos$V1[1]-0.01, y = pos$V1[2]-0.11,
                      label = paste(text,"\n","Point of Contact \n i.e., Coef of",
                                    "alpha=",fractions(a)),size=3)+
    xlab(expression(beta[1]))+
    ylab(expression(beta[2]))+
    ggtitle(paste("alpha =",as.character(fractions(a))))+
    theme(legend.position="none")
}
# $\alpha=0$ - Ridge
p1 <- plot_alpha(alpha=0,restrict=(0.21^2)/2,beta1_range=0.21,
                 annot=c(0.15,-0.25,0.205,-0.05))
p1 <- p1 + ggtitle(expression(paste(alpha, "=0 (Ridge)")))
```

```
# $\alpha=1/9$
p2 <- plot_alpha(alpha=1/9,restrict=0.046,beta1_range=0.22,
                 annot =c(0.15,-0.25,0.212,-0.02))
p2 <- p2 + ggtitle(expression(paste(alpha, "=1/9")))
# $\alpha=1/5$
p3 <- plot_alpha(alpha=1/5,restrict=0.063,beta1_range=0.22,
                 annot=c(0.13,-0.25,0.22,0))
p3 <- p3 + ggtitle(expression(paste(alpha, "=1/5")))
# $\alpha=1/2$
p4 <- plot_alpha(alpha=1/2,restrict=0.123,beta1_range=0.22,
                 annot=c(0.12,-0.25,0.22,0))
p4 <- p4 + ggtitle(expression(paste(alpha, "=1/2")))
# $\alpha=3/4$
p5 <- plot_alpha(alpha=3/4,restrict=0.17,beta1_range=0.22,
                 annot=c(0.12,-0.25,0.22,0))
p5 <- p5 + ggtitle(expression(paste(alpha, "=3/4")))
# $\alpha=1$ - LASSO
t=0.22
K = seq(0,t,length.out = 50)
fills = data.frame(x=c(-rev(K),K),
                   y1=c(rev(t-K),c(t-K)),y2=c(-rev(t-K),-c(t-K)))
p6 <- base +
  geom_segment(aes(x = 0, y = t, xend = t, yend = 0),
               colour = "salmon1",alpha=0.1,size=0.2)+
  geom_segment(aes(x = 0, y = t, xend = -t, yend = 0),
               colour = "salmon1",alpha=0.1,size=0.2)+
  geom_segment(aes(x = 0, y = -t, xend = t, yend = 0),
               colour = "salmon1",alpha=0.1,size=0.2)+
  geom_segment(aes(x = 0, y = -t, xend = -t, yend = 0),
               colour = "salmon1",alpha=0.1,size=0.2)+
  geom_polygon(data = fills, aes(x, y1),fill = "red", alpha = 0.2)+
  geom_polygon(data = fills, aes(x, y2), fill = "red", alpha = 0.2)+
  geom_segment(aes(x = 0.12 , y = -0.25, xend=0.22, yend=0),colour="magenta",
               arrow = arrow(length=unit(0.30,"cm")),alpha=0.8)+
  ggplot2::annotate("text", x = 0.11, y = -0.36,
    label = "(0.22,0)\n Point of Contact \n i.e Coef of LASSO",size=3) +
  xlab( expression(beta[1]))+
  ylab( expression(beta[2]))+
  theme(legend.position="none")+
  ggtitle(expression(paste(alpha, "=1 (LASSO)")))
```

Then, let's add the six feasible regions corresponding to $\alpha = 0$ (Ridge), $\alpha = \frac{1}{9}$, $\alpha = \frac{1}{5}$, $\alpha = \frac{1}{2}$, $\alpha = \frac{3}{4}$ and $\alpha = 1$ (LASSO). Figure 11.12 provides some intuition into the continuum from Ridge to LASSO regularization. The feasible regions are drawn as ellipse contours of the SSE in *red*. Curves around the corresponding feasible regions represent the *boundary of the constraint function* $\frac{1-\alpha}{2}\|\beta\|_2^2 + \alpha\|\beta\|_1 \leq t$. In this example, β_2 shrinks to 0 for $\alpha = \frac{1}{5}$, $\alpha = \frac{1}{2}$, $\alpha = \frac{3}{4}$ and $\alpha = 1$.

We observe that it is almost impossible for the contours of Ridge regression to touch the circle at any of the coordinate axes. This is also true in higher dimensions (nD), where the L_1 and L_2 metrics are unchanged and the 2D ellipse representations of the feasibility regions become hyper-ellipsoidal shapes. Generally, as α goes from 0 to 1. The coefficients of more features tend to shrink towards 0. This specific property makes LASSO useful for variable selection.

By Lagrangian duality, any solution of $\min_\beta \|Y - X\beta\|_2^2 + \lambda\|\beta\|_2$ and $\min_\beta \|Y - X\beta\|_1 + \lambda\|\beta\|_1$ must also represent a solution to the corresponding

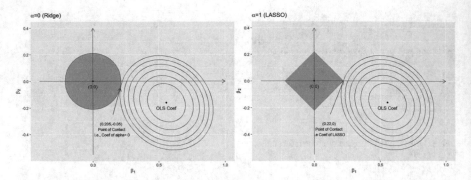

Fig. 11.12 A 2D simulation showing the feasibility regions corresponding to the Euclidean (Ridge) and diamond (LASSO) topologies. This figure explains the ability of LASSO regularization to shrink and annihilate coefficients paired with features associated with coordinate axes. The SSE concentric elliptical contours show the corresponding penalty regions

Ridge ($\widehat{\beta}^{RR}$) or LASSO ($\widehat{\beta}^{L}$) optimization problems

$$\min_{\beta} \|Y - X\beta\|_2^2, \text{ subject to } \|\beta\|_2 \le \left\|\widehat{\beta}^{RR}\right\|_2,$$

$$\min_{\beta} \|Y - X\beta\|_1, \text{ subject to } \|\beta\|_1 \le \left\|\widehat{\beta}^{L}\right\|_1,$$

Suppose we actually know the values of $\left\|\widehat{\beta}^{RR}\right\|_2$ and $\left\|\widehat{\beta}^{L}\right\|_1$, then we can pictorially represent the optimization problem and illustrate the complementary model-fitting, variable selection, and shrinkage of the Ridge and LASSO regularization.

The topologies of the solution (*domain*) regions are different for Ridge and LASSO. Ridge regularization corresponds with ball topology and LASSO with diamond topology. This is because the solution regions are defined by $\|\beta\|_2 \le \left\|\widehat{\beta}^{RR}\right\|_2$ and $\|\beta\|_1 \le \left\|\widehat{\beta}^{L}\right\|_1$, respectively.

On the other hand, the topology of the *fidelity term* $\|Y - X\beta\|_2^2$ is ellipsoidal, centered at the OLS estimate, $\widehat{\beta}^{OLS}$. To solve the optimization problem, we look for the tightest contour around $\widehat{\beta}^{OLS}$ that hits the solution domain (ball for Ridge or diamond for LASSO). This intersection point would represent the solution estimate $\widehat{\beta}$. As the LASSO domain space (l_1 unit ball) has these corners, the solution estimate $\widehat{\beta}$ is likely to be at the corners. Hence, LASSO solutions tend to include many zeroes, whereas Ridge regression solutions (constraint set is a round ball) may not annihilate many of the variables. Let's compare the feasibility regions corresponding to *Ridge* (top, $p1$) and *LASSO* (bottom, $p6$) regularization (Fig. 11.12).

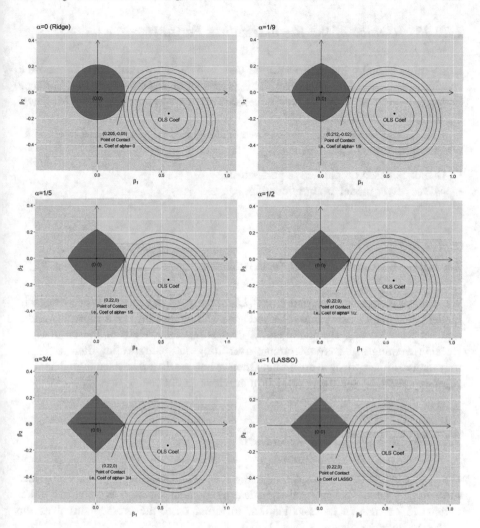

Fig. 11.13 A collage of 6 alpha values showing the progression of the feasibility penalty regions from Ridge to LASSO

```
plot(p1) # ridge
plot(p6) # lasso
```

Finally, we can also plot the *progression* of the SSE concentric elliptical contours from Ridge to LASSO. This composite *plot is intense* and may take several minutes to render! (Fig. 11.13)

```
library("gridExtra")
grid.arrange(p1, p2, p3, p4, p5, p6, nrow=3)
```

11.2.18   Choice of the Regularization Parameter

Efficiently obtaining the entire solution path is nice, but we still have to choose a specific λ regularization parameter. This is critical as λ controls the bias-variance tradeoff. Traditional model selection methods rely on various metrics like Mallows' C_p, AIC, BIC, and adjusted R^2.[14]

Internal statistical validation (cross-validation) is a popular modern alternative, which offers some of these benefits

- Choice is based on predictive performance
- Makes fewer model assumptions
- Wider applicability.

11.2.19   Cross-validation Motivation

We discussed statistical internal *cross-validation* (CV) in Chap. 9. When assessing model performance using a regularized approach, we would like a separate validation set for choosing the parameter λ controlling the weight of the regularizer. Reusing training sets may encourage overfitting and using testing data to pick λ may underestimate the true error rate. Often, when we do not have enough data for a separate validation set, cross-validation provides an alternative strategy.

11.2.20   n-Fold Cross-validation

We have already seen examples of using cross-validation, e.g., Chap. 9 provides more details about this internal statistical assessment strategy. We can use either automated or manual cross-validation. In either case, the protocol involves the following iterative steps:

1. Randomly split the training data into n parts ("folds")
2. Fit a model using data in $n - 1$ folds for multiple λs
3. Calculate some prediction quality metrics (e.g., MSE, accuracy) on the last remaining fold, see Chap. 9
4. Repeat the process and average the prediction metrics across iterations

Common choices of n are 5, 10, and N ($n = N$, the sample size, corresponds to leave-one-out CV). The *one standard error* rule suggests choosing a λ value corresponding to a model with the smallest number of parameters, which has MSE within one standard error of the minimum MSE.

---

[14] https://doi.org/10.1007/s13571-015-0096-0

11.2.21   LASSO 10-Fold Cross-validation

Now, let's apply an internal statistical cross-validation to assess the quality of the LASSO and Ridge models, based on our Parkinson's disease case study (Figs. 11.14 and 11.15). Recall our split of the PD data into training (yTrain and XTrain) and testing (yTest and XTest) sets.

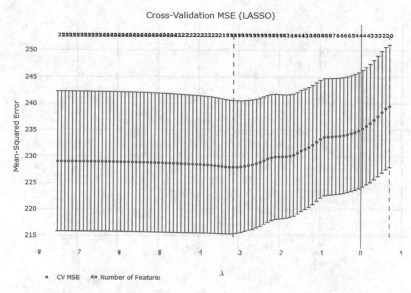

Fig. 11.14 LASSO model cross-validation MSE (vertical axis) vs. regularization parameter

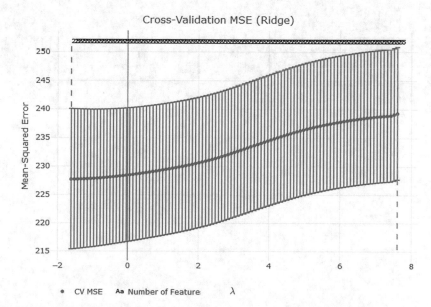

Fig. 11.15 Ridge model cross-validation MSE (vertical axis) vs. regularization parameter

```
plotCV.glmnet <- function(cv.glmnet.object, name="") {
  df <- as.data.frame(cbind(x=log(cv.glmnet.object$lambda),
      y=cv.glmnet.object$cvm, errorBar=cv.glmnet.object$cvsd),
      nzero=cv.glmnet.object$nzero)
  featureNum <- cv.glmnet.object$nzero
  xFeature <- log(cv.glmnet.object$lambda)
  yFeature <- max(cv.glmnet.object$cvm)+max(cv.glmnet.object$cvsd)
  dataFeature <- data.frame(featureNum, xFeature, yFeature)
  plot_ly(data = df) %>%
    # add error bars for each CV-mean at log(lambda)
    add_trace(x = ~x, y = ~y, type = 'scatter', mode = 'markers',
        name = 'CV MSE', error_y = ~list(array = errorBar)) %>%
    # add the lambda-min and lambda 1SD vertical dash lines
    add_lines(data=df, x=c(log(cv.glmnet.object$lambda.min),
log(cv.glmnet.object$lambda.min)),
              y=c(min(cv.glmnet.object$cvm)-max(df$errorBar),
max(cv.glmnet.object$cvm)+max(df$errorBar)),
              showlegend=F, line=list(dash="dash"), name="lambda.min",
              mode = 'lines+markers') %>%
    add_lines(data=df, x=c(log(cv.glmnet.object$lambda.1se),
              log(cv.glmnet.object$lambda.1se)),
              y=c(min(cv.glmnet.object$cvm)-max(df$errorBar),
              max(cv.glmnet.object$cvm)+max(df$errorBar)),
              showlegend=F, line=list(dash="dash"), name="lambda.1se") %>%
    # Add Number of Features Annotations on Top
    add_trace(dataFeature, x = ~xFeature, y = ~yFeature, type = 'scatter',
        name="Number of Features",
        mode = 'text', text = ~featureNum, textposition = 'middle right',
        textfont = list(color = '#000000', size = 9)) %>%
    layout(title = paste0("Cross-Validation MSE (", name, ")"),
                    xaxis = list(title=paste0("log(",TeX("\\lambda"),")")),
                    side="bottom", showgrid=TRUE), # type="Log"
                    hovermode = "x unified", legend = list(orientation='h'),
                    yaxis = list(title = cv.glmnet.object$name,
                              side="left", showgrid = TRUE))
}
#### 10-fold cross validation ####
# LASSO
library("glmnet")
library(doParallel)
cl <- makePSOCKcluster(6)
registerDoParallel(cl)
set.seed(seed)  # set seed for LASSO (10-fold) cross validation
cvLASSO = cv.glmnet(XTrain, yTrain, alpha = 1, parallel=TRUE)
plotCV.glmnet(cvLASSO, "LASSO")
```

```
# Report MSE LASSO
predLASSO <- predict(cvLASSO, s = cvLASSO$lambda.1se, newx = XTest)
testMSE_LASSO <- mean((predLASSO - yTest)^2); testMSE_LASSO
## [1] 233.183
plotCV.glmnet <- function(cv.glmnet.object, name="") {
  df <- as.data.frame(cbind(x=log(cv.glmnet.object$lambda),
               y=cv.glmnet.object$cvm, errorBar=cv.glmnet.object$cvsd),
               nzero=cv.glmnet.object$nzero)
  featureNum <- cv.glmnet.object$nzero
  xFeature <- log(cv.glmnet.object$lambda)
  yFeature <- max(cv.glmnet.object$cvm)+max(cv.glmnet.object$cvsd)
  dataFeature <- data.frame(featureNum, xFeature, yFeature)
  plot_ly(data = df) %>%
    # add error bars for each CV-mean at Log(Lambda)
    add_trace(x = ~x, y = ~y, type = 'scatter', mode = 'markers',
        name = 'CV MSE', error_y = ~list(array = errorBar)) %>%
    # add the Lambda-min and Lambda 1SD vertical dash lines
    add_lines(data=df, x=c(log(cv.glmnet.object$lambda.min),
            log(cv.glmnet.object$lambda.min)),
            y=c(min(cv.glmnet.object$cvm)-max(df$errorBar),
max(cv.glmnet.object$cvm)+max(df$errorBar)),
        showlegend=F, line=list(dash="dash"), name="lambda.min",
        mode='lines+markers') %>%
    add_lines(data=df, x=c(log(cv.glmnet.object$lambda.1se),
            log(cv.glmnet.object$lambda.1se)),
            y=c(min(cv.glmnet.object$cvm)-max(df$errorBar),
            max(cv.glmnet.object$cvm)+max(df$errorBar)),
        showlegend=F, line=list(dash="dash"), name="lambda.1se") %>%
    # Add Number of Features Annotations on Top
    add_trace(dataFeature, x = ~xFeature, y = ~yFeature, type = 'scatter',
        name="Number of Features",
        mode = 'text', text = ~featureNum, textposition = 'middle right',
        textfont = list(color = '#000000', size = 9)) %>%
    layout(title = paste0("Cross-Validation MSE (", name, ")"),
            xaxis = list(title=paste0("log(",TeX("\\lambda"),")"),
            side="bottom", showgrid=TRUE), # type="log"
            hovermode = "x unified", legend = list(orientation='h'),
            yaxis = list(title = cv.glmnet.object$name, side="left",
                    showgrid = TRUE))
}
#### 10-fold cross validation #### Ridge Regression
set.seed(seed)  # set seed (10-fold) cross validation for Ridge Regression
cvRidge = cv.glmnet(XTrain, yTrain, alpha = 0, parallel=TRUE)
plotCV.glmnet(cvRidge, "Ridge")

# Report MSE Ridge
predRidge <- predict(cvRidge, s = cvRidge$lambda.1se, newx = XTest)
testMSE_Ridge <- mean((predRidge - yTest)^2); testMSE_Ridge
## [1] 233.183
stopCluster(cl)
```

Note that the `predict()` method applied to `cv.gmlnet` or `glmnet` fore-casting models is effectively a function wrapper to `predict.gmlnet()`. According to what you would like to get as a *prediction output*, you can use `type="..."` to specify one of the following types of prediction outputs

- `type="link"`, reports the linear predictors for "binomial," "multinomial," "poisson," or "cox" models; for "gaussian" models it gives the fitted values.
- `type="response"`, reports the fitted probabilities for "binomial" or "multinomial", fitted mean for "poisson" and the fitted relative-risk for "cox"; for "gaussian" type "response" is equivalent to type "link".
- `type="coefficients"`, reports the coefficients at the requested values for s. Note that for "binomial" models, results are returned only for the class corresponding to the second level of the factor response.
- `type="class"`, applies only to "binomial" or "multinomial" models, and produces the class label corresponding to the maximum probability.
- `type="nonzero"`, returns a list of the indices of the nonzero coefficients for each value of s.

11.2.22   Stepwise OLS (Ordinary Least Squares)

For a fair comparison, let's also obtain an OLS stepwise model selection, which we saw earlier.

```
dt = as.data.frame(cbind(yTrain,XTrain))
ols_step <- lm(yTrain ~., data = dt)
ols_step <- step(ols_step, direction = 'both', k=2, trace = F)
summary(ols_step)
```

We use `direction=both` for both *forward* and *backward* selection and choose an optimal and consistent model. The driving information criterion is specified by the parameter $k = 2$ (for AIC) and $k = \log (n)$ (for BIC). Then, we use the `ols_step` model to predict the outcome Y for some new test data.

```
betaHatOLS_step = ols_step$coefficients
var_step <- colnames(ols_step$model)[-1]
XTestOLS_step = cbind(rep(1, nrow(XTest)), XTest[,var_step])
predOLS_step = XTestOLS_step%*%betaHatOLS_step
testMSEOLS_step = mean((predOLS_step - yTest)^2)
# Report MSE OLS Stepwise feature selection
testMSEOLS_step
## [1] 243.939
```

Alternatively, we can predict the outcomes directly using the `predict()` function, and we can confirm that the manual and automated results are identical.

```
pred2 <- predict(ols_step,as.data.frame(XTest))
any(pred2 == predOLS_step)
## [1] TRUE
```

11.2.23 Final Models

Let's identify the most important (predictive) features, which can then be interpreted in the context of the specific data.

```
# Determine final models, Extract Coefficients
# OLS coefficient estimates
betaHatOLS = fitOLS$coefficients
# LASSO coefficient estimates
betaHatLASSO = as.double(coef(fitLASSO, s=cvLASSO$lambda.1se))  # s is Lambda
# Ridge  coefficient estimates
betaHatRidge = as.double(coef(fitRidge, s=cvRidge$lambda.1se))
# Test Set MSE, calculate predicted values
XTestOLS = cbind(rep(1, nrow(XTest)), XTest) # add intercept to test data
predOLS = XTestOLS%*%betaHatOLS
predLASSO = predict(fitLASSO, s = cvLASSO$lambda.1se, newx = XTest)
predRidge = predict(fitRidge, s = cvRidge$lambda.1se, newx = XTest)
# calculate test set MSE
testMSEOLS = mean((predOLS - yTest)^2)
testMSELASSO = mean((predLASSO - yTest)^2)
testMSERidge = mean((predRidge - yTest)^2)
```

Figure 11.16 shows a rank-ordered list of the key predictors of the clinical outcome variable (*total UPDRS, y <- data1$UPDRS_part_I + data1$UPDRS_part_II + data1$UPDRS_part_III*).

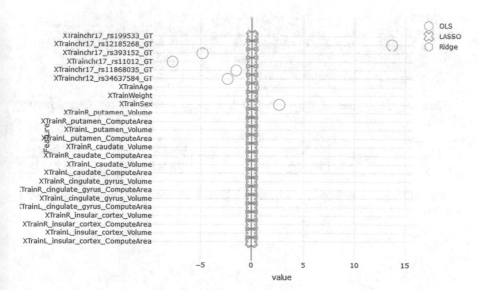

Fig. 11.16 Contrasting the model coefficient estimates corresponding to OLS, Ridge, and LASSO. Interactive exploration using the code allows magnification of the dynamic SVG plot near $x = 0$. This shows more detailed differences of the parameters estimated by the three different models

```
# Plot Regression Coefficients
library("arm")
par(mar=c(2, 13, 1, 1))    # extra large left margin
varNames <- colnames(data1[ , !(names(data1) %in% drop_features)]); varNames;
length(varNames)
df <- as.data.frame(cbind(Feature=attributes(betaHatOLS)$names[2:26],
    OLS=betaHatOLS[2:26], LASSO=betaHatLASSO[2:26], Ridge=betaHatRidge[2:26]))
data_long <- gather(df, Method, value, OLS:Ridge, factor_key=TRUE)
data_long$value <- as.numeric(data_long$value)
# Note that Plotly will automatically order your axes by the order that is
present in the data
# When using character vectors - order is alphabetic; in case of factors the
order is by levels.
# To override this behavior, specify categoryorder and categoryarray for the
appropriate axis in the layout
formY <- list(categoryorder = "array", categoryarray = df$Feature)
plot_ly(data_long, x=~value, y=~Feature, type="scatter", mode="markers",
        marker=list(size=20), color=~Method, symbol=~Method,
        symbols=c('circle-open','x-open','hexagon-open')) %>%
  layout(yaxis = formY)
```

11.2.24   Model Performance

We next quantify the performance of the models.

```
# Test Set MSE Table, create table as data frame
MSETable = data.frame(OLS=testMSEOLS, OLS_step=testMSEOLS_step,
                      LASSO=testMSELASSO, Ridge=testMSERidge)
# convert to markdown
kable(MSETable, format="pandoc", caption="Test Set MSE",
      align=c("c", "c", "c", "c"))
```

Here are the results of the corresponding MSE results for the four different models.

OLS	OLS_step	LASSO	Ridge
247.3367	243.939	233.183	233.183

We can also compare the features selected by different models as salient variables.

```
var_step = names(ols_step$coefficients)[-1]
var_lasso = colnames(XTrain)[which(coef(fitLASSO,s=cvLASSO$lambda.min)!=0)-1]
intersect(var_step, var_lasso)
##  [1] "L_insular_cortex_ComputeArea"  "L_insular_cortex_Volume"
##  [3] "R_insular_cortex_Volume"       "L_cingulate_gyrus_ComputeArea"
##  [5] "R_cingulate_gyrus_Volume"      "L_caudate_Volume"
##  [7] "L_putamen_ComputeArea"         "L_putamen_Volume"
##  [9] "R_putamen_ComputeArea"         "Sex"
## [11] "Weight"                        "Age"
## [13] "chr17_rs11868035_GT"           "chr17_rs11012_GT"
## [15] "chr17_rs393152_GT"             "chr17_rs12185268_GT"
coef(fitLASSO, s = cvLASSO$lambda.min)
## 26 x 1 sparse Matrix of class "dgCMatrix"
##                                           s1
## (Intercept)                    1.7349137426
## L_insular_cortex_ComputeArea  -0.0031461632
## L_insular_cortex_Volume        0.0007428576
## R_insular_cortex_ComputeArea   .
## R_insular_cortex_Volume       -0.0007386605
## L_cingulate_gyrus_ComputeArea  0.0060323275
## L_cingulate_gyrus_Volume       .
## R_cingulate_gyrus_ComputeArea -0.0004655064
## R_cingulate_gyrus_Volume      -0.0009788965
## L_caudate_ComputeArea          .
## L_caudate_Volume              -0.0031007230
## R_caudate_ComputeArea          .
## R_caudate_Volume              -0.0007081574
## L_putamen_ComputeArea         -0.0099013352
## L_putamen_Volume               0.0038351119
## R_putamen_ComputeArea          0.0056737358
## R_putamen_Volume               .
## Sex                            2.6406206813
## Weight                         0.0577691358
## Age                            0.1642627834
## chr12_rs34637584_GT            2.1268900512
## chr17_rs11868035_GT           -1.4279120508
## chr17_rs11012_GT              -6.6808710487
## chr17_rs393152_GT             -3.3231021784
## chr17_rs12185268_GT           10.9433767653
## chr17_rs199533_GT              .
```

Stepwise variable selection for OLS selects 12 variables, whereas LASSO with the best λ selects 9 salient variables. There are 6 variables common for both OLS and LASSO.

11.2.25   Summary

Traditional linear models are useful but also have their shortcomings:

- Prediction accuracy may be suboptimal.
- Model interpretability may be challenging (especially when a large number of features are used as regressors).
- Stepwise model selection may improve the model performance and add some interpretations, but still may not be optimal.

Regularization adds a penalty term to the estimation and has the following benefits:

- Enables exploitation of the *bias-variance* tradeoff
- Provides flexibility on specifying penalties to allow for continuous variable selection
- Allows incorporation of prior knowledge

11.3   Knockoff Filtering (FDR-Controlled Feature Selection)

11.3.1   Simulated Knockoff Example

Variable selection that controls the false discovery rate (FDR) of *salient features* can be accomplished in different ways. The *knockoff* filtering represents one strategy for controlled variable selection.[15] To show the usage of knockoff.filter, we start with a synthetic dataset constructed so that the true coefficient vector β has only a few nonzero entries.

The essence of the knockoff filtering is based on the following three-step process:

- Construct the decoy features (knockoff variables), one for each real observed feature. These act as controls for assessing the importance of the real variables.
- For each feature, X_j, compute the knockoff statistic, W_j, which measures the importance of the variable, relative to its decoy counterpart, $\tilde{X}_j$. This *importance* is measured by comparing the corresponding parameter estimates, $\widehat{\beta}_{X_j}$ and $\widehat{\beta}_{\tilde{X}_j}$, obtained via regularized linear modeling (e.g., LASSO).
- Determine the overall knockoff threshold. This is computed by rank-ordering the W_j statistics (from large to small), walking down the list of W_j's, selecting variables X_j corresponding to positive W_j's, and terminating this search the last time the ratio of negative to positive W_j's is below the default FDR q value, e.g., $q = 0.10$.

Mathematically, we consider X_j to be *unimportant* (i.e., peripheral or extraneous) if the conditional distribution of Y given $X_1, \cdots, X_p$ does not depend on X_j. Formally, X_j is unimportant if it is conditionally independent of Y given all other features, X_{-j}:

$$Y \perp X_j \mid X_{-j}.$$

We want to generate a Markov blanket of Y, such that the smallest set of features J satisfies this condition. Further, to make sure we do not make too many mistakes, we search for a set $\widehat{S}$ controlling the false discovery rate (FDR)

---

[15] https://doi.org/10.1214/18-AOS1755

$$\text{FDR}\left(\widehat{S}\right) = E\left(\frac{\#j \in \widehat{S} : x_j \text{ unimportant}}{\#j \in \widehat{S}}\right) \le q \text{ (e.g.10\%).}$$

Let's look at one simulation example.

```
# Problem parameters
n = 1000           # number of observations
p = 300            # number of variables
k = 30             # number of variables with nonzero coefficients
amplitude = 3.5    # signal amplitude (for noise level = 1)
# Problem data
X = matrix(rnorm(n*p), nrow=n, ncol=p)
nonzero = sample(p, k)
beta = amplitude * (1:p %in% nonzero)
y.sample <- function() X %*% beta + rnorm(n)
```

To begin with, we will invoke the knockoff.filter() method using the default settings.

```
# install.packages("knockoff")
library(knockoff)
y = y.sample()
result = knockoff.filter(X, y)
print(result)
## Selected variables:
##  [1]   2  14  21  25   30  42  47  51  61  80  81  82  96 112 127 152 157 164 172
## [20] 174 178 186 206 213 227 254 258 274 282 295
```

The false discovery proportion (fdp) can be computed as follows.

```
fdp <- function(selected) sum(beta[selected] == 0) / max(1, length(selected))
fdp(result$selected)
## [1] 0.0625
```

This yields an approximate FDR of 0.10.

The default settings of the knockoff filter uses a test statistic based on LASSO—knockoff.stat.lasso_signed_max, which computes the W_j statistics that quantify the discrepancy between a real (X_j) and a decoy, knockoff ($\tilde{X}_j$), feature coefficient estimates:

$$W_j = \max\left(X_j, \tilde{X}_j\right) \times \text{sign}\left(X_j - \tilde{X}_j\right).$$

Effectively, the W_j statistics measures how much more important the variable X_j is relative to its decoy counterpart $\tilde{X}_j$. The strength of the importance of X_j relative to $\tilde{X}_j$ is measured by the magnitude of W_j. The knockoff package includes several other test statistics, with appropriate names prefixed by *knockoff.stat*. For instance, we can use a statistic based on forward selection (*fs*) and a lower target FDR of 0.10.

```
result = knockoff.filter(X, y, fdr = 0.10, statistic = stat.glmnet_coefdiff)
# Old: statistic=knockoff.stat.fs)
#knockoff::stat.forward_selection        Importance statistics based on forward
selection
#knockoff::stat.glmnet_coefdiff    Importance statistics based on a GLM with
cross-validation
#knockoff::stat.glmnet_lambdadiff        Importance statistics based on a GLM
#knockoff::stat.glmnet_lambdasmax       GLM statistics for knockoff
#knockoff::stat.lasso_coefdiff     Importance statistics based the lasso with
cross-validation
#knockoff::stat.lasso_coefdiff_bin      Importance statistics based on
regularized logistic regression with cross-validation
#knockoff::stat.lasso_lambdadiff         Importance statistics based on the lasso
#knockoff::stat.lasso_lambdadiff_bin       Importance statistics based on
regularized logistic regression
#knockoff::stat.lasso_lambdasmax        Penalized linear regression statistics
for knockoff
#knockoff::stat.lasso_lambdasmax_bin        Penalized logistic regression
statistics for knockoff
#knockoff::stat.random_forest      Importance statistics based on random forests
# knockoff::stat.sqrt_lasso     Importance statistics based on the square-root
lasso
#knockoff::stat.stability_selection      Importance statistics based on stability
selection
#knockoff::verify_stat_depends     Verify dependencies for chosen statistics)
fdp(result$selected)
```

One can also define additional test statistics, complementing the ones included in the package already. For instance, below we show how we can implement the following test-statistics

$$W_j = \left\| X^t \cdot y \right\| - \left\| \tilde{X}^t \cdot y \right\|.$$

```
new_knockoff_stat <- function(X, X_ko, y) {
  abs(t(X) %*% y) - abs(t(X_ko) %*% y)
}
result = knockoff.filter(X, y, statistic = new_knockoff_stat)
# print indices of selected features
print(sprintf("Number of KO-selected features: %d", length(result$selected)))
## [1] "Number of KO-selected features: 25"
cat("Indices of KO-selected features: ", result$selected)
## Indices of KO-selected features:   2 14 25 30 42 47 51 80 82 96 112 127 152 157
172 174 178 206 213 227 254 258 274 282 295
fdp(result$selected)
```

11.3.2   Knockoff Invocation

The knockoff.filter function is a wrapper around several simpler functions that (1) construct knockoff variables (*knockoff.create*); (2) compute the test statistic W (various functions with prefix *knockoff.stat*); and (3) compute the threshold for variable selection (*knockoff.threshold*).

The high-level function *knockoff.filter* will automatically normalize the columns of the input matrix (unless this behavior is explicitly disabled). However, all other functions in this *package assume that the columns of the input matrix have unitary Euclidean norm.*

11.3.3 PD Neuroimaging-Genetics Case Study

Let's illustrate controlled variable selection via knockoff filtering using the real PD dataset.

The goal is to determine which imaging, genetics, and phenotypic covariates are associated with the clinical diagnosis of PD. The dataset is available at the DSPA case study archive site.

Preparing the Data
The dataset consists of clinical, genetics, and demographic measurements. To evaluate our results, we will compare diagnostic predictions created by the model for the *UPDRS scores* and the *ResearchGroup* factor variable.

Fetching and Cleaning the Data
First, we download the data and read it into data frames.

```
data1 <-
    read.table('https://umich.instructure.com/files/330397/download?download_frd=1',
               sep=",", header=T)
# For now, let's just ignore incomplete cases
data1.completeRowIndexes <- complete.cases(data1)
prop.table(table(data1.completeRowIndexes))
## data1.completeRowIndexes
##     FALSE      TRUE
## 0.3452381 0.6547619
data2 <- data1[data1.completeRowIndexes, ]
Dx_label  <- data2$ResearchGroup; table(Dx_label)
## Dx_label
## Control      PD   SWEDD
##     121     897     137
```

Preparing the Design Matrix
We now construct the design matrix X and the response vector Y. The features (columns of X) represent covariates that will be used to explain the response Y.

```
# Construct preliminary design matrix.
# define response and predictors
Y <- data1$UPDRS_part_I + data1$UPDRS_part_II + data1$UPDRS_part_III
table(Y)   # Show Clinically relevant classification
Y <- Y[data1.completeRowIndexes]
drop_features <- c("FID_IID", "ResearchGroup", "UPDRS_part_I",
                   "UPDRS_part_II", "UPDRS_part_III")
X <- data1[ , !(names(data1) %in% drop_features)]
X = as.matrix(X)
X <- X[data1.completeRowIndexes, ]; dim(X)  ## [1] 1155   26
summary(X)
mode(X) <- 'numeric'
Dx_label <- Dx_label[data1.completeRowIndexes]; length(Dx_label)
## [1] 1155
```

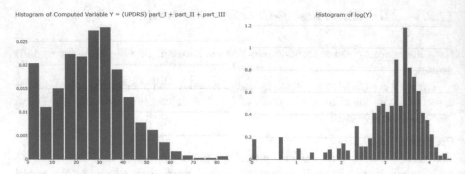

Fig. 11.17 Histograms of the computed outcome feature (Parkinson's disease outcome), linear scale (left) and log scale (right)

Preparing the Response Vector

The knockoff filter is designed to control the FDR under Gaussian noise. A quick inspection of the response vector shows that it is highly non-Gaussian (Fig. 11.17).

```
h <- hist(Y, breaks='FD', plot = F)
plot_ly(x = h$mids, y = h$density, type = "bar") %>%
    layout(bargap=0.1, title="Histogram of Computed Variable Y = (UPDRS)
            part_I + part_II + part_III")
# hist(Log(Y), breaks='FD')
h <- hist(log(Y), breaks='FD', plot = F)
plot_ly(x = h$mids, y = h$density, type = "bar") %>%
    layout(bargap=0.1, title="Histogram of log(Y)")
```

A `log-transform` may sometimes be helpful to stabilize the response variable.

For *binary outcome variables*, or *ordinal categorical variables*, we can employ the `logistic curve` to transform the polytomous outcomes into real values. The Logistic curve is $y = f(x) = \frac{1}{1+e^{-x}}$, where y and x represent probability and quantitative-predictor values, respectively. A slightly more general form is: $y = f(x) = \frac{K}{1+e^{-x}}$, where the covariate $x \in (-\infty, \infty)$ and the response $y \in [0, K]$.

Running the Knockoff Filter

We now run the knockoff filter along with the Benjamini–Hochberg (BH) procedure for controlling the false-positive rate of feature selection. Before running either selection procedure, remove rows with missing values, reduce the design matrix by removing predictor columns that do not appear frequently (e.g., at least three times in the sample), and remove any columns that are duplicates.

```
library(knockoff)
Y <- data1$UPDRS_part_I + data1$UPDRS_part_II + data1$UPDRS_part_III
table(Y)   # Show Clinically relevant classification
Y <- as.matrix(Y[data1.completeRowIndexes]); colnames(Y) <- "y"
mode(Y)
drop_features <- c("FID_IID", "ResearchGroup", "UPDRS_part_I",
                   "UPDRS_part_II", "UPDRS_part_III")
X <- data1[ , !(names(data1) %in% drop_features)]
X = as.matrix(X)
X <- X[data1.completeRowIndexes,]; dim(X); mode(X)
View(cbind(X,Y))
# Direct call to knockoff filtering
fdr <- 0.4
set.seed(1234)
result = knockoff.filter(X, Y, fdr=fdr, knockoffs=create.second_order);
print(result$selected) # Old: knockoffs='equicorrelated')
## L_cingulate_gyrus_ComputeArea        R_putamen_ComputeArea
##                             5                           15
##                        Weight                          Age
##                            18                           19
##             chr17_rs11868035_GT
##                            21
# knockoff::create.fixed          Fixed-X knockoffs
# knockoff::create.gaussian       Model-X Gaussian knockoffs
# knockoff::create.second_order       Second-order Gaussian knockoffs
# knockoff::create.solve_asdp         Relaxed optimization for fixed-X and
Gaussian knockoffs
# knockoff::create.solve_equi         Optimization for equi-correlated fixed-X and
Gaussian knockoffs
# knockoff::create.solve_sdp      Optimization for fixed-X and Gaussian knockoffs
# knockoff::create_equicorrelated        Create equicorrelated fixed-X knockoffs.
# knockoff::create_sdp         Create SDP fixed-X knockoffs.
# knockoff::create.vectorize_matrix      Vectorize a matrix into the SCS format
names(result$selected)
## [1] "L_cingulate_gyrus_ComputeArea" "R_putamen_ComputeArea"
## [3] "Weight"                        "Age"
## [5] "chr17_rs11868035_GT"
knockoff_selected <- names(result$selected)
# Run BH (Benjamini-Hochberg)
k = ncol(X)
lm.fit = lm(Y ~ X - 1) # no intercept
p.values = coef(summary(lm.fit))[,4]
cutoff = max(c(0, which(sort(p.values) <= fdr * (1:k) / k)))
BH_selected = names(which(p.values <= fdr * cutoff / k))
knockoff_selected; BH_selected
## [1] "L_cingulate_gyrus_ComputeArea" "R_putamen_ComputeArea"
## [3] "Weight"                        "Age"
## [5] "chr17_rs11868035_GT"
##  [1] "XL_insular_cortex_ComputeArea"  "XL_insular_cortex_Volume"
##  [3] "XL_cingulate_gyrus_ComputeArea" "XL_putamen_ComputeArea"
##  [5] "XL_putamen_Volume"              "XR_putamen_ComputeArea"
##  [7] "XSex"                           "XWeight"
##  [9] "XAge"                           "Xchr17_rs11868035_GT"
## [11] "Xchr17_rs11012_GT"              "Xchr17_rs393152_GT"
## [13] "Xchr17_rs12185268_GT"
```

```
list(Knockoff = knockoff_selected, BHq = BH_selected)
## $Knockoff
## [1] "L_cingulate_gyrus_ComputeArea"  "R_putamen_ComputeArea"
## [3] "Weight"                         "Age"
## [5] "chr17_rs11868035_GT"
## $BHq
##  [1] "XL_insular_cortex_ComputeArea"  "XL_insular_cortex_Volume"
##  [3] "XL_cingulate_gyrus_ComputeArea" "XL_putamen_ComputeArea"
##  [5] "XL_putamen_Volume"              "XR_putamen_ComputeArea"
##  [7] "XSex"                           "XWeight"
##  [9] "XAge"                           "Xchr17_rs11868035_GT"
## [11] "Xchr17_rs11012_GT"              "Xchr17_rs393152_GT"
## [13] "Xchr17_rs12185268_GT"
# Alternatively, for more flexible Knockoff invocation
set.seed(1234)
knockoffs = function(X) create.gaussian(X, 0, Sigma=diag(dim(X)[2]))
# identify var-covar matrix Sigma of rank equal to the number of features
stats = function(X, Xk, y) stat.glmnet_coeffdiff(X, Xk, y, nfolds=10)
# The Output X_k is an n-by-p matrix of knockoff features
result = knockoff.filter(X, Y, fdr=fdr, knockoffs=knockoffs,
                         statistic=stats); print(result$selected)
## L_cingulate_gyrus_ComputeArea         R_putamen_ComputeArea
##                             5                            15
##                           Age          chr17_rs11868035_GT
##                            19                            21
##          chr17_rs12185268_GT
##                            24
# Housekeeping: remove the "X" prefixes in the BH_selected list of features
for(i in 1:length(BH_selected)) {
  BH_selected[i] <- substring(BH_selected[i], 2)
}
intersect(BH_selected,knockoff_selected)
## [1] "L_cingulate_gyrus_ComputeArea"  "R_putamen_ComputeArea"
## [3] "Weight"                         "Age"
## [5] "chr17_rs11868035_GT"
```

We see that there are some features that are selected by both methods suggesting these variables may be indeed important.

11.4   Practice Problems

Readers may practice different types of variable selection methods using the SOCR_Data_AD_BiomedBigMetadata on SOCR website. This is a smaller dataset that has 744 observations and 63 variables. Here we utilize DXCURREN or current diagnostics as the class variable.

First, import the dataset.

```
library(rvest)
wiki_url <- read_html("https://wiki.socr.umich.edu/index.php/SOCR_Data_AD_BiomedBigMetadata")
html_nodes(wiki_url, "#content")
alzh <- html_table(html_nodes(wiki_url, "table")[[1]])
summary(alzh)
```

The data summary shows that we have several factor variables. After converting their type to numeric, we find some missing data. We can manage this issue by selecting only the complete observation of the original dataset or by using multivariate imputation, see Chap. 2.

```
chrtofactor<-c(3, 5, 8, 10, 21:22, 51:54)
alzh[alzh=="."] <- NA  # replace all missing "." values with "NA"
alzh[chrtofactor]<-data.frame(apply(alzh[chrtofactor], 2, as.numeric))
alzh<-alzh[complete.cases(alzh), ]
```

For simplicity, we can eliminate the missing data and work with the residual 408 complete observations, or alternatively employ multiple imputation to complete several chains of the data. Next, we can apply the Boruta method for feature selection and report the rank-ordered features clearly identifying confirmed salient variables.

```
set.seed(123)
train<-Boruta(DXCURREN~.-SID, data=alzh, doTrace=0)
print(train)
```

Chapter 12
Big Longitudinal Data Analysis

The time-varying (longitudinal) characteristics of large information flows represent a special case of the complexity, dynamic, and multiscale nature of big biomedical data, which we discussed in the beginning introduction and motivation. Previously, in Chap. 3, we saw space-time (4D) functional magnetic resonance imaging (fMRI) data, and in Chap. 10, we discussed streaming data, which also has a natural temporal dimension.

In this chapter, we will expand our ML/AI predictive data analytic strategies specifically for analyzing longitudinal data. We will interrogate datasets that track homologous information, across subjects, units, or locations, over a period of time. In the first part of the chapter, we will present classical approaches including time-series analysis, forecasting using autoregressive integrated moving average (ARIMA) models, structural equation models (SEM), and longitudinal data analysis via linear mixed models. In the second part, we will discuss recent AI methods for time-series analysis and forecasting including recurrent neural networks (RNN) and long short-term memory (LSTM) networks.

12.1 Classical Time-Series Analytic Approaches

12.1.1 Information theoretic model evaluation criteria

The Akaike information criterion (AIC) and the Bayesian information criterion (BIC) are metrics that quantify the fit of different (typically) regression models. The AIC is calculated by the formula $AIC = 2k - 2\ ln(L)$, *where* k *is the number of parameters estimated in the model, and* $ln(L)$ *is the log-likelihood of the model. In essence, the AIC quantifies how likely the model is, given the observed data (in terms of the likelihood value). Suppose we have estimated several different regression models, the optimal model corresponds to the smallest AIC value, i.e., the model with the lowest AIC yields the best fit (highest likelihood, relative to the*

number of model parameters). The sign of the AIC does not matter, the lower the
AIC value, the better the model fit.

Similarly, the *BIC* is calculated by the formula $BIC = k\ ln(n) - 2ln(L)$, where n is
the number of data points, k is the number of parameters estimated in the model, and
$ln(L)$ is the log-likelihood of the model. Lower *BIC* values correspond to higher
likelihoods ($2ln(L)$) and lower penalty terms ($k\ ln(n)$); i.e., better models.

12.1.2   Time-Series Analysis

Time-series analysis relies on models like ARIMA (Autoregressive integrated moving average)[1] that utilize past longitudinal information to predict near future outcomes. Time-series data tend to track univariate, sometimes multivariate, processes
over a continuous time interval. The stock market, e.g., daily closing value of the
Dow Jones Industrial Average index,[2] or electroencephalography (EEG) data[3]
provide examples of such longitudinal datasets (time-series).

The basic concepts in time-series analysis include the following:

- The characteristics of *(second-order) stationary time-series* (e.g., the first two
  moments are stable over time) do not depend on the time at which the series
  process is observed.
- *Differencing*—a transformation applied to time-series data to make it stationary.
  Differences between consecutive time-observations may be computed by
  $y'_t = y_t - y_{t-1}$. Differencing removes the level changes in the time-series, elim-
  inates trend, reduces seasonality, and stabilizes the mean of the time-series.
  Differencing the time-series repeatedly may yield a stationary time-series. For
  example, a second-order differencing:

$$
\begin{aligned}
y''_t &= y'_t - y'_{t-1} \\
&= (y_t - y_{t-1}) - (y_{t-1} - y_{t-2}). \\
&= y_t - 2y_{t-1} + y_{t-2}
\end{aligned}
$$

- *Seasonal differencing* is computed as a difference between one observation and
  its corresponding observation in the previous epoch, or season (e.g., annually,
  there are $m = 4$ seasons in a cycle), like in this example

$$
y'''_t = y_t - y_{t-m} \quad m = \text{number of seasons.}
$$

- The differenced data may then be used to estimate an ARMA model.

---

[1] https://doi.org/10.2307/2346970
[2] https://doi.org/10.3905/jwm.2000.320332
[3] https://doi.org/10.1038/s41597-019-0104-

We will use the Beijing air quality PM2.5 dataset as an example to demonstrate the analysis process. This dataset measures air pollutants—PM2.5 particles in micrograms per cubic meter[4] for 8 years (2008–2016). It measures the *hourly average of the number of particles that are of size 2.5 microns (PM2.5)* once per hour in Beijing, China. Let's first import the dataset into R.

```
beijing.pm25<-
    read.csv("https://umich.instructure.com/files/1823138/download?download_frd=1")
summary(beijing.pm25)
##      Index              Site             Parameter          Date..LST.
## Min.    :    1    Length:69335       Length:69335       Length:69335
## 1st Qu.:17335    Class :character    Class :character    Class :character
## Median :34668    Mode  :character    Mode  :character    Mode  :character
## Mean    :34668
## 3rd Qu.:52002
## Max.    :69335
##       Year            Month              Day               Hour
## Min.    :2008    Min.    : 1.000    Min.    : 1.00    Min.    : 0.0
## 1st Qu.:2010    1st Qu.: 4.000    1st Qu.: 8.00    1st Qu.: 5.5
## Median :2012    Median : 6.000    Median :16.00    Median :11.0
## Mean    :2012    Mean    : 6.407    Mean    :15.73    Mean    :11.5
## 3rd Qu.:2014    3rd Qu.: 9.000    3rd Qu.:23.00    3rd Qu.:17.5
## Max.    :2016    Max.    :12.000    Max.    :31.00    Max.    :23.0
##      Value            Duration          QC.Name
## Min.    :-999.00    Length:69335       Length:69335
## 1st Qu.:  22.00    Class :character    Class :character
## Median :  63.00    Mode  :character    Mode  :character
## Mean    :  24.99
## 3rd Qu.: 125.00
## Max.    : 994.00
```

The `Value` column records PM2.5 AQI (Air Quality Index) for 8 years. We observe that there are some missing data in the `Value` column. By looking at the `QC.Name` column, we have about 6.5% (~4408) of the observations with missing values. One way of solving the missingness is to replace them with the corresponding variable mean. In practical applications, some of the more powerful data imputation methods we discussed earlier should be used.

```
beijing.pm25[beijing.pm25$Value==-999, 9] <- NA
beijing.pm25[is.na(beijing.pm25$Value), 9] <-
            floor(mean(beijing.pm25$Value, na.rm = T))
```

Here we first reassign the missing values into NA labels. Then we replace all NA labels with the *mean* computed using all nonmissing observations. Note that the floor() function casts the arithmetic averages as integer numbers, which is needed as AQI values are expected to be whole numbers.

Now, let's observe the trend of hourly average PM2.5 across 1 day. You can see a significant pattern: The PM2.5 level peaks in the afternoons and is the lowest in the early mornings and exhibits approximate periodic boundary conditions (these patterns oscillate daily) (Fig. 12.1).

---

[4]https://doi.org/10.1016/j.scitotenv.2006.08.041

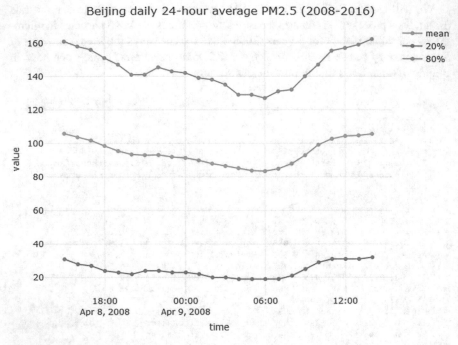

Fig. 12.1 A short fragment of the smoothed average trend of the Beijing P2.5 hourly data with confidence bands

```
library(plotly)
library(ggplot2)
id = 1:nrow(beijing.pm25)
mat = matrix(0,nrow=24,ncol=3)
stat = function(x) {  c(mean(beijing.pm25[iid,"Value"]),
                          quantile(beijing.pm25[iid,"Value"],c(0.2,0.8)))
}
for (i in 1:24) {  iid = which(id%%24==i-1);  mat[i,] = stat(iid)  }
mat <- as.data.frame(mat)
colnames(mat) <- c("mean","20%","80%")
mat$time <-
        readr::parse_datetime(beijing.pm25$Date..LST., "%m/%d/%Y %h:%M")[1:24]
require(reshape2)
dt <- melt(mat, id="time")
plot_ly(data = dt, x=~time, y=~value, color = ~variable, type="scatter",
        mode="markers+lines") %>%
  layout(title="Beijing daily 24-hour average PM2.5 (2008-2016)")
```

Are there any daily or monthly trends? We can start the data interrogation by building an ARIMA model and examining detailed patterns in the data.

Step 1: Plot Time-Series
To begin with, we can visualize the overall trend by plotting PM2.5 values against time. This can be achieved using the `plyr` package (Fig. 12.2).

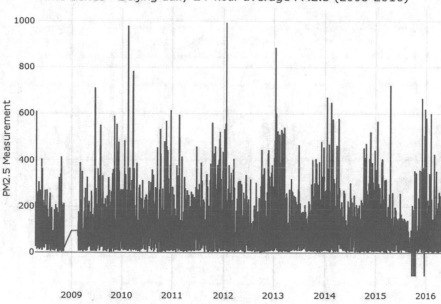

Fig. 12.2 The raw Beijing P2.5 hourly data is much more noisy, incomplete, and nonstationary

```
library(plyr)
ts <- ts(beijing.pm25$Value, start=1, end=69335, frequency=1)  # ts.plot(ts)
dateTime <- readr::parse_datetime(beijing.pm25$Date..LST., "%m/%d/%Y %h:%M")
tsValue <- ifelse(beijing.pm25$Value>=0, beijing.pm25$Value, -100)
df <- as.data.frame(cbind(dateTime=dateTime, tsValue=tsValue))
plot_ly(x=~dateTime, y=~tsValue, type="scatter", mode="lines") %>%
  layout(
    title = "Time Series - Beijing daily 24-hour average PM2.5 (2008-2016)",
    xaxis = list(title = "date"), yaxis=list(title="PM2.5 Measurement"))
```

The dataset is recorded hourly, and the 8-year time interval includes about 69,335 hours of records. Therefore, we start at the first hour and end with 69,335th hour. Each hour has a univariate PM2.5 AQI value measurement, so $frequency = 1$. From this time-series plot, we observe that the data has some extreme peaks and many AQI (air quality index) values around 200 (which are considered "very unhealthy").

The original plot seems to have no trend at all. Remember we have our measurements in hours. Will there be any difference if we use monthly average instead of hourly reported values? In this case, we can use Simple Moving Average (SMA) technique to smooth the original graph., using the R-package TTR (Fig. 12.3).

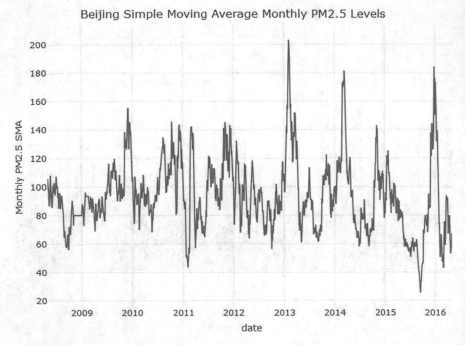

Fig. 12.3 Monthly averaged Beijing P2.5 data still show relatively high levels of noise and some variability trends

```
# install.packages("TTR")
library(TTR)
bj.month <- SMA(tsValue, n=720)
plot_ly(x=~dateTime, y=~bj.month, type="scatter", mode="lines") %>%
  layout(title = "Beijing Simple Moving Average Monthly PM2.5 Levels",
         xaxis = list(title = "date"), yaxis=list(title="Monthly PM2.5 SMA"))
```

We chose the lag smoothing parameter to be $n = 24 \times 30 = 720$. It seems that for the first 4 years (or approximately 35,040 hours) the AQI fluctuates less than the last 5 years. Let's see what happens if we use *exponentially-weighted moving average* (EMA) of the data, instead of using the *arithmetic mean* (SMA). The pattern seems less obvious in this graph. Here we used an exponential smoothing ratio of $2/(n + 1)$ (Fig. 12.4).

```
bj.month <- EMA(tsValue, n=1, ratio = 2/(720+1))
plot_ly(x=~dateTime, y=~tsValue, type="scatter", mode="lines", opacity=0.2,
        name="Observed") %>%
  add_trace(x=~dateTime, y=~SMA(tsValue, n=720), type="scatter",
            mode="lines", opacity=1.0, name="SMA") %>%
  add_trace(x=~dateTime, y=~bj.month, type="scatter", mode="lines",
            name="EMA") %>% # line = list(dash = 'dot')
  layout(title = "Beijing PM2.5 Levels with EMA and SMA Smoothing",
         xaxis = list(title = "date"), yaxis=list(title="PM2.5 Values"))
```

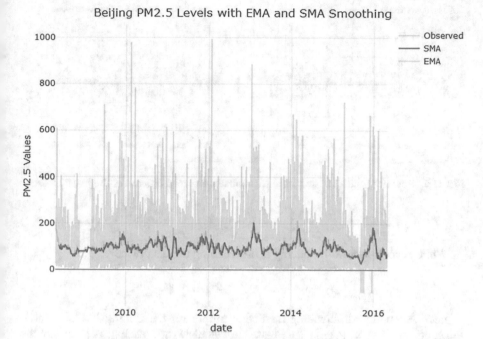

Fig. 12.4 EMA and SMA smoothing of the Beijing P2.5 data

Step 2: Find Proper Parameter Values for ARIMA Model

ARIMA models have two components—autoregressive part (AR) and moving average part (MA). An $ARMA(p, d, q)$ model is a model with p terms in AR and q terms in MA, and d representing the order difference, where differencing is used to make the original dataset approximately stationary. If we denote by L the *lag operator*, by ϕ_i the parameters of the autoregressive part of the model, by θ_i the parameters of the moving average part, and by ϵ_t error terms, then the $ARMA(p, d, q)$ has the following analytical form:

$$\left(1 - \sum_{i=1}^{p} \phi_i L^i\right)(1 - L)^d X_t = \left(1 + \sum_{i=1}^{q} \theta_i L^i\right)\epsilon_t.$$

Check the Differencing Parameter

First, let's try to determine the parameter d. To make the data stationary on the mean (remove any trend), we can use first differencing or second-order differencing. Mathematically, first differencing is taking the difference between two adjacent data points

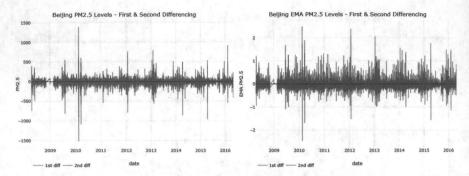

Fig. 12.5 Row (left) and EMA-smoothed (right) first and second differences (Beijing P2.5 data)

$$y_t' = y_t - y_{t-1}.$$

While second-order differencing is differencing the data twice

$$y_t^* = y_t' - y_{t-1}' = y_t - 2y_{t-1} + y_{t-2}.$$

Let's see which differencing method is proper for the Beijing PM2.5 dataset. Function diff() in R base can be used to calculate differencing. We can plot the differences by plot.ts() or using plot_ly(). As neither of the differences series appears quite stationary, we can consider using some smoothing techniques on the data like we did above (bj.month <− SMA(ts, $n = 720$)). Let's see if smoothing by exponentially weighted mean (EMA) can help make the data approximately stationary (Fig. 12.5).

```
bj.diff2 <- diff(tsValue, differences=2)
bj.diff  <- diff(tsValue, differences=1)
plot_ly(x=~dateTime[2:length(dateTime)], y=~bj.diff, type="scatter",
        mode="lines", name="1st diff", opacity=0.5) %>%
  add_trace(x=~dateTime[3:length(dateTime)], y=~bj.diff2, type="scatter",
            mode="lines", name="2nd diff", opacity=0.5)  %>%
  layout(title = "Beijing PM2.5 Levels - First & Second Differencing",
         legend=list(orientation='h'), xaxis=list(title="date"),
         yaxis=list(title="PM2.5"))
bj.diff  <- diff(bj.month, differences=1)
bj.diff2 <- diff(bj.month, differences=2)
plot_ly(x=~dateTime[2:length(dateTime)], y=~bj.diff, type="scatter",
        mode="lines", name="1st diff", opacity=0.5) %>%
  add_trace(x=~dateTime[3:length(dateTime)], y=~bj.diff2, type="scatter",
            mode="lines",
            name="2nd diff", opacity=0.5)  %>%
  layout(title = "Beijing EMA PM2.5 Levels - First & Second Differencing",
         legend = list(orientation='h'),
         xaxis = list(title = "date"), yaxis=list(title="EMA PM2.5"))
```

The EMA-filtered graphs have tempered variance and appear pretty stationary with respect to the first two moments, i.e., mean and variance.

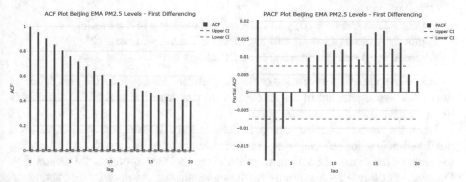

Fig. 12.6 Autocorrelation factor (ACF) and partial autocorrelation factor (PACF) plots. Mind the scale of the vertical axes and the departure correlation factors' departure outside the confidence bands

Identifying the AR and MA Parameters

To decide the auto-regressive (AR) and moving average (MA) parameters in the model we need to create *autocorrelation factor (ACF)* and *partial autocorrelation factor (PACF) plots*. PACF may suggest a value for the AR-term parameter p, and ACF may help us determine the MA-term parameter q. We plot the ACF and PACF, we use approximately stationary time series `bj.diff` objects. The dash lines on the ACF/PACF plots indicate the bounds on the correlation values beyond which the auto-correlations are considered statistically significantly different from zero. Correlation values outside the confidence lines could suggest nonpurely random, i.e., correlated, parts in the longitudinal signal (Fig. 12.6).

```
acf1 <- acf(bj.diff, lag.max = 20, main="ACF", plot=F)
ci <- qnorm((1 + 0.95)/2)/sqrt(length(bj.diff))  # 95% CI
plot_ly(x=~acf1$lag[,1,1], y=~acf1$acf[,1,1], type = "bar", name="ACF") %>%
  # add CI lines
  add_lines(x=~c(acf1$lag[1,1,1],acf1$lag[length(acf1$lag),1,1]),y=~c(ci,ci),
            mode="lines", name="Upper CI", line=list(dash='dash')) %>%
add_lines(x=~c(acf1$lag[1,1,1],acf1$lag[length(acf1$lag),1,1]),y=~c(-ci,-ci),
          mode="lines", name="Lower CI", line=list(dash='dash')) %>%
  layout(bargap=0.8, xaxis=list(title="lag"), yaxis=list(title="ACF"),
         title="ACF Plot Beijing EMA PM2.5 Levels - First Differencing")
pacf1 <- pacf(ts(bj.diff), lag.max = 20, main="PACF", plot=F)
plot_ly(x = ~pacf1$lag[,1,1], y = ~pacf1$acf[,1,1], type = "bar",
        name="PACF") %>%
  # add CI lines
add_lines(x=~c(pacf1$lag[1,1,1],acf1$lag[length(pacf1$lag),1,1]),y=~c(ci,ci),
          mode="lines", name="Upper CI", line=list(dash='dash')) %>%
add_lines(x=~c(acf1$lag[1,1,1],acf1$lag[length(acf1$lag),1,1]),y=~c(-ci,-ci),
          mode="lines", name="Lower CI", line=list(dash='dash')) %>%
  layout(bargap=0.8, xaxis=list(title="lag"),yaxis=list(title="Partial ACF"),
         title="PACF Plot Beijing EMA PM2.5 Levels - First Differencing")
```

Notes:

- A pure AR model ($p = 0$) will have a cut off at lag q in the PACF.
- A pure MA model ($q = 0$) will have a cut off at lag p in the ACF.
- ARIMA(p, q) will (eventually) have a decay in both.

All ACF spikes appear outside of the insignificant zone in the *ACF plot*, whereas only a few are significant in the *PACF plot*. In this case, the best ARIMA model is likely to have both AR and MA parts.

Next, we can examine for seasonal effects in the data using `stats::stl()`, a flexible function for decomposing and forecasting the series, which uses averaging to calculate the seasonal component of the series and then subtracts the seasonality. Decomposing the series and removing the seasonality can be done by subtracting the seasonal component from the original series using `forecast::seasadj()`. The frequency parameter in the `ts()` object specifies the periodicity of the data or the number of observations per period, e.g., 30 (for monthly smoothed daily data) (Fig. 12.7).

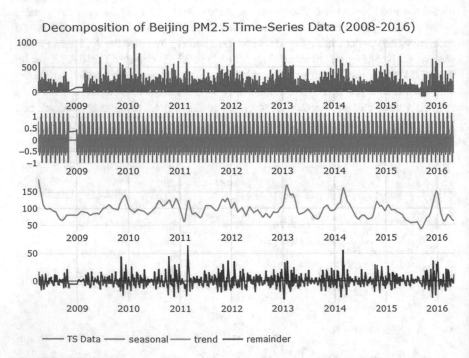

Fig. 12.7 Beijing data—decomposing the time-series into seasonal and trend effects

```
count_ma = ts(bj.month, frequency=30*24)
decomp = stl(count_ma, s.window="periodic")
deseasonal_count <- forecast::seasadj(decomp)
plot_ly(x=~dateTime, y=~tsValue, type="scatter", mode="lines") %>%
  layout(
    title = "Time Series - Beijing daily 24-hour average PM2.5 (2008-2016)",
    xaxis = list(title = "date"), yaxis=list(title="PM2.5 Measurement"))
figTS_Data     <- plot_ly(x=~dateTime, y=~tsValue, type="scatter",
                          mode="lines", name="TS Data")
figSeasonal    <- plot_ly(x=~dateTime, y=~decomp$time.series[,1],
                          type='scatter', mode='lines', name="seasonal")
figTrend       <- plot_ly(x=~dateTime, y=~decomp$time.series[,2],
                          type='scatter', mode='lines', name="trend")
figRemainder   <- plot_ly(x=~dateTime, y=~decomp$time.series[,3],
                          type='scatter', mode='lines', name="remainder")
fig <- subplot(figTS_Data, figSeasonal, figTrend, figRemainder, nrows=4) %>%
  layout(title = list(text =
           "Decomposition of Beijing PM2.5 Time-Series Data (2008-2016)"),
         hovermode = "x unified", legend = list(orientation='h'))
```

The augmented Dickey–Fuller (ADF) test,[5] tseries::adf.test can be used to examine the time-series stationarity. The null hypothesis is that the *series is nonstationary*. The ADF test quantifies if the change in the series can be explained by a lagged value and a linear trend. Nonstationary series can be *corrected* by differencing to remove trends or cycles.

```
tseries::adf.test(count_ma, alternative = "stationary")
##  Augmented Dickey-Fuller Test
## Dickey-Fuller = -8.0304, Lag order = 41, p-value = 0.01
## alternative hypothesis: stationary
tseries::adf.test(bj.diff, alternative = "stationary")
##  Augmented Dickey-Fuller Test
## Dickey-Fuller = -29.187, Lag order = 41, p-value = 0.01
## alternative hypothesis: stationary
```

We see that we can reject the null and therefore, there is no statistically significant nonstationarity in the bj.diff time-series.

Step 3: Build an ARIMA Model

As we have some evidence suggesting $d = 1$, the auto.arima() function in the forecast package can help us to find the optimal estimates for the remaining pair parameters of the ARIMA model, p and q (Fig. 12.8).

---

[5] https://doi.org/10.1016/0165-1765(92)90022-Q

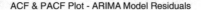

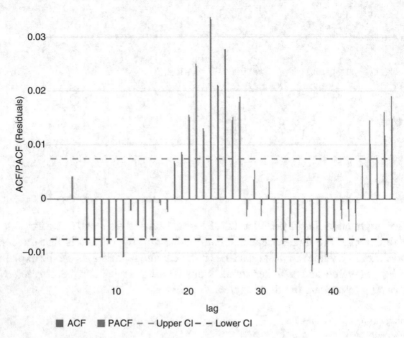

Fig. 12.8 ARIMA(4,1,0) model residuals—ACF and PACF plots

```
# install.packages("forecast")
library(forecast)
fit <- auto.arima(bj.month, approx=F, trace = F); fit
## ARIMA(4,1,0)
## Coefficients:
##          ar1      ar2      ar3      ar4
##       1.0218  -0.0492  -0.0129  -0.0102
## s.e.  0.0038   0.0054   0.0054   0.0038
## sigma^2 = 0.004629:  log likelihood = 87976.49
## AIC=-175943    AICc=-175943    BIC=-175897.2
acf1 <- Acf(residuals(fit), plot = F)
ci <- qnorm((1 + 0.95)/2)/sqrt(length(bj.diff))
pacf1 <- Pacf(residuals(fit), plot = F)
plot_ly(x = ~acf1$lag[-1,1,1], y = ~acf1$acf[-1,1,1], type = "bar", # ACF
        name="ACF") %>%
  add_trace(x=~pacf1$lag[-1,1,1], y=~pacf1$acf[-1,1,1], type="bar", # PACF
            name="PACF") %>%
  # add CI lines
  add_lines(x=~c(acf1$lag[2,1,1],acf1$lag[length(acf1$lag),1,1]),y=~c(ci,ci),
            mode="lines", name="Upper CI", line=list(dash='dash')) %>%
add_lines(x=~c(acf1$lag[2,1,1],acf1$lag[length(acf1$lag),1,1]),y=~c(-ci,-ci),
          mode="lines", name="Lower CI", line=list(dash='dash')) %>%
  layout(bargap=0.8, title="ACF & PACF Plot - ARIMA Model Residuals",
         xaxis=list(title="lag"), yaxis=list(title="ACF/PACF (Residuals)"),
         hovermode = "x unified", legend = list(orientation='h'))
```

Finally, the optimal model determined by the stepwise selection is ARIMA (4, 1, 0). We can also use external information to fit ARIMA models. For example, if we want to add the month information, in case we suspect a seasonal change in PM2.5 AQI, we can fit a different model, e.g., *ARIMA*(2, 1, 0) model.

```
fit1 <- auto.arima(bj.month, xreg=beijing.pm25$Month, approx=F,trace=F); fit1
## Regression with ARIMA(4,1,0) errors
## Coefficients:
##          ar1      ar2      ar3      ar4     xreg
##       1.0218  -0.0492  -0.0129  -0.0102  -0.0021
## s.e.  0.0038   0.0054   0.0054   0.0038   0.0015
## sigma^2 = 0.004629:  log likelihood = 87977.47
## AIC=-175942.9   AICc=-175942.9   BIC=-175888
fit3 <- arima(bj.month, order = c(2, 1, 0))
fit3
## Coefficients:
##          ar1      ar2
##       1.0237  -0.0725
## s.e.  0.0038   0.0038
## sigma^2 estimated as 0.004631: log likelihood = 87954.05, aic = -175902.1
```

We want the model AIC and BIC to be as small as possible. This model is actually worse than the last model without Month predictor in terms of AIC and BIC. Also, the coefficient is very small and not significant (*t*-test). Thus, we can remove the Month term.

We can examine further the ACF and the PACF plots and the residuals to determine the model quality. When the model order parameters and structure are correctly specified, we expect no significant autocorrelations present in the model residual plots.

```
plot_ly(x=~dateTime, y=~residuals(fit), type="scatter", mode="lines") %>%
  # add CI Lines
  add_lines(x=~c(dateTime[1], dateTime[length(dateTime)]), y=~c(1.96, 1.96),
            mode="lines", name="Upper CI", line=list(dash='dash')) %>%
  add_lines(x=~c(dateTime[1], dateTime[length(dateTime)]), y=~c(-1.96,-1.96),
            mode="lines", name="Lower CI", line=list(dash='dash')) %>%
  layout(title = "Beijing PM2.5: ARIMA(2, 1, 0) Model Residuals",
         xaxis = list(title = "date"), yaxis=list(title="Residuals"),
         hovermode = "x unified")
acf1 <- Acf(residuals(fit), plot = F)
ci <- qnorm((1 + 0.95)/2)/sqrt(length(bj.diff))
pacf1 <- Pacf(residuals(fit), plot = F)
plot_ly(x = ~acf1$lag[-1,1,1], y = ~acf1$acf[-1,1,1], type = "bar",
        name="ACF")  %>%   # ACF
  add_trace(x = ~pacf1$lag[-1,1,1], y = ~pacf1$acf[-1,1,1], type = "bar",
            name="PACF") %>%   # PACF
  # add CI Lines
  add_lines(x=~c(acf1$lag[2,1,1],acf1$lag[length(acf1$lag),1,1]),y=~c(ci,ci),
            mode="lines", name="Upper CI", line=list(dash='dash')) %>%
add_lines(x=~c(acf1$lag[2,1,1],acf1$lag[length(acf1$lag),1,1]),y=~c(-ci,-ci),
          mode="lines", name="Lower CI", line=list(dash='dash')) %>%
  layout(bargap=0.8, title="ACF & PACF Plot - ARIMA Model Residuals",
         xaxis=list(title="lag"), yaxis=list(title="ACF/PACF (Residuals)"),
         hovermode = "x unified", legend = list(orientation='h'))
```

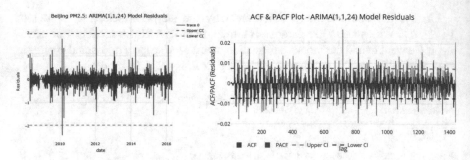

Fig. 12.9 ARIMA(1,1,24) model quality plots

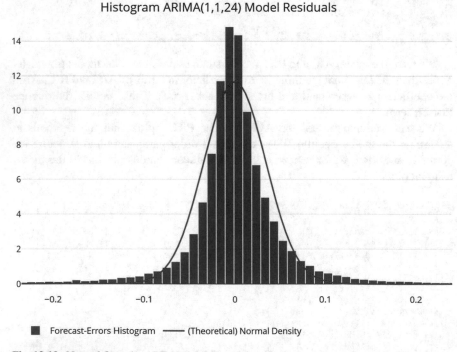

Fig. 12.10 Normal fit to the ARIMA(1,1,24) model residuals

There is a clear pattern present in ACF/PACF plots suggesting that the model residuals repeat with an approximate lag of 12 or 24 months. We may try a modified model with different parameters, e.g., $p = 24$ or $q = 24$. We can define a new `displayForecastErrors()` function to show a histogram of the forecasted errors (Figs. 12.9 and 12.10).

```
fit24 <- arima(deseasonal_count, order=c(1,1,24)); fit24
## Call:
## arima(x = deseasonal_count, order = c(1, 1, 24))
## Coefficients:
##          ar1     ma1     ma2     ma3     ma4     ma5     ma6     ma7
##       0.9501  0.0479  0.0159  0.0020 -0.0032 -0.0061 -0.0137 -0.0119
## s.e. 0.0032  0.0049  0.0049  0.0048  0.0047  0.0046  0.0045  0.0044
##          ma8     ma9    ma10    ma11    ma12    ma13    ma14    ma15
##      -0.0127 -0.0096 -0.0086 -0.0124 -0.0038 -0.0052 -0.0058 -0.0043
## s.e. 0.0044  0.0043  0.0042  0.0042  0.0041  0.0041  0.0041  0.0041
##         ma16    ma17    ma18    ma19    ma20    ma21    ma22    ma23    ma24
##       0.0018  0.0007  0.0088  0.009  0.0147  0.0215  0.0078  0.0247  0.0109
## s.e. 0.0041  0.0041  0.0040  0.004  0.0040  0.0040  0.0040  0.0040  0.0039
## sigma^2 estimated as 0.004669:  log likelihood = 87670.15, aic = -175288.3
plot_ly(x=~dateTime, y=~residuals(fit24), type="scatter", mode="lines") %>%
  # add CI Lines
  add_lines(x=~c(dateTime[1], dateTime[length(dateTime)]), y=~c(1.96, 1.96),
            mode="lines", name="Upper CI", line=list(dash='dash')) %>%
  add_lines(x=~c(dateTime[1], dateTime[length(dateTime)]), y=~c(-1.96,-1.96),
            mode="lines", name="Lower CI", line=list(dash='dash')) %>%
  layout(title = "Beijing PM2.5: ARIMA(1,1,24) Model Residuals",
    xaxis = list(title = "date"), yaxis=list(title="Residuals"),
    hovermode = "x unified")
acf1 <- Acf(residuals(fit24), plot = F)
ci <- qnorm((1 + 0.95)/2)/sqrt(length(bj.diff))
pacf1 <- Pacf(residuals(fit24), plot = F)
plot_ly(x = ~acf1$lag[-1,1,1], y = ~acf1$acf[-1,1,1], type = "bar",
        name="ACF") %>%    # ACF
  add_trace(x = ~pacf1$lag[-1,1,1], y = ~pacf1$acf[-1,1,1], type = "bar",
        name="PACF") %>%   # PACF
  # add CI Lines
  add_lines(x=~c(acf1$lag[2,1,1],acf1$lag[length(acf1$lag),1,1]),y=~c(ci,ci),
            mode="lines", name="Upper CI", line=list(dash='dash')) %>%
add_lines(x=~c(acf1$lag[2,1,1],acf1$lag[length(acf1$lag),1,1]),y=~c(-ci,-ci),
            mode="lines", name="Lower CI", line=list(dash='dash')) %>%
  layout(bargap=0.8, title="ACF & PACF Plot - ARIMA(1,1,24) Model Residuals",
         xaxis=list(title="lag"), yaxis=list(title="ACF/PACF (Residuals)"),
         hovermode = "x unified", legend = list(orientation='h'))

displayForecastErrors <- function(forecastErrors)  {
    # Generate a histogram of the Forecast Errors
    binsize <- IQR(forecastErrors)/4
    sd    <- sd(forecastErrors)
    min   <- min(forecastErrors) - sd
    max   <- max(forecastErrors) + sd
    # Generate 5K normal(0,sd) RVs
    norm <- rnorm(5000, mean=0, sd=sd)
    min2 <- min(norm)
    max2 <- max(norm)
    if (min2 < min) { min <- min2 }
    if (max2 > max) { max <- max2 }
    # Plot red histogram of the forecast errors
    bins <- seq(min, max, binsize)
    histForecast <- hist(forecastErrors, breaks=bins, plot = F)
    histNormal <- hist(norm, plot=FALSE, breaks=bins)
    plot_ly(x = histForecast$mids, y = histForecast$density, type = "bar",
            name="Forecast-Errors Histogram") %>%
        add_lines(x=histNormal$mids/2, y=2*dnorm(histNormal$mids, 0, sd),
                type="scatter", mode="lines",
                name="(Theoretical) Normal Density") %>%
        layout(bargap=0.1, title="Histogram ARIMA(1,1,24) Model Residuals",
                legend = list(orientation = 'h'))
}
displayForecastErrors(residuals(fit24))
```

Step 4: Forecasting with ARIMA Model

Now, we can use our models to make predictions for future PM2.5 AQI. We will use the function `forecast()` to make predictions. In this function, we have to specify the number of periods we want to forecast. Note that the data has been smoothed. Let's make predictions for the next month or July 2016. Then there are $24 \times 30 = 720$ hours, so we specify a horizon h = 720 (Fig. 12.11).

```
ts.forecasts<-forecast(fit, h=720)
# extend time for 30 days (hourly predictions), k=720 hours
forecastDates <- seq(as.POSIXct("2016-05-01 00:00:00 UTC"),
                     as.POSIXct("2016-05-30 23:00:00 UTC"), by = "hour")
plot_ly(x=~dateTime, y=~ts.forecasts$model$fitted, type="scatter",
        mode="lines", name="Observed") %>%
  # add CI lines
  add_lines(x=~forecastDates, y=~ts.forecasts$mean, mode="lines",
            name="Mean Forecast", line=list(size=5)) %>%
  add_lines(x=~forecastDates, y=~ts.forecasts$lower[,1], mode="lines",
            name="Lower 80%", line=list(dash='dash')) %>%
  add_lines(x=~forecastDates, y=~ts.forecasts$lower[,2], mode="lines",
            name="Lower 95%", line=list(dash='dot')) %>%
  add_lines(x=~forecastDates, y=~ts.forecasts$upper[,1], mode="lines",
            name="Upper 80%", line=list(dash='dash')) %>%
  add_lines(x=~forecastDates, y=~ts.forecasts$upper[,2], mode="lines",
            name="Upper 95%", line=list(dash='dot')) %>%
  layout(title = paste0("Beijing PM2.5: Forecast using ",
                        ts.forecasts$method, " Model"),
    xaxis = list(title = "date"), yaxis=list(title="PM2.5"),
    hovermode = "x unified", legend = list(orientation='h'))
```

When plotting the forecasted values with the original smoothed data, we include only the last 5 months in the original smoothed data to see the predicted values clearer. The shaded regions indicate ranges of expected errors. The darker (inner) region represents by *80% confidence range* and the lighter (outer) region bounds by the *95% interval*. Obviously near-term forecasts have tighter ranges of expected errors, compared to longer-term forecasts where the variability naturally expands.

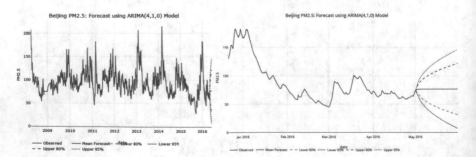

Fig. 12.11 ARIMA(1,1,24) model prediction

12.1.2.1 Autoregressive Integrated Moving Average Extended/Exogenous (ARIMAX) Model

The classical ARIMA model makes prediction of a univariate outcome based only on the past values of the specific forecast variable. It assumes that future values of the outcome linearly depend on an additive representation of the effects of its previous values and some stochastic components.

The extended, or exogenous feature, (vector-based) time-series model (ARIMAX)[6] allows forecasting of the univariate outcome based on multiple independent (predictor) variables. Similar to going from simple linear regression to multivariate linear models, *ARIMAX* generalizes the *ARIMA* model accounting for autocorrelation present in residuals of the linear regression to improve the accuracy of a time-series forecast. ARIMAX models, also called dynamic regression models, represent a combination of ARIMA, regression, and single-input-single-output transfer function models.

When there are no covariates, traditional time-series $y_1, y_2, \ldots, y_n$ can be modeled by ARMA(p, q) model

$$y_t = \phi_1 y_{t-1} + \phi_2 y_{t-2} + \cdots + \phi_p y_{t-p} - \left(\theta_1 \epsilon_{t-1} + \theta_2 \epsilon_{t-2} + \cdots + \theta_q \epsilon_{t-q}\right) + \epsilon_t,$$

where $\epsilon_t \sim N(0, 1)$ is a white Gaussian noise.

The extended dynamic time-series model, ARIMAX, adds the covariates to the right-hand side

$$y_t = \left(\sum_{k=1}^{K} \beta_k x_{k,t}\right) + \phi_1 y_{t-1} + \phi_2 y_{t-2} + \cdots + \phi_p y_{t-p}$$
$$- \left(\theta_1 \epsilon_{t-1} + \theta_2 \epsilon_{t-2} + \cdots + \theta_q z_{t-q}\right) + \epsilon_t,$$

where $x_{k,t}$ is the value of the kth covariate at time t and β_k is its regression coefficient.

In the ARIMAX models, the interpretation of the covariate coefficient, β_k, is somewhat different from the linear modeling case; β_k does not really represent the effect of increasing $x_{k,t}$ by 1 on y_t. The coefficients β_k may be interpreted as conditional effects of the predictor x_k on the prior values of the response variable, y, as the right-hand side of the equation includes lagged values of the response variable.

Using the short-hand back-shift operator representation, the ARMAX model is

---

[6] https://doi.org/10.1109/PESGM.2014.6939802

$$\phi(B)y_t = \left(\sum_{k=1}^{K} \beta_k x_{k,t}\right) + \theta(B)\epsilon_t.$$

Alternatively,

$$y_t = \sum_{k=1}^{K} \left(\frac{\beta_k}{\phi(B)} x_{k,t}\right) + \frac{\theta(B)}{\phi(B)}\epsilon_t,$$

where $\phi(B) = 1 - (\phi_1 B + \phi_2 B + \cdots + \phi_p B^p)$ and $\theta(B) = 1 - (\theta_1 B + \theta_2 B + \cdots + \theta_q B^q)$.

The auto-regressive coefficients get mixed up with both the covariate and the error terms. To clarify these effects, we can look at the regression models with ARMA errors

$$y_t = \sum_{k=1}^{K} \left(\frac{\beta_k}{\phi(B)} x_{k,t}\right) + \eta_t,$$

$$\eta_t = (\phi_1 \eta_{t-1} + \phi_2 \eta_{t-2} + \cdots + \phi_p \eta_{t-p}) - (\theta_1 \epsilon_{t-1} + \theta_2 \epsilon_{t-2} + \cdots + \theta_q z_{t-q} + \epsilon_t).$$

In this formulation, the regression coefficients have a more natural interpretation. Both formulations lead to the same model-based forecasting, but the second one helps with explication and interpretation of the effects.

The back-shift model formulation is

$$y_t = \sum_{k=1}^{K} \left(\frac{\beta_k}{\phi(B)} x_{k,t}\right) + \frac{\theta(B)}{\phi(B)}\epsilon_t,$$

and transfer function models generalize both of these models

$$y_t = \sum_{k=1}^{K} \left(\frac{\beta_k(B)}{v(B)} x_{k,t}\right) + \frac{\theta(B)}{\phi(B)}\epsilon_t.$$

This representation models the lagged effects of covariates (by the $\beta_k(B)$ back-shift operator) and allows for decaying effects of covariates (by the $v(B)$ back-shift operator).

The Box-Jenkins method for selecting the orders of a transfer function model is often challenging in practice.[7]

To estimate the ARIMA errors when dealing with nonstationary data, we can replace $\phi(B)$ with $\nabla^d \phi(B)$, where $\nabla = (1 - B)$ is the differencing operator. This accomplishes both differencing in y_t and x_t prior to fitting ARIMA models with

---

[7] https://doi.org/10.1002/for.3980030307

errors. For model consistency and to avoid spurious regression effects, we do need to *difference* all variables before we estimate models with nonstationary errors.

There are alternative R functions to implement ARIMAX models, e.g., `fore-cast::arima()`, `forecast::Arima()`, and `forecast::auto.arima()` fit extended ARIMA models with multiple covariates and error terms. Remember that there are differences in the signs of the moving average coefficients between the alternative model parameterization formulations. Also, the `TSA::arimax()` function fits the *transfer function model*, not the ARIMAX model.

12.1.2.2   Simulated ARIMAX Example

Let's look at one ARIMAX simulated example representing a 4D synthetic dataset covering $t = 700$ days of records (from "2016-05-01 00:00:00 EDT" to "2018-03-31 00:00:00 EDT"), i.e., 100 weeks of observations, Y = time-series values (volume of customers) and X = (weekday, Holiday, day) exogenous variables (Figs. 12.12, 12.13 and 12.14).

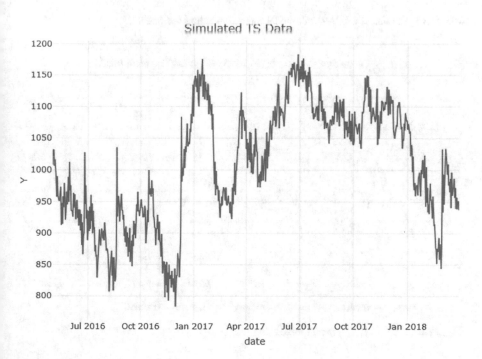

Fig. 12.12   Simulated time-series data

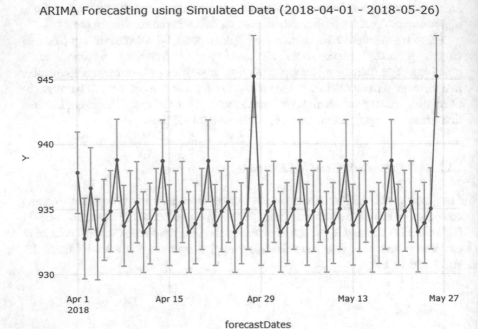

Fig. 12.13 Simulated data ARIMA model forecasting with error bands

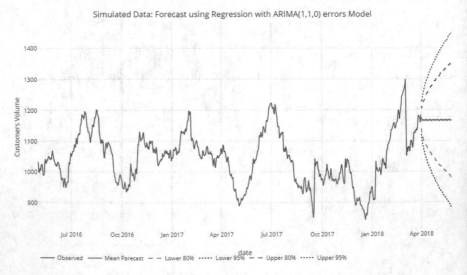

Fig. 12.14 ARIMA(1,1,0) model forecasting

```
library(forecast)
# create the 4D synthetic data, t=700 days, 100 weeks,
# Y=eventArrivals (customers), X=(weekday, NewYearsHoliday, day)
weeks <- 100
days <- 7*weeks
# define holiday effect (e.g., more customers go to stores to shop)
holidayShopping <- rep(0, days)
y <- rep(0, days)
for (i in 1:days) {
  if (i %% 28 == 0) holidayShopping[i] = 1  # Binary feature: Holiday
  else holidayShopping[i] = 0
  # Outcome (Y)
  if (i %% 56 == 0) y[i] = rpois(n=1, lambda=1500)
  else y[i] = rpois(n=1, lambda=1000)
  if (i>2) y[i] = (y[i-2] + y[i-1])/2 + rnorm(n=1, mean=0, sd=20)
  if (i %% 56 == 0) y[i] = rpois(n=1, lambda=1050)
}
# extend time for "days", k=700 days
forecastDates <- seq(as.POSIXct("2016-05-01 00:00:00 UTC"),
                     length.out = days, by = "day")
plot_ly(x=~forecastDates, y=~y, type="scatter", mode="lines",
        name="Y=eventArrivals", line=list(size=5)) %>%
  layout(title = paste0("Simulated TS Data"), hovermode = "x unified",
         xaxis = list(title = "date"), yaxis=list(title="Y"))

synthData <- data.frame(eventArrivals = y, # expected number of arrivals=1000
                        weekday = rep(1:7, weeks),     # weekday indicator variable
                        Holiday = holidayShopping, # Binary feature: Holiday
                        day=1:days)  # day indicator
# Create matrix of numeric predictors
covariatesX <- cbind(weekday = model.matrix(~as.factor(synthData$weekday)),
                     Day = synthData$day,
                     Holiday=synthData$Holiday)
# Generate prospective covariates for external validation/prediction
pred_length <- 56
newCovX <- cbind(weekday =
                 model.matrix(~as.factor(synthData$weekday[1:pred_length])),
                 Day = synthData$day[1:pred_length],
                 Holiday=synthData$Holiday[1:pred_length])
# Remove the intercept
synthX_Data <- covariatesX[,-1]
# Rename columns
colnames(synthX_Data)<-c("Mon","Tue","Wed","Thu","Fri","Sat","Day","Holiday")
colnames(newCovX) <- c("Intercept", colnames(synthX_Data)); colnames(newCovX[,-
1])
# Response (Y) to be modeled as a time-series, weekly oscillations (7-days)
observedArrivals <- ts(synthData$eventArrivals, frequency=7)
# Estimate the ARIMAX model, remove day-index (7)
fitArimaX <- auto.arima(observedArrivals, xreg=synthX_Data[,-7]); fitArimaX
## Regression with ARIMA(1,1,0) errors
## Coefficients:
##          ar1      Mon     Tue      Wed     Thu      Fri     Sat  Holiday
##      -0.5352  -2.9695  0.5318  -5.0786  -2.3569  -1.5485  -0.2679  7.0597
## s.e.  0.0323   2.8401  2.5769   2.9355   2.9356   2.5829   3.0733  4.7087
## sigma^2 = 624.9:  log likelihood = -3237.92
## AIC=6493.84   AICc=6494.1   BIC=6534.79
```

```r
# Predict prospective arrivals, remove Intercept (1) and day-index (8)
predArrivals <- predict(fitArimaX, n.ahead = pred_length,
                            newxreg = newCovX[,-c(1,8)])
forecastDates <- seq(as.POSIXct("2018-04-01 EDT"),
                       length.out = pred_length, by = "day")
df <- as.data.frame(cbind(x=forecastDates, y=predArrivals$pred,
                       errorBar=predArrivals$pred))
plot_ly(data = df) %>%     # add error bars for each CV-mean at Log(Lambda)
    add_trace(x = ~forecastDates, y = ~y, type = 'scatter',
            mode = 'markers+lines',
            name = 'CV MSE', error_y = ~list(array = errorBar/300,
            color="green", opacity=0.5)) %>%
    layout(title = paste0("ARIMA Forecasting using Simulated Data (",
            forecastDates[1], " - ", forecastDates[pred_length], ")"),
            hovermode = "x unified",  # xaxis2 = ax,
            yaxis = list(title = 'Y',   side="left", showgrid = TRUE))


trainingDates <- seq(as.POSIXct("2016-05-01 00:00:00 UTC"),
                 length.out = days, by = "day")
# extend time for 56 days of forward prediction
forecastDates <- seq(as.POSIXct("2018-04-01 EDT"),
                       length.out = pred_length, by = "day")
ts.forecasts <- forecast(fitArimaX, xreg = newCovX[,-c(1,8)])
plot_ly(x=~trainingDates, y=~ts.forecasts$model$fitted, type="scatter",
        mode="lines", name="Observed") %>%
  # add CI lines
  add_lines(x=~forecastDates, y=~ts.forecasts$mean, mode="lines",
            name="Mean Forecast", line=list(size=5)) %>%
  add_lines(x=~forecastDates, y=~ts.forecasts$lower[,1], mode="lines",
            name="Lower 80%", line=list(dash='dash')) %>%
  add_lines(x=~forecastDates, y=~ts.forecasts$lower[,2], mode="lines",
            name="Lower 95%", line=list(dash='dot')) %>%
  add_lines(x=~forecastDates, y=~ts.forecasts$upper[,1], mode="lines",
            name="Upper 80%", line=list(dash='dash')) %>%
  add_lines(x=~forecastDates, y=~ts.forecasts$upper[,2], mode="lines",
            name="Upper 95%", line=list(dash='dot')) %>%
  layout(title = paste0("Simulated Data: Forecast using ",
                        ts.forecasts$method, " Model"),
    xaxis = list(title = "date"), yaxis=list(title="Customers Volume"),
    hovermode = "x unified", legend = list(orientation='h'))
```

There are also Vector Autoregressive Moving-Average Time-Series (VARMA) models that can be used to fit multivariate linear time-series for stationary processes.[8]

12.1.2.3 Google Trends Analytics

We can use dynamic Google Trends data to retrieve information, identify temporal patterns and motifs due to various human experiences, conduct time-series analyses, and forecast future trends. If we retrieve data for multiple terms (keywords or phrases) over different periods of time and across geographic locations, the problem can certainly get complex. We will utilize the R packages gtrendsR and prophet.

```r
# install.packages("prophet", "devtools", "gtrendsR")
library(gtrendsR)
```

---

[8]https://doi.org/10.1016/j.neucom.2018.04.011

```
library(ggplot2)
library(prophet)
```

Let's search *Google Trends* for big data, data science, predictive analytics, and Artificial Intelligence in the USA over the past 10 years, Fig. 12.15. Note that a time span can be specified via:

- "now 1-H": Last hour
- "now 4-H": Last 4 hours
- "now 1-d": Last day
- "now 7-d": Last 7 days
- "today 1-m": Past 30 days
- "today 3-m": Past 90 days
- "today 12-m": Past 12 months
- "today+5-y": Last 5 years (default)
- "all": Since the beginning of Google Trends (2004)
- "Y-m-d Y-m-d": Time span between two dates (e.g., "2012-06-22 2022-06-21").

```
DSPA_trends_US <- gtrends(c("big data", "data science",
                "predictive analytics", "Artificial Intelligence"),
                geo=c("US"), gprop="web", time="2012-06-22 2022-06-21")[[1]]
plot_ly(data = DSPA_trends_US, x=~date, y=~hits, type="scatter",
        mode="lines", color=~keyword, name=~keyword) %>%
  layout(title = "USA: Google Trends (big data, Data Science,
                Predictive Analytics): 2012-2022",
    xaxis=list(title = "date"), yaxis=list(title="Phrase Search Frequency"),
    hovermode = "x unified", legend = list(orientation='h'))
```

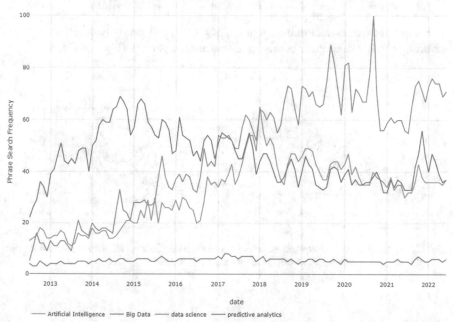

Fig. 12.15 Dynamic Google Trends plot illustrating the temporal changes in various search queries

Similarly, we can also examine *global* geographic trends in searches for "data science", e.g., US, China, UK, etc., by specifying geo = c("US","CN","GB"), gprop = "web". Such plots may expose interesting patterns, trends, and behaviors.

Next, we can use the prophet package to automatically identify patterns and provide forecasts of future searches. The prophet() function call requires the input data-frame to have columns "ds" and "y" representing the time-series dates and values, respectively. *Prophet* implements an additive time-series forecasting model with nonlinear trends fit with annual, weekly, and daily seasonality, plus holiday effects.

```
US_ts <- DSPA_trends_US[which(DSPA_trends_US$keyword == "data science"),
                        names(DSPA_trends_US) %in% c("date","hits")]
US_ts$hits <- as.numeric(US_ts$hits)
colnames(US_ts) <-c("ds","y")
US_ts_prophet <- prophet(US_ts, weekly.seasonality=TRUE)
```

To generate forward looking predictions, we will use the method predict() (Fig. 12.16).

```
future_df <- make_future_dataframe(US_ts_prophet, periods = 730)
US_ts_prophet_pred <- predict(US_ts_prophet, future_df)
plot_ly(x=~US_ts_prophet_pred$ds, y=~US_ts_prophet_pred$yhat, type="scatter",
        mode="markers+lines", name="Prophet Model") %>%
  add_trace(x=~US_ts_prophet_pred$ds, y=~US_ts_prophet_pred$yhat_lower,
            type="scatter", mode="lines", name="Lower Limit") %>%
  add_trace(x=~US_ts_prophet_pred$ds, y=~US_ts_prophet_pred$yhat_upper,
            type="scatter", mode="lines", name="Upper Limit") %>%
  layout(title = "Prophet Additive TS Model", xaxis = list(title = "date"),
         yaxis=list(title="TS Value (data science)"),
         hovermode = "x unified", legend = list(orientation='h'))
```

Finally, we can extract daily, monthly, quarterly, and yearly patterns, along with widening profit model error bands for distance time periods (Fig. 12.17).

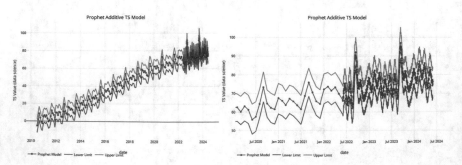

Fig. 12.16 Time-series *prophet* model-based prediction using 2010–2022 data to forecast 2 years of expected future "data science" websearch patterns (US trends)

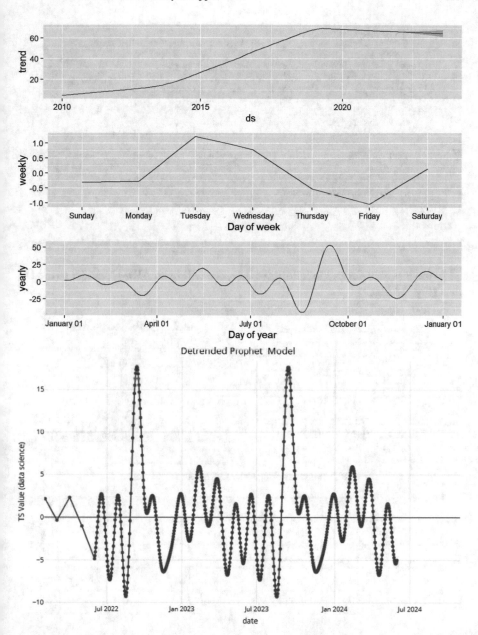

Fig. 12.17 Visualization of *prophet* model patterns. (Top) global model trajectory with weekly and daily trends. (Bottom) Detrended forward *prophet* model forecast for 2 years

```
prophet_plot_components(US_ts_prophet, US_ts_prophet_pred)
plot_ly(x=~US_ts_prophet_pred$ds, y=~US_ts_prophet_pred$trend,
        type="scatter", mode="markers+lines", name="Prophet Model") %>%
  add_trace(x=~US_ts_prophet_pred$ds, y=~US_ts_prophet_pred$trend_lower,
            type="scatter", mode="lines", name="Lower Limit") %>%
    add_trace(x=~US_ts_prophet_pred$ds, y=~US_ts_prophet_pred$trend_upper,
            type="scatter", mode="lines", name="Upper Limit") %>%
  layout(title = "Prophet Model Trend", xaxis = list(title = "date"),
         yaxis=list(title="TS Value (data science)"),
         hovermode = "x unified", legend = list(orientation='h'))

plot_ly(x=~US_ts_prophet_pred$ds, y=~US_ts_prophet_pred$yearly, type="scatter",
mode="markers+lines", name="Prophet Model") %>%
  # add_trace(x=~US_ts_prophet_pred$ds, y=~US_ts_prophet_pred$yearly_lower,
type="scatter", mode="lines", name="Lower Limit") %>%
  # add_trace(x=~US_ts_prophet_pred$ds, y=~US_ts_prophet_pred$yearly_upper,
type="scatter", mode="lines", name="Upper Limit") %>%
  layout(title = "Detrended Prophet  Model",
    xaxis = list(title = "date"), yaxis=list(title="TS Value (data science)"),
hovermode = "x unified", legend = list(orientation='h'))
```

In the last time-series modeling example, we will fit an ARIMA model to the US data (Fig. 12.18).

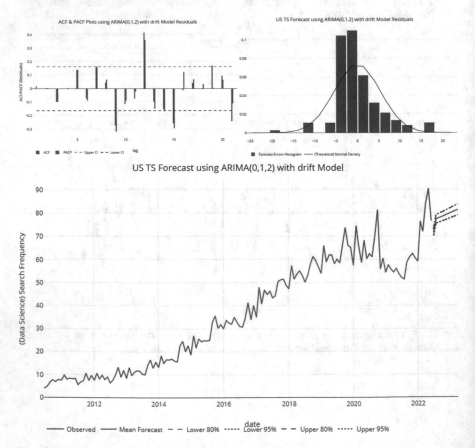

Fig. 12.18 US time-series ARIMA(0,1,2) model

```r
library(forecast)
fit_US_ts <- auto.arima(US_ts$y, approx=F, trace = F); fit_US_ts
acf1 <- Acf(residuals(fit_US_ts), plot = F) # Acf(residuals(fit_US_ts))
ci <- qnorm((1 + 0.95)/2)/sqrt(length(US_ts$y))  # 95% CI
pacf1 <- Pacf(residuals(fit_US_ts), plot = F)           # ACF & PACF
plot_ly(x=~acf1$lag[-1,1,1], y=~acf1$acf[-1,1,1], type="bar",name="ACF") %>%
  add_trace(x=~pacf1$lag[-1,1,1],y=~pacf1$acf[-1,1,1],type="bar",name="PACF") %>%
  # add CI Lines
  add_lines(x=~c(acf1$lag[2,1,1], acf1$lag[length(acf1$lag),1,1]), y=~c(ci, ci),
            mode="lines", name="Upper CI", line=list(dash='dash')) %>%
  add_lines(x=~c(acf1$lag[2,1,1], acf1$lag[length(acf1$lag),1,1]), y=~c(-ci,-ci),
            mode="lines", name="Lower CI", line=list(dash='dash')) %>%
  layout(bargap=0.8, xaxis=list(title="lag"),
         yaxis=list(title="ACF/PACF (Residuals)"),
         title=paste0("ACF & PACF Plots using ", fit_US_ts_forecasts$method,
                      " Model Residuals"),
         hovermode = "x unified", legend = list(orientation='h'))
displayForecastErrors <- function(forecastErrors)  {
    binsize <- IQR(forecastErrors)/4 # Generate a histogram of Forecast Errors
    sd   <- sd(forecastErrors)
    min  <- min(forecastErrors) - sd
    max  <- max(forecastErrors) + sd
    norm <- rnorm(5000, mean=0, sd=sd)  # Generate 5K normal(0,sd) RVs
    min2 <- min(norm);    max2 <- max(norm)
    if (min2 < min) { min <- min2 }
    if (max2 > max) { max <- max2 }
    # Plot red histogram of the forecast errors
    bins <- seq(min, max, length.out = 20)  # binsize)
    histForecast <- hist(forecastErrors, breaks=bins, plot = F)
    histNormal <- hist(norm, plot=FALSE, breaks=bins)
    plot_ly(x = histForecast$mids, y = histForecast$density, type = "bar",
            name="Forecast Errors Histogram") %>%
        add_lines(x=histNormal$mids, y=dnorm(histNormal$mids, 0, sd),
            type="scatter", mode="lines", name="(Theoretical) Normal Density") %>%
        layout(bargap=0.1, legend = list(orientation = 'h'),
               title=paste0("US TS Forecast using ", fit_US_ts_forecasts$method,
                            " Model Residuals"))
}
displayForecastErrors(residuals(fit_US_ts))
fit_US_ts_forecasts <- forecast(fit_US_ts, h=10, level=20)
forecastDates <- seq(as.POSIXct("2022-06-28 GMT"), length.out=10, by = "month")
plot_ly(x=~US_ts$ds, y=~fit_US_ts_forecasts$fitted, type="scatter",
        mode="lines", name="Observed") %>%
  add_lines(x=~forecastDates, y=~fit_US_ts_forecasts$mean, mode="lines",
            name="Mean Forecast", line=list(size=5)) %>%  # add CI Lines
  add_lines(x=~forecastDates, y=~fit_US_ts_forecasts$lower[,1], mode="lines",
            name="Lower 80%", line=list(dash='dash')) %>%
  add_lines(x=~forecastDates, y=~fit_US_ts_forecasts$lower[,1], mode="lines",
            name="Lower 95%", line=list(dash='dot')) %>%
  add_lines(x=~forecastDates, y=~fit_US_ts_forecasts$upper[,1], mode="lines",
            name="Upper 80%", line=list(dash='dash')) %>%
  add_lines(x=~forecastDates, y=~fit_US_ts_forecasts$upper[,1], mode="lines",
            name="Upper 95%", line=list(dash='dot')) %>%
layout(title=paste0("US TS Forecast using ",fit_US_ts_forecasts$method," Model"),
    xaxis = list(title = "date"), legend=list(orientation='h'),
    hovermode = "x unified", yaxis=list(title="(Data Science) Search Frequency"))
```

12.1.3   *Structural Equation Modeling (SEM)-Latent Variables*

Time-series analysis provides an effective strategy to interrogate longitudinal uni-variate data. What happens if we have multiple, potentially associated, measurements recorded at each time point?

SEM is a general multivariate statistical analysis technique that can be used for causal modeling and inference, path analysis, confirmatory factor analysis (CFA), covariance structure modeling, and correlation structure modeling. This method allows *separation of observed and latent variables*. Other standard statistical procedures may be viewed as special cases of SEM, where statistical significance may be less important, and covariances are the core of structural equation models.

Latent variables are features that are not directly observed but may be inferred from the actually observed variables. In other words, a combination or transformation of observed variables can create latent features, which may help us reduce the dimensionality of data. Also, SEM can address multicollinearity issues when we fit models because we can combine some high collinearity variables to create a single (latent) variable, which can then be included into the model.

12.1.3.1   Foundations of SEM

SEMs consist of two complementary components—a *path model*, quantifying specific cause-and-effect relationships between observed variables, and a *measurement model*, quantifying latent linkages between unobservable components and observed variables. The LISREL (LInear Structural RELations) framework represents a unifying mathematical strategy to specify these linkages.[9]

The most general kind of SEM is a structural regression path model with latent variables, which accounts for measurement errors of observed variables. *Model identification* determines whether the model allows for unique parameter estimates and may be based on model degrees of freedom ($df_M \geq 0$) or a known scale for every latent feature. If ν represents the number of observed variables, then the total degrees of freedom for a SEM, $\frac{\nu(1+\nu)}{2}$, corresponds to the number of variances and unique covariances in a variance–covariance matrix for all the features, and the model degrees of freedom, $df_M = \frac{\nu(1+\nu)}{2} - l$, where l is the number of estimated parameters.

Examples include the following:

- *Just-identified model* ($df_M = 0$) with unique parameter estimates.
- *Over-identified model* ($df_M > 0$) desirable for model testing and assessment.
- *Under-identified model* ($df_M < 0$) is not guaranteed unique solutions for all parameters. In practice, such models occur when the effective degrees of freedom are reduced due to two or more highly correlated features, which presents

---

[9]https://doi.org/10.1017/CBO9780511617799

problems with parameter estimation. In these situations, we can exclude or combine some of the features boosting the degrees of freedom.

The latent variables' *scale* property reflects their unobservable, not measurable, characteristics. The latent scale, or unit, may be inferred from one of its observed constituent variables, e.g., by imposing a unit loading identification constraint fixing at 1.0 the factor loading of one observed variable.

An SEM model with appropriate *scale* and degrees of freedom conditions may be identifiable subject to Bollen's two-step identification rule.[10] When both the CFA path components of the SEM model are identifiable, then the whole SR model is identified, and model fitting can be initiated.

- For the confirmatory factor analysis (CFA) part of the SEM, identification requires (1) a minimum of two observed variables for each latent feature, (2) independence between measurement errors and the latent variables, and (3) independence between measurement errors.
- For the path component of the SEM, ignoring any observed variables used to measure latent variables, model identification requires: (1) errors associated with endogenous latent variables to be uncorrelated, and (2) all causal effects to be unidirectional.

The LISREL representation can be summarized by the following matrix equations:

$$\text{Measurement model component} \begin{cases} x = \Lambda_x \xi + \delta, \\ y = \Lambda_y \eta + \epsilon \end{cases}.$$

The path model component is

$$\eta = B\eta + \Gamma \xi + \zeta,$$

where $x_{p \times 1}$ is a vector of observed *exogenous variables* representing a linear function of $\xi_{j \times 1}$ vector of *exogenous latent variables*, $\delta_{p \times 1}$ is a *vector of measurement error*, Λ_x is a $p \times j$ matrix of factor loadings relating x to ξ, $y_{q \times 1}$ is a vector of observed *endogenous variables*, $\eta_{k \times 1}$ is a vector of *endogenous latent variables*, $\epsilon_{q \times 1}$ is a vector of *measurement error for the endogenous variables*, and Λ_y is a $q \times k$ matrix of factor loadings relating y to η. Let's also denote the two variance–covariance matrices, $\Theta_\delta (p \times p)$ and $\Theta_\epsilon (q \times q)$ representing the variance–covariance matrices among the measurement errors δ and ϵ, respectively. The third equation describing the LISREL path model component as relationships among latent variables includes $B_{k \times k}$ a matrix of path coefficients describing the *relationships among endogenous latent variables*, $\Gamma_{k \times j}$ as a matrix of path coefficients representing the *linear effects of exogenous variables on endogenous variables*, $\zeta_{k \times 1}$ as a vector of *errors of*

---

[10] https://doi.org/10.1002/9781118619179

endogenous variables, and the corresponding two variance–covariance matrices $\Phi_{j \times j}$ of the *latent exogenous variables*, and $\Psi_{k \times k}$ of the *errors of endogenous variables*.

The basic statistic for a typical SEM implementation is based on covariance structure modeling and model fitting relies on optimizing an objective function, $\min f(\Sigma, S)$, representing the difference between the model-implied variance–covariance matrix, Σ, predicted from the causal and noncausal associations specified in the model, and the corresponding observed variance–covariance matrix S, which is estimated from observed data. The objective function, $f(\Sigma, S)$ can be estimated as follows.[11]

In general, causation implies correlation, suggesting that if there is a causal relationship between two variables, there must also be a systematic relationship between them. Specifying a set of theoretical causal paths, we can reconstruct the model-implied variance–covariance matrix, Σ, from total effects and unanalyzed associations. The LISREL strategy specifies the following mathematical representation

$$\Sigma = \begin{vmatrix} \Lambda_y A (\Gamma \Phi \Gamma' + \Psi) A' \Lambda_y' + \Theta_\epsilon & \Lambda_y A \Gamma \Phi \Lambda_x' \\ \Lambda_x \Phi \Gamma' A' \Lambda_y' & \Lambda_x \Phi \Lambda_x' + \Theta_\delta \end{vmatrix},$$

where $A = (I - B)^{-1}$. This representation of Σ does not involve the observed and latent exogenous and endogenous variables, x, y, ξ, η. Maximum likelihood estimation (MLE) may be used to obtain the Σ parameters via iterative searches for a set of optimal parameters minimizing the element-wise deviations between Σ and S.

The process of optimizing the objective function $f(\Sigma, S)$ can be achieved by computing the log likelihood ratio, i.e., comparing the likelihood of a given fitted model to the likelihood of a perfectly fit model. MLE estimation requires multivariate normal distribution for the endogenous variables and Wishart distribution for the observed variance–covariance matrix, S.

Using MLE estimation simplifies the objective function to

$$f(\Sigma, S) = \ln |\Sigma| + \mathrm{tr}\left(S \times \Sigma^{-1}\right) - \ln |S| - \mathrm{tr}\left(SS^{-1}\right),$$

where tr() is the trace of a matrix. The optimization of $f(\Sigma, S)$ also requires independent and identically distributed observations, and positive definite matrices. The iterative MLE optimization generates estimated variance–covariance matrices and path coefficients for the specified model. More details on model assessment, using Root Mean Square Error of Approximation (RMSEA) and Goodness of Fit Index, and the process of defining a priori SEM hypotheses are available in.[12]

---

[11] https://doi.org/10.1017/CBO9781139979573
[12] https://doi.org/10.1155/2012/263953

12.1.3.2   SEM Components

The R *Lavaan* package uses the following SEM syntax to represent relationships between variables. We can follow the following structure to specify Lavaan models

Formula type	Operator	Explanation
Latent variable definition	=~	Is measured by
Regression	~	Is regressed on
(Residual) (co)variance	~~	Is correlated with
Intercept	~1	Intercept

For example, in R, we can write the following model

```
model<- ' # regressions
```

$$y1 + y2 \sim f1 + f2 + x1 + x2$$
$$f1 \sim f2 + f3$$
$$f2 \sim f3 + x1 + x2$$

```
# latent variable definitions
```

$$f1 = \sim y1 + y2 + y3$$
$$f2 - \sim y4 + y5 + y6$$
$$f3 = \sim y7 + y8 + y9 + y10$$

```
# variances and covariances
```

$$y1 \sim\sim y1$$
$$y1 \sim\sim y2$$
$$f1 \sim\sim f2$$

```
# intercepts
```

$$y1 \sim 1$$
$$f1 \sim 1$$

```
'
```

Note that the two apostrophe "'" symbols (in the beginning and ending of a model description) are very important in the R-syntax.

12.1.3.3   Case Study—Parkinson's Disease (PD)

Let's use the PPMI dataset in our class file as an example to illustrate SEM model fitting.

Step 1: Collecting Data

The Parkinson's disease data represent a realistic simulation case study to examine associations between clinical, demographic, imaging, and genetics variables for Parkinson's disease. This is an example of big data for investigating important neurodegenerative disorders.

Step 2: Exploring and Preparing the Data

Now, we can import the dataset into R and recode the `ResearchGroup` variable into a binary variable.

```
par(mfrow=c(1, 1))
PPMI <- read.csv("https://umich.instructure.com/files/330397/download?download_frd=1")
summary(PPMI)
PPMI$ResearchGroup <- ifelse(PPMI$ResearchGroup=="Control", "1", "0")
```

This large dataset has 1746 observations and 31 variables with missing data in some of them. A lot of the variables are highly correlated. You can inspect high correlation using *heat maps*, which reorders these covariates according to correlations to illustrate clusters of high correlations (Fig. 12.19).

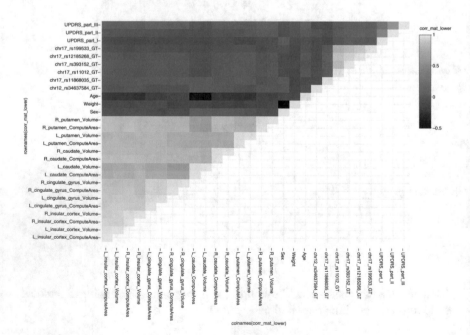

Fig. 12.19   Parkinson's disease data feature correlation heatmap.

```
pp_heat <- PPMI[complete.cases(PPMI), -c(1, 20, 31)]
corr_mat = cor(pp_heat)    # Remove upper triangle
corr_mat_lower = corr_mat
corr_mat_lower[upper.tri(corr_mat_lower)] = NA
# Melt correlation matrix and make sure order of factor variables is correct
corr_mat_melted = melt(corr_mat_lower)
colnames(corr_mat_melted) <- c("Var1", "Var2", "value")
corr_mat_melted$Var1=factor(corr_mat_melted$Var1, levels=colnames(corr_mat))
corr_mat_melted$Var2=factor(corr_mat_melted$Var2, levels=colnames(corr_mat))
plot_ly(x =~colnames(corr_mat_lower), y = ~rownames(corr_mat_lower),
        z = ~corr_mat_lower, type = "heatmap")
```

And there are some specific correlations worth pointing out.

```
cor(PPMI$L_insular_cortex_ComputeArea, PPMI$L_insular_cortex_Volume)
## [1] 0.9837297
cor(PPMI$UPDRS_part_I, PPMI$UPDRS_part_II, use = "complete.obs")
## [1] 0.4027434
cor(PPMI$UPDRS_part_II, PPMI$UPDRS_part_III, use = "complete.obs")
## [1] 0.5326681
```

One way to solve this is to create some latent variables. We can consider the following model.

```
model1<-
  ' Imaging =~ L_cingulate_gyrus_ComputeArea +
L_cingulate_gyrus_Volume+R_cingulate_gyrus_ComputeArea+R_cingulate_gyrus_Volume+R
_insular_cortex_ComputeArea+R_insular_cortex_Volume
    UPDRS=~UPDRS_part_I+UPDRS_part_II+UPDRS_part_III
    DemoGeno =~ Weight+Sex+Age
    ResearchGroup ~ Imaging + DemoGeno + UPDRS
  '
```

Here we try to create three latent variables—Imaging, DemoGeno and UPDRS. Let's fit a SEM model using cfa() (confirmatory factor analysis) function. Before fitting the data, we need to scale our dataset. However, we don't need to scale our binary response variable. We can use the following chunk of code to do the job.

```
Mydata <- scale(PPMI[, -c(1,20,31)]) # avoid scaling ID, Dx, Time
mydata <- data.frame(PPMI$FID_IID, mydata, cbind(PPMI$time_visit,
PPMI$ResearchGroup))
colnames(mydata)[1]  <- "FID_IID"
colnames(mydata)[30] <- "time_visit"
colnames(mydata)[31] <- "ResearchGroup"
```

Step 3: Fitting a Model on the Data
Now, we can start to build the model. The cfa() function we will use shortly belongs to the lavaan R-package.

```
# install.packages("Lavaan", "pbivnorm")
library(lavaan)
# Lavaan requires all variables to be ordered
mydata$ResearchGroup <- as.ordered(mydata$ResearchGroup)
mydata$time_visit <- as.ordered(mydata$time_visit)
# See Lavaan's protocol for handling categorical engo/exogen covariates
fit <- lavaan::cfa(model1, data=mydata, estimator = "PML")
```

The output includes some warning messages. Both our covariance and error term matrices are not positive definite. Nonpositive definite matrices can cause the estimates of our model to be biased. There are many factors that can lead to this problem. In this case, we might create some latent variables that are not a good fit for our data. Let's try to delete the DemoGeno latent variable. We can add Weight, Sex, and Age directly to the regression model.

```
model2 <-
    ' # (1) Measurement Model
    Imaging =~  L_cingulate_gyrus_ComputeArea +
      L_cingulate_gyrus_Volume+R_cingulate_gyrus_ComputeArea +
      R_cingulate_gyrus_Volume+
      R_insular_cortex_ComputeArea+R_insular_cortex_Volume
    UPDRS =~  UPDRS_part_I  +UPDRS_part_II + UPDRS_part_III
    # (2) Regressions
    ResearchGroup ~ Imaging + UPDRS +Age+Sex+Weight
    '
```

When fitting model2, the warning messages are gone. We can see that falsely adding a latent variable can cause those matrices to be not positive definite. Currently, the lavaan functions sem() and cfa() are the same.

```
fit2 <- lavaan::cfa(model2, data=mydata, optim.gradient = "numerical")
summary(fit2, fit.measures=TRUE)
##    Estimator                                   DWLS
##    Optimization method                         NLMINB
##    Number of model parameters                  34
##
##                                          Used        Total
##    Number of observations                1206        1764
## Model Test User Model:
##                                      Standard       Robust
##    Test Statistic                    467.329      328.737
##    Degrees of freedom                     60           60
##    P-value (Chi-square)                0.000        0.000
##    Scaling correction factor                        1.602
##    Shift parameter                                 37.049
##         simple second-order correction
## Model Test Baseline Model:
##    Test statistic                 10440.212     3566.398
##    Degrees of freedom                     45           45
##    P-value                             0.000        0.000
##    Scaling correction factor                        2.952
## User Model versus Baseline Model:
##    Comparative Fit Index (CFI)         0.961        0.924
##    Tucker-Lewis Index (TLI)            0.971        0.943
##    Robust Comparative Fit Index (CFI)                  NA
##    Robust Tucker-Lewis Index (TLI)                     NA
```

```
## Root Mean Square Error of Approximation:
##   RMSEA                                            0.075        0.061
##   90 Percent confidence interval - lower           0.069        0.055
##   90 Percent confidence interval - upper           0.081        0.067
##   P-value RMSEA <= 0.05                             0.000        0.003
##   Robust RMSEA                                                      NA
## Parameter Estimates:
## Latent Variables:
##                    Estimate  Std.Err  z-value  P(>|z|)
##   Imaging =~
##     L_cnglt_gyr_CA    1.000
##     L_cnglt_gyrs_V    0.988    0.010   97.026    0.000
##     R_cnglt_gyr_CA    0.984    0.017   56.291    0.000
##     R_cnglt_gyrs_V    0.975    0.018   54.140    0.000
##     R_nslr_crtx_CA    0.951    0.023   41.932    0.000
##     R_nslr_crtx_Vl    0.930    0.023   40.375    0.000
##   UPDRS =~
##     UPDRS_part_T      1.000
##     UPDRS_part_II     1.990    0.148   13.436    0.000
##     UPDRS_part_III    2.032    0.155   13.111    0.000
## Regressions:
##                    Estimate  Std.Err  z-value  P(>|z|)
##   ResearchGroup ~
##     Imaging           0.003    0.044    0.068    0.946
##     UPDRS            -3.376    0.231  -14.632    0.000
##     Age              -0.042    0.045   -0.920    0.358
##     Sex              -0.063    0.058   -1.095    0.274
##     Weight           -0.023    0.059   -0.389    0.697
## Covariances:
##                    Estimate  Std.Err  z-value  P(>|z|)
##   Imaging ~~
##     UPDRS             0.036    0.013    2.876    0.004
## Intercepts:
##                    Estimate  Std.Err  z-value  P(>|z|)
##    .L_cnglt_gyr_CA    0.057    0.034    1.689    0.091
##    .L_cnglt_gyrs_V    0.058    0.030    1.898    0.058
##    .R_cnglt_gyr_CA    0.054    0.035    1.554    0.120
##    .R_cnglt_gyrs_V    0.055    0.031    1.793    0.073
##    .R_nslr_crtx_CA    0.059    0.041    1.449    0.147
##    .R_nslr_crtx_Vl    0.061    0.033    1.843    0.065
##    .UPDRS_part_I     -0.002    0.043   -0.056    0.956
##    .UPDRS_part_II    -0.002    0.037   -0.059    0.953
##    .UPDRS_part_III   -0.005    0.029   -0.178    0.858
##    .ResearchGroup     0.000
##     Imaging           0.000
##     UPDRS             0.000
## Thresholds:
##                    Estimate  Std.Err  z-value  P(>|z|)
##     ResearchGrp|t1    1.253    0.049   25.770    0.000
## Variances:
##                    Estimate  Std.Err  z-value  P(>|z|)
##    .L_cnglt_gyr_CA    0.022    0.002    8.980    0.000
##    .L_cnglt_gyrs_V    0.043    0.003   12.553    0.000
##    .R_cnglt_gyr_CA    0.065    0.004   17.426    0.000
##    .R_cnglt_gyrs_V    0.081    0.004   21.883    0.000
##    .R_nslr_crtx_CA    0.090    0.006   16.278    0.000
##    .R_nslr_crtx_Vl    0.119    0.005   23.890    0.000
##    .UPDRS_part_I      0.849    0.028   30.547    0.000
##    .UPDRS_part_II     0.443    0.021   21.152    0.000
##    .UPDRS_part_III    0.401    0.021   18.911    0.000
##    .ResearchGroup    -0.586
##     Imaging           0.922    0.050   18.313    0.000
##     UPDRS             0.139    0.019    7.250    0.000
```

12.1.3.4 Outputs of Lavaan SEM

In the output of our model, we have information about how to create these two latent variables (Imaging, UPDRS) and the estimated regression model. Specifically, it gives the following information.

1. First six lines in the header contain the following information:

   • Lavaan version number.
   • Lavaan converge info (normal or not), and # iterations needed.
   • The number of observations that were effectively used in the analysis.
   • The number of missing patterns identified, if any.
   • The estimator that was used to obtain the parameter values (here: ML).
   • The model test statistic, the degrees of freedom, and a corresponding p-value.

2. Next, we have the Model test baseline model and the value for the SRMR.
3. The last section contains the parameter estimates, standard errors (if the information matrix is expected or observed, and if the standard errors are standard, robust, or based on the bootstrap). Then, it tabulates all free (and fixed) parameters that were included in the model. Typically, first the latent variables are shown, followed by covariances and (residual) variances. The first column (Estimate) contains the (estimated or fixed) parameter value for each model parameter; the second column (Std.err) contains the standard error for each estimated parameter; the third column (Z-value) contains the Wald statistic (which is simply obtained by dividing the parameter value by its standard error), and the last column contains the p-value for testing the null hypothesis that the parameter equals zero in the population.

12.1.4 Longitudinal Data Analysis—Linear Mixed Model

As mentioned earlier, longitudinal studies take measurements for the same individual repeatedly through a period of time. Under this setting, we can measure the change after a specific treatment. However, the measurements for the same individual may be correlated with each other. Thus, we need special models that deal with this type of internal interdependencies.

If we use the latent variable UPDRS (created in the output of the SEM model) rather than the research group as our response, we can conduct a longitudinal analysis.

12.1.4.1 Mean Trend

According to the output of model fit, our latent variable UPDRS is a combination of three observed variables-UPDRS_part_I, UPDRS_part_II, and

UPDRS_part_III. We can visualize how average UPDRS differ in different research groups over time; this graph is not shown as it's not very informative, there is no clear pattern emerging.

```
mydata$UPDRS <-
mydata$UPDRS_part_I+1.890*mydata$UPDRS_part_II+2.345*mydata$UPDRS_part_III
mydata$Imaging <- mydata$L_cingulate_gyrus_ComputeArea +
    0.994*mydata$L_cingulate_gyrus_Volume+
    0.961*mydata$R_cingulate_gyrus_ComputeArea+
    0.955*mydata$R_cingulate_gyrus_Volume+
    0.930*mydata$R_insular_cortex_ComputeArea+
    0.920*mydata$R_insular_cortex_Volume
```

The above script stored UPDRS and Imaging variables into mydata. We can use ggplot2 or plotly for data visualization, e.g., plot UPDRS or Imaging across time-visits, blocking for gender. Exploring the group-level and longitudinal graphs may provide more intuition (these graphs are not shown here).

```
sexCast <- as.factor(ifelse(mydata$Sex>0, "Male", "Female"))
mydata$time_visit <- factor(mydata$time_visit,
        levels = c("0","3","6","9","12","18","24","30","36","42","48","54"))
plot_ly(data=mydata, x=~time_visit, y=~UPDRS, color=~sexCast, type="box") %>%
    layout(title="Parkinson's Disease UPDRS across Time", boxmode = "group")
plot_ly(data=mydata, x=~time_visit, y = ~Imaging, color = ~sexCast,
    type = "box") %>%
layout(title="Parkinson's Disease Imaging Score across Time",boxmode="group")
```

We will use the aggregate() function to get the mean, minimum, and maximum of UPDRS for each time point. Then, we will use separate colors for the two research groups and examine their mean trends.

```
# calculate all column means and SDs based on the time_visit column
means <- aggregate( . ~time_visit, data=mydata, mean)
errorBars <- aggregate( . ~time_visit, data=mydata, sd)
plot_ly(x = ~means$time_visit, y = ~means$UPDRS, type = 'scatter',
        mode = 'markers', name = 'UPDRS', marker=list(size=20),
        error_y = ~list(array = errorBars$UPDRS, color = 'black')) %>%
  layout(xaxis=list(title="time_visit"), yaxis=list(title="UPDRS"))
plot_ly(x = ~means$time_visit, y = ~means$Imaging, type = 'scatter',
        mode = 'markers', name = 'Imaging', marker=list(size=20),
        error_y = ~list(array = errorBars$Imaging, color = 'gray')) %>%
  layout(xaxis=list(title="time_visit"), yaxis=list(title="Imaging"))
```

Despite slight overlaps in some lines, the resulting graph illustrates better the mean differences between the two cohorts. The control group (1) appears to have relative lower means and tighter ranges compared to the PD patient group (0). However, we need further data interrogation to determine if this visual (EDA) evidence translates into statistically significant group differences.

Generally speaking, we can always use the *General Linear Modeling (GLM)* framework. However, GLM may ignore the individual differences. So, we can try to fit a *Linear Mixed Model (LMM)* to incorporate different intercepts for each individual participant. Consider the following GLM

$$UPDRS_{ij} \sim$$
$$\beta_0 + \beta_1 * Imaging_{ij} + \beta_2 * ResearchGroup_i +$$
$$\beta_3 * time_{visit_j} + \beta_4 * ResearchGroup_i * time_{visit_j} + \beta_5 * Age_i +$$
$$\beta_6 * Sex_i + \beta_7 * Weight_i + \epsilon_{ij}$$

If we fit a different intercept for each individual (indicated by FID_IID), we obtain the following LMM model

$$UPDRS_{ij} \sim$$
$$\beta_0 + \beta_1 * Imaging + \beta_2 * ResearchGroup + \beta_3 * time_{visit_j} +$$
$$\beta_4 * ResearchGroup_i * time\_visit_j + \beta_5 * Age_i + \beta_6 * Sex_i + \beta_7 * Weight_i + b_i + \epsilon_{ij}$$

The LMM actually has two levels:

Stage 1

$$Y_i = Z_i \beta_i + \epsilon_i,$$

where both Z_i and β_i are matrices.

Stage 2
The second level allows fitting random effects in the model

$$\beta_i = A_i * \beta + b_i.$$

In essence, we can express the full model in matrix form

$$Y_i = X_i * \beta + Z_i * b_i + \epsilon_i.$$

In this case study, we only consider random intercept and avoid including random slopes, however the model can indeed be extended by setting $Z_i = 1$ in the model. Let's compare the two models (GLM and LMM). One R package implementing LMM is `lme4` (Fig. 12.20).

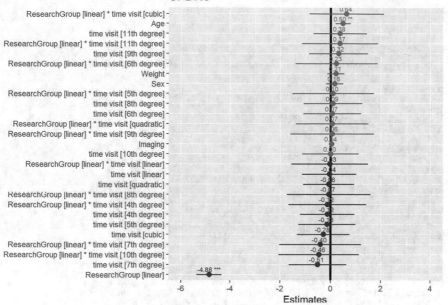

Fig. 12.20 Parkinson's disease linear mixed effect model parameter estimates with confidence limits

```
#install.packages("lme4", "arm")
library(lme4)
library(arm)
#GLM
model.glm <- glm(UPDRS ~ Imaging +ResearchGroup*time_visit +Age +Sex +Weight,
                 data=mydata)
summary(model.glm)
## Coefficients:
##                             Estimate Std. Error t value Pr(>|t|)
## (Intercept)                -2.750810   0.174359 -15.777  < 2e-16 ***
## Imaging                     0.038506   0.019088   2.017   0.0439 *
## ResearchGroup.L            -4.894215   0.247615 -19.765  < 2e-16 ***
## time_visit.L                0.047769   0.596729   0.080   0.9362
## time_visit.Q               -0.027248   0.567875  -0.048   0.9617
## time_visit.C               -0.359290   0.577376  -0.622   0.5339
## time_visit^4               -0.074992   0.601325  -0.125   0.9008
## time_visit^5               -0.159437   0.622539  -0.256   0.7979
## time_visit^6               -0.007191   0.622665  -0.012   0.9908
## time_visit^7               -0.496948   0.633565  -0.784   0.4330
## time_visit^8                0.084922   0.622229   0.136   0.8915
## time_visit^9                0.291171   0.606517   0.480   0.6313
## time_visit^10              -0.032783   0.606037  -0.054   0.9569
## time_visit^11               0.338666   0.588468   0.576   0.5651
## Age                         0.559043   0.109960   5.084 4.29e-07 ***
## Sex                         0.141882   0.121838   1.165   0.2444
## Weight                      0.187597   0.119023   1.576   0.1153
## ResearchGroup.L:time_visit.L  -0.124803   0.843722  -0.148   0.8824
## ResearchGroup.L:time_visit.Q   0.072158   0.802935   0.090   0.9284
## ResearchGroup.L:time_visit.C   0.737085   0.816353   0.903   0.3668
## ResearchGroup.L:time_visit^4  -0.169526   0.850553  -0.199   0.8421
## ResearchGroup.L:time_visit^5   0.128390   0.881095   0.146   0.8842
## ResearchGroup.L:time_visit^6   0.279808   0.880722   0.318   0.7508
## ResearchGroup.L:time_visit^7  -0.482036   0.895889  -0.538   0.5906
## ResearchGroup.L:time_visit^8  -0.076597   0.879914  -0.087   0.9306
## ResearchGroup.L:time_visit^9   0.126178   0.857781   0.147   0.8831
## ResearchGroup.L:time_visit^10 -0.422469   0.857066  -0.493   0.6222
## ResearchGroup.L:time_visit^11  0.503690   0.833222   0.605   0.5456
```

```
#LMM
model.lmm <- lmer(UPDRS ~ Imaging+ResearchGroup*time_visit +Age +Sex +Weight+
            (1|FID_IID), data=mydata)
summary(model.lmm)
## Linear mixed model fit by REML ['lmerMod']
## Random effects:
##  Groups    Name         Variance Std.Dev.
##  FID_IID  (Intercept) 8.006    2.830
##  Residual              3.420    1.849
## Number of obs: 1206, groups:  FID_IID, 440
## Fixed effects:
##                                Estimate Std. Error t value
## (Intercept)                   -2.7546183  0.1789582 -15.393
## Imaging                        0.0448035  0.0271733   1.649
## ResearchGroup.L               -4.8848129  0.2548364 -19.168
## time_visit.L                  -0.0430196  0.5503313  -0.078
## time_visit.Q                  -0.0632548  0.5191771  -0.122
## time_visit.C                  -0.2775249  0.5360783  -0.518
## time_visit^4                  -0.1219084  0.5562893  -0.219
## time_visit^5                  -0.1298668  0.5813000  -0.223
## time_visit^6                   0.0664629  0.5881864   0.113
## time_visit^7                  -0.5073520  0.5864765  -0.865
## time_visit^8                   0.0937665  0.5983303   0.157
## time_visit^9                   0.3177891  0.6011728   0.529
## time_visit^10                  0.0006156  0.5754803   0.001
## time_visit^11                  0.3775198  0.5422331   0.696
## Age                            0.4993501  0.1553835   3.214
## Sex                            0.1577211  0.1776827   0.888
## Weight                         0.2137695  0.1752609   1.220
## ResearchGroup.L:time_visit.L  -0.0309263  0.7784538  -0.040
## ResearchGroup.L:time_visit.Q   0.0653420  0.7341262   0.089
## ResearchGroup.L:time_visit.C   0.6385781  0.7578530   0.843
## ResearchGroup.L:time_visit^4  -0.1183248  0.7866613  -0.150
## ResearchGroup.L:time_visit^5   0.1004386  0.8246079   0.122
## ResearchGroup.L:time_visit^6   0.2331817  0.8323577   0.280
## ResearchGroup.L:time_visit^7  -0.3977826  0.8293361  -0.480
## ResearchGroup.L:time_visit^8  -0.0727112  0.8460313  -0.086
## ResearchGroup.L:time_visit^9   0.0645356  0.8498876   0.076
## ResearchGroup.L:time_visit^10 -0.4617512  0.8141553  -0.567
## ResearchGroup.L:time_visit^11  0.3704408  0.7688145   0.482
#install.packages('sjPlot')
library('sjPlot')
plot_model(model.lmm, vline = "black", sort.est = TRUE, transform = NULL,
            show.values=TRUE, value.offset=0.5, dot.size=2.5, value.size=2.5)
```

Note that we use the notation `ResearchGroup*time_visit` that is same as `ResearchGroup+time_visit+ResearchGroup*time_visit` where R will include both terms and their interaction into the model. According to the model outputs, the LMM model has a relatively smaller AIC. In terms of AIC, LMM may represent a better model fit than GLM.

12.1.4.2   Modeling the Correlation

In the reported summary of the LMM model, we can see a section called `Correlation of Fixed Effects`. The original model made no assumption about the correlation (unstructured correlation). In R, we usually have the following four types of correlation models.

- *Independence*: no correlation

$$\begin{pmatrix} 1 & 0 & 0 \\ 0 & 1 & 0 \\ 0 & 0 & 1 \end{pmatrix}.$$

- *Exchangeable*: correlations are constant across measurements

$$\begin{pmatrix} 1 & \rho & \rho \\ \rho & 1 & \rho \\ \rho & \rho & 1 \end{pmatrix}.$$

- *Autoregressive order 1 (AR(1))*: correlations are stronger for closer measurements and weaker for more distanced measurements

$$\begin{pmatrix} 1 & \rho & \rho^2 \\ \rho & 1 & \rho \\ \rho^2 & \rho & 1 \end{pmatrix}.$$

- *Unstructured*: correlation is different for each occasion

$$\begin{pmatrix} 1 & \rho_{1,2} & \rho_{1,3} \\ \rho_{1,2} & 1 & \rho_{2,3} \\ \rho_{1,3} & \rho_{2,3} & 1 \end{pmatrix}.$$

In the LMM model, the output also seems unstructured. So, we needn't worry about changing the correlation structure. However, if the output under unstructured correlation assumption looks like an exchangeable or AR(1) structure, we may consider changing the LMM correlation structure accordingly.

12.1.5 *Generalized Estimating Equations (GEE)*

Much like the generalized linear mixed models (GLMM), generalized estimating equations (GEE) may be utilized for longitudinal data analysis. If the response is a binary variable like `ResearchGroup`, we need to use the *General Linear Mixed Model (GLMM)* instead of *LMM*. Although GEE represents the marginal model of GLMM, GLMM and GEE are actually different.

In situations where the responses are discrete, there may not be a uniform or systematic strategy for dealing with the joint multivariate distribution of $Y_i = \{(Y_{i,1}, Y_{i,2}, \cdots, Y_{i,n})\}^T$. That's where the GEE method comes into play as it's based on the concept of estimating equations. It provides a general approach for analyzing discrete and continuous responses with marginal models.

GEE is applicable when

1. β, a generalized linear model regression parameter, characterizes systematic variation across covariate levels.
2. The data represents repeated measurements, clustered data, multivariate response.
3. The correlation structure is a nuisance feature of the data.

Notation

- Response variables: $\{Y_{i,1}, Y_{i,2}, \cdots, Y_{i,n_i}\}$, where $i \in [1, N]$ is the index for clusters or subjects, and $j \in [1, n_i]$ is the index of the measurement within cluster/subject.
- Covariate vector: $\{X_{i,1}, X_{i,2}, \cdots, X_{i,n_i}\}$.

The primary focus of GEE is the estimation of the *mean model* $E(Y_{i,j}|X_{i,j}) = \mu_{i,j}$, where

$$g(\mu_{i,j}) = \beta_0 + \beta_1 X_{i,j}(1) + \beta_2 X_{i,j}(2) + \beta_3 X_{i,j}(3) + \cdots + \beta_p X_{i,j}(p) = X_{i,j} \times \beta.$$

This mean model can be any generalized linear model. For example: $P(Y_{i,j} = 1|X_{i,j}) = \pi_{i,j}$ (marginal probability, as we don't condition on any other variables)

$$g(\mu_{i,j}) = \ln\left(\frac{\pi_{i,j}}{1 - \pi_{i,j}}\right) = X_{i,j} \times \beta.$$

Since the data could be clustered (e.g., within subject, or within unit), we need to choose a correlation model. Let

$$V_{i,j} = \text{var}(Y_{i,j}|X_i),$$
$$A_i = \text{diag}(V_{i,j}),$$

the paired correlations are denoted by

$$\rho_{i,j,k} = \text{corr}(Y_{i,j}, Y_{i,k}|X_i),$$

the correlation matrix

$$R_i = (\rho_{i,j,k}), \text{for all } j \text{ and } k,$$

and the paired predictor-response covariances are

$$V_i = \text{cov}(Y_i|X_i) = A_i^{1/2} R_i A_i^{1/2}.$$

Assuming different correlation structures in the data naturally leads to alternative models, see examples above.

GEE Summary
- GEE is a semi-parametric technique because:

  - The specification of a mean model, $\mu_{i,j}(\beta)$, and a correlation model, $R_i(\alpha)$, does not identify a complete probability model for Y_i.
  - The model $\{\mu_{i,j}(\beta), R_i(\alpha)\}$ is semi-parametric since it only specifies the first two multivariate moments (mean and covariance) of Y_i. Higher order moments are not specified.

- Without an explicit likelihood function, to estimate the parameter vector β, (and perhaps the covariance parameter matrix $R_i(\alpha)$) and perform valid statistical inference that takes the dependence into consideration, we need to construct an unbiased estimating function:

  - $D_i(\beta) = \frac{\partial \mu_i}{\partial \beta}$, the partial derivative, w.r.t. β, of the mean model for subject i.
  - $D_i(j, k) = \frac{\partial \mu_{i,j}}{\partial \beta_k}$, the partial derivative, w.r.t. the kth regression coefficient (βk), of the mean model for subject i and measurement (e.g., time point) j.

  Estimating (cost) function

$$U(\beta) = \sum_{i=1}^{N} D_i^T(\beta) V_i^{-1}(\beta, \alpha)\{Y_i - \mu_i(\beta)\}$$

and solving the Estimating Equations leads to parameter estimating solutions

$$0 = U\left(\widehat{\beta}\right) = \left[\sum_{i=1}^{N} \underbrace{D_i^T\left(\widehat{\beta}\right)}_{\text{scale}} \underbrace{\left(V_i^{-1}\widehat{\beta}, \alpha\right)}_{\text{variance weight}} \underbrace{\left(Y_i - \mu_i\left(\widehat{\beta}\right)\right)}_{\text{model mean}}\right].$$

Scale: a change of scale term transforming the scale of the mean, μ_i, to the scale of the regression coefficients (covariates).

Variance weight: the inverse of the variance–covariance matrix is used to weight in the data for subject i, i.e., giving more weight to differences between observed and expected values for subjects that contribute more information.

Model mean: specifies the mean model, $\mu_i(\beta)$, compared to the observed data, Y_i. This fidelity term minimizes the difference between actually-observed and mean-expected (within the i-th cluster/subject).

12.1.5.1 GEE Versus GLMM

There is a difference in the interpretation of the model coefficients between GEE and GLMM. The fundamental difference between GEE and GLMM is in the target of inference: population-average vs. subject-specific. For instance, consider an example where the observations are dichotomous outcomes (Y), e.g., single Bernoulli trials or death/survival of a clinical procedure, that are grouped/clustered into hospitals and units within hospitals, with N additional demographic, phenotypic, imaging, and genetics predictors. To model the failure rate between genders (males vs. females) in a hospital, where all patients are spread among different hospital units (or clinical teams), let Y represent the binary response (death or survival).

In GLMM, the model will be pretty similar to the LMM model

$$\log \left(\frac{P(Y_{ij}=1)}{P(Y_{ij}=0)} | X_{ij}, b_i \right) = \beta_0 + \beta_1 x_{ij} + b_i + \epsilon_{ij}.$$

The only difference between GLMM and LMM in this situation is that GLMM used a *logit link* for the binary response. With GEE, we don't have random intercept or slope terms

$$\log \left(\frac{P(Y_{ij}=1)}{P(Y_{ij}=0)} | X_{ij}, b_i \right) = \beta_0 + \beta_1 x_{ij} + \epsilon_{ij}.$$

In the marginal model (GEE), we are ignoring differences among hospital-units and just aim to obtain population (hospital-wise) rates of failure (patient death) and its association with patient gender. The GEE model fit estimates the odds ratio representing the population-averaged (hospital-wide) odds of failure associated with patient gender. Thus, parameter estimates $(\hat{\beta})$ from GEE and GLMM models may differ because they estimate different things.

12.1.6   PD/PPMI Case Study: SEM, GLMM, and GEE Modeling

Let's use the PD/PPMI dataset (05_PPMI_top_UPDRS_Integrated_LongFormat1. csv) to show longitudinal SEM, GEE, and GLMM data modeling.

Exploratory Data Analytics

```
library(lavaan)
# data   05_PPMI_top_UPDRS_Integrated_LongFormat1.csv (dim(myData) 1764  31)
dataPD <-
  read.csv("https://umich.instructure.com/files/330397/download?download_frd=1",
            header = TRUE)
# dichotomize the "ResearchGroup" variable
dataPD$ResearchGroup <- ifelse(dataPD$ResearchGroup == "Control", 1, 0)
head(dataPD)
```

Next we can display the histogram of patients' number of visits and plot the
UPDRS_Part_I values across time for patients with different genotypes
(*chr17_rs11868035_GT*).

```
library(plotly)
plot_ly(x = ~dataPD$time_visit, type = "histogram", nbinsx = 10) %>%
  layout(title="PD - PPMI Data", bargap=0.1,
         xaxis=list(title="Number of Visits"), yaxis=list(title="Frequency"))
# factorize the categorical features
dataPD_new <- dataPD
dataPD_new$ResearchGroup <- factor(dataPD_new$ResearchGroup)
dataPD_new$Sex <- factor(dataPD_new$Sex)
dataPD_new$chr12_rs34637584_GT <- factor(dataPD_new$chr12_rs34637584_GT)
dataPD_new$chr17_rs11868035_GT <- factor(dataPD_new$chr17_rs11868035_GT)
dataPD_new %>%
    group_by(chr17_rs11868035_GT) %>%
    do(p=plot_ly(., x=~time_visit, y=~UPDRS_part_I, color=~FID_IID,
        name=~paste0("pat=",FID_IID), type="scatter",mode="markers+lines") %>%
        layout(annotations = list(text = ~paste0("GT=",chr17_rs11868035_GT),
                               xref = "x", yref = "y", x=20, y=10)) %>%
        hide_colorbar()) %>% subplot(nrows=2, shareX=TRUE, shareY = TRUE) %>%
  layout(title="Patients UPDRS_part_I by chr17_rs11868035_GT")
```

SEM

Let's define a SEM model (model1) with three latent variables (*Imaging*,
DemoGeno, and *UPDRS*), a single regression relation, and use the lavaan::
sem() method to estimate the model (Fig. 12.21).

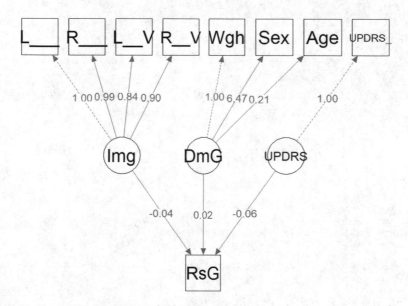

Fig. 12.21 Graphical representation of the PD structural equation model

```r
library(reshape2)  # convert the long-to-wide data format to unwind the time
subsetPD <- dataPD[, c("FID_IID","L_insular_cortex_ComputeArea",
    "R_insular_cortex_ComputeArea","L_cingulate_gyrus_ComputeArea",
    "R_cingulate_gyrus_ComputeArea","L_putamen_Volume" ,
    "R_putamen_Volume", "Sex", "Weight" , "ResearchGroup" , "Age" ,
    "chr12_rs34637584_GT", "chr17_rs11868035_GT",
    "UPDRS_part_I", "UPDRS_part_II", "UPDRS_part_III", "time_visit"
  )]
subsetPD$time_visit <-  c("T1","T2","T3","T4")   # convert all times to 1:4
# First Wide to Long for UPDRS variable.names
subsetPD_long <- melt(subsetPD, id.vars = c("FID_IID",
     "L_insular_cortex_ComputeArea", "R_insular_cortex_ComputeArea",
     "L_cingulate_gyrus_ComputeArea", "R_cingulate_gyrus_ComputeArea",
     "L_putamen_Volume", "R_putamen_Volume", "Sex", "Weight",
     "ResearchGroup", "Age", "chr12_rs34637584_GT", "chr17_rs11868035_GT",
     "time_visit"
   ),  variable.name = "UPDRS", value.name = "UPDRS_value"
 )
# Need to concatenate 2 columns "UPDRS" & "time_visit"
subsetPD_long$UPDRS_Time <-
  do.call(paste, c(subsetPD_long[c("UPDRS", "time_visit")], sep = "_"))


# remove the old "UPDRS" & "time_visit" columns
subsetPD_long1 <-
  subsetPD_long[,!(names(subsetPD_long) %in% c("UPDRS", "time_visit"))]
# Convert Long to Wide format
library(reshape2)
subsetPD_wide <- dcast(subsetPD_long,
    FID_IID + L_insular_cortex_ComputeArea + R_insular_cortex_ComputeArea +
    L_cingulate_gyrus_ComputeArea + R_cingulate_gyrus_ComputeArea +
    L_putamen_Volume + R_putamen_Volume + Sex + Weight + ResearchGroup +
    Age + chr12_rs34637584_GT + chr17_rs11868035_GT ~ UPDRS_Time,
    value.var = "UPDRS_value", fun.aggregate = mean
  )
# SEM modeling
model1 <- '
# latent variable definitions - defining how the latent variables are "manifested
by" a set of observed
# (or manifest) variables, aka "indicators"
# (1) Measurement Model
Imaging =~ L_cingulate_gyrus_ComputeArea + R_cingulate_gyrus_ComputeArea +
L_putamen_Volume + R_putamen_Volume
DemoGeno =~ Weight+Sex+Age
UPDRS =~ UPDRS_part_I_T1
# UPDRS =~ UPDRS_part_II_T1 + UPDRS_part_II_T2 + UPDRS_part_II_T3 +
UPDRS_part_II_T4
# (2) Regressions
ResearchGroup ~ Imaging + DemoGeno + UPDRS
'
summary(subsetPD_wide)
# selective scale features (e.g., avoid scaling Subject ID's)
dataPD2 <- as.data.frame(cbind(scale(subsetPD_wide[, !(
    names(subsetPD_wide) %in% c("FID_IID","Sex","ResearchGroup",
      "chr12_rs34637584_GT", "chr17_rs11868035_GT") )]),
    subsetPD_wide[, (names(subsetPD_wide) %in% c("FID_IID","Sex",
      "ResearchGroup", "chr12_rs34637584_GT", "chr17_rs11868035_GT") )]))
summary(dataPD2)
sem(model1, data = dataPD2, estimator = "MLM")
# Check the SEM model covariances
```

```
fitSEM1@SampleStats@cov
…
summary(fitSEM1)

…
inspect(fitSEM1, "r2")   # lavInspect()
## L_cingulate_gyrus_ComputeArea R_cingulate_gyrus_ComputeArea
##                         0.975                          0.932
##             L_putamen_Volume              R_putamen_Volume
##                         0.687                          0.789
##                        Weight                           Sex
##                        -0.038                        -7.399
##                           Age              UPDRS_part_I_T1
##                        -0.002                          1.000
##                 ResearchGroup
##                         0.049
# install.packages("semPlot")
library(semPlot)
semPlot::semPaths(fitSEM1, intercept = FALSE, whatLabel = "est",
  residuals=FALSE, exoCov=FALSE, edge.label.cex=1.0, label.cex=1.5,sizeMan=8)
```

GLMM

```
# scale some features
dataPD_new$L_cingulate_gyrus_ComputeArea <-
                    scale(dataPD_new$L_cingulate_gyrus_ComputeArea)
dataPD_new$L_cingulate_gyrus_Volume <-
                    scale(dataPD_new$L_cingulate_gyrus_Volume)
dataPD_new$R_cingulate_gyrus_ComputeArea <-
                    scale(dataPD_new$R_cingulate_gyrus_ComputeArea)
dataPD_new$R_cingulate_gyrus_Volume <-
                    scale(dataPD_new$R_cingulate_gyrus_Volume)
dataPD_new$R_insular_cortex_ComputeArea <-
                    scale(dataPD_new$R_insular_cortex_ComputeArea)
dataPD_new$R_insular_cortex_Volume<-scale(dataPD_new$R_insular_cortex_Volume)
# define the outcome UPDRS and imaging latent feature
dataPD_new$UPDRS <- dataPD_new$UPDRS_part_I+1.890*dataPD_new$UPDRS_part_II +
               2.345*dataPD_new$UPDRS_part_III
dataPD_new$Imaging <- dataPD_new$L_cingulate_gyrus_ComputeArea  +
  0.994*dataPD_new$L_cingulate_gyrus_Volume+
  0.961*dataPD_new$R_cingulate_gyrus_ComputeArea+
  0.955*dataPD_new$R_cingulate_gyrus_Volume+
  0.930*dataPD_new$R_insular_cortex_ComputeArea+
  0.920*dataPD_new$R_insular_cortex_Volume
model.glmm <- glmer(ResearchGroup~UPDRS+Imaging+Age+Sex+Weight+(1|FID_IID),
                    data=dataPD_new, family="binomial")
arm::display(model.glmm)
```

```
## glmer(formula = ResearchGroup ~ UPDRS + Imaging + Age + Sex +
##     Weight + (1 | FID_IID), data = dataPD_new, family = "binomial")
##             coef.est coef.se
## (Intercept) -58.42     0.00
## UPDRS        -3.37     0.00
## Imaging       1.89     0.00
## Age           0.88     0.00
## Sex2          1.37     0.00
## Weight        0.66     0.00
## Error terms:
##  Groups    Name        Std.Dev.
##  FID_IID   (Intercept) 50.44
##  Residual              1.00
## ---
## number of obs: 1206, groups: FID_IID, 440
## AIC = 96.8, DIC = -81.9
## deviance = 0.4
dataPD_new$predictedGLMM <- predict(model.glmm, newdata=dataPD_new[1:1764,
        !(names(dataPD_new) %in% c("ResearchGroup", "UPDRS_part_II_T4"))],
        allow.new.levels=T, type="response")  # Lme4::predict.merMod()
# factorize the predictions
dataPD_new$predictedGLMM <- factor(ifelse(dataPD_new$predictedGLMM<0.5,
                                          "0", "1"))
# compare overall GLMM-predicted values against observed ResearchGroup labels
caret::confusionMatrix(dataPD_new$predictedGLMM, dataPD_new$ResearchGroup)
## Confusion Matrix and Statistics
##           Reference
## Prediction    0    1
##          0 1079    0
##          1    0  127
##                Accuracy : 1
##                  95% CI : (0.9969, 1)
##     No Information Rate : 0.8947
##     P-Value [Acc > NIR] : < 2.2e-16
##                   Kappa : 1
##             Sensitivity : 1.0000
##             Specificity : 1.0000
##          Pos Pred Value : 1.0000
##          Neg Pred Value : 1.0000
##              Prevalence : 0.8947
##          Detection Rate : 0.8947
##    Detection Prevalence : 0.8947
##       Balanced Accuracy : 1.0000
table(dataPD_new$predictedGLMM, dataPD_new$ResearchGroup)
```

GEE

We can use several alternative R packages to fit and interpret GEE models, e.g., gee and geepack. Below we will demonstrate GEE modeling of the PD data using gee.

```
library(gee)
# Full GEE model
gee.fit <- gee(ResearchGroup~Imaging+Age+Sex+Weight+UPDRS_part_I,
            data=dataPD_new, family = "binomial", id = FID_IID,
            corstr = "exchangeable", scale.fix = TRUE)
##   (Intercept)        Imaging            Age           Sex2         Weight
## -0.9612274596 -0.0463517707 -0.0099415181 -0.0605950335 -0.0009592125
##   UPDRS_part_I
## -0.5866705844
# reduced model (-UPDRS_part_I)
gee.fit2 <- gee(ResearchGroup~Imaging+Age+Sex+Weight, data=dataPD_new,
        family="binomial", id=FID_IID, corstr="exchangeable", scale.fix=TRUE)
##   (Intercept)        Imaging            Age           Sex2         Weight
##   0.106938489 -0.039306507 -0.010051002 -0.295100962 -0.003659216
summary(gee.fit)
## Call:
## gee(formula = ResearchGroup ~ Imaging + Age + Sex + Weight +
##      UPDRS_part_I, id = FID_IID, data = dataPD_new, family = "binomial",
##      corstr = "exchangeable", scale.fix = TRUE)
## Coefficients:
##                  Estimate  Naive S.E.   Naive z  Robust S.E.   Robust z
## (Intercept)   -0.493190613 0.919383685 -0.5364361 1.012978539 -0.4868717
## Imaging       -0.043221623 0.017254202 -2.5049912 0.018888781 -2.2882166
## Age           -0.010064377 0.009939440 -1.0125698 0.011859148 -0.8486593
## Sex2          -0.111662440 0.252935779 -0.4414656 0.271071683 -0.4119296
## Weight        -0.001522845 0.006949881 -0.2191181 0.007416382 -0.2053353
## UPDRS_part_I  -0.458581284 0.086798874 -5.2832631 0.072854390 -6.2944907
## Working Correlation
##           [,1]      [,2]      [,3]      [,4]
## [1,] 1.0000000 0.2538755 0.2538755 0.2538755
## [2,] 0.2538755 1.0000000 0.2538755 0.2538755
## [3,] 0.2538755 0.2538755 1.0000000 0.2538755
## [4,] 0.2538755 0.2538755 0.2538755 1.0000000
# Individual Wald test and confidence intervals for each covariate
predictors <- coef(summary(gee.fit))
gee.fit.CI <- with(as.data.frame(predictors),
                cbind(lwr=Estimate-1.96*predictors[, 4], est=Estimate,
                upr=Estimate+1.96*predictors[, 4]))
rownames(gee.fit.CI) <- rownames(predictors)
gee.fit.CI
##                      lwr          est          upr
## (Intercept)  -2.47862855 -0.493190613  1.492247323
## Imaging      -0.08024363 -0.043221623 -0.006199612
## Age          -0.03330831 -0.010064377  0.013179554
## Sex2         -0.64296294 -0.111662440  0.419638058
## Weight       -0.01605895 -0.001522845  0.013013264
## UPDRS_part_I -0.60137589 -0.458581284 -0.315786678
# exponentiate the interpret the results as "odds", instead of log-odds
UPSRS_est <- coef(gee.fit)["UPDRS_part_I"]
UPDRS_se <- summary(gee.fit)$coefficients["UPDRS_part_I", "Robust S.E."]
exp(UPSRS_est + c(-1, 1) * UPDRS_se * qnorm(0.975))
## [1] 0.5480585 0.7292131
```

The results show that the estimated UPDRS-assessment effect of the clinical diagnosis (ResearchGroup) taken from the GEE model exchangeable structure (summary(gee.fit)$working.correlation) is -0.458. We can use the robust standard errors (Robust S.E.) to compute the associated 95% confidence interval, $[-0.65; -0.33972648]$.

Finally, remember that in the binomial/logistic outcome modeling, these effect-size estimates are on a log-odds scale. Interpretation of the results is simpler if we exponentiate the values to get the effects in terms of (simple raw) odds. This gives a UPDRS effect of 0.632 and a corresponding 95% confidence interval of [0.548; 0.729]. This CI clearly excludes the origin and suggests a strong association between UPDRS_part_I (nonmotor experiences of daily living) and ResearchGroup (clinical diagnosis).

The three models are not directly comparable because they are so intrinsically different. The table below reports the AIC, but we can also compute other model-quality metrics, for SEM, GLMM, and GEE.

```
AIC(fitSEM1)
AIC(model.glmm)
# install.packages("MuMIn")
library("MuMIn")
# to rank several models based on QIC: model.sel(gee.fit, gee.fit2, rank=QIC)
QIC(gee.fit)
```

Methods	SEM	GLMM	GEE
AIC	4871	96.8	773.9

12.2   Network-Based Approaches

This setion expands our model-based predictive data analytic strategies for analyzing longitudinal data to include model-free techniques. In the first part, we discussed datasets that track the same type of information, for the same subjects, units, or locations, over a period of time. Specifically, we presented classical approaches such as time-series analysis, forecasting using autoregressive integrated moving average (ARIMA) models, structural equation models (SEM), and longitudinal data analysis via linear mixed models. Next, we will present neural-network methods for time-series analysis, including recurrent neural networks (RNN) and long short-term memory (LSTM) Networks.

12.2.1   Background

The time-varying (longitudinal) characteristics of large information flows represent a special case of the complexity, dynamic, and multiscale nature of big biomedical data that we discussed in the Introduction (Chap. 1). In Chap. 2, we saw (4D) space-time functional magnetic resonance imaging (fMRI) data, and in Chap. 10 we discussed streaming data, which also has a natural temporal dimension.

12.2.2 *Recurrent Neural Networks (RNN)*

Earlier, in Chap. 6, we briefly outlined the ideas behind neural networks. Later, in Chap. 14, we will expand this to deep neural networks. Let's now focus on one specific type of neural networks—recursive NN. RNN are a special kind of neural networks that can be applied to predicting the behavior of sequential longitudinal data. An example is forecasting the trends of a periodic sequence. In general, RNN may be memory intensive as they try to keep all past events in memory. Long short-term memory (LSTM) blocks represent a basic building unit for the RNN layers (Fig. 12.22).

LSTM tends to yield better results and utilizes less computer resources, e.g., memory. A LSTM block consists of a cell, an input gate, an output gate, and a forget gate. This allows each cell in the NN to "remember" values over specific time intervals, which explains the *short-memory* in LSTM. The three cell gates mimic the action of a classical artificial neuronal cell part of a multilayer feed-forward network. The gates rely on an activation function that computes a weighted action-potential sum.

Recurrent neural networks address the need to harvest prior knowledge into "learning" new patterns, which has traditionally been a challenge in machine learning. RNN's utilize loops to allow knowledge persistence. Following the Gers–Schmidhuber–Cummins model,[13] the expressions below illustrate the equations describing the LSTM block forward pass with a forget gate (Fig. 12.23).

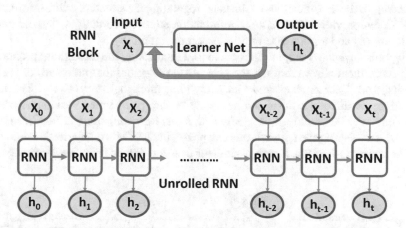

Fig. 12.22 Schematic representation of recurrent neural networks

---

[13] https://doi.org/10.1162/089976600300015015

$$f_t = \sigma_g\left(W_f x_t + U_f h_{t-1} + b_f\right)$$
$$i_t = \sigma_g\left(W_i x_t + U_i h_{t-1} + b_i\right)$$
$$o_t = \sigma_g\left(W_o x_t + U_o h_{t-1} + b_o\right)$$
$$c_t = f_t \circ c_{t-1} + i_t \circ \sigma_c\left(W_c x_t + U_c h_{t-1} + b_c\right)$$
$$h_t = o_t \circ \sigma_h(c_t).$$

In this model:

- $c_0 = 0$ and $h_0 = 0$ are initial values.
- The math operator $\circ$ denotes the matrix-based Hadamard product.
- Subscript $_t$ denotes time (as an iteration step).
- Superscripts ^{d} and ^{h} refer to the number of input features and number of hidden units.
- $x_t \in \mathbb{R}^d$ is the input vector to the LSTM block.
- $f_t \in \mathbb{R}^h$ is the activation vector for the *forget gate*.
- $i_t \in \mathbb{R}^h$ is the activation vector for the *input gate*.
- $o_t \in \mathbb{R}^h$ is the activation vector for the *output gate*.
- $h_t \in \mathbb{R}^h$ is the output vector of the LSTM block.
- $c_t \in \mathbb{R}^h$ is the cell state vector.
- $W \in \mathbb{R}^{h \times d}$, $U \in \mathbb{R}^{h \times h}$ and $b \in \mathbb{R}^h$ represent the weight matrices and bias vector parameters that will be learned during the training phase.

Cell states in LSTM networks, represented as horizontal lines running at the bottom of the LSTM node diagram, aggregates feedback from the entire chain via linear operations. LSTM nodes can add or remove information from the cell state according to the specifications of the gates regulating the structure of the information flow. Gates provide control for the information stream according to sigmoid neural net layers (σ) and a pointwise multiplication operation ($\times$).

Sigmoid layers (σ) output numbers in $[0, 1]$ indicating the throughout proportion each component allows through the gate. At the extremes, output values of zero or one indicate "gate is shut" and "let everything through," respectively. The three LSTM gates directly control the cell state at the given time. Various activation functions may be employed, e.g., *sigmoid*, *hyperbolic tangent*, rectified linear unit (*ReLU*), etc. During the network training phase, the LSTM's total error is minimized on the training data via iterative gradient descent. Either using back-propagation

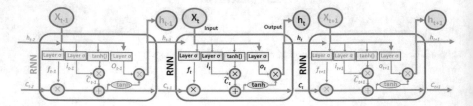

Fig. 12.23 Forward pass with a forget gate for a long short-term memory network

through time, or utilizing the derivative of the error with respect to time, we can derive/change the weights at each iteration (epoch). Note that then the spectral radius of $W < 1$, $\lim_{n \to \infty}(W^n) = 0$. Thus, when gradient descent optimization is used, the error gradients may quickly become trivial (0) with time.

However, with LSTM blocks, the error values are back-propagated from the output, and the total error is kept in the LSTM memory. This continuous error feedback is transferred to each of the gates, which helps in the learning of the gate threshold level. Thus, back-propagation effectively allows the LSTM unit to remember values over long periods of time.

There are also alternative strategies to train the LSTM network, e.g., combining artificial evolution for the *weights to the hidden units* and pseudo-inverse, or support vector machines, for *weights to the output units*. Reinforced LSTM nets may also be trained by policy gradient methods, evolution strategies, or genetic algorithms. Finally, stacks of LSTM networks may be trained by connectionist temporal classification (CTC).[14] This involves finding RNN weight matrices that, using the input sequences, maximize the probability of the outcome labels in the corresponding training datasets, which yields joint alignment and recognition.

12.2.3 Tensor Format Representation

The ability of LSTM RNN to recognize patterns and maintain the state over the length of the time-series are useful for prediction tasks. Time-series typically include correlation between consecutive versions of lagged segments of the time-series. The LSTM recurrent architecture models the persistence of the states by communicating updates between weight estimates across each epoch iteration. RNNs are enhanced by the LSTM cell architecture and facilitate long term persistence in addition to short term memory.

In RNN models, the predictors (X) are represented as tensors, specifically, 3D-array with dimensions samples × timesteps × features.

- Dimension 1: represents the number of samples
- Dimension 2: is the number of time steps (lags)
- Dimension 3: is the number of predictors (1 if univariate or n if multivariate predictors)

The outcome (Y) is also a tensor, however it is univariate and is represented by a 2D-array of dimensions: *samples* × *timesteps*, where the two dimensions are (1) the *number of samples* (D1), and (2) the *number of time steps in a lag* (D2). Thus, the product $D1 \times D2$ is the total sample-size. The proportion of the training set length to the testing set length must be an integer.

---

[14] https://doi.org/10.1007/978-3-642-24797-2_7

For example, suppose we have a total of 1000 observations that are stacked in sets of 200 time points, per lag, 5 time steps (5 lags), and two features (bivariate predictor-vector). Then, the RNN/LSTM input format will be a 3-tensor of dimensions (200, 5, 2).

The *batch size* is the number of training examples in one forward/backward pass of a RNN before a weight update. The choice of batch size requires that these proportions are integral: $\frac{\text{training length}}{\text{batch size}}$, $\frac{\text{testing length}}{\text{batch size}}$. A *time step* is the number of lags included in the training and testing datasets. The *epochs* are the total number of forward-backward pass iterations. Typically, a larger number of epochs improves model performance, unless overfitting occurs at which time the validation accuracy or loss may revert.

For example, if we have daily data over 10 years, we can choose a prediction of window *3650* days (365 days × 10 years). Suppose we use the auto-correlation function (ACF) and determine that the best auto-correlation is seasonal, i.e., 91 (quarterly). We need to make sure that the autocorrelation period is evenly divisible by the forecasting range. If necessary, we may increase the forecasting period. We can select a batch size of 30 time points (days), which should evenly divide the number of testing and training observations. We may also select time steps = 1, to indicate we are only using one lag, and set epochs = 300, which we can adjust to balance the tradeoff between bias and precision. Let's look at a couple of RNN examples.

12.2.4 Simulated RNN Case Study

In this example, we will try to predict a trigonometric function (X) from a noisy wave function (Y). The RNN model is expected to accurately estimate the phase shift of the oscillatory wave functions as well as generate an output (X) that represents a denoised version of the input (Y). The synthetic training dataset represents 25 oscillations each of which containing 50 point samples.

For simplicity, all data are renormalized to the unit interval [0, 1]. In general, all neural networks work best when the data are prenormalized to ensure convergence and biased results. We can use any number of hidden layers, number of neurons, and epochs (learning iterations) (Figs. 12.24 and 12.25).

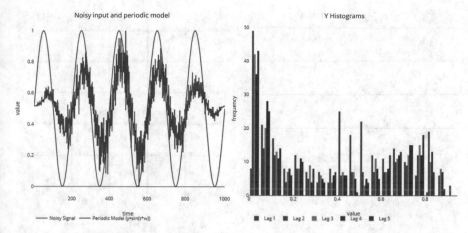

Fig. 12.24 Simulated noisy data from an oscillatory model (left) and RNN model distributions (right)

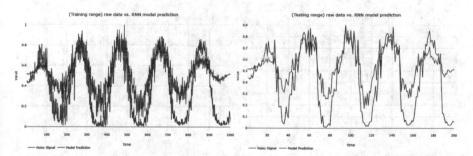

Fig. 12.25 Original noisy data and RNN model prediction over the training range (left) and testing range (right)

```r
# install.packages("rnn")
library("rnn")
set.seed(1234)
# Set oscillatory wave frequency, period, and phase
f <- 5
w <- 2*pi*f
phase <- -pi/8 # offset the real outcome signal
# Note: period of sin(t*w+phase) is 1/10, thus, lag=50
# Create input and output sequences, which are different in terms of
# phase (offset of -pi/3), quadratic amplitude tau=tau(t), and noise N(0,0.3)
n=1000
seq_step= 1.0/n
t <- seq(seq_step, 1, by=seq_step)
tau <- (-4) * (t) * (t-1); length(tau) # plot(t, tau)
## [1] 1000
# x <- sin(t*w+phase) + rnorm(1000, 0, 0.3)  # input
x <- tau * (sin(t*w+phase) + rnorm(1000, 0, 0.3))  # input
y <- sin(t*w)                              # output
# For example, suppose we have a total 1,000 observations that are stacked in
# samples of 200 time-points (per lag), 5 time steps (5 lags), and 1 feature
# (univariate predictor-vector). Then, the RNN/LSTM input format will be a 3-tensor
# of dimensions (100, 10, 1).
X <- matrix(x, nrow = 200, ncol = 5)
Y <- matrix(y, nrow = 200, ncol = 5)
dim(X); dim(Y) ## [1] 200   5
# Plot noisy waves
library(plotly)
plot_ly(x=~c(1:length(as.vector(X))), y=~as.vector(X), type="scatter",
        mode="lines", name="Noisy Signal") %>%
  add_trace(x=~c(1:length(as.vector(X))), y=~as.vector(Y),
            name="Periodic Model (y=sin(t*w))") %>%
  layout(title="Noisy input and periodic model",
         xaxis=list(title="time"), yaxis=list(title="value"),
         legend = list(orientation='h'))
# RNN requires standardization in the interval 0 - 1
min_x <- min(X); min_y <- min(Y); max_x <- max(X); max_y <- max(Y)
# Generic transformation:
# forward (scale), for raw data, and reverse (unscale), for predicted data
my.scale <- function (x, forward=TRUE, input=TRUE) {
  if (input && forward) {           # X=Input==predictors & Forward scaling
    x <- (x - min_x) / (max_x - min_x)
  } else if (input && !forward) {   # X=Input==predictors & Reverse scaling
    x <- x * (max_x - min_x) + min_x
  } else if (!input && forward) {   # X=Output==response & Forward scaling
    x <- (x - min_y) / (max_y - min_y)
  } else if (!input && !forward) {  # X=Output==response & Reverse scaling
    x <- x * (max_y - min_y) + min_y
  }
  return (x)
}
```

```
# Save these transform parameters; center/scale, so we can invert the transforms
# after we get the predicted values
X <- my.scale(X, forward=TRUE, input=TRUE)
Y <- my.scale(Y, forward=TRUE, input=FALSE)
# random 80-20% train-test split
set.seed(1234)
train_index <- sample(seq_len(nrow(X)), size = 0.8*nrow(X))
# Train the RNN model using only the training data
set.seed(1234)
model_rnn <- rnn::trainr(Y = Y[train_index,],
                X = X[train_index,], learningrate = 0.06,
                hidden_dim = 200, learningrate_decay =0.99,
                numepochs = 100, network_type = "rnn")
# Predicted RNN values
pred_Y <- predictr(model_rnn, X)
plot_ly(x=~pred_Y[,1], type="histogram", name="Lag 1") %>%
  add_histogram(x=~pred_Y[,2], name="Lag 2") %>%
  add_histogram(x=~pred_Y[,3], name="Lag 3") %>%
  add_histogram(x=~pred_Y[,4], name="Lag 4") %>%
  add_histogram(x=~pred_Y[,5], name="Lag 5") %>%
  layout(title="Y Histograms",
         xaxis=list(title="value"), yaxis=list(title="frequency"),
         legend = list(orientation='h'))
```

```
plot_ly(x=~c(1:length(as.vector(Y))), y=~as.vector(X), type="scatter",
        mode="lines", name="Noisy Signal") %>%
  add_trace(x=~c(1:length(as.vector(pred_Y))), y=~as.vector(pred_Y),
            name="Model Prediction") %>%
  layout(title="(Training range) raw data vs. RNN model prediction",
         xaxis=list(title="time"), yaxis=list(title="value"),
         legend = list(orientation='h'))
# Plot predicted vs actual timeseries using only the testing data
plot_ly(x=~c(1:length(as.vector(Y[-train_index, ]))),
        y=~as.vector(X[-train_index, ]),
        type="scatter", mode="lines", name="Noisy Signal") %>%
  add_trace(x=~c(1:length(as.vector(pred_Y[-train_index, ]))),
            y=~as.vector(pred_Y[-train_index, ]),name="Model Prediction") %>%
  layout(title="(Testing range) raw data vs. RNN model prediction",
         xaxis=list(title="time"), yaxis=list(title="value"), legend =
list(orientation='h'))
```

Notice the learning process expressed indirectly as progressive improvement of the RNN prediction (blue curve) over the time span. Three specific (longitudinally expressed) characteristics of the forecasting are clearly shown:

- The improved amplitude, signal intensity magnitude
- Reduced level of noise
- Reduction of the phase offset (initial phase was $\frac{\pi}{8}$)

12.2.5   Climate Data Study

Let's use the 2009–2017 Climate Data from the Max Planck Institute in Jena, Germany to demonstrate time-series analysis via RNN. In a nutshell, this sequence data represents a time-series recorded at the Weather Station at the Max Planck

Institute for Biogeochemistry in Jena, Germany. The data include date-time and 14 climate measurements/features (e.g., atmospheric pressure, temperature, and humidity), which are recorded every 10 minutes over 9 years. We will start by ingesting the large climate data (~50 MB).

```
# Download the climate data
clim_data_url <-"https://umich.instructure.com/files/8014703/download?download_frd=1"
clim_data_zip_file <- tempfile(); download.file(clim_data_url,
                                               clim_data_zip_file,mode="wb")
climate_data <- read.csv(unzip(clim_data_zip_file))
dim(climate_data);  head(climate_data)
## [1] 473111       15
##    Date_Time p_mbar T_degC Tpot_K Tdew_degC rh_percent VPmax_mbar Pact_mbar
## 1 1/1/2009 0:10 996.52  -8.02 265.40     -8.90       93.3       3.33      3.11
## 2 1/1/2009 0:20 996.57  -8.41 265.01     -9.28       93.4       3.23      3.02
## 3 1/1/2009 0:30 996.53  -8.51 264.91     -9.31       93.9       3.21      3.01
## 4 1/1/2009 0:40 996.51  -8.31 265.12     -9.07       94.2       3.26      3.07
## 5 1/1/2009 0:50 996.51  -8.27 265.15     -9.04       94.1       3.27      3.08
## 6 1/1/2009 1:00 996.50  -8.05 265.38     -8.78       94.4       3.33      3.14
##    VPdef_mbar sh_g_kg H2OC_mmol_mol rho_g_m3 wv_m_s max_wv_m_s wd_deg
## 1        0.22    1.94          3.12 1307.75   1.03       1.75  152.3
## 2        0.21    1.89          3.03 1309.80   0.72       1.50  136.1
## 3        0.20    1.88          3.02 1310.24   0.19       0.63  171.6
## 4        0.19    1.92          3.08 1309.19   0.34       0.50  198.0
## 5        0.19    1.92          3.09 1309.00   0.32       0.63  214.3
## 6        0.19    1.96          3.15 1307.86   0.21       0.63  192.7
unlink(clim_data_zip_file)
```

Prior to modeling the data using RNN, we can try some exploratory analytics (Figs. 12.26 and 12.27).

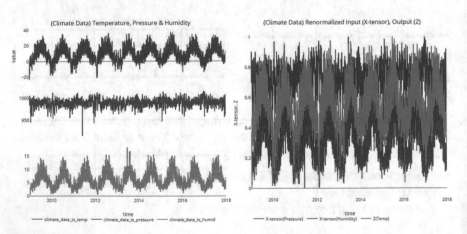

Fig. 12.26 Climate data temperature, atmospheric pressure, and humidity—raw data (left) and normalized data (right)

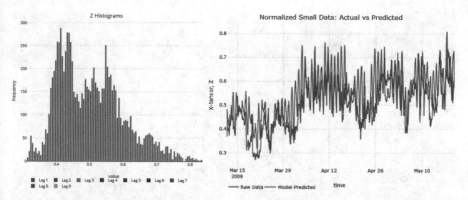

Fig. 12.27 RNN model of climate data—lag histogram frequencies (left) and model prediction vs. expected outcome (right)

```
climate_time <- as.POSIXct(climate_data$Date_Time, format = "%d/%m/%Y %H:%M")
head(climate_time)
## [1] "2009-01-01 00:10:00 EST" "2009-01-01 00:20:00 EST"
## [3] "2009-01-01 00:30:00 EST" "2009-01-01 00:40:00 EST"
## [5] "2009-01-01 00:50:00 EST" "2009-01-01 01:00:00 EST"
# install.packages("zoo")
library("zoo")
# define each time series separately
anyDuplicated(climate_time) # there are some 9517 duplicated date-time points
climate_data_ts_temp <- zoo(climate_data$T_degC[!duplicated(climate_time)],
                            climate_time[!duplicated(climate_time)])
climate_data_ts_pressure <-
                    zoo(climate_data$p_mbar[!duplicated(climate_time)],
                        climate_time[!duplicated(climate_time)])
climate_data_ts_humid <- zoo(climate_data$sh_g_kg[!duplicated(climate_time)],
                            climate_time[!duplicated(climate_time)])
# aggregate TS object including all individual time-series for each feature
climate_data_ts_aggregate = cbind(climate_data_ts_temp,
                            climate_data_ts_pressure, climate_data_ts_humid)
x_len <- dim(climate_data_ts_aggregate)[1]
pl1 <- plot_ly(x=~climate_time[!duplicated(climate_time)],
              y=~climate_data_ts_aggregate[, 1],type="scatter", mode="lines",
              name=colnames(climate_data_ts_aggregate)[1]) %>%
  layout(hovermode = "x unified")
pl2 <- plot_ly(x=~climate_time[!duplicated(climate_time)],
              y=~climate_data_ts_aggregate[, 2], type="scatter", mode="lines",
              name=colnames(climate_data_ts_aggregate)[2]) %>%
  layout(hovermode = "x unified")
pl3 <- plot_ly(x=~climate_time[!duplicated(climate_time)],
              y=~climate_data_ts_aggregate[, 3], type="scatter", mode="lines",
              name=colnames(climate_data_ts_aggregate)[3]) %>%
  layout(hovermode = "x unified")
subplot(pl1, pl2, pl3, nrows=3, shareX = TRUE, titleX = TRUE) %>%
```

```r
  layout(title="(Climate Data) Temperature, Pressure & Humidity",
         xaxis=list(title="time"), yaxis=list(title="value"),
         legend = list(orientation='h'))
# Recall: Bivariate Input=(X,Y); Univariate Outcome (Z)
X <- climate_data_ts_pressure
Y <- climate_data_ts_humid
Z <- climate_data_ts_temp
# RNN requires standardization in the interval 0 - 1
min_x <- min(X); min_y <- min(Y); min_z <- min(Z)
max_x <- max(X); max_y <- max(Y); max_z <- max(Z)
# Generic transformation:
# forward (scale), for raw data, and reverse (unscale), for predicted data
my.scale <- function (x, forward=TRUE, input="X") {
  if (input=="X" && forward) {          # X=Input==predictors & Forward scaling
    x <- (x - min_x) / (max_x - min_x)
  } else if (input=="X" && !forward) {# X=Input==predictors & Reverse scaling
    x <- x * (max_x - min_x) + min_x
  } else if (input=="Y" && forward) { # Y=Input==predictors & Forward scaling
    x <- (x - min_y) / (max_y - min_y)
  } else if (input=="Y" && !forward) {# Y=Input==predictors & Reverse scaling
    x <- x * (max_y - min_y) + min_y
  } else if (input=="Z" && forward) {# Z=Output==predictors & Forward scaling
    x <- (x - min_z) / (max_z - min_z)
  } else if (input=="Z" && !forward){# Z=Output==predictors & Reverse scaling
    x <- x * (max_z - min_z) + min_z
  }
  return (x)
}
X <- my.scale(X, forward=TRUE, input="X")
Y <- my.scale(Y, forward=TRUE, input="Y")
Z <- my.scale(Z, forward=TRUE, input="Z")
X <- matrix(X, nrow = 52560, ncol = 9)
Y <- matrix(Y, nrow = 52560, ncol = 9)
Z <- matrix(Z, nrow = 52560, ncol = 9)
X_tensor <- array(0, dim=c(52560,9,2))
X_tensor[,,1] <- X
X_tensor[,,2] <- Y
dim(X_tensor); dim(Z) ## [1] 52560    9    2
# Plot the time courses of Input (predictor) tensor & Output (Z) time-series
X_ts <- zoo(as.vector(X_tensor[ , , 1]),
                      climate_time[!duplicated(climate_time)])
Y_ts <- zoo(as.vector(X_tensor[ , , 2]),
                      climate_time[!duplicated(climate_time)])
Z_ts <- zoo(as.vector(Z[ , ]), climate_time[!duplicated(climate_time)])
x_len <- dim(X_ts)[1]
plot_ly(x=~climate_time[!duplicated(climate_time)], y=~X_ts,
        type="scatter", mode="lines", name="X-tensor(Pressure)") %>%
  add_trace(x=~climate_time[!duplicated(climate_time)], y=~Y_ts,
        type="scatter", mode="lines", name="X-tensor(Humidity)")  %>%
  add_trace(x=~climate_time[!duplicated(climate_time)], y=~Z_ts,
        type="scatter", mode="lines", name="Z(Temp)")  %>%
  layout(title="(Climate Data) Renormalized Input (X-tensor), Output (Z)",
         xaxis=list(title="time"), yaxis=list(title="X-tensor, Z"), legend =
list(orientation='h'))
```

```
# Train the RNN model using only the training data
# Running the full model is extremely computationally expensive:
#  model_rnn <- rnn::trainr(Y=Z[train_index,], X=X_tensor[train_index, , ])
# We run a reduced model as a demo, only learning on 1:10000, 1 (yr1) time
set.seed(1234)
model_rnn <- rnn::trainr(Y=Z[1:10000, ], X=X_tensor[1:10000, , ],
                 learningrate=0.06, hidden_dim=32, learningrate_decay=0.99,
                 numepochs = 3, network_type = "rnn")
# Predicted RNN values
pred_Z <- predictr(model_rnn, X_tensor[10001:20000, , ])
pl <- plot_ly()
for (i in 1:dim(pred_Z)[2]) {
 pl <- pl %>% add_trace(x=~pred_Z[,i],type="histogram",name=paste0("Lag ",i))
}
pl <- pl %>%
  layout(title="Z Histograms",
         xaxis=list(title="value"), yaxis=list(title="frequency"),
         legend = list(orientation='h'))
pl
x_sample <- climate_time[!duplicated(climate_time)]
x1_sample <- x_sample[10001:20000]
plot_ly(x=~x1_sample, y=~as.vector(Z[10001:20000, 1]),
         type="scatter", mode="lines", name="Raw Data") %>%
  add_trace(x=~x1_sample, y=~as.vector(pred_Z[ , 1]),
         type="scatter", mode="lines", name="Model Predicted")  %>%
  layout(title="Normalized Small Data: Actual vs Predicted",
         xaxis=list(title="time"), yaxis=list(title="X-tensor, Z"), legend =
list(orientation='h'))
```

These results can be significantly improved, by extending the scope of the learning; here we only used 10,000 points (about 10 weeks of data) to learn. In addition, only 10 epochs were used to quickly complete the learning, prediction, and plotting operations. Readers may run the experiment with a larger sample-size, modify the `rnn::trainr()` method parameters, and try to plot observed vs. predicted outcomes (temperature in Celsius). What conclusions can be drawn from this RNN forecasting?

12.2.5.1   Examine the ACF

The Autocorrelation Function (ACF) determines the self-correlation within the time-series by identifying similar repeats or lagged versions of itself. The `stats::acf()` function computes the ACF values for all lags and plots the results. We can also obtain the raw ACF values for the time-series using a new function `my_acf()` (Fig. 12.28).

```
acf(climate_data_ts_temp, lag.max = 52560)
```

The ACF is useful to identify that we have autocorrelation exceeding 0.5 beyond the lag 52,560 (corresponding to annual measures). We can theoretically use this high autocorrelation lag to develop an LSTM model.

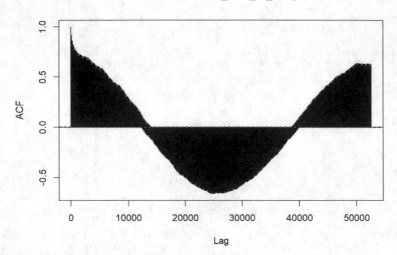

Fig. 12.28   Climate data autocorrelation function (ACF)

We can employ *backtesting* as time-series modeling cross-validation (CV). Cross validation (Chap. 9) allows assessment of the model performance and evaluation of the statistical reliability using data subsampling. To quantify the expected accuracy level and error range, we can iteratively split the complete dataset into training data and a complementary validation set. As time-series have intrinsic auto-correlation, they are distinct from cross-sectional data, so modified cross validation strategies are needed. In particular, the special time dependency on previous time samples has to be accounted for when developing a time-series CV sampling strategy. The simplest way to design a time-series CV approach is to use an offset window, e.g., one lag wide, to select sequential subsamples. This type of strategy is called *backtesting*. This strategy suggests that the time-series CV splits the longitudinal data into multiple contiguous sequences offset by lag-windows, which facilitates testing and validation of past, current, and prospective (in time) observations.

We can employ the rsample package to perform time-series sampling, cross-validation, and backtesting. In our *Climate Data*, one sampling strategy may use 2 years of data (initial $105,120 = 24 \times 6 \times 365 \times 2$ observations, each 10-minutes apart) as a training set. The sequence of time points, covering the third year, will include $105,121 : 157,681$) and will serve as a validation/testing dataset.

```
library(ggplot2)
df_Temp_Time <- data.frame(Z=climate_data$T_degC[!duplicated(climate_time)],
                           t=as.Date(climate_time[!duplicated(climate_time)]))
plot_ly(data=df_Temp_Time, x=~t, y=~Z,
        type="scatter", mode="lines", name="Raw Data") %>%
  layout(title="2009-2017 Temperature (Full Data Set)",
         xaxis=list(title="time"), yaxis=list(title="T_degC"),
         legend = list(orientation='h'))
```

12.2.6   Keras-Based Multicovariate LSTM Time-Series Analysis and Forecasting

The LSTM RNN model may be appropriate if there is evidence of periodicity in the data with autocorrelation that can be estimated using the autocorrelation function (ACF). LSTM uses the autocorrelation estimate to make forward series predictions. For instance, to generate a 1-year *batch forecasting*, we can create a single pass prediction (batch mode) across the entire forecast time domain. This is different from the more traditional time point–based prediction, which can also be used to iteratively estimate a sequence of predictions on prospective time points (intervals). Of course, batch prediction requires that the autocorrelation lag is bigger than the 1 year (365 days, or 52,560 10-minute time increments that the *Climate Data* is actually acquired at).

12.2.6.1   Using Keras to Model Stateful LSTM Time-Series

Recurrent neural networks are typically affected by *gradient vanishing*, which in ML refers to the reduction of the gradient during the process of interactively training the artificial RNN using backpropagation and gradient-based learning. At each learning epoch, the updates of the neural networks' weights are proportional to the magnitude of the *gradient of the error function*, relative to the current weights. The ranges of the activation function values, e.g., hyperbolic tangent, include zero, e.g., $(-1, 1)$ or $[0, 1)$, and the use of chain rule in the backpropagation process may lead to multiplication of n by small, or trivial, numbers. Thus, the gradient estimates of the "front" layers in an n-layer RNN yield to exponential decrease in the gradient (error signal) w.r.t. n, which in turn, leads to very slow training.

Stateful LSTM networks allow fine control over resetting the internal state of the LSTM network, which avoids the gradient vanishing by replacing update multiplication by *addition* when computing the candidate weights at each iteration. This additive update of the state of every cell in the network prevents the rapid decay of the gradient.

Statefulness is a property that determines if the network cell states are reset at each recursive iteration. *Stateless* models reset all cell states at each sequence, whereas *stateful* models propagate the cell states to the next batch; the state of the sample, X_i, located at index i, will be used in the computation of the sample $X_{i + bs}$ in the next batch, where bs is the batch size, i.e., no shuffling is applied. In practice, the `stateful` argument is a Boolean. The default is `stateful = False`, all cell states are reset at the next batch. In this situation, `keras` shuffles (i.e., permutes) the samples in the input matrix X and the dependencies between X_i and $X_{i + 1}$ are lost.

However, when `stateful = True`, the last state for each sample at index *i* in a batch is used as the initial state of the following batch for the same sample index *i*. Building the input matrix *X* is important. Its *shape* depends on `nb_samples`, `timesteps`, `input_dim`, and `batch_size`, which must divide `nb_samples`. A LSTM model with ratio `nb_samples/batch_size` will receive this many blocks of samples, compute each output (number of timesteps for each sample), average the gradients, and propagate it to update the weight parameters vector.

```
# install.packages("keras")
# install.packages("devtools")
# devtools::install_github("rstudio/keras")
library(keras)
```

Here is an example of building a single `keras` stateful LSTM model using a single sample. It's simpler to merge the training and testing datasets into a single long-format dataset, including a separate column specifying the data type—*training* or *testing*. We need to re-specify the *tbl_time* object during the `bind_rows()` step.

```
# install.packages("tidyverse")
# library("tidyverse")
df_train <- as.numeric(df_Temp_Time[1:10000, 1])
df_test <- as.numeric(df_Temp_Time[10001:20000, 1])
```

The LSTM model assumptions include standardized (centered and scaled) input.

```
df_train.std <- scale(df_train)
df_test.std <- scale(df_test)
```

Save the standardizing transformation, so that later we would be able to transform back the results into the domain of the original data.

```
mean.train <- mean(df_train); sd.train <- sd(df_train)
mean.test <- mean(df_test); sd.test <- sd(df_test)
c("TRAIN: center" = mean.train, "TRAIN: SD" = sd.train)
## TRAIN: center      TRAIN: SD
##      -0.996869       5.134751
c("TEST: center" = mean.test, "TEST: SD" = sd.test)
## TEST: center      TEST: SD
##      9.785808       5.693495
```

12.2.6.2 Definitions

To build an LSTM network, let's clarify the basic terms in the architecture.

- *Tensor Format*: The predictors (*X*) are 3D arrays of dimensions $[D_1 = \text{samples},$ $D_2 = \text{timesteps}, D_3 = \text{features}]$, where D_1 is the length of values, D_2 is the number of time steps (lags), and D_3 is the number of predictors (1 if univariate, or n if multivariate).

- *Outcomes/Targets*: (y) is a 2D Array of dimensions: $[D_1 = $ samples, $D_2 = $ timesteps].
- *Training/Testing*: The training and testing length must be evenly divisible (e.g., $\frac{\text{training length}}{\text{testing length}}$ must be an integer).
- *Batch Size*: This represents the number of training examples in one forward/ backward pass of the RNN prior to a weight update. The batch size must be evenly divisible into both the training and the testing lengths.
- *Time Steps*: The time step is the number of lags included in the training/ testing set.
- *Epochs*: The epochs represent the total number of forward/backward pass iterations. Higher number of epochs tends to improve model performance, unless overfitting occurs; however, it's more computationally intense.

12.2.6.3 Keras Modeling of Time-Series Data

Let's try to fit a stateful RNN model for a time-series problem on a subset of the *Climate Data*, covering 2 years of data. For training, we will use the initial $105,120 = 24 \times 6 \times 365 \times 2$ observations, each 10 minutes apart, the third year of observations including 105,121 and 157,681 that will serve as a validation and testing dataset (Fig. 12.29).

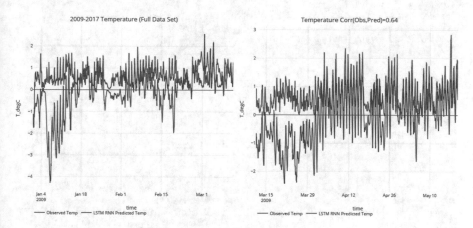

Fig. 12.29 Observed and RNN-predicted temperature

```r
# for stateful LSTM rnn, tsteps can be set to 1
tsteps <- 1
batch_size <- 25
epochs <- 25
# number of elements ahead that are used to make the prediction
lahead <- 1
# Prep the data
df_Temp_Humid_Time <-
                data.frame(C=climate_data$T_degC[!duplicated(climate_time)],
                      H=climate_data$rh_percent[!duplicated(climate_time)],
                      T=as.Date(climate_time[!duplicated(climate_time)]))
df_Temp_train  <- as.numeric(df_Temp_Humid_Time[1:10000, 1])
df_Temp_test   <- as.numeric(df_Temp_Humid_Time[10001:20000, 1])
df_Humid_train <- as.numeric(df_Temp_Humid_Time[1:10000, 2])
df_Humid_test  <- as.numeric(df_Temp_Humid_Time[10001:20000, 2])
# The LSTM model assumptions include standardized (centered & scaled) input
df_Temp_train.std <- scale(df_Temp_train); df_Temp_test.std <-
scale(df_Temp_test)
df_Humid_train.std <- scale(df_Humid_train)
df_Humid_test.std <- scale(df_Humid_test)
x <- as.POSIXct(climate_data$Date_Time, format = "%d/%m/%Y %H:%M")
# Reformat the data as a 3D tensor, see above
df_Temp_train.std.tensor <- array(data = df_Temp_train.std,
                            dim = c(dim(df_Temp_train.std)[1], 1))
df_Humid_train.std.tensor <- array(data=df_Humid_train.std, dim =
c(dim(df_Humid_train.std)[1], 1,1))
y <- df_Temp_train.std.tensor; x <- df_Humid_train.std.tensor
dim(x); dim(y); summary(x); summary(y)
# model formulation
model.2 <- keras_model_sequential()
model.2 %>%
  layer_lstm(units = 50, input_shape = c(tsteps, 1), batch_size = batch_size,
              return_sequences = TRUE, stateful = TRUE) %>%
  layer_lstm(units = 50, return_sequences = FALSE, stateful = TRUE) %>%
  layer_dense(units = 1)
model.2 %>% compile(loss = 'mse', optimizer = 'rmsprop')
### Iterative model fitting on training data
for (i in 1:epochs) {
  model.2 %>% fit(x, y, batch_size = batch_size,
                  epochs = 1, verbose = 1, shuffle = FALSE)
  model.2 %>% reset_states()
}



# Predict (standardized) Temp (C) using (standardized) Humidity (Time=1:10K)
predicted_output <- model.2 %>% predict(x, batch_size = batch_size)
x1 <- as.POSIXct(climate_data$Date_Time, format = "%d/%m/%Y %H:%M")
plot_ly(x=~x1[1:10000], y=~y[ , 1], type="scatter", mode="lines",
        name="Observed Temp") %>%
  add_trace(x=~x1[1:10000], y=~predicted_output[ , 1],
            name="LSTM RNN Predicted Temp") %>%
  layout(title="2009-2017 Temperature (Full Data Set)",
         xaxis=list(title="time"), yaxis=list(title="T_degC"),
         legend = list(orientation='h'))
### Prospective Forecast/Predict Temp using Humidity (time: 10001 - 20000)
x_test <- array(data=df_Humid_test.std, dim=c(dim(df_Humid_test.std)[1],1,1))
y_test <- array(data=df_Temp_test.std, dim = c(dim(df_Temp_test.std)[1], 1))
predicted_output_test <- model.2 %>% predict(x_test, batch_size = batch_size)
plot_ly(x=~x1[10001:20000], y=~y_test[ , 1], type="scatter",
        mode="lines", name="Observed Temp") %>%
  add_trace(x=~x1[10001:20000], y=~predicted_output_test[ , 1],
            name="LSTM RNN Predicted Temp") %>%
  layout(title=paste0("Temperature Corr(Obs,Pred)=", round(cor(y_test[,1],
predicted_output_test[,1]), 2)),
         xaxis=list(title="time"), yaxis=list(title="T_degC"),
         legend = list(orientation='h'))
```

12.2.6.4 Keras Modeling of Image Classification Data (CIFAR10)

The CIFAR-10 dataset includes common images along with human derived class-labels. Specifically, CIFAR-10 contains 60,000 color images of size 32×32, each labeled in 10 different classes: *airplanes, cars, birds, cats, deer, dogs, frogs, horses, ships, and trucks*. There are 6000 images of each class. Each class label is represented as a nominal factor (from 0 to 9), representing the ground truth (human labeling of each image). These labels are included in the file *batches.meta. mat*. Let's try to build a keras deep learning model that can predict the image class labels (Figs. 12.30 and 12.31).

```
library(keras)
# 1. define model parameters
batch_size <- 50
epochs <- 4    # increase the epochs to improve the results
data_augmentation <- TRUE
# 2. prepare the data
# run ?dataset_cifar10 for more info (provided with keras distribution)
cifar10 <- dataset_cifar10()
# 3. scale RGB values in test and train inputs to [0; 1] range
x_train <- cifar10$train$x/255
x_test <- cifar10$test$x/255
y_train <- to_categorical(cifar10$train$y, num_classes = 10)
y_test <- to_categorical(cifar10$test$y, num_classes = 10)
class_labels <- c("airplanes", "cars", "birds", "cats", "deer", "dogs",
                  "frogs", "horses", "ships", "trucks")
y_class_label <- rep("", dim(y_train)[1]); str(y_class_label)
for (i in 1:dim(y_train)[1]) {
  # dim(y_train) is 50000(images) * 10 (class-label-indicators)
  for (j in 1:dim(y_train)[2]) {
    if (y_train[i,j] == 1)
      y_class_label[i] <- class_labels[j]
  }
}
# 4. Visualize some of the images
library("imager")
dim(x_train)    # [1] 50000    32    32     3
# first convert the CSV data (one row per image, 42,000 rows)
N <- 4      # array_3D[index, x, y, RGB]
array_3D <- array(x_train[1001:(1000+N), , , 1], c(4, 32, 32, 3))
mat_2D <- t(matrix(array_3D[1, , , 1], nrow = 32, ncol = 32))
plot(as.cimg(mat_2D))
pretitle <- function(index) {
  sprintf("Image: %d, true label: %s", index, y_class_label[index])
}
op <- par(mfrow = c(2,2), oma = c(5,4,0,0) + 0.1, mar = c(0,0,1,1) + 0.1)
img_3D <- as.cimg(array_3D[N, , , 1], 32, 32, 1)
for (k in 1:N) {
  img_3D <- as.cimg(t(matrix(array_3D[k, , , 1], nrow = 32, ncol = 32)))
  plot(img_3D, k, xlim = c(0,32), ylim = c(32,0), axes=F, ann=T,
main=pretitle(1000+k))
}
```

Image: 1001, true label: trucks   **Image: 1002, true label: deer**

Image: 1003, true label: cats   **Image: 1004, true label: birds**

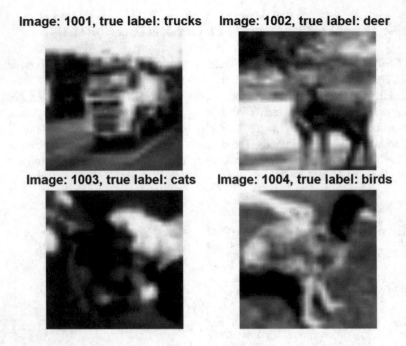

Fig. 12.30 A sample of images (and their corresponding class labels) from the CIFAR-10 archive

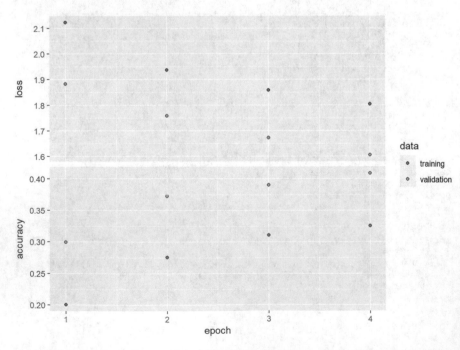

Fig. 12.31 Initial phases (four epochs) of the RNN model fitting—objective function optimization (loss on top) and the model performance (accuracy on bottom). Higher number of iterations will significantly enhance the results

```r
# 5. define a sequential LSTM rNN model #### Initialize sequential model
model.3 <- keras_model_sequential()
model.3 %>%
  # First hidden 2D convolutional layer of 32x32 pixel 2D images
  layer_conv_2d(filter = 32, kernel_size = c(4,4), padding = "same",
    input_shape = c(32, 32, 3) ) %>%
  layer_activation("relu") %>%
  # Second hidden layer
  layer_conv_2d(filter = 32, kernel_size = c(4,4)) %>%
  layer_activation("relu") %>%
  # Use max pooling
  layer_max_pooling_2d(pool_size = c(2,2)) %>%
  layer_dropout(0.25) %>%
  # add 2 additional hidden 2D convolutional layers
  layer_conv_2d(filter = 32, kernel_size = c(4,4), padding = "same") %>%
  layer_activation("relu") %>%
  layer_conv_2d(filter = 32, kernel_size = c(4,4)) %>%
  layer_activation("relu") %>%
  # Use max pooling again
  layer_max_pooling_2d(pool_size = c(2,2)) %>%
  layer_dropout(0.25) %>%
  # Flatten max filtered output into feature vector and feed into dense layer
  layer_flatten() %>%
  layer_dense(512) %>%
  layer_activation("relu") %>%
  layer_dropout(0.5) %>%
  # Outputs from dense layer are projected onto 10-unit output layer
  layer_dense(10) %>%
  layer_activation("softmax")

opt <- optimizer_rmsprop(learning_rate = 0.0001, decay = 1e-6)

### Compile the model (i.e., specify loss function, optimizer, and metrics)
model.3 %>% compile(loss = "categorical_crossentropy",
  optimizer = opt, metrics = "accuracy")

# 6. Model training
if(!data_augmentation){
  history <- model.3 %>% fit(
    x_train, y_train,
    batch_size = batch_size,
    epochs = epochs,
    validation_data = list(x_test, y_test),
    shuffle = TRUE
  )
} else {
    datagen <- image_data_generator(
    rotation_range = 20,
    width_shift_range = 0.2,
```

```r
    height_shift_range = 0.2,
    horizontal_flip = TRUE
  )
  datagen %>% fit_image_data_generator(x_train)
  history <- model.3 %>% fit(
    flow_images_from_data(x_train, y_train, datagen, batch_size = batch_size),
    steps_per_epoch = as.integer(20000/batch_size),
    # increase the iterations (steps_per_epoch) to improve the results
    epochs = epochs,
    validation_data = list(x_test, y_test)
  )
}

# 7. Validation: illustrate the relation between real and predicted class Labels
# Generate the 10 * 10 confusion matrix to
pred_prob <- predict(object = model.3, x = x_test)
y_pred_class_label <- rep("", dim(y_test)[1]); str(y_pred_class_label)
for (i in 1:dim(y_test)[1]) { # dim(y_test)=10000(images)*10 (class-Label-indicators)
  for (j in 1:dim(y_test)[2]) {
    if(j==1) j_max = 1
    else if (pred_prob[i,j] > pred_prob[i, j_max]) j_max = j
  }
  y_pred_class_label[i] <- class_labels[j_max]
}
y_test_class_label <- rep("", dim(y_test)[1]); str(y_test_class_label)
for (i in 1:dim(y_test)[1])
  for (j in 1:dim(y_test)[2]) {
    if (y_test[i,j] == 1)
      y_test_class_label[i] <- class_labels[j]
  }
}
length(y_test_class_label)==length(y_pred_class_label)
table(y_pred_class_label, y_test_class_label)
caret::confusionMatrix(as.factor(y_pred_class_label),
as.factor(y_test_class_label))

# 7. Plot algorithm convergence history  # plot(history, type="L")
time <- 1:epochs
hist_df <- data.frame(time=time, loss=history$metrics$loss,
            acc=history$metrics$accuracy, valid_loss=history$metrics$val_loss,
            valid_acc=history$metrics$val_accuracy)
plot_ly(hist_df, x = ~time)  %>%
  add_trace(y = ~loss, name = 'training loss', type="scatter", mode='lines') %>%
  add_trace(y = ~acc, name='training accuracy', type="scatter",
            mode='lines+markers') %>%
  add_trace(y = ~valid_loss, name = 'validation loss', type="scatter",
            mode = 'lines+markers') %>%
  add_trace(y = ~valid_acc, name = 'validation accuracy', type="scatter",
            mode = 'lines+markers') %>%
  layout(title="CIFAR-10 Classificaiton - NN Model Performance",
            legend = list(orientation = 'h'), yaxis=list(title="metric"))

# 8. Plot heatmap of actual and predicted CIFAR-10 class Labels
heat <- table(factor(y_pred_class_label), factor(y_test_class_label))
plot_ly(x =~class_labels, y = ~class_labels, z = ~matrix(heat, 10,10),
    name="NN Model Performance", hovertemplate=paste('<i>Matching</i>: %{z:.0f}',
        '<br><b>True</b>: %{x}<br>', '<b>Pred</b>: %{y}'),
        colors = 'Reds', type = "heatmap") %>%
  layout(title="CIFAR-10 Predicated vs. True Image Class Labels",
        xaxis=list(title="Actual Image Class"),
        yaxis=list(title="Predicted Image Class"))
```

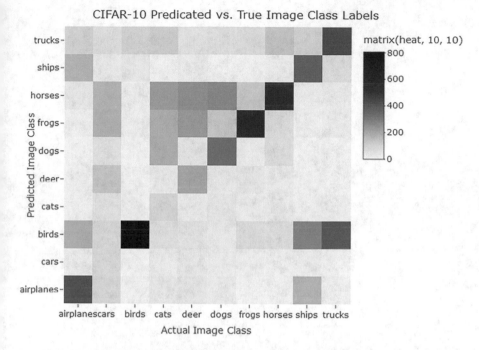

Fig. 12.32 Heatmap of actual (horizontal axis) and predicted (vertical axis) image class labels (CIFAR-10 data)

Although the prediction accuracy may only be around 0.38, this is pretty good as the expected random classifier accuracy is just 0.1 (1 out of 10 classes). The heatmap shows the predominant agreement between real image class labels and their predicted counterparts, see the main diagonal of the confusion matrix shown on Fig. 12.32.

Additional examples illustrating the practical use of keras are included in Chap. 14.

Chapter 13
Function Optimization

Most data-driven scientific inference, qualitative, quantitative, and visual analytics involve formulating, understanding the behavior of, and optimizing objective (cost) functions. Presenting the mathematical foundations of representation and interrogation of diverse spectra of objective functions provides mechanisms for obtaining effective solutions to complex big data problems. (Multivariate) *function optimization* (minimization or maximization) is the process of searching for arguments $x_1, x_2, x_3, \cdots, x_n$ that either minimize or maximize the multivariate cost (objective) function $f(x_1, x_2, x_3, \cdots, x_n)$. In this chapter, we will specifically discuss (1) constrained and unconstrained optimization; (2) Lagrange multipliers; (3) linear, quadratic, and (general) nonlinear programming; and (4) data denoising.

13.1 General Optimization Approach

In its most general framework, most continuous optimization algorithms involve iteratively traversing the domain and assessing the change of the objective function. The process may start by specifying the initial conditions or randomly choosing the starting point in the domain, the traversal pattern, and the iterative update scheme to estimate the cost-function. The last part is computed step-wise using a fixed update mechanism that leads to the iterative estimation of the next domain point. The updating function typically involves the relative change of the objective function, e.g., gradient computed at past and current locations. *Gradient descent optimization* relies on updates computed using the negative gradient, whereas the updating of the points in *momentum-based optimization*, an alternative to stochastic gradient descent, uses a scaled exponential moving average of the gradients. The main differences between alternative optimization algorithms are the *objective function* and the *update protocol*. The pseudocode shown in Table 13.1 defines the general algorithmic framework for unconstrained continuous optimization. Following the (random or seeded) initialization of the algorithm (x_o) in the domain of the objective function, we traverse the domain by iteratively updating the current location (x_i) step-by-step using a predefined *learning rate*, or step-size, (γ), a momentum decay factor (α), a *functor* (ϕ) of the objective function (f), and its gradient (∇f), as well as the current location (x_{i-1}) and all the past locations $\left(\{x_j\}_{j=o}^{i-1} \right)$.

Various performance metrics may be used to drive the learning in the optimization process. Such loss metrics reward good optimizers or penalize bad optimizers, respectively. When minimizing an objective function, the loss representing the sum of the objective values over all iterations, i.e., the cumulative regret, leads to good optimizers that converge rapidly.

13.1.1   First-Order Gradient-Based Optimization

First-order gradient-based methods for solving unconstrained optimization problems are applicable for twice continuously differentiable (multivariate) functions. The solutions $x^* \in \mathbb{R}^n$ satisfy:

- The gradient (vector) of the objective function at x^*, $\nabla f(x^*) = 0$, i.e., $\frac{\partial f(x^*)}{\partial x_j} = 0, \forall 1 \le j \le n$.
- The Hessian matrix of the objective function at x^* is positive definite, $\nabla^2 f(x^*) > 0$, i.e., $u' \nabla^2 f(x^*) u > 0$, $\forall u \in \mathbb{R}^n - \{0\}$, where the *prime* notation, $'$, denotes the transpose (matrix or vector).

Gradient-based optimization involves four steps:

- Set iteration index $k = 0$, choose a starting point x_o, and specify a convergence criterion,
- Check if convergence conditions are as follows: satisfied; If yes, stop and declare current location x_k as the solution; if not, continue.
- Propose a step direction (descent direction in $\mathbb{R}^n$) by defining a vector $\nu_k \in \mathbb{R}^n \backslash \{0\}$ that reduces the value of the objective function relative to its value at the current location x_k.
- Calculate the step-size, $a_k > 0$, in the direction ν_k that yields $f(x_k + a_k \nu_k) < f(x_k)$.
- Update the current solution $x_k \rightarrow x_{k+1} = x_k + a_k \nu_k$ and the iteration index $k \rightarrow (k+1)$ and continue repeating the process (step 2).

Different gradient-based methods may utilize alternative strategies to calculating the descent direction (step 3) or the estimation of the step-size, learning-rate, in step 4. For instance:

- The *steepest descent method* (gradient descent) uses the normalized negative gradient vector as the search direction at each iteration. Specifically, the search direction is $\nu_k = \frac{\nabla f(x_k)}{\|\nabla f(x_k)\|^2}$ and the step-size is $a_k = \arg\min_a f(x_k - a\nu_k)$.

Table 13.1 Outline of a generic optimization pseudo algorithm

Generic initialization	Objective function $f(\cdot)$
Iterator	for $i = 1, 2, 3, \cdots$ do
	$\Delta x = \phi\left(\{x_j,\ f(x_j),\ \nabla f(x_j)\}_{j=0}^{i-1}\right) =$
	gradient descent : $\qquad\qquad \phi(\cdot) = -\gamma \nabla f(x_{i-1})$
	stochastic gradient descent : $\phi(\cdot) = -\gamma \nabla f(x_{i-1}) + \xi(i-1)$, $\xi(i-1)$ is stochastic noise
	momentum method : $\qquad\quad \phi(\cdot) = -\gamma \left(\displaystyle\sum_{j=0}^{i-1} \alpha^{(i-j-1)} \nabla f(x_j)\right)$
	neural net ML : $\qquad\qquad \phi(\cdot) : W_{ij}^{\text{layer}} = W_{ij}^{\text{layer}} - \gamma \dfrac{\partial J}{\partial W_{ij}^{\text{layer}}},$ $J =$ NN error, $W_{ij}^{\text{layer}} =$ weight coefficients
Stopping condition	If stopping criterion is met $\qquad$ return location x_{i-1}
	Otherwise $\qquad\qquad\qquad\qquad$ update the location $x_i = x_{i-1} + \Delta x$
for loop end	

- The *conjugate descent method* attempts to move more directly towards the optimum by taking into account the history of the prior gradients. Although there are many alternative formulations, the general search direction is computed by

$$
\nu_k = \begin{cases} -\nabla f(x_k) & \text{if } k = 0 \\ -\nabla f(x_k) + \gamma_k \nu_{k-1} & \text{if } k > 0 \end{cases},
$$

where one option for the coefficients is the Fletcher–Reeves estimate $\gamma_k = \frac{\|\nabla f(x_k)\|^2}{\|\nabla f(x_{k-1})\|^2}$. The learning-rate is a number that satisfies

$$
\begin{cases} f(x_k) - f(x_k + a_k \nu_k) \geq -\delta a_k (\nabla f(x_k))' \nu_k \\ \|(\nabla f(x_k + a_k \nu_k))'\|^2 \leq -\sigma (\nabla f(x_k))' \nu_k \end{cases},
$$

for some pair of positive real values $0 < \delta < \sigma < 1$.

13.1.2 Second-Order Hessian-Based Optimization

Second-, and higher-order, optimization methods require more intensive calculations of the *search direction* and *step-size* that typically involve the Hessian matrix.

13.1.2.1 Newton's Method

The Newton's method[1] is often an improvement over first-order gradient descent optimization methods as it also utilizes the second-order Hessian to estimate the search descent direction and the learning rate, as follows:

- The descent direction is computed by $\nu_k = [\nabla^2 f(x_k)]^{-1} \times [\nabla f(x_k)]$.
- The learning-rate is calculated by $a_k = \arg \min_a f(x_k - a\nu_k)$.

13.1.2.2 Broyden–Fletcher–Goldfarb–Shanno (BFGS) Method

The Hessian matrix computation is generally expensive and there are several alternatives to the brute-force Newton's method that improve the computational efficiency. The Broyden–Fletcher–Goldfarb–Shanno (BFGS) method[2] represents one

---

[1] https://doi.org/10.1137/1037125
[2] https://doi.org/10.1016/0009-2614(85)80574-1

such alternative using the gradient to *approximate* the inverse of the Hessian matrix $H_k^{-1} = \left[\nabla^2 f(x_k)\right]^{-1}$ at each iteration index k and at each point x_k

$$H_k^{-1} = \left[\nabla^2 f(x_k)\right]^{-1} = \left(I_{n \times n} - \frac{s_k y_k'}{s_k' y_k}\right) \times H_{k-1}^{-1} \times \left(I_{n \times n} - \frac{s_k y_k'}{s_k' y_k}\right) + \frac{s_k y_k'}{s_k' y_k},$$

where the s and y vectors are defined by $s_x = x_k - x_{k-1}$ and $y_k = \nabla f(x_k) - \nabla f(x_{k-1})$.

13.1.3   Gradient-Free Optimization

As we saw above, gradient-based methods heavily rely on information about the gradient and the Hessian of the objective-function to estimate both the search-direction and the learning-rate. This makes such techniques applicable only to cost functions that have multiple continuous derivatives. Alternative strategies are required for solving more elaborate optimization problems involving multivariate objective functions that may not be continuous, differentiable, or possessing multiple minima.

The Nelder–Mead method[3] represents an example of a convex simplex technique that yields effective and computationally tractable solutions to complex unconstrained optimization problems. Simulated annealing (SANN)[4] is an alternative strategy that tracks the proximity of the initial point to the optimal point. It can't always guarantee a global minimum is reached since the iterative dynamics mimic physical cooling of a material in a heath bath, a process that allows uphill and downhill search-directional moves. Most simulated annealing implementations utilize the Metropolis algorithm, which simulates the change in the system energy subject to the cooling process. The optimization tends to converge to a final frozen steady state with a low energy.

13.2   Free (Unconstrained) Optimization

Unconstrained function optimization refers to searching for extrema without restrictions for the domain of the cost function, $\Omega \ni \{x_i\}$. The extreme value theorem[5] suggests that a solution to the free optimization processes, $\min_{x_1, x_2, x_3, \cdots, x_n} f(x_1, x_2, x_3, \cdots, x_n)$ or $\max_{x_1, x_2, x_3, \cdots, x_n} f(x_1, x_2, x_3, \cdots, x_n)$, may be obtained by a gradient vector descent method. This means that

---

[3] https://doi.org/10.1080/00401706.1975.10489269
[4] https://doi.org/10.1126/science.220.4598.671
[5] https://doi.org/10.1007/s11590-012-0587-0

we can minimize/maximize the objective function by finding solutions to $\nabla f = \left\{ \frac{\partial f}{\partial x_1}, \frac{\partial f}{\partial x_2}, \cdots, \frac{\partial f}{\partial x_n} \right\} = \{0, 0, \cdots, 0\}$. Solutions to this equation, $x_1, \cdots, x_n$, will present candidate (local) minima and maxima.

In general, identifying critical points using gradients or tangent planes, where the partial derivatives are trivial, may not be sufficient to determine the *extrema* (*minima* or *maxima*) of multivariate objective functions. Some critical points may represent inflection points, or local extrema that are far from the global *optimum* of the objective function. The eigenvalues of the Hessian matrix, which includes the second-order partial derivatives at the critical points, provide clues to pinpoint extrema. For instance, invertible Hessian matrices that are positive definite (i.e., all eigenvalues are positive) yield a local minimum at the critical point, whereas negative definite Hessians (i.e., all eigenvalues are negative) at the critical point suggests that the objective function has a local maximum. Hessians with both positive and negative eigenvalues yield a saddle point for the objective function at the critical point where the gradient is trivial.

There are two complementary strategies to avoid being trapped in *local* extrema. First, we can run many iterations with different initial vectors. At each iteration, the objective function may achieve a (local) maximum/minimum/saddle point. Finally, we select the overall minimal (or maximal) value from all iterations. Another adaptive strategy involves either adjusting the step sizes or accepting solutions *in probability* (e.g., simulated annealing is one example of an adaptive optimization).

13.2.1 Example 1: Minimizing a Univariate Function (Inverse-CDF)

The cumulative distribution function (CDF) of a real-valued random process X, also known as the distribution function of X, represents the probability that the random variable X does not exceed a certain level. Mathematically speaking, the CDF of X is $F_X(x) = P(X \leq x)$. Recall the Chap. 1 discussions of Uniform, Normal, Cauchy, Binomial, Poisson, and other discrete and continuous distributions. Try the Probability Distributome *navigator* and explore the dynamic representations of density and distribution functions included in the Distributome *calculators*.

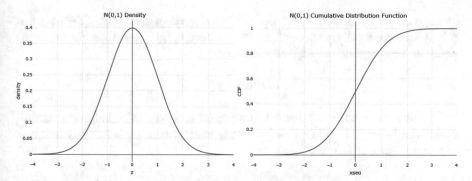

Fig. 13.1 Normal density (left) and cumulative distribution (right) functions

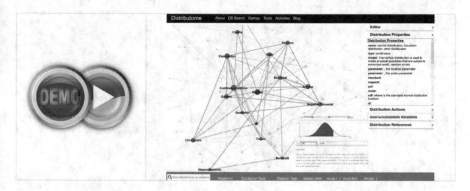

http://distributome.org/V3/

For each $p \in [0, 1]$, the *inverse distribution function*, also called *quantile function* (e.g., qnorm), yields the critical value (x) at which the probability of the random variable is less than or equal to the given probability (p). When the CDF F_X is continuous and strictly increasing, the value of the inverse CDF at p, $F^{-1}(p) = x$, is the unique real number x such that $F(x) = p$. Below, we will plot the probability density function (PDF) and the CDF for *Normal* distribution in R (Fig. 13.1).

```r
library(plotly)
par(mfrow=c(1,2), mar=c(3,4,4,2))
z <- seq(-4, 4, 0.1)  # points from -4 to 4 in 0.1 steps
q <- seq(0.001, 0.999, 0.001)  # prob quantiles, 0.1% to 99.9% in 0.1% steps
dStandardNormal <- data.frame(Z=z, Density=dnorm(z, mean=0, sd=1),
                              Distribution=pnorm(z, mean=0, sd=1))
z <- seq(-4, 4, 0.01)
density<-dnorm(z, 0, 1)
plot_ly(x=~z, y=~density, type="scatter", mode="lines",
        name="N(0,1) Density") %>% layout(title="N(0,1) Density")
# Compute the CDF
xseq <- seq(-4, 4, 0.01); CDF <- pnorm(xseq, 0, 1)
plot_ly(x=~xseq, y=~CDF, type="scatter", mode="lines", name="N(0,1) CDF") %>%
  layout(title="N(0,1) Cumulative Distribution Function")
```

Suppose we are interested in computing, or estimating, the inverse-CDF from first principles. Specifically, to invert the CDF, we need to be able to solve the following equation (representing our objective function)

$$CDF(x) - p = 0.$$

The `stats::uniroot` and `stats::nlm` R functions do *nonlinear minimization* of a function *f* using a Newton–Raphson algorithm. Let's test that optimization using $N(\mu = 100, \sigma = 20)$.

```
set.seed(1234)
x <- rnorm(1000, 100, 20)
pdf_x <- density(x)
# Interpolate the density, the values returned when input x values are outside
[min(x): max(x)] should be trivial
f_x <- approxfun(pdf_x$x, pdf_x$y, yleft=0, yright=0)
cdf_x <- function(x) { # Manual computation of CDF by numeric integration
  v <- integrate(f_x, -Inf, x)$value
  if (v<0) v <- 0
  else if(v>1) v <- 1
  return(v)
}
# Finding the roots of the inverse-CDF function by hand (CDF(x)-p=0)
invcdf <- function(p){
  uniroot(function(x){cdf_x(x) - p}, range(x))$root
  # alternatively, can use nlm(function(x){cdf_x(x) - p}, 0)$estimate
  # minimum - the value of the estimated minimum of f.
  # estimate - the point at which the minimum value of f is obtained.
}
invcdf(0.5)
## [1] 99.16995
# We can validate that the inverse-CDF is correctly computed: F^{-1}(F(x))==x
cdf_x(invcdf(0.8))
## [1] 0.8
```

The ability to compute exactly, or at least estimate, the inverse-CDF function is important for many reasons. For instance, generating random observations from a specified probability distribution (e.g., normal, exponential, or gamma distribution) is an important task in many scientific studies. One approach for such random number generation from a specified distribution evaluates the inverse CDF at random uniform $u \sim U(0, 1)$ values. Recall that in Chap. 10, we showed an example of generating random uniform samples using atmospheric noise. This is just one example of the key ability to estimate the inverse CDF function quickly, efficiently, and reliably.

Let's see why inverting the CDF using random uniform data works. Consider the cumulative distribution function (CDF) of a probability distribution from which we are interested in sampling. If the CDF has a closed form analytic expression and is invertible, then we can generate a random sample from that distribution by evaluating the inverse CDF at u, where $u \sim U(0, 1)$. This is possible since a continuous CDF, F, is a one-to-one mapping of the domain of the CDF (range of X) into the interval $[0, 1]$. Therefore, if U is a uniform random variable on $[0, 1]$, then

$X = F^{-1}(U)$ has the distribution F. Suppose $U \sim Uniform[0, 1]$, then $P(F^{-1}(U) \leq x) = P(U \leq F(x))$, by applying F to both sides of this inequality, since F is monotonic. Thus, $P(F^{-1}(U) \leq x) = F(x)$, since $P(U \leq u) = u$ for uniform random variables.

13.2.2   Example 2: Minimizing a Bivariate Function

Let's look at the function $f(x_1, x_2) = (x_1 - 3)^2 + (x_2 + 4)^2 + x_1 x_2$. We define the function in R and utilize the optim function to obtain the extrema points in the support of the objective function and/or the extrema values at these critical points. Everyone can optimize in memory or by hand the simpler objective function $g(x_1, x_2) = (x_1 - 3)^2 + (x_2 + 4)^2$, which attains its minimum (0) at $x_1 = 3$ and $x_2 = -4$.

```
require("stats")
f <- function(x) { (x[1] - 3)^2 + (x[2] +4)^2 + x[1]*x[2]}
initial_x <- c(0, -1)
x_optimal <- optim(initial_x, f, method="CG") # performs minimization
x_min <- x_optimal$par
# x_min contains the domain values where the (local) minimum is attained
x_min   # critical point/vector
## [1]   6.666667 -7.333335
x_optimal$value  # extrema value of the objective function
## [1] -24.33333
```

The function optim() supports six alternative optimization strategies:

- *Nelder–Mead*: The Nelder–Mead method is robust but relatively slow. It works reasonably well for nondifferentiable functions.
- *BFGS*: Broyden–Fletcher–Goldfarb–Shanno quasi-Newton method (also known as a variable metric algorithm), uses function values and gradients to build up a picture of the surface to be optimized.
- *CG*: conjugate gradients method[6] is fragile but successful in larger optimization problems because it's unnecessary to save large matrices.
- *L-BFGS-B*[7]: allows box constraints.
- *SANN*: a variant of simulated annealing, belonging to the class of stochastic global optimization methods.
- *Brent*: Brent's method[8] applies to one-dimensional problems only. It's useful in cases where optim() is used inside other functions where only the method argument can be specified.

Let's first visualize the objective function (when running the code, the interactive 3D plot allows stereotactic manipulation of the scene using the mouse) (Fig. 13.2)

---

[6] https://doi.org/10.1002/wics.13
[7] https://doi.org/10.1145/279232.279236
[8] https://doi.org/10.1016/S0096-3003(02)00190-X

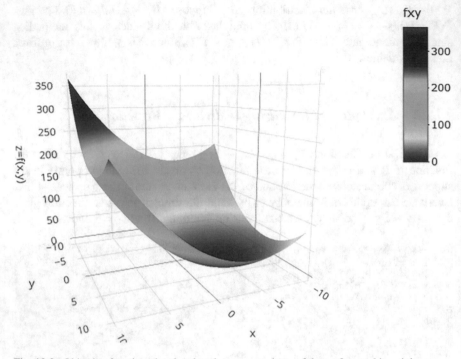

Fig. 13.2 Objective function plot showing the concave shape of the surface and its minimum

$$f(x_1, x_2) = (x_1 - 3)^2 + (x_2 + 4)^2.$$

```
library(magrittr, plotly)
grid_length <- 101   # define the function on a grid (matrix n*n)
f_function <- function(A) { # input bivariate matrix n*2 (x1, x2)
  A <- matrix(A, ncol=2)
  z <- (A[, 1]-3)^2 + (A[, 2]+4)^2 # or the second function + A[, 1] * A[, 2]
  return(z)
}
# define the 2D grid to plot function over
x <- seq(-10, 10, length = grid_length)
y <- seq(-10, 10, length = grid_length)
A <- as.matrix(expand.grid(x, y))
colnames(A) <- c("x", "y")
# evaluate function
z <- f_function(A)
# put x, y and z values in a data.frame for plotting
df <- data.frame(A, z)
z_label <- list(title = "z=f(x,y)")
fxy = matrix(z, grid_length,grid_length)
myPlot <- plot_ly(x=~x, y=~y, z=~fxy, type="surface",
            colors = colorRamp(rainbow(8)), opacity=0.9, hoverinfo="none") %>%
  layout(scene = list(zaxis=z_label))
myPlot
```

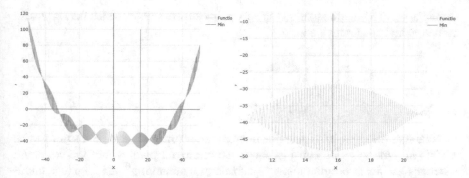

Fig. 13.3 Global (left) and magnified local (right) oscillatory behaviors of the objective function

13.2.3 Example 3: Using Simulated Annealing to Find the Maximum of an Oscillatory Function

Consider the function $f(x) = 10 \sin (0.3x) \times \sin (1.3x^2) - 0.00002x^4 + 0.3x + 35$. Maximizing $f()$ is equivalent to minimizing $-f()$. Let's plot this oscillatory function, and then find and report its critical points and extrema values, Fig. 13.3.

The function $\text{optim}()$ returns two important results:

- par: the best set of domain parameters found to optimize the function
- value: the extreme values of the function corresponding to par

```
funct_osc <- function (x) {
  -(10*sin(0.3*x)*sin(1.3*x^2) - 0.00002*x^4 + 0.3*x+35)
}
res <- optim(16, funct_osc, method = "SANN",
             control = list(maxit = 20000, temp = 20, parscale = 20))
res$par    ## [1] 15.66167
res$value  ## [1] -48.49418
library("plotly")
x <- seq(-50, 50, 0.01);    y <- funct_osc(x)
df <- as.data.frame(cbind(x,y))
plot_ly(data=df, x = ~x, y = ~y, name = 'Function',
        type = 'scatter', mode = 'lines', line = list(width = 0.2)) %>%
  add_segments(x = res$par, xend = res$par, y = -50, yend = 100,
               name = 'Min', line = list(width = 1.0))
```

13.3 Constrained Optimization

13.3.1 Equality Constraints

When there are support restrictions, dependencies, or other associations between the domain variables $x_1, x_2, \ldots, x_n$, constrained optimization needs to be applied. For example, we can have k equations specifying these restrictions, which may represent certain model constraints, e.g.,

$$\begin{cases} g_1(x_1, \ x_2, \ \ldots, \ x_n) = 0 \\ \qquad\qquad \vdots \\ g_k(x_1, \ x_2, \ \ldots, \ x_n) = 0 \end{cases}.$$

Note that the right-hand sides of these equations may always be assumed to be trivial (0), otherwise we can just move the nontrivial parts within the constraint functions g_i. Linear programming,[9] quadratic programming,[10] and Lagrange multipliers[11] may be used to solve such equality-constrained optimization problems.

13.3.2   *Lagrange Multipliers*

We can merge the equality constraints within the objective function ($f \to f^*$). Lagrange multipliers represents a typical solution strategy that turns the *constrained* optimization problem ($\min_x f(x)$ subject to $g_i(x_1, x_2, \ldots, x_n) = 0$, $1 \leq i \leq k$), into an *unconstrained* optimization problem:

$$f^*(x_1, x_2, \ \ldots, \ x_n; \lambda_1, \lambda_2, \ \ldots, \ \lambda_k) = f(x_1, x_2, \ \ldots, \ x_n) + \sum_{i=1}^{k} \lambda_i g_i(x_1, x_2, \ \ldots, \ x_n).$$

Then, we can apply traditional unconstrained optimization schemas, e.g., extreme value theorem, to minimize the unconstrained problem

$$f^*(x_1, x_2, \ \ldots, \ x_n; \lambda_1, \lambda_2, \ \ldots, \ \lambda_k) = f(x_1, x_2, \ \ldots, \ x_n) + \lambda_1 g_1(x_1, x_2, \ \ldots, \ x_n)$$
$$+ \cdots + \lambda_k g_k(x_1, x_2, \ \ldots, \ x_n).$$

This represents an unconstrained optimization problem using Lagrange multipliers.

The solution of the constrained problem is also a solution to

---

[9] https://doi.org/10.1007/978-3-030-03243-2_648-1

[10] https://doi.org/10.1093/imamat/7.1.76

[11] https://doi.org/10.1073/pnas.42.10.767

$$\nabla f^* = \left[\underbrace{\frac{\partial f}{\partial x_1}, \frac{\partial f}{\partial x_2}, \cdots, \frac{\partial f}{\partial x_n}}_{\text{initial variables}}; \underbrace{\frac{\partial f}{\partial \lambda_1}, \frac{\partial f}{\partial \lambda_2}, \cdots, \frac{\partial f}{\partial \lambda_k}}_{\text{Lagrange multipliers}} \right] = [0, 0, \cdots, 0].$$

13.3.3 Inequality Constrained Optimization

There are no general solutions for arbitrary inequality constraints; however, partial solutions do exist when some restrictions on the form of constraints are present.

When both the constraints and the objective function are `linear functions` of the domain variables, then the problem can be solved by linear programming.

13.3.3.1 Linear Programming (LP)

LP works when the objective function is a linear function. The constraint functions are also linear combinations of the same variables. Consider the following elementary (`minimization`) example

$$\min_{x_1, x_2, x_3} \left(-3x_1 - 4x_2 - 3x_3 \right)$$

subject to:

$$\begin{cases} 6x_1 + 2x_2 + 4x_3 & \leq 150 \\ x_1 + x_2 + 6x_3 & \geq 0 \\ 4x_1 + 5x_2 + 4x_3 & = 40 \end{cases}$$

The exact solution is $x_1 = 0$, $x_2 = 8$, $x_3 = 0$, and can be computed using the package `lpSolveAPI` to set up the constraint problem and the generic `solve()` method to find its solutions.

```
# install.packages("lpSolveAPI")
library(lpSolveAPI)
lps.model <- make.lp(0, 3) # define 3 variables
# add the constraints as a matrix of linear coefficients, relations and RHS
add.constraint(lps.model, c(6, 2, 4), "<=", 150)
add.constraint(lps.model, c(1, 1, 6), ">=",   0)
add.constraint(lps.model, c(4, 5, 4), "=" ,  40)
# set objective function (default: find minimum)
set.objfn(lps.model, c(-3, -4, -3))
solve(lps.model)  ## [1] 0
# Retrieve the values of the variables from a solved linear program model
get.variables(lps.model)
# check against the exact solution x_1 = 0, x_2 = 8, x_3 = 0
## [1] 0 8 0
get.objective(lps.model) # get optimal (min) value ## [1] -32
```

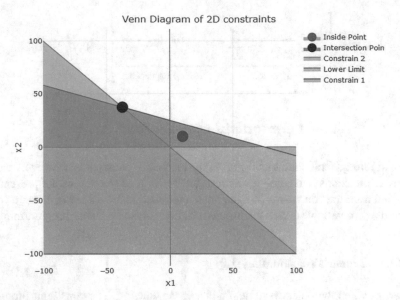

Fig. 13.4 2D schematic of linear programming constraints

In lower dimensional problems, we can also plot the constraints to graphically demonstrate the corresponding support restriction. For instance, here is an example of a simpler 2D constraint and its Venn diagrammatic representation (Fig. 13.4)

$$
\begin{cases}
x_1 & \leq \dfrac{150 - 2x_2}{6} \\
x_1 & \geq -x_2
\end{cases}.
$$

```
x = seq(-100, 100, by=1)
y = (150-2*x)/6
plot_ly(x = ~x, y = ~y, type = 'scatter', mode = 'lines',
        fill = 'tonexty', opacity=0.2, name="Constrain 1") %>%
  add_trace(x = ~x, y = -100, type = 'scatter', mode = 'lines',
            opacity=0.2, name="Lower Limit") %>%
  add_trace(x = ~x, y = ~(-x), type = 'scatter', mode = 'lines',
            fill = 'tonexty', opacity=0.2, name="Constrain 2") %>%
  add_markers(x=-150/4, y=150/4, mode='markers', marker=list(size=20),
              name="Intersection Point") %>%
  add_markers(x=10, y=10, mode='markers', marker=list(size=20),
              name="Inside Point") %>%
  layout(title="Venn Diagram of 2D constraints",
         xaxis = list(title = 'x1'), yaxis = list(title = 'x2'))
```

Here is another example of maximization of a trivariate cost function

$$f(x_1, x_2, x_3) = 3x_1 + 4x_2 - x_3$$

subject to

$$\begin{cases} -x_1 + 2x_2 + 3x_3 & \le 16 \\ 3x_1 - x_2 - 6x_3 & \ge 0 \\ x_1 - x_2 & \le 2 \end{cases}.$$

```r
lps.model2 <- make.lp(0, 3)
add.constraint(lps.model2, c(-1, 2, 3), "<=", 16)
add.constraint(lps.model2, c(3, -1, -6), ">=", 0)
add.constraint(lps.model2, c(1, -1, 0), "<=", 2)
set.objfn(lps.model2, c(3, 4, -1), indices = c(1, 2, 3))
lp.control(lps.model2, sense='max')       # changes to max: 3 x1 + 4 x2 - x3
solve(lps.model2)              # 0 suggests that this solution convergences
## [1] 0
get.variables(lps.model2) # get point of maximum
## [1] 20 18  0
get.objective(lps.model2) # get optimal (max) value
## [1] 132
```

In 3D we can utilize the `rgl::surface3d()` method to display the constraints. This output is suppressed, as it can only be interpreted via the pop-out 3D rendering window.

```r
library("rgl")
library("rglwidget")  # install.packages("rglwidget")
n <- 100
x <- y <- seq(-500, 500, length = n)
region <- expand.grid(x = x, y = y)
z1 <- matrix(((150 -2*region$x -4*region$y)/6), n, n)
z2 <- matrix(-region$x + 6*region$y, n, n)
z3 <- matrix(40 -5*region$x - 4*region$y, n, n)
# open3d()
surface3d(x, y, z1, back='line', front='line', col='red', lwd=1.5, alpha=0.4)
surface3d(x, y, z2, back='line',front='line',col='orange',lwd=1.5, alpha=0.4)
surface3d(x, y, z3, back='line',front='line', col='blue', lwd=1.5, alpha=0.4)
axes3d()
rglwidget() # use rglwidget() to embed an interactive 3D plot into HTML
```

We can also use `plot_ly` to display the linear constraints (planes) in 3D. Again, the generated 3D scene facilitates interactive manipulations (e.g., zoom, pan, rotation, glyph metadata exploration) (Fig. 13.5).

```r
#define the regular x,y grid (in 2D)
n <- 100
x <- y <- seq(-500, 500, length = n)
region <- expand.grid(x = x, y = y)
# define the z values for all three 2D planes
z1 <- matrix(((150 -2*region$x -4*region$y)/6), n, n)
z2 <- matrix(-region$x + 6*region$y, n, n)
z3 <- matrix(40 -5*region$x - 4*region$y, n, n)
### Compute and Plot the unique 3D point of the 3 intersecting planes
library(geometry)
library(pracma)
# plane normals and their unitary counterparts
n1 <- c(2,4,6); n2 <- c(1,-6,1); n3 <- c(5,4,1)
n1 <- n1/sqrt(dot(n1,n1)); n2 <- n2/sqrt(dot(n2,n2));
n3 <- n3/sqrt(dot(n3,n3))
# Points on the panes
P1 <- c(0,0,150/6); P2 <- c(0,0,0); P3 <- c(0,0,-40)
# compute the normalizing determinant of the normals matrix
det <- det(as.matrix(cbind(n1, n2, n3)))
# unique point of intersection
intersectPoint <- (dot(P1,n1)*cross(n2,n3) + dot(P2,n2)*cross(n3,n1) +
                   dot(P3,n3)*cross(n1,n2))/det
iP <- c(round(intersectPoint[1], 3), round(intersectPoint[2], 3),
        round(intersectPoint[3], 3))
paste0("Intersection point of all 3 Planes is (", iP[1], ",", iP[2], ",",
       iP[3], "!)")
## [1] "Intersection point of all 3 Planes is (-15.5,2.2,28.7!)"
library(plotly)
plot_ly() %>%
  # 1. Add 3 vectors representing the paired intersections (there are 3 of these)
of any pair of planes
  add_trace(x=c(iP[1], iP[1]+400*cross(n1,n2)[2]), y=c(iP[2],
          iP[2]+400*cross(n1,n2)[1]), z=c(iP[3], iP[3]+400*cross(n1,n2)[3]),
          type="scatter3d", mode="lines", name="Planes 1-2",
          line=list(color = "orange", width=40), opacity=1.0) %>%
  add_trace(x=c(iP[1], iP[1]+400*cross(n1,n3)[2]), y=c(iP[2],
          iP[2]+400*cross(n1,n3)[1]), z=c(iP[3], iP[3]+400*cross(n1,n3)[3]),
          type="scatter3d", mode="lines", name="Planes 1-3",
          line=list(color = "gray", width=40), opacity=1.0) %>%
  add_trace(x=c(iP[1], iP[1]+400*cross(n2,n3)[2]), y=c(iP[2],
          iP[2]+400*cross(n2,n3)[1]), z=c(iP[3], iP[3]+400*cross(n2,n3)[3]),
          type="scatter3d", mode="lines", name="Planes 2-3",
          line=list(color = "blue", width=40), opacity=1.0) %>%
  # 2. Add all 3 planes
  add_trace(x=~x, y=~y, z=~z1, name="Plane 1",
      colors = c("blue", "red"), type="surface", opacity=0.3) %>%
  add_trace(x=~x, y=~y, z=~z2, type="surface", name="Plane 2",
            colors = "green", opacity=0.3) %>%
  add_trace(x=~x, y=~y, z=~z3, type="surface", name="Plane 3",
            colors = "orange", opacity=0.3) %>%
  # 3. Add common intersection point
  add_trace(x=~intersectPoint[1], y=~intersectPoint[2], z=~intersectPoint[3],
          type="scatter3d", mode="markers", name="Common Intersection Point",
          marker=list(color = "blue", size=30), opacity=1.0) %>%
  layout(title="Hyperplane constraints in 3D", legend=list(orientation='h'),
        scene=list(aspectmode = "manual", aspectratio = list(x=1, y=1, z=1),
        xaxis = list(title = "X"), yaxis = list(title = "Y"),
        zaxis = list(title = "ZA"))) %>% hide_colorbar()
```

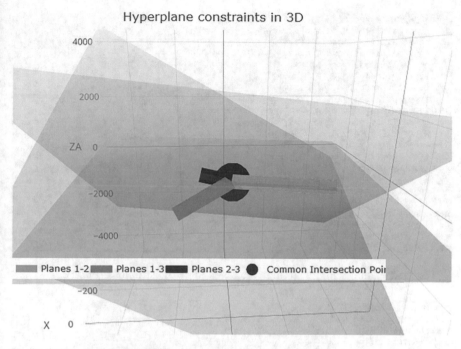

Fig. 13.5 3D schematic of linear programming constraints

It is possible to restrict the domain type to contain only solutions that are as follows:

- *Integers*, which makes it an Integer Linear Programming (ILP)
- *Binary/Boolean* values (BLP)
- *Mixed* types, Mixed Integer Linear Programming (MILP)

Some examples are included below.

13.3.3.2 Mixed Integer Linear Programming (MILP)

Let's demonstrate MILP with an example where the type of x_1 is unrestricted, x_2 is dichotomous (binary), and x_3 is restricted to be an *integer*.

```
lps.model <- make.lp(0, 3)
add.constraint(lps.model, c(6, 2, 4), "<=", 150)
add.constraint(lps.model, c(1, 1, 6), ">=", 0)
add.constraint(lps.model, c(4, 5, 4), "=", 40)
set.objfn(lps.model, c(-3, -4, -3))
set.type(lps.model, 2, "binary")
set.type(lps.model, 3, "integer")
get.type(lps.model) # This is Mixed Integer Linear Programming (MILP)
## [1] "real"    "integer" "integer"
set.bounds(lps.model, lower=-5, upper=5, columns=c(1))
# give names to columns and restrictions
dimnames(lps.model) <- list(c("R1", "R2", "R3"), c("x1", "x2", "x3"))
print(lps.model)
solve(lps.model)
## [1] 0
get.objective(lps.model)
## [1] -30.25
get.variables(lps.model)
## [1] 4.75 1.00 4.00
get.constraints(lps.model)
## [1] 46.50 29.75 40.00
```

The next example limits all three variables to be dichotomous (*binary*).

```
lps.model <- make.lp(0, 3)
add.constraint(lps.model, c(1, 2, 4), "<=", 5)
add.constraint(lps.model, c(1, 1, 6), ">=", 2)
add.constraint(lps.model, c(1, 1, 1), "=",  2)
set.objfn(lps.model, c(2, 1, 2))
set.type(lps.model, 1, "binary")
set.type(lps.model, 2, "binary")
set.type(lps.model, 3, "binary")
print(lps.model)
solve(lps.model)
## [1] 0
get.variables(lps.model)
## [1] 1 1 0
```

13.3.4   Quadratic Programming (QP)

QP can be used for second-order (quadratic) objective functions, but the constraint functions are still linear combinations of the domain variables. A matrix formulation of the problem can be expressed as minimizing an objective function

$$f(X) = \frac{1}{2}X^{\mathrm{T}}DX - d^{\mathrm{T}}X,$$

where X is a vector $[x_1, x_2, \ldots, x_n]^{\mathrm{T}}$, D is a symmetric positive-definite matrix of weights of each association pair, x_i, x_j, and d is a vector of the linear weights for each individual feature, x_i. The $\frac{1}{2}$ coefficient ensures that the weights matrix D is symmetric and each x_i, x_j combination pair is unique. This cost function is subject to the constraints

$$AX \ [=|\ge] \ b,$$

where the first k constraints may represent equalities ($=$) and the remaining ones are inequalities ($\ge$), and b is a constant vector constraining the right-hand side (RHS).

Here is an example of a QP *objective function* and its R optimization

$$f(x_1, x_2, x_3) = x_1^2 - x_1 x_2 + x_2^2 + x_2 x_3 + x_3^2 - 5x_2 + 3x_3.$$

We can rewrite f in a slightly modified form to explicitly specify the parameters (D and d)

$$f(x_1, x_2, x_3) = \frac{1}{2} \underbrace{\left(2x_1^2 - 2x_1 x_2 + 2x_2^2 + 2x_2 x_3 + 2x_3^2\right)}_{X^T D X} - \underbrace{(5x_2 - 3x_3)}_{d^T X}.$$

The symmetric positive definite matrix, D, and the linear weights, d, are as follows:

$$D = \begin{pmatrix} 2 & -1 & 0 \\ -1 & 2 & 1 \\ 0 & 1 & 2 \end{pmatrix}, \ d = (0, 5, -3)^t.$$

The optimization is subject to the following constraints ($A_{eq} X = b_{eq}$ and $AX \le b$)

$$-4x_1 - 3x_2 = -8$$
$$2x_1 + x_2 = 2 \ .$$
$$2x_2 - x_3 \ge 0$$

```
library(quadprog)
Dmat         <- matrix(c( 2, -1, 0,
                         -1, 2, 1,
                          0, 1, 2), 3, 3)
dvec         <- c(0, 5, -3)
Amat         <- matrix(c(-4, -3, 0,
                          2, 1, 0,
                          0, 2, -1), 3, 3)
bvec         <- c(-8, 2, 0)
n.eqs        <- 2 # the first two constraints are equalities
sol <- solve.QP(Dmat, dvec, Amat, bvec=bvec, meq=2)
sol$solution # get the (x1, x2, x3) point of minimum
## [1] -1.0  4.0 -3.5
sol$value  # get the actual cost function minimum
## [1] -11.25
```

The minimum value, -11.25, of the QP solution is attained at $x_1 = -1, x_2 = 4,$ $x_3 = -3.5$. Let's double check the solution.

```
ef <- function(X, D, d, A) { 1/2 * t(X) %*% D %*% X - t(d) %*% X  }
ef_man <- function(x) {
  (1/2)*(2*x[1]^2-2*x[1]*x[2]+2*x[2]^2+2*x[2]*x[3]+2*x[3]^2)-(5*x[2]-3*x[3])
}
X1 <- c(-1.0,  4.0, -3.5); X2 <- c(-2.5, 6, 0)
ef(X1, Dmat, dvec, Amat); ef(X2, Dmat, dvec, Amat)
##          [,1]
## [1,] -11.25
##          [,1]
## [1,] 27.25
ef_man(X1); ef_man(X2)
## [1] -11.25
## [1] 27.25
```

When D is a positive definite matrix, i.e., $X^{\mathrm{T}}DX > 0$, for all nonzero X, the QP problem may be solved in polynomial time. Otherwise, the QP problem is NP-hard. In general, even if D has only one negative eigenvalue, the QP problem is still NP-hard.[12] The QP function `solve.QP()` expects a positive definite matrix D.

13.4 General Nonlinear Optimization

The package `Rsolnp` provides a special function `solnp()`, which solves the general nonlinear programming problem

$$\min_x f(x)$$

subject to

$$g(x) = 0$$
$$l_h \leq h(x) \leq u_h,$$
$$l_x \leq x \leq u_x$$

where $f(x)$, $g(x)$, $h(x)$ are all smooth functions.

13.4.1 Dual Problem Optimization

Duality in math really just means having two complementary ways to think about an optimization problem. The *primal problem* represents an optimization challenge in terms of the original decision variable x. The *dual problem*, also called *Lagrange dual*, searches for a lower bound of a minimization problem or an upper bound for a maximization problem. In general, the primal problem may be difficult to analyze, or

---

[12] https://doi.org/10.1007/BF00365407

solve directly, because it may include nondifferentiable penalty terms, e.g., l_1 norms, recall LASSO/Ridge regularization in Chap. 11. Hence, we turn to the corresponding *Lagrange dual problem* where the solutions may be more amenable, especially for convex functions that satisfy the following inequality

$$f(\lambda x + (1 - \lambda)y) \le \lambda f(x) + (1 - \lambda)f(y).$$

13.4.1.1   Motivation

Suppose we want to borrow money, x, from a bank, or lender, and $f(x)$ represents the borrowing cost to us. There are natural "design constraints" on money lending. For instance, there may be a cap in the interest rate, $h(x) \le b$, or we can have many other constraints on the loan duration. There may be multiple lenders, including self-funding, that may "charge" us $f(x)$ for lending us x. *Lenders' goals are to maximize profits*. Yet, they can't charge you more than the prime interest rate plus some premium based on your credit worthiness. Thus, for a given fixed λ, a lender may make us an offer to lend us x aiming to minimize

$$f(x) + \lambda \times h(x).$$

If this cost is not optimized, i.e., minimized, you may be able to get another loan y at lower cost $f(y) < f(x)$, and the funding agency loses your business. If the cost/ objective function is minimized, the lender may maximize their profit by varying λ and still get us to sign on the loan.

The customer's strategy represents a *game theoretic interpretation* the *primal problem*, whereas the *dual problem* corresponds to the strategy of the lender.

In solving complex optimization problems, *duality* is equivalent to the existence of a saddle point of the Lagrangian. For convex problems, the double-dual is *equivalent* to the primal problem. In other words, applying the convex conjugate (Fenchel transform)[13] twice returns the *convexification* of the original objective function, which is the same as the original function in most situations.

The *dual of a vector space* is defined as the space of all continuous linear functionals on that space. Let $X = \mathbb{R}^n$, $Y = \mathbb{R}^m$, $f : X \to \mathbb{R}$, and $h : X \to Y$. Consider the following optimization problem

---

[13] https://doi.org/10.1090/noti788

$$\min_x f(x)$$

subject to

$$x \in X$$

$$h(x) \leq 0$$

Then, this *primal problem* has a corresponding *dual problem*

$$\min_\lambda \inf_{x \in X} (f(x) + \langle \lambda, \ h(x) \rangle)$$

subject to

$$\lambda_i \geq 0, \forall 0 \leq i \leq m$$

The parameter $\lambda \in \mathbb{R}^m$ is an element of the dual space of Y, i.e., Y^*, since the inner product $\langle \lambda, h(x) \rangle$ is a *continuous linear functional on Y*. Here Y is finite dimensional, and by the Riesz representation theorem,[14] Y^* is isomorphic to Y. Note that in general, for infinite dimensional spaces, Y and Y^* are not guaranteed to be isomorphic.

13.4.1.2   Example 1: Linear Example

Minimize $f(x, y) = 5x - 3y$, constrained by $x^2 + y^2 = 136$, which has a minimum value of -68 attained at $(-10, 6)$. We will use the $\texttt{Rsolnp::solnp()}$ method in this example.

```
# install.packages("Rsolnp")
library(Rsolnp)
fn1 <- function(x) {  5*x[1] - 3*x[2]  }
# constraint z1: x^2+y^2=136
eqn1 <- function(x) {
  z1=x[1]^2 + x[2]^2
  return(c(z1))
}
constraints = c(136)
x0 <- c(1, 1) # setup initial values
sol1 <- solnp(x0, fun = fn1, eqfun = eqn1, eqB = constraints)
## Iter: 1 fn: 37.4378    Pars:  30.55472 38.44528
## Iter: 2 fn: -147.9181     Pars:  -6.57051 38.35517
...
## Iter: 9 fn: -68.0000  Pars:  -10.00000   6.00000
## solnp--> Completed in 9 iterations
sol1$values[10]   # sol1$values contains all steps of the iteration algorithm and
the last value is the min value
## [1] -68
sol1$pars
## [1] -10    6
```

[14] https://doi.org/10.2307/2037423

13.4.1.3   Example 2: Quadratic Example

Minimize $f(x, y) = 4x^2 + 10y^2 + 5$ subject to the inequality constraint $0 \le x^2 + y^2 \le 4$, which has a minimum value of 5 attained at the origin $(0, 0)$.

```
fn2 <- function(x) {    4*x[1]^2 + 10*x[2]^2 +5  }
# constraint z1: x^2+y^2 <= 4
ineq2 <- function(x) {
  z1=x[1]^2 + x[2]^2
  return(c(z1))
}
lh <- c(0)
uh <- c(4)
x0 = c(1, 1) # setup initial values
sol2 <- solnp(x0, fun = fn2, ineqfun = ineq2, ineqLB = lh, ineqUB=uh)
## solnp--> Completed in 15 iterations
sol2$values
##  [1] 19.000000  7.869675  5.645626  5.160388  5.040095  5.010024  5.002506
##  [8]  5.000627  5.000157  5.000039  5.000010  5.000002  5.000001  5.000000
## [15]  5.000000  5.000000
sol2$pars
## [1]  1.189207e-04 -4.976052e-08
```

There are a number of parameters that control the `solnp` procedure. For instance, TOL defines the tolerance for optimality (which impacts the convergence) and `trace=0` turns off the printing of the results at each iteration.

```
ctrl <- list(TOL=1e-15, trace=0)
sol2 <- solnp(x0, fun = fn2, ineqfun = ineq2, ineqLB = lh, ineqUB=uh,
control=ctrl)
sol2$pars
## [1]  1.402813e-08 -5.015532e-08
```

13.4.1.4   Example 3: More Complex Nonlinear Optimization

Let's try to minimize

$$f(X) = -x_1 x_2 x_3$$

subject to

$$4x_1 x_2 + 2x_2 x_3 + 2x_3 x_1 = 100$$
$$1 \le x_i \le 10, i = 1, 2, 3$$

```
fn3 <- function(x, ...)   {  -x[1]*x[2]*x[3]  }
eqn3 <- function(x, ...)  {  4*x[1]*x[2]+2*x[2]*x[3]+2*x[3]*x[1] }
constraints3 = c(100)
lx <- rep(1, 3)
ux <- rep(10, 3)
pars <- c(2, 1, 7) # setup: Try alternative starting-parameter vector (pars)
ctrl <- list(TOL=1e-6, trace=0)
sol3 <- solnp(pars, fun=fn3, eqfun=eqn3, eqB = constraints3,
              LB=lx, UB=ux, control=ctrl)
sol3$values
## [1] -14.00000 -37.77774 -33.33337 -33.33340 -32.05189 -43.52798 -46.70522
## [8] -48.10927 -48.11252 -48.11252
sol3$pars
## [1] 2.886751 2.886751 5.773505
```

The nonlinear optimization is sensitive to the initial parameters (pars), especially when the objective function is not smooth or if there are many local minima. The function gosolnp() may be employed to generate initial (guesstimates of the) parameters.

13.4.1.5   Example 4: Another Linear Example

Let's try another minimization of a linear objective function $f(x, y, z) = 4y - 2z$ subject to

$$2x - y - z = 2$$
$$x^2 + y^2 = 1$$

```
fn4 <- function(x) {  4*x[2] - 2*x[3]   }
# constraint z1: 2x-y-z  = 2
# constraint z2: x^2+y^2 = 1
eqn4 <- function(x){
  z1=2*x[1] - x[2] - x[3]
  z2=x[1]^2 + x[2]^2
  return(c(z1, z2))
}
constraints4 <- c(2, 1)
x0 <- c(1, 1, 1)
ctrl <- list(trace=0)
sol4 <- solnp(x0, fun = fn4, eqfun = eqn4, eqB = constraints4, control=ctrl)
sol4$values
## [1]   2.000000  -5.078795 -11.416448  -5.76405  -3.58489  -3.2245 -3.2112
## [8]  -3.211103  -3.211103
sol4$pars
## [1]   0.55470019 -0.83205030 -0.05854932
```

The linear algebra and matrix computing Chap. 3 and the regularized parameter estimation in Chap. 11 provide additional examples of least squares parameter estimation, regression and regularization.

13.5   Manual Versus Automated Lagrange Multiplier Optimization

Let's manually implement the Lagrange multipliers procedure and then compare the results to some optimization examples obtained by automatic R function calls. The latter strategies may be more reliable, efficient, flexible, and rigorously validated. The manual implementation provides a more direct and explicit representation of the actual optimization strategy.

We will test a simple example of an objective function

$$f(x, y, z) = 4y - 2z + x^2 + y^2,$$

subject to two constraints

$$2x - y - z = 2$$
$$x^2 + y^2 + z = 1.$$

The R package numDeriv may be used to calculate numerical approximations of partial derivatives.

```
# define the main Lagrange Multipliers Optimization strategy from scratch
require(numDeriv)
lagrange_multipliers <- function(x, f, g) {
    # Objective/cost function, f, and constraints, g
    k <- length(x)
    l <- length(g(x))
    # Compute the derivatives
    grad_f <- function(x) { grad(f, x) }
    # g, representing multiple constraints, is a vector-valued function: its
first derivative is a matrix
    grad_g <- function(x) { jacobian(g, x) }
    # The Lagrangian is a scalar valued function:
    #    L(x, lambda) = f(x) - lambda * g(x)
    #    whose first derivative roots give the optimal solutions
    #    h(x, lambda) = c( f'(x) - lambda * g'(x), - g(x) ).
    h <- function(y) {
        c(grad_f(y[1:k]) - t(y[-(1:k)]) %*% grad_g(y[1:k]), -g(y[1:k]))
    }
    # To find the roots of the first derivative, we can use Newton's method:
    # iterate   y <- y - h'(y)^{-1} h(y)   until convergence criterion is met
    # e.g., (\delta <= 1e-6)
    grad_h <- function(y) { jacobian(h, y) }
    y <- c(x, rep(0, l))
    previous <- y + 1
    while(sum(abs(y-previous)) > 1e-6) {
        previous <- y
        y <- y - solve( grad_h(y), h(y) )
    }
    y[1:k]
}
x <- c(0, 0, 0)
```

```r
# Define the objective cost function
fn4 <- function(x) {   4*x[2] - 2*x[3] + x[1]^2+ x[2]^2   }
# check the derivative of the objective function
grad(fn4, x)
## [1]  0  4 -2
eqn4 <- function(x){
  z1=2*x[1] - x[2] - x[3] -2
  z2=x[1]^2 + x[2]^2 + x[3] -1
  return(c(z1, z2))
}
# Check the Jacobian of the constraints
jacobian(eqn4, x)
##      [,1] [,2] [,3]
## [1,]    2   -1   -1
## [2,]    0    0    1
# Call the Lagrange-multipliers solver
# check one step of the algorithm
k <- length(x)
l <- length(eqn4(x));
h <- function(x) {
   c(grad(fn4, x[1:k])-t(-x[(1:2)]) %*% jacobian(eqn4,x[1:k]),-eqn4(x[1:k]))
}
jacobian(h, x)
##       [,1] [,2]           [,3]
## [1,]     4    0  0.000000e+00
## [2,]    -1    2  5.482583e-15
## [3,]    -1    1  0.000000e+00
## [4,]    -2    1  1.000000e+00
## [5,]     0    0 -1.000000e+00
# Lagrange-multipliers solver for f(x, y, z) subject to g(x, y, z)
params <- lagrange_multipliers(x, fn4, eqn4); params
## [1]  0.3416408 -1.0652476 -0.2514708
fn4(params)
## [1] -2.506578
```

Now, let's double-check the above manual optimization results against the automatic solnp() solution minimizing

$$f(x, y, z) = 4y - 2z + x^2 + y^2$$

subject to

$$2x - y - z = 2$$
$$x^2 + y^2 = 1$$

```r
library(Rsolnp)
fn4 <- function(x) { 4*x[2] - 2*x[3] + x[1]^2+ x[2]^2  }
eqn4 <- function(x) {
  z1=2*x[1] - x[2] - x[3]
  z2=x[1]^2 + x[2]^2 + x[3]
  return(c(z1, z2))
}
constraints4 <- c(2, 1)
x0 <- c(1, 1, 1)
ctrl <- list(trace=0)
sol4 <- solnp(x0, fun = fn4, eqfun = eqn4, eqB = constraints4, control=ctrl)
sol4$values
## [1]  4.0 -0.1146266 -5.9308852 -3.7035124 -2.5810141 -2.5069444 -2.5065779
## [8] -2.5065778 -2.5065778
sol4$pars
## [1]  0.3416408 -1.0652476 -0.2514709
```

We obtain identical results from both the manual and the automated experiments identifying the optimal (x, y, z) coordinates minimizing the objective function $f(x, y, z) = 4y - 2z + x^2 + y^2$.

Optimization approach	function call	arg_x	arg_y	arg_z	min_value
Manual	`lagrange_multipliers (x, fn4, eqn4)`	0.34164	−1.065	−0.2515	−2.5066
Automated	`solnp(x0, fun = fn4, eqfun = eqn4, eqB = con-straints4, control=ctrl)`	0.34164	−1.065	−0.2515	−2.5066

13.6   Data Denoising

Suppose we are given x_{noisy} with n noise-corrupted data points. The noise may be additive ($x_{\text{noisy}} \sim x + \epsilon$) or not additive. We may be interested in denoising the signal and recovering a version of the original (unobserved) dataset x, potentially as a smoother representation of the original (uncorrupted) process. Smoother signals suggest less (random) fluctuations between neighboring data points.

One objective function we can design to denoise the observed signal, x_{noisy}, may include a *fidelity term* and a *regularization term*; see the regularized linear modeling, Chap. 11. Total variation denoising assumes that for each time point t, the observed noisy data is

$$\underbrace{x_{\text{noisy}}(t)}_{\text{observed signal}} \sim \underbrace{x(t)}_{\text{native signal}} + \underbrace{\epsilon(t)}_{\text{random noise}} .$$

To recover the *native signal*, $x(t)$, we can optimize ($\text{argmin}_x f(x)$) the following objective cost function:

$$f(x) = \underbrace{\frac{1}{2} \sum_{t=1}^{n-1} \| y(t) - x_{\text{noisy}}(t) \|^2}_{\text{fidelity term}} + \underbrace{\lambda \sum_{t=2}^{n-1} |x(t) - x(t-1)|}_{\text{regularization term}},$$

where λ is the regularization smoothness parameter, $\lambda \to 0 \Rightarrow y \to x_{\text{noisy}}$. Minimizing $f(x)$ provides a minimum total-variation solution to the data denoising problem.

Below is an example illustrating total variation (TV) denoising using a simulated noisy dataset. We start by generating an oscillatory noisy signal. Then, we compute several smoothed versions of the noisy data (using *LOESS*, locally estimated scatterplot smoothing), plot the initial and smoothed signals, and define and optimize

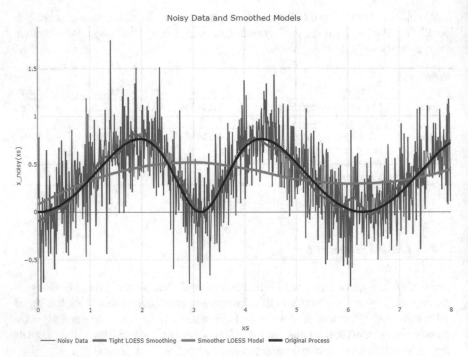

Fig. 13.6 Simulated noisy oscillatory data with several smoothing models

the TV denoising objective function, which is a mixture of a fidelity term and a regularization term (Fig. 13.6).

```
n  <- 1000
x <- rep(0, n)
xs <- seq(0, 8, len=n)    # seq(from = 1, to = 1, length)
noise_level = 0.3  # sigma of the noise, try varying this noise-level
# here is where we add the zero-mean noise
set.seed(1234)
x_noisy <- function (x) {
  sin(x)^2/(1.5+cos(x)) + rnorm(length(x), 0, noise_level)
}
# initialize the manual denoised signal
x_denoisedManu <- rep(0, n)
df <- as.data.frame(cbind(xs, x_noisy(xs)))
# loess fit a polynomial surface determined by numerical predictors,
# using local fitting
poly_model1 <- loess(x_noisy(xs) ~ xs, span=0.1, data=df) # tight model
poly_model2 <- loess(x_noisy(xs) ~ xs, span=0.9, data=df) # smoother model
plot_ly() %>%
  add_trace(x=~xs, y=~x_noisy(xs), type="scatter", mode="lines",
            name="Noisy Data") %>%
  add_trace(x=~xs, y=~poly_model1$fitted, type="scatter", mode="lines",
            line=list(width=5), name="Tight LOESS Smoothing") %>%
  add_trace(x=~xs, y=~poly_model2$fitted, type="scatter", mode="lines",
            line=list(width=5), name="Smoother LOESS Model") %>%
  add_trace(x=~xs, y=~sin(xs)^2/(1.5+cos(xs)), type="scatter", mode="lines",
            line=list(width=5), name="Original Process") %>%
  layout(title="Noisy Data and Smoothed Models",legend=list(orientation='h'))
```

Next, let's initiate the parameters, define the objective function and optimize it. We will estimate the parameters that minimize the cost function as a mixture of fidelity and regularization terms (Fig. 13.7).

```r
# initialization of parameters
betas_0 <- c(0.3, 0.3, 0.5, 1)
betas <- betas_0
x_denoised <- function(x, betas) {  # Denoised model
  if (length(betas) != 4) {
print(paste0("Error!!! length(betas)=",length(betas)," != 4!!! Exiting ..."))
    break();
  }
  return((betas[1]*sin(betas[2]*x)^2)/(betas[3]+cos(x)))
}
library(Rsolnp)
fidelity <- function(x, y) {  sqrt((1/length(x)) * sum((y - x)^2))  }
regularizer <- function(betas) {  reg <- 0
  for (i in 1:(length(betas-1))) { reg <- reg + abs(betas[i])  }
  return(reg)
}
# Objective Function
objective_func <- function(betas)  {
  fid <- fidelity(x_noisy(xs), x_denoised(xs, betas))
  reg <- abs(betas[4])*regularizer(betas)
  error <- fid + reg
  # uncomment to track the iterative optimization state
  # print(paste0(".... Fidelity =", fid, " ... Regularizer = ", reg, " ...
TotalError=", error))
  # print(paste0(".....betas=(",round(betas[1],3),",",round(betas[2],3),",",
  #       round(betas[3],3),",", round(betas[4],3), ")"))
  return(error)
}
# inequality constraint forcing the regularization parameter lambda=beta[4]>0
inequalConstr <- function(betas)  {   betas[4]  }
inequalLowerBound <- 0; inequalUpperBound <- 100
set.seed(121)
sol_lambda <- solnp(betas_0, fun = objective_func, ineqfun = inequalConstr,
            ineqLB=inequalLowerBound, ineqUB=inequalUpperBound, control=ctrl)
# report the optimal parameter estimates (betas)
sol_lambda$pars
## [1] 2.5649689 0.9829681 1.7605481 0.9895268
# Reconstruct the manually-denoised signal using the optimal betas
betas <- sol_lambda$pars
x_denoisedManu <- x_denoised(xs, betas)
print(paste0("Final Denoised Model:", round(betas[1],3), "*sin(",
            round(betas[2],3), "*x)^2/(", round(betas[3],3), "+cos(x)))"))
## [1] "Final Denoised Model:2.565*sin(0.983*x)^2/(1.761+cos(x))"
plot_ly() %>%
  add_trace(x=~xs, y=~x_noisy(xs), type="scatter", mode="lines",
            name="Noisy Data") %>%
  add_trace(x=~xs, y=~x_denoisedManu/2, type="scatter", mode="lines",
            name="Manual denoising", line=list(width=5)) %>%
  add_trace(x=~xs, y=~sin(xs)^2/(1.5+cos(xs)), type="scatter", mode="lines",
            line=list(width=5), name="Original Process") %>%
 layout(title="Noisy Data and Smoothed Models", legend=list(orientation='h'))
```

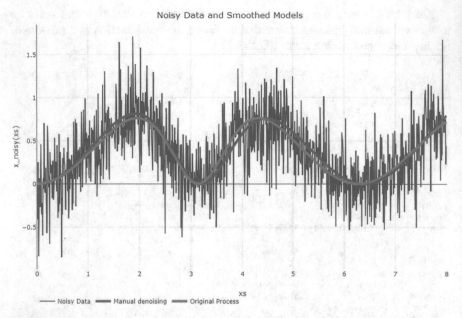

Fig. 13.7 Simulated noisy data along with the original (noiseless) signal and a denoising model

Finally, we can validate our manual denoising protocol against the automated TV denoising using the R package tvd[15] (Fig. 13.8).

```
# install.packages("tvd")
library("tvd")
lambda_0 <- 0.5
x_denoisedTVD <- tvd1d(x_noisy(xs), lambda_0, method = "Condat")
# lambda_o is the total variation penalty coefficient
# method is a string indicating the algorithm to use for denoising
plot_ly() %>%
  add_trace(x=~xs, y=~x_noisy(xs), type="scatter", mode="lines",
            name="Noisy Data", opacity=0.3) %>%
  add_trace(x=~xs, y=~x_denoisedManu/2, type="scatter", mode="lines",
            name="Manual Denoising", line=list(width=5)) %>%
  add_trace(x=~xs, y=~poly_model1$fitted, type="scatter", mode="lines",
            name="LOESS Smoothing", line=list(width=5)) %>%
  add_trace(x=~xs, y=~sin(xs)^2/(1.5+cos(xs)), type="scatter", mode="lines",
            line=list(width=5), name="Original Process") %>%
  add_trace(x=~xs, y=~x_denoisedTVD, type="scatter", mode="lines",
            name="TV Denoising", line=list(width=5)) %>%
 layout(title="Noisy Data and Smoothed Models", legend=list(orientation='h'))
```

---

[15] https://doi.org/10.1109/LSP.2013.2278339

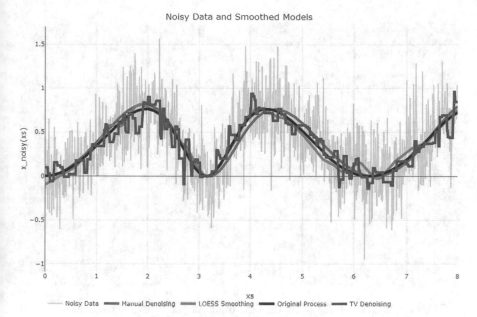

Fig. 13.8 Noisy data along with several alternative denoising models

13.7   Sparse Matrices

In Chap. 3, we saw the power of linear algebra and matrix computing. Often, we need new data structures to efficiently store *big* but *sparse* matrices, whose elements are mostly trivial (zero). Dense matrices have mostly nontrivial elements, whereas sparse matrices contain mostly trivial elements. The *sparsity of a matrix* is the proportion of nonzero elements. Even if the original data are not sparse, some data preprocessing may result in sparse data structures. Various techniques to store and process sparse matrices are included in the R package `Matrix`.

Here is an example of a large 15,000 × 15,000 but sparse diagonal matrix (*SM*) compared to a standard diagonal matrix (*D*) of the same size.

```
# install.packages("plyr")
library("Matrix")
memory.limit(50000) # increase the RAM allocation
n = 15000
SM = sparseMatrix(1:n, 1:n, x = 1)
D = diag(1, n, n)
# Check the sizes of the SM and D:
object.size(SM); object.size(D)
## 241504 bytes
## 1800000216 bytes
# Try to invert these matrices to see the differences (SM is more efficient)
solve(SM)[1:10, 1:10] # skip this is very intensive: solve(D)[1:10, 1:10]
## 10 x 10 sparse Matrix of class "dgCMatrix"
##  [1,] 1 . . . . . . . . .
##  [2,] . 1 . . . . . . . .
##  [3,] . . 1 . . . . . . .
##  [4,] . . . 1 . . . . . .
##  [5,] . . . . 1 . . . . .
##  [6,] . . . . . 1 . . . .
##  [7,] . . . . . . 1 . . .
##  [8,] . . . . . . . 1 . .
##  [9,] . . . . . . . . 1 .
## [10,] . . . . . . . . . 1
```

The size of the matrix D is 10, 000 times larger than SM even though both represent $n \times n$ matrices. The difference is that information is sorted differently in *sparse* matrices, where identical values that appear multiple times are only stored once, along with pointers to the matrix locations with the same value.

13.8 Parallel Computing

Parallel computing is useful for many processes where the algorithm can be partitioned into smaller jobs that can be run in parallel on different computing cores with results integrated at the end, e.g., Monte-Carlo simulations,[16] machine learning tasks, separable transformations. We can create a virtual cluster of computing nodes where each core runs independently, and the resulting information pieces are aggregated at the end. Let's try a simple calculation of the mean.

```
n = 200000
sapply(1:n, mean)[1:20]
##  [1]  1  2  3  4  5  6  7  8  9 10 11 12 13 14 15 16 17 18 19 20
```

Let's create a private computing cluster using four of the available eight cores and rerun the same script using parallel processing via the R `parallel` package.

---

[16]https://doi.org/10.1088/0031-9155/51/13/R17

```
library("parallel")
detectCores()  # check the number of available cores
## [1] 8
clust = makeCluster(4) # construct a cluster of 4 cores
parSapply(clust, 1:n, mean)[1:20] # swap sapply() with parSapply()
##  [1]  1  2  3  4  5  6  7  8  9 10 11 12 13 14 15 16 17 18 19 20
stopCluster(clust)
```

Once done, we should always stop the clusters and release the system resources to avoid memory leaks. Most computers include multiple processors which can be utilized to optimize the calculations and speed-up performance. Never request, or use, all cores, as this will halt the machine, and do not expect to achieve performance improvement directly proportional to the number of cores used, as there is multi-thread communication overhead.

13.9 Foundational Methods for Function Optimization

Function optimization may not always be possible, i.e., finding *exact* minima or maxima of a function is not always analytically tractable. However, there are iterative algorithms to compute *approximate* solutions to such function optimization problems.

13.9.1 Basics

Let's recall the following Newtonian principles for a given *objective* or *cost* function* $f : \mathbb{R}^n \to \mathbb{R}$, which we want to optimize, i.e., we are looking for solution (s) $x^* = \arg\min_x f(x)$.

- Maximizing f is the same as minimizing $-f$, as $\mathrm{argmax}_x f(x) = \arg\min_x -f(x)$.
- If ψ is strictly increasing (e.g., log, x^2, $\exp(x)$), then

$$\arg\min{}_x f(x) = \arg\min{}_x \psi(f(x)).$$

- The *accuracy* (bias) measures how close we get to the optimum point x^*.
- The *convergence speed* reflects how quickly (in terms of the number of iterations) we get towards x^*.
- The *computational complexity* captures how expensive it is to perform a single iteration.
- For 1D functions ($n = 1$), if f is smooth, then x^* is a *local optimum* implies that $f'(x^*) = 0$. The sign of the second derivative determines if the optimum is minimum ($f''(x^*) > 0$) or maximum ($f''(x^*) < 0$).
- In $\mathbb{R}^n$, for smooth $f : \mathbb{R}^n \to \mathbb{R}$, then at (local) optimal points, $\nabla f(x^*) = 0$, where the

gradient of f is the vector of all partial derivatives $\nabla f(x) = \begin{pmatrix} \dfrac{\partial f(x)}{\partial x_1} \\[6pt] \dfrac{\partial f(x)}{\partial x_2} \\[6pt] \vdots \\[6pt] \dfrac{\partial f(x)}{\partial x_n} \end{pmatrix}$.

- In higher dimensions, the second derivative is represented as the Hessian matrix, $\nabla^2 f$, which is defined at each point x by $\nabla^2 f(x) = \left[\nabla^2 f(x)\right]_{ij} = \frac{\partial^2 f(x)}{\partial x_i \partial x_j}$. At a local minimum x^*, the Hessian is positive definite ($v^{\mathrm{T}} \nabla^2 f(x^*) v > 0$, for all v), for minima, or negative-definite ($v^{\mathrm{T}} \nabla^2 f(x^*) v < 0$, for all v), for maxima.

13.9.2   Gradient Descent

Let's recall the relation between function changes (rise), relative to changes in the argument (run), gradients, and derivatives. The derivative of a function is defined as the limit of the rise over the run

$$f'(x_0) = \lim_{x \to x_0} \frac{f(x) - f(x_0)}{x - x_0}.$$

Thus, when x is close to x_0, a first-order (linear) approximation of the function at x is obtained by $f(x) \approx f(x_0) + f'(x_0)(x - x_0)$. This linear approximation allows us to approximate (locally) the function extrema by moving down the slope, or gradient, $f'(x_0)$. The higher-dimensional analogue is similar, for $x \sim x_0 \in \mathbb{R}^n$, $f(x) \approx f(x_0) + \nabla f(x_0)^{\mathrm{T}}(x - x_0)$. Effectively, all smooth functions look linear in a small neighborhood around each domain point (including the extrema points). In addition, the gradient $\nabla f(x_0)$ points in the direction of fastest ascent. Therefore, to optimize f, we move in the direction given by $- \nabla f(x_0)$. Recall that the inner product of two vectors, $\langle a, b \rangle$, is defined by $\langle a, b \rangle = a^{\mathrm{T}} b = \sum_{i=1}^{n} a_i b_i$.

13.9.2.1   Gradient Descent Pseudo Algorithm

Here is a simple illustrative gradient descent algorithm for minimizing f by iteratively moving in the direction of the negative gradient.

1. (*Initialization*): Start with initial guess $x_{(0)}$, a step size η (aka *learning rate*), and a threshold (tolerance level),

2. (*Iterative Update*) For $k = 1, 2, 3, \cdots$:

- Compute the gradient $\nabla f(x_{(k-1)})$
- If gradient is close to zero (stopping criterion threshold), then stop, otherwise continue
- Update $x_{(k)} = x_{(k-1)} - \eta \nabla f(x_{(k-1)})$

3. Return the final $x_{(k)}$ as an approximate solution x^*.

13.9.2.2 Example

Let's demonstrate a simple example performing gradient descent optimization.

```r
# install.packages("numDeriv")
library(numDeriv)          # to access the gradient calculation function: grad()
gradDescent=function(f,x0,max.iter=500,stepSize=0.01,stoppingCriterion=0.001) { n
= length(x0)
  xmat = matrix(0, nrow=n, ncol=max.iter)
  xmat[,1] = x0
  for (k in 2:max.iter) {
    # Calculate the current gradient
    currentGrad = grad(f, xmat[,k-1])
    # Check Stopping criterion
    if (all(abs(currentGrad) < stoppingCriterion)) { k = k-1; break  }
    # Move in the opposite direction of the gradient
    xmat[,k] = xmat[,k-1] - stepSize * currentGrad
  }
  xmat = xmat[,1:k]        # remove the initial guess (x0)
  # return final solution, solution path, min.value, and number of iterations
  return(list(x=xmat[,k], xmat=xmat, min.val=f(xmat[,k]), k=k))
}
```

Let's try one of the earlier examples, $\min f(x_1, x_2) = \min \{(x_1 - 3)^2 + (x_2 + 4)^2\}$, which we previously solved using `optim()`.

```r
# Define the function
f <- function(x) { (x[1] - 3)^2 + (x[2] +4)^2 }
initial_x <- c(0, -1)
x_optimal <- optim(initial_x, f, method="CG") # performs minimization
x_min <- x_optimal$par
# x_min contains the domain values where the (local) minimum is attained
x_min    # critical point/vector
## [1]  3 -4
x_optimal$value
## [1] 8.450445e-15
# call the gradient descent optimizer
x0 = c(0, 0)
optim.f = gradDescent(f, x0)
optim.f$x    # local min x
## [1]  2.999626 -3.999502
optim.f$min.val   # optimal value
## [1] 3.882821e-07
optim.f$k   # number of iterations
## [1] 446
```

We can also display a 3D scene visualizing alternative solution paths corresponding to different starting points of the optimization process.

```
surface = function(f, from.x=0, to.x=1, from.y=0, to.y=1, n.x=30, n.y=30,
                   theta=5, phi=80, ...) {
  x.seq = seq(from=from.x,to=to.x,length.out=n.x)  # Build the 2d grid
  y.seq = seq(from=from.y,to=to.y,length.out=n.y)
  plot.grid = expand.grid(x.seq,y.seq)
  z.vals = apply(plot.grid,1,f)
  z.mat = matrix(z.vals,nrow=n.x)
  # Plot with the persp function
  orig.mar = par()$mar # Save the original margins
  par(mar=c(1,1,1,1))   # Make the margins small
  r = persp(x.seq,y.seq,z.mat,theta=theta,phi=phi,...)
  par(mar=orig.mar) # Restore the original margins
  invisible(r)
}
x <- seq(from=-2, to=5, length.out=100)
y <- seq(from=-6, to=5, length.out=100)
z_fun <- function(x,y) { return((x - 3)^2 + (y +4)^2 ) }
z <- outer(x, y, FUN="z_fun")
plot_ly() %>%
  add_trace(x=x, y=y, z=t(z), type="surface", opacity=0.7,
            showlegend = FALSE, name="Function Surface") %>%
  add_markers(x = optim.f$x[1], y = optim.f$x[2], z = f(optim.f$x),
              type = 'scatter3d', mode = 'markers', opacity = 1,
       marker=list(size=20, color="red"), name='Minimum (f)', showlegend=F) %>%
  add_trace(x=c(optim.f$x[1], optim.f$x[1]), y=c(optim.f$x[2],optim.f$x[2]),
            z = c(f(optim.f$x),f(optim.f$x)+80), type = 'scatter3d',
            mode = 'lines', opacity = 1, line=list(width=4, color="orange"),
            name = 'Min Projection', showlegend=F) %>%
  layout(title="Graphical Representation of a Quadratic Function
               Optimization") %>% hide_colorbar()
```

13.9.2.3 Summary of Gradient Descent

There are pros and cons of using gradient descent optimization.
Advantages of Gradient Descent:

- Simple and intuitive.
- Easy to implement.
- Iterations are usually computationally efficient (involving estimation of the gradient).

Disadvantages:

- The algorithm may be slow and may get trapped into left-right alternating patterns when $\nabla f(x)$ are of very different sizes.
- It may require a long time to converge to the optimum.

For some functions, getting close to the optimum $(x_{(k)} \sim x^*$, where $f(x_{(k)}) - f(x*) \leq \epsilon$, may require a large number of iterations, $k \approx 1/\epsilon$. However, for smoother functions this may require $k \approx \log(1/\epsilon)$ iterations.

13.9.3 Convexity

There are substantial differences between convex function optimization over convex sets and nonconvex function optimization over nonconvex domains. The *convexity* assumptions make optimization problems much easier than the general nonconvex space optimization problems since (1) local extrema must be global extrema in convex spaces, and (2) first-order conditions sufficient conditions for optimality.[17]

Let's reexamine our simple quadratic convex optimization problem

$$\min f(x_1, x_2) = \min \left\{ (x_1 - 3)^2 + (x_2 + 4)^2 \right\}.$$

We can plot a number of gradient descent pathways starting with different initial conditions. If they all merge into each other (convergence), this would suggest robustness and reproducibility of the optimization (Fig. 13.9).

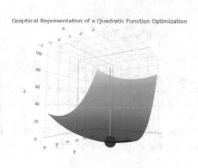

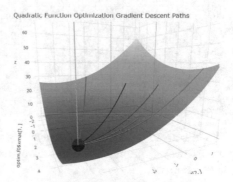

Objective function surface

Examples of alternative solution paths converging to unique (optimal) solution

Fig. 13.9 Examples of solution trajectories corresponding to quadratic function optimization with different initializations

[17] https://doi.org/10.1137/1035044

```
x0 = c(0,0);   optim.f0 = gradDescent(f,x0)
x1 = c(-2,-2); optim.f1 = gradDescent(f,x1)
x2 = c(2,1);   optim.f2 = gradDescent(f,x2)
x3 = c(3,-1);  optim.f3 = gradDescent(f,x3)
x4 = c(4,2);   optim.f4 = gradDescent(f,x4)
x <- seq(from=-2, to=5, length.out=100)
y <- seq(from=-5, to=2, length.out=100)
z_fun <- function(x,y) { return((x - 3)^2 + (y +4)^2 ) }
z <- outer(x, y, FUN="z_fun")
plot_ly() %>%
  add_trace(x=x, y=y, z=t(z), type="surface", opacity=0.7,
            showlegend = FALSE, name="Function Surface") %>%
  add_markers(x = optim.f$x[1], y = optim.f$x[2], z = f(optim.f$x),
            type = 'scatter3d', mode = 'markers', opacity=1, showlegend=F,
            marker = list(size=20, color="red"), name='Minimum (f)') %>%
  add_trace(x=c(optim.f$x[1], optim.f$x[1]),
            y=c(optim.f$x[2],optim.f$x[2]), z=c(f(optim.f$x),f(optim.f$x)+80),
            type = 'scatter3d', mode = 'lines', opacity = 1, showlegend=F,
            line = list(width=4, color="orange"), name='Min Projection') %>%
  # Add Solution Paths
  add_trace(x = ~optim.f0$xmat[1,], y = ~optim.f0$xmat[2,],
            z = apply(optim.f0$xmat,2,f),
            type = 'scatter3d', mode = 'lines', opacity = 1,
            line = list(width = 5), name='Solution Path 1', showlegend=F) %>%
  add_trace(x = ~optim.f1$xmat[1,], y = ~optim.f1$xmat[2,],
            z = apply(optim.f1$xmat,2,f), showlegend=F,
            type = 'scatter3d', mode = 'lines', opacity = 1,
            line = list(width = 5), name = 'Solution Path 2') %>%
  add_trace(x = ~optim.f2$xmat[1,], y = ~optim.f2$xmat[2,],
            z = apply(optim.f2$xmat,2,f), showlegend=F,
            type = 'scatter3d', mode = 'lines', opacity = 1,
            line = list(width = 5), name = 'Solution Path 3') %>%
  add_trace(x = ~optim.f3$xmat[1,], y = ~optim.f3$xmat[2,],
            z = apply(optim.f3$xmat,2,f), showlegend=F,
            type = 'scatter3d', mode = 'lines', opacity = 1,
            line = list(width = 5), name = 'Solution Path 4') %>%
  add_trace(x = ~optim.f4$xmat[1,], y = ~optim.f4$xmat[2,],
            z = apply(optim.f4$xmat,2,f), showlegend=F,
            type = 'scatter3d', mode = 'lines', opacity = 1,
            line = list(width = 5), name = 'Solution Path 5') %>%
  layout(title="Quadratic Function Optimization Gradient Descent Paths") %>%
  hide_colorbar()
```

So, all iterative solution pathways in this convex problem lead to the optimal point. However, problems are not always convex, and this process can be significantly disrupted.

Let's look at another example,

$$\min_{x=(x_1,\ x_2)} f_1(x) = \min\left(\left(\frac{1}{2}x_1^2 - \frac{1}{4}x_2^2 + 3\right) \times \cos\left(2x_1 + 1 - e^{x_2}\right)\right).$$

In this nonconvex optimization problem, different initial conditions (starting points) lead to divergent solution trajectories and different optima points. Different optimization trajectories may either smoothly approach the local minima (surface sulci or gyral valleys), rapidly switch between neighboring surface slopes, or even jump across different crests (Fig. 13.10).

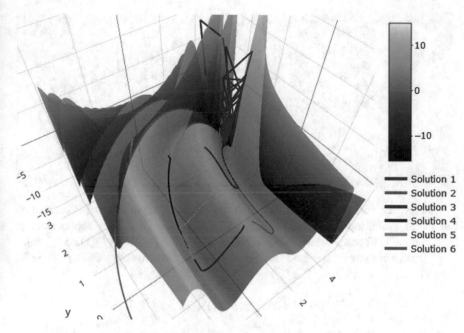

Fig. 13.10 Examples of solution trajectories corresponding to nonconvex function optimization with different initializations. Running this experiment interactively in RStudio allows dynamic exploration of the 3D scene

```
f1=function(x) { return((1/2*x[1]^2-1/4*x[2]^2+3)*cos(2*x[1]+1-exp(x[2]))) }
x0 = c(0.5,0.5);      optim.f0 = gradDescent(f1,x0,stepSize=0.01)
x1 = c(-0.1,-1.3);    optim.f1 = gradDescent(f1,x1,stepSize=0.01,max.iter=400)
x2 = c(-0.5,-1.3);    optim.f2 = gradDescent(f1,x2,stepSize=0.01,max.iter=400)
x3 = c(-0.2,1.4);     optim.f3 = gradDescent(f1,x3,stepSize=0.01,max.iter=400)
x4 = c(-0.5,-0.5);    optim.f4 = gradDescent(f1,x4,stepSize=0.01,max.iter=400)
x5 = c(-1.7, 1.45);   optim.f5 = gradDescent(f1,x5,stepSize=0.01,max.iter=400)
# Show the f1 optimization space, and plot all gradient descent pathways
library(magrittr); library(plotly)
radius <- 2
x <- seq(from=-2*radius, to=2*radius+1, by=0.05)
y <- seq(from=-radius, to=radius+1, by=0.05)
z_fun <- function(x,y) { return((1/2*x^2-1/4*y^2+3)*cos(2*x+1-exp(y))) }
z <- outer(x, y, FUN="z_fun")
plot_ly() %>%
  add_trace(x=x, y=y, z=t(z), type="surface", opacity=0.7,
            showlegend = FALSE) %>%
  add_trace(x = optim.f0$xmat[1,], y = optim.f0$xmat[2,],
            z = apply(optim.f0$xmat,2,f1),
            type = 'scatter3d', mode = 'lines', opacity = 1,
            line = list(width = 4, color = "red"), name = 'Solution 1') %>%
  add_trace(x = optim.f1$xmat[1,], y = optim.f1$xmat[2,],
            z = apply(optim.f1$xmat,2,f1),
            type = 'scatter3d', mode = 'lines', opacity = 1,
            line = list(width = 4, color = "green"), name = 'Solution 2') %>%
  add_trace(x = optim.f2$xmat[1,], y = optim.f2$xmat[2,],
```

```
            z = apply(optim.f2$xmat,2,f1),
            type = 'scatter3d', mode = 'lines', opacity = 1,
            line = list(width = 4, color = "blue"), name = 'Solution 3') %>%
  add_trace(x = optim.f3$xmat[1,], y = optim.f3$xmat[2,],
            z = apply(optim.f3$xmat,2,f1),
            type = 'scatter3d', mode = 'lines', opacity = 1,
            line = list(width = 4, color = "purple"), name='Solution 4') %>%
  add_trace(x = optim.f4$xmat[1,], y = optim.f4$xmat[2,],
            z = apply(optim.f4$xmat,2,f1),
            type = 'scatter3d', mode = 'lines', opacity = 1,
            line = list(width = 4, color = "orange"), name='Solution 5') %>%
  add_trace(x = optim.f5$xmat[1,], y = optim.f5$xmat[2,],
            z = apply(optim.f5$xmat,2,f1),
            type = 'scatter3d', mode = 'lines', opacity = 1,
            line = list(width = 4, color = "gray"), name='Solution 6')
```

Clearly, the nonconvex problem has divergent solution pathways that depend on the initial conditions and the topology of the space. Convexity represents the fundamental difference between these two optimization problems ($f(x)$ and $f_1(x)$).

If $f(x)$ is a convex real-valued function defined on a convex domain $D, f: D \to \mathbb{R}$, then $\forall x_1, x_2 \in D$ and $\forall t \in [0, 1]$

$$f(tx_1 + (1-t)x_2) \leq tf(x_1) + (1-t)f(x_2).$$

The convex optimization problem is to find a point $x^* \in D$ for which $f(x)$ is optimized, i.e., $f(x^*) \leq f(x), \forall x \in D$. In finite-dimensional normed spaces, the Hahn-Banach theorem[18] provides theoretical necessary and sufficient conditions for optimality. Duality theory[19] generalizes the classical linear programming problem to more complex situations and provides effective computational methods.

Notes
- All extrema of convex functions are global, i.e., there are no local extrema. Optimization of convex problems is of polynomial complexity.
- Gradient descent optimization provides solutions to most smooth convex functions, subject to selecting appropriate numeric parameters (step-size, i.e., *learning rate*)
- Gradient descent may often fail for nonconvex functions, where moving downhill locally may not always lead to the optimum,
- Nonconvex optimization is an NP-hard problem and is much harder in general to solve.

---

[18] https://doi.org/10.1016/S0166-8641(96)00142-3

[19] https://doi.org/10.1057/jors.2009.81

13.9.4   Foundations of the Newton–Raphson's Method

As a second-order method, Newton–Raphson optimization[20] is a bit more sophisticated than gradient descent and may also be more accurate. Let's recall the *second-order Taylor expansion* of functions

$$f(x) \approx f(x_0) + f'(x_0)(x - x_0) + \frac{1}{2}f''(x_0)(x - x_0)^2.$$

This represents a more accurate approximation of $f(x)$ near x_0. This directly generalizes to the multivariate case, $f(x) : D \subset \mathbb{R}^n \to \mathbb{R}$:

$$f(x) \approx \underbrace{f(x_0)}_{c,\text{constant}} + \underbrace{\nabla f(x_0)^{\mathrm{T}} \left(\overbrace{x - x_0}^{y} \right)}_{b^{\mathrm{T}}y,\text{linear term}} + \underbrace{\frac{1}{2}(x - x_0)^{\mathrm{T}} \nabla^2 f(x_0)(x - x_0)}_{\frac{1}{2}y^{\mathrm{T}}Hy,\text{quadratic term}}.$$

The basic idea of the Newton–Raphson method is to repeatedly expand the second-order Taylor representation of the objective function, reduce the size of the quadratic term on the right-hand side, and iterate.

The generic quadratic form $q(y) = c + b^{\mathrm{T}}y + \frac{1}{2}y^{\mathrm{T}}Hy$ is *minimized* when its gradient is trivial (as a vector), $\nabla q(y) = b^{\mathrm{T}} + Hy = 0$. Hence, given that H is positive definite and its inverse exists, $\underbrace{y}_{x - x_0} = -H^{-1}\underbrace{b^{\mathrm{T}}}_{\nabla f(x_0)^{\mathrm{T}}}$. Therefore, assuming we are at location $x_{(k-1)}$, the inductive step in the Newton's optimization scheme provides a mechanism to navigate to the next state point $x_{(k)}$ (in $\mathbb{R}^n$) via

$$x_{(k)} = x_{(k-1)} - \overbrace{\eta}^{\text{learning rate}} H^{-1}\nabla f\left(x_{(k-1)}\right)^{\mathrm{T}}.$$

Note that the *learning rate*, η, could be constant or can depend on the iteration index, i.e., $\eta = \eta_k$. Also, recall that the gradient vectors for real-valued *linear* $l : \mathbb{R}^n \to \mathbb{R}$ and *quadratic* $q : \mathbb{R}^n \to \mathbb{R}$ functions are given by

$$l(x) = \underbrace{b^{\mathrm{T}}x}_{\text{scalar}} \equiv x^{\mathrm{T}}b \quad \to \quad \nabla l(x) = b,$$

$$q(x) = \underbrace{x^{\mathrm{T}}Ax}_{\text{scalar}} \quad \to \quad \nabla q(x) = A^{\mathrm{T}}x + Ax.$$

---

[20] https://doi.org/10.1137/1037125

Similarly, for *vector-valued functions*, $f : \mathbb{R}^n \to \mathbb{R}^m$, $x = (x_1, x_2, \cdots, x_n)^T$, $f(x) = (f_1(x), f_2(x), \cdots, f_m(x))^T$, and $f(x) \approx f(x_0) + J_f(x_0)(x - x_0)$, where the $m \times n$ *Jacobian matrix*, $J_f(x)$, represents the first-order partial derivatives of the components of f, i.e., $\left(J_f(x)\right)_{i=1,j=1}^{m,n} = \left(\frac{\partial f_i(x)}{\partial x_j}\right)_{i=1,j=1}^{m,n}$.

13.9.4.1 Newton–Raphson Method Pseudocode

Repeat the formulation and minimization of the quadratic approximation to f.

1. Start with initial solution guess $x_{(0)}$, a step-size η (learning step), and a tolerance level (ϵ).
2. Iterate for $k = 1, 2, 3, \cdots$:

   - Compute the gradient (vector for real-valued functions, or Jacobian matrix for vector-valued functions) $g = \nabla f(x_{(k-1)})$ and the Hessian matrix $H = \nabla^2 f(x_{(k-1)})$
   - If gradient is close to zero ($\|g\| < \epsilon$), then stop, otherwise continue
   - Update the solution to $x_{(k)} = x_{(k-1)} - \eta H^{-1} g$

3. Return final $x_{(k)}$ as an approximate solution x^*.

13.9.4.2 Advantages and Disadvantages of the Newton–Raphson Method

Advantages:

- Converges faster to a solution than gradient descent, because jointly, the Hessian and gradient together point in a more reliable direction than the gradient does alone.
- For nice functions, the expected number of iterations to get $f(x_{(k)}) - f(x^*) \leq \epsilon$, is $k \approx \log\log(1/\epsilon)$ iterations.
- Typically, it requires fewer iterations than gradient descent.
- For quadratic functions, it converges in just one step.

Disadvantages:

- In principle, each Newton iteration is much more expensive than its gradient descent counterpart than a single gradient descent update. Requires inverting the Hessian.
- If the Hessian isn't invertible (or is close to singular), the algorithm may fail.

13.9.5   *Stochastic Gradient Descent*

Recall from Chap. 4, that to estimate the linear regression coefficients on p variables, we minimize the fidelity term

$$f(\beta) = \frac{1}{n} \sum_{i=1}^{n} \left(y_i - x_i^T \beta \right)^2.$$

For observed responses y_i and predictors x_i, $i = 1, \cdots, n$, the fidelity represents the standard least squares loss. When n, p are reasonable in size, then we can just solve this using linear algebra:

$$\beta^* = \left(X^T X \right)^{-1} X^T y,$$

where $X_{n \times p}$ (design) predictor matrix (with ith row x_i), and $y_{n \times 1}$ is the response vector (with ith component y_i).

For extreme sample or parameter sizes, e.g., when $n = 10^k$, it may be difficult to compute $X^T X$, which will impede the computational solution. Gradient descent may work, but may also be expensive, because the gradient $\nabla f(\beta) = \frac{1}{n} \sum_{i=1}^{n} x_i \left(x_i^T \beta - y_i \right)$ involves a sum of n terms.

This problem leads to the development of *stochastic methods* that overcome that challenge of large-scale statistical optimization. The idea is to simplify the calculations so that each time we need to compute a complex gradient or a Hessian, we can approximate it by a simpler analogue computed by *random estimation.*

For instance, instead of updating the solution using

$$\beta - t\nabla f(\beta) = \beta - \frac{t}{n} \sum_{i=1}^{n} x_i \left(x_i^T \beta - y_i \right),$$

for each time, t, a process that may be prohibitively expensive, we can update the solution by

$$\beta - tg = \beta - \frac{t}{m} \sum_{i \in I} x_i \left(x_i^T \beta - y_i \right).$$

The range of the sum above is reduced to $I \subset \{1, 2, \ldots, n\}$, which represents a random subset of $\{1, \ldots, n\}$ of size $|I| = m \ll n$. In other words, we replace the *full gradient* by a stochastic gradient estimate

$$g = \frac{1}{m} \sum_{i \in I} x_i \left(x_i^T \beta - y_i \right).$$

Note that the latter is an unbiased estimate of the former and is computed over just m data points. This is much more computationally efficient when m is relatively small. In general, stochastic gradient descent makes rapid *initial* progress in minimizing the objective function at the start. However, it may also take longer to get to highly accurate solutions at the end.

13.9.5.1   Stochastic Gradient Descent Pseudocode

Let's demonstrate the pseudocode implementation of stochastic gradient descent for high-dimensional data with a large number of predictors, p. For both statistical as well as optimization reasons, a complete search over all p regression parameters may be impractical. In a statistical sense, doing a full search may yield bad estimates (e.g., with high variance), and in a computational sense, the algorithm may be very expensive and slow to converge. Therefore, when we have a large number of features ($p \gg 10^m$), it's likely that most of the predictors may be less important and only a few may be salient features. We can ignore the small effects by shrinking them to zero, just like we did in Chap. 11 for regularized linear modeling. Below is an example of a *sparse* stochastic gradient descent pseudocode.

1. Start with initial guess $\beta^{(0)}$, step-size η, and tolerance level ϵ.
2. For $k = 1, 2, 3, \cdots :$

   - Randomly shuffle indices of the cases and select the reduced index set, $I \subset \{1, 2, \ldots, n\}$.
   - Approximate the true gradient $\nabla f(\beta^{(k-1)})$, by $g = \frac{1}{m} \sum_{i \in I} x_i \left(x_i^T \beta - y_i \right)$.
   - Check if gradient is close to zero; if so stop, otherwise continue.
   - Update $\beta^{(k)} = \beta^{(k-1)} - \eta \nabla f(\beta^{(k-1)})$.
   - Correct $\beta^{(k)}$ by thresholding the small components to zero.

3. Return final $\beta^{(k)}$ as approximate solution β^*.

Note that if all β get simultaneously smaller as we shrink the smaller coefficients to zero, this will guarantee the converge of the algorithm and will ultimately yield the *LASSO* solution.

13.9.6   Simulated Annealing (SANN)

Simulated annealing is another approach for *probabilistic* approximation of the global optimum of an objective function over a large domain (search space). It is very effective for discrete search spaces and for problems where quick identification of an approximate global optimum is more important than finding an accurate local optimum. *Annealing* is a term used in metallurgy to control repeated heating and cooling of materials to increase the size or reduce defects in the materials. In SANN, the *simulation of annealing* refers to finding approximations of the global minimum of a cost function with a large number of variables. This process involves equilibration (annealing) and a simulated walk through the solution space to slow decrease in the probability of accepting worse solutions compared to previously censored solutions.

13.9.6.1   SANN Pseudocode

Below is a simulated annealing pseudocode that starts from a state s_o and continues until a maximum of k_{max} steps are completed. At each step, the `neighbor(s)` call generates a randomly chosen neighbor of a given state s, and `random(0, 1)` returns a random Uniform distribution value. The annealing schedule is defined by `temperature(r)`, which yields the temperature to use, given the fraction r of the time budget that has been expended so far.

1. Initialize the algorithm by setting $s = s_o$.
2. For $k \in \{0, \ldots, k_{max}\}$:

    – $T \leftarrow \text{temperature}(k/k_{max})$.
    – Pick a random neighbor, $s_{new} \leftarrow \text{neighbor(s)}$.
    – If $P(E(s), E(s_{new}), T) \geq \text{random}(0, 1)$, then $s \leftarrow s_{new}$.

3. Output: the final state, s.

Below is a SANN example optimizing the objective function

$$f(x_1, x_2) = (x_1 - 3)^2 + (x_2 + 4)^2.$$

```
f <- function(x) { (x[1] - 3)^2 + (x[2] +4)^2 }
initial_x <- c(0, -1)
x_optimal <- optim(initial_x, f, method="SANN") # Simulated Annealing min
x_min <- x_optimal$par
# x_min contains the domain values where the (local) minimum is attained
x_min    # critical point/vector
## [1]   2.997603 -3.994186
x_optimal$value
## [1] 3.954959e-05
```

13.10   Hands-On Examples

The examples below illustrate some basic approaches and technical skills necessary to formulate and solve practical optimization problems. These also draw direct parallels between problem formulations and their corresponding mathematical representations, computational algorithm implementations, and validation of analytical and numerical solutions.

13.10.1   Example 1: Healthcare Manufacturer Product Optimization

To improve the return on investment for their shareholders, a healthcare manufacturer needs to optimize their production line. The organization's data-analytics team is tasked with determining the optimal production quantities of two products to maximize the company's bottom line. The pair of core company products include the following:

- A new noninvasive colonoscopy testkit (CTK)[21] that retails at $339 per kit
- A novel statistical data obfuscation software tool (DataSifter)[22] that enables the secure sharing of sensitive data, which costs $399 per year

The production cost of the healthcare company to make, and support each of these products is $195 per CTK set and $225 per DataSifter License. Additional company operational fixed costs include $400, 000 per year. In competitive market conditions, the number of sales of these healthcare products (a testkit and a software license) does affect the sale prices. Assume for each product, the sales price drops by one cent ($0.01) for each additional item sold. There is also an association between the sales of the CTK and DataSifter products.

The company's historical sales suggest that the CTK unit price is reduced by an additional $0.003 for each DataSifter license purchased. Similarly, the price for the DataSifter license decreases by $0.004 for each CTK sold. These product price fluctuations are due to partnerships with wholesale vendors and package deals with academic and research institutions. The healthcare manufacturer believes that stable market conditions, constant production and support of their two flagship products, along with these above assumptions, would maximize the volume of sales. The key question the analytics team needs to resolve is: what is the optimal level of production? That is, *how many units of each type of product should the healthcare company plan to manufacture and support (this includes R&D and product support) to maximize the company profit?*

---

[21] https://doi.org/10.1177/0969141315584694

[22] https://doi.org/10.1177/17483026211065379

Let's first translate the problem formulation into a mathematical optimization framework using this notation:

- s_1: the number of CTK units produced annually by the healthcare company, $s_1 \geq 0$
- s_2: the number of DataSifter licenses issued/sold each year, $s_2 \geq 0$
- p_1: the CTK sale price per unit ($)
- p_2: the DataSifter price per license ($)
- C: the R&D plus manufacturing costs ($/year)
- R: total sales revenue ($/year)
- P: total profit from all sales ($/year)

The provided market estimates result in the following model equations

$$p_1 = 339 - 0.01s_1 - 0.003s_2$$
$$p_2 = 399 - 0.004s_1 - 0.01s_2$$
$$R = s_1 p_1 + s_2 p_2$$
$$C = 400{,}000 + 195s_1 + 225s_2$$
$$P = R - C$$

By plugging in and expressing P as a function of s_1 and s_2, the objective cost function (*profit*) is a nonlinear function of the two product sales (s_1, s_2)

$$f = P(s_1, s_2) = -400{,}000 + 144s_1 + 174s_2 - 0.01s_1^2 - 0.01s_2^2 - 0.007s_1s_2.$$

13.10.1.1 Unconstrained Optimization

Let's assume there are no constraints other than, s_1, $s_2 \geq 0$. To solve the unconstrained optimization problem, find the s_1 and s_2 sales numbers that maximize the profit (P) in the first quadrant, $\{P = (s_1, s_2) \in \mathbb{R}^2 | s_i \geq 0\}$. To identify candidate extreme point (s_1, s_2) that maximizes P, we set the partial derivatives to zero and solve the following linear system of equations

$$\frac{\partial P}{\partial s_1} = 144 - 0.02s_1 - 0.007s_2 = 0$$
$$\frac{\partial P}{\partial s_2} = 174 - 0.007s_1 - 0.02s_2 = 0$$

The unique solution is $(s_1^o, s_2^o) = (4{,}735.7, 043)$, which yields a maximum profit value $P^o(s_1^o, s_1^o) = 553{,}641$. As $s_i^o \geq 0$, the solution is indeed in the feasible region (first planar quadrant). To examine the type of extremum (min or max), let's inspect the (symmetric) Hessian matrix, $H_P(s_1^o, s_2^o)$, including the second-order derivatives of the Profit

$$H_P\left(s_1^o, s_2^o\right) = \begin{bmatrix} \dfrac{\partial^2 P}{\partial s_1^2} & \dfrac{\partial^2 P}{\partial s_1 \partial s_2} \\[3mm] \dfrac{\partial^2 P}{\partial s_2 \partial s_1} & \dfrac{\partial^2 P}{\partial s_2^2} \end{bmatrix} = \begin{bmatrix} -0.02 & -0.007 \\ -0.007 & -0.02 \end{bmatrix}.$$

As the problem is convex, a sufficient condition for *maximizing* the profit at $\left(s_1^o, s_2^o\right) = (4, 735, 7, 043)$ is that the Hessian, $H_P\left(s_1^o, s_2^o\right)$, is *negative semi-definite*, i.e., $X^T H_P\left(s_1^o, s_2^o\right) X \le 0$, for all 2D vectors $X = (x_1, x_2)$, where $x_1, x_2 \ge 0$

$$X^T H_P\left(s_1^0, s_2^0\right) X = [x_1 \; x_2] \begin{bmatrix} -0.02 & -0.007 \\ -0.007 & -0.02 \end{bmatrix} \begin{bmatrix} x_1 \\ x_2 \end{bmatrix}$$

$$= [x_1 \; x_2] \begin{bmatrix} -0.02x_1 & -0.007x_2 \\ -0.007x_1 & -0.02x_2 \end{bmatrix} =$$

$$= -0.02{x_1}^2 - 0.041x_1 x_2 - 0.02{x_2}^2 \le 0, \; \forall x_1, x_2 \ge 0.$$

Let's display a 3D surface plot of the profit objective function, $P(s_1, s_2)$. As you move the mouse over the interactive surface, note that profit *isolines* form closed curves surrounding the maximum at $\left(s_1^o, s_2^o\right) = (4735, 7043)$ (Fig. 13.11).

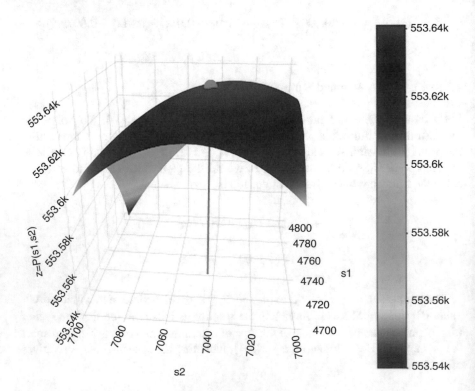

Fig. 13.11 Unconstrained optimization of healthcare manufacturer return on investment

```
grid_length <- 101
Profit_function <- function(x) { # input bivariate x is a matrix n*2
  x <- matrix(x, ncol=2)
  z <- -400000 + 144*x[ ,1] + 174*x[ ,2] - 0.01*x[ ,1]^2 - 0.01*x[ ,2]^2
       - 0.007*x[ ,1]*x[ ,2]
  return(z)
}
# define 2D grid to plot f=P around optimal value (s1^o,s2^o)=(4,735,7,043)
x <- seq(4700, 4800, length = grid_length)
y <- seq(7000, 7100, length = grid_length)
A <- as.matrix(expand.grid(x, y))
colnames(A) <- c("s1", "s2")
z <- Profit_function(A)   # evaluate function
df <- data.frame(A, z)    # put X and y values in a data.frame for plotting
library(plotly)
x_label <- list(title = "s1")
y_label <- list(title = "s2")
z_label <- list(title = "z=P(s1,s2)")
# Define vertical Line at arg_Max{Profit}
count <- 300
xl <- c(); yl <- c(); zl <- c()
for (i in 1:count) {   xl <- 4735; yl <- 7043 }
zl <- seq(553541, 553641, length.out=count)
vert_line <- data.frame(xl, yl, zl)
myPlotly <- plot_ly(x=~x, y=~y, z=~matrix(z, grid_length,grid_length),
                    type="surface", colors = colorRamp(rainbow(8)),
                    opacity=1.0, hoverinfo="none") %>%
  add_trace(vert_line, x=~xl, y=~yl, z=~zl, type='scatter3d', mode='lines',
            line = list(width = 4, color = "gray",
                    colorscale = list(c(0,'gray'), c(1,'black')))) %>%
  # add a Ball centered at arg_max
  add_trace(x=4735, y=7043, z=553641, type="scatter3d", mode="markers") %>%
  layout(scene = list(xaxis=x_label, yaxis=y_label, zaxis=z_label),
         showlegend = FALSE)
myPlotly
```

13.10.1.2   Constrained Optimization

Next, we will explore more realistic scenarios where the company has *limited resources* restricting the number of products that can annually be produced and supported to $0 \le s_1 \le 5000$, $0 \le s_2 \le 8000$, and $0 \le s_1 + s_2 \le 10,000$.

Note that the current optimum production plan that maximizes the profit already satisfies the first two constraints, $\left(s_1^o = 4735 \le 5000 \right.$ and $s_2^o = 7043 \le 8000$. However, it violates the last constraint $s_1^o + s_2^o = 4735 + 7043 = 11,778 \ge 10,000$. Thus, the global Profit maximum point is not outside the *feasible region* and the *constraint problem optimal* (max Profit) must be on the boundary of the convex domain. We will apply nonlinear constrained optimization to maximize the Profit

$$f = P(s_1, s_2) = -400,000 + 144s_1 + 174s_2 - 0.01s_1^2 - 0.01s_2^2 - 0.007s_1s_2$$

subject to

$$\text{constraint}(s_1, s_2) : s_1 + s_2 - 10,000 = 0.$$

13.10.1.3 Manual Solution

Let's first solve the problem by hand using first-principles. We can translate the primary problem to a dual problem using Lagrange multipliers. The *dual Profit function* will be $P^*(s_1, s_2, \lambda) = P(s_1, s_2) + \lambda \times \text{constraint}(s_1, s_2)$. To optimize it, we set $\nabla P^* = 0$, which yields $\nabla P = -\lambda \nabla \text{constraint}$, i.e.,

$$\frac{\partial}{\partial s_1}: \quad 144 - 0.02s_1 - 0.007s_2 \quad = \quad -\lambda$$

$$\frac{\partial}{\partial s_2}: \quad 174 - 0.007s_1 - 0.02s_2 \quad = \quad -\lambda$$

We can substitute λ to get a single linear relation between s_1 and s_2, $-0.013s_1 + 0.013s_2 = 30$. Pairing this linear equation with the additional boundary constraint ($s_1 + s_2 = 10,000$) yields a system of *two* linear equations with *two* unknowns (s_1, s_2), which may have a unique solution that maximizes the Profit objective function given all the restrictions on the operations of the healthcare company

$$-0.013s_1 \quad + \quad 0.013s_2 \quad = \quad 30$$
$$s_1 \quad \quad + \quad s_2 \quad = \quad 10,000$$

Substituting s_2, or s_1, from the second constraint equation into the first one yields a (argmin) solution

$$(s_1', s_2') = (3, 846, 6, 154),$$

with a corresponding Profit value $P'(3846, 6154) = 532, 308$. The latter profit is *less* than the *global* profit maximum at $(s_1^o, s_2^o) = (4, 735, 7, 043)$. Recall that the global maximum profit was

$$P^o(s_1^o, s_1^o) = P^o(4735, 7043) = 553,641.$$

13.10.1.4 R-Based Automated Solution

Next we will solve the constraint optimization problem using `Rsolnp::solnp()` and confirm that the two approaches yield the same results—maximum profit subject to production limitations for the CTK and the DataSifter healthcare products. Recall the formulation of this quadratic Profit optimization problem and its linear constraint

$$f = P(s_1, s_2) = -400{,}000 + 144s_1 + 174s_2 - 0.01s_1^2 - 0.01s_2^2 - 0.007s_1 s_2$$

$$\min_{(s_1,\, s_2)} \left(-P(s_1,\ s_2) \right) = \max_{(s_1,\, s_2)} P(s_1, s_2),$$

subject to

$$\text{constraint}(s_1, s_2) : s_1 + s_2 \leq 10{,}000.$$

Mind that in the earlier *manual solution*, we used multivariate calculus knowledge to argue that extrema must occur at points where the gradient of the Profit objective is trivial, *or* at points of discontinuity or nondifferentiability, *or* on the boundary. Hence, the constraint used equality, $\text{constraint}(s_1, s_2) : s_1 + s_2 = 10{,}000$. Here, as we are using the generic nonlinear optimization, we need to specify the *real (inequality) constraint*

$$\text{constraint}(s_1, s_2) : s_1 + s_2 \leq 10{,}000.$$

```
library(Rsolnp)
# define objective profit to minimize
Profit_function <- function(x) { # input bivariate x is a matrix n*2
  x <- matrix(x, ncol=2)
  z <- -(-400000 + 144*x[ ,1] + 174*x[ ,2] - 0.01*x[ ,1]^2 - 0.01*x[ ,2]^2
        - 0.007*x[ ,1]*x[ ,2])
  return(z)
}
# constraints s1, s2 >=0, and z1: s1 + s2 <= 10,000
ineqn1 <- function(x) {
  z1=x[1];  z2=x[2];  z3=x[1] + x[2];  return(c(z1, z2, z3))
}
lh <- c(0, 0, 0)                    # x1, x2 and x1 + x2 >-0
uh <- c(10000, 10000, 10000)        # x1, x2 and x1 + x2 <= 10,000
x0 = c(4000, 5000) # setup initial values
sol2 <- solnp(x0, fun=Profit_function, ineqfun=ineqn1, ineqLB=lh, ineqUB=uh)
## Iter: 3 fn: -532307.6918  Pars:   3846.26334 6153.73664
## solnp--> Completed in 3 iterations
cat("Max Profit=$",-sol2$values[length(sol2$values)],"\n") #Last optimal value
## Max Profit = $ 532307.7
cat ("Location of Profit Max = (s1(#CTK)=", sol2$pars[1],
     ", s2(#DataSifter)=", sol2$pars[2], ")!\n")  # argmin (s1,s2)
## Location of Profit Max = (s1(#CTK)=3846.263 , s2(#DataSifter)=6153.737 )!
```

13.10.2   Example 2: Optimization of the Booth's Function

Find the extrema of the Booth's function $f(x, y) = (x + 2y - 7)^2 + (2x + y - 5)^2$ on the square $S = \{(x, y) \in \mathbb{R}^2 | -10 \le x, y \le 10\}$. For brevity, the resulting 3D surface plot is intentionally excluded.

```
grid_length <- 101
Booth_function <- function(A) { # input bivariate x is a matrix n*2
  A <- matrix(A, ncol=2)
  z <- ((A[,1] + 2*A[,2] -7)^2 + (2*A[,1]+A[,2] - 5)^2)
  return(z)
}
x <- seq(-10, 10, length = grid_length) # define the 2D grid to plot f over
y <- seq(-10, 10, length = grid_length)
A <- as.matrix(expand.grid(x, y))
colnames(A) <- c("x", "y")
z <- Booth_function(A)   # evaluate function
df <- data.frame(A, z)   # put X and y values in a data.frame for plotting
library(plotly)
z_label <- list(title = "z=f(x,y)")
myPlotly <- plot_ly(x=~x, y=~y, z=~matrix(z, grid_length,grid_length),
                    type="surface", colors = colorRamp(rainbow(8)),
                    opacity=1.0, hoverinfo="none") %>%
            layout(scene = list(zaxis=z_label))
myPlotly
```

13.10.3   Example 3: Extrema of the Bivariate Goldstein–Price Function

Minimize and maximize the *Goldstein–Price* function

$$f(x, y) = \left(1 + (x + y + 1)^2 (19 - 14x + 3x^2 - 14y + 6xy + 3y^2)\right)$$
$$\times \left(30 + (2x - 3y)^2 (18 - 32x + 12x^2 + 48y - 36xy + 27y^2)\right).$$

We can use the method `optim()`, with Nelder-Mead, Simulated Annealing, and conjugate gradient optimization strategies, to report a table with the extrema points and corresponding functional values. The basic invocation protocol is (Fig. 13.12)

```
NM_min <- optim(c(1,1), GP_function, method = "Nelder-Mead").
```

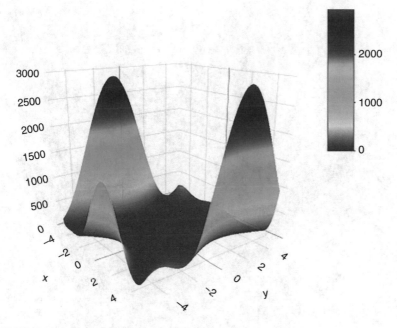

Fig. 13.12 Optimization of the Goldstein–Price function

```
GP_function <- function(A) { # input bivariate x is a matrix n*2
  A <- matrix(A, ncol=2)
  x <- A[ , 1]
  y <- A[ , 2]
  # calculate the function value for each row of x
  z_xy <- ((1+(x+y+1)^2*(19-14*x+3*x^(2)-14*y+6*x*y+3*y^(2))))*
    (30+(2*x-3*y)^2*(18-32*x+12*x^2+48*y-36*x*y+27*y^2))/(10^5)
  # return function value
  return(z_xy)
}
x <- seq(-5, 5, length = grid_length)
y <- seq(-5, 5, length = grid_length)
# plot the function
A <- as.matrix(expand.grid(x, y))
colnames(A) <- c("x", "y")
# evaluate function
z <- GP_function(A); length(z) ## [1] 10201
df <- data.frame(A, z)
# plot the function
library(plotly)
myPlotly <- plot_ly(x=~x, y=~y, z=~matrix(df$z, grid_length,grid_length),
             type="surface", colors=colorRamp(rainbow(8)), opacity=0.9) %>%
  layout(scene = list(zaxis=z_label))
myPlotly
```

13.10.4   Example 4: Bivariate Oscillatory Function

Determine the extrema of a complicated oscillatory function (Fig. 13.13)

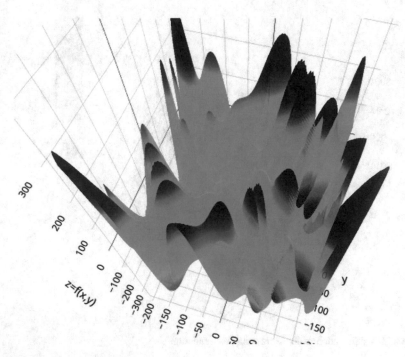

Fig. 13.13 Optimization of a highly oscillatory function

$$f(x, y) = -(y+50)\cos\left(\sqrt{|y+x+50|}\right) - x\sin\left(\sqrt{|x-y-50|}\right).$$

```
BO_function <- function(A) {
  A <- matrix(A, ncol=2)
  x <- A[ , 1]
  y <- A[ , 2]
  # calculate the function value for each row of x
  z_xy <- -(y+50)*cos(sqrt(abs(y+x+50)))-x*sin(sqrt(abs(x-(y+50))))
  return(z_xy)
}
x <- seq(-200, 200, length = grid_length)
y <- seq(-200, 200, length = grid_length)
A <- as.matrix(expand.grid(x, y))
colnames(A) <- c("x", "y")
# evaluate function
z <- BO_function(A)
# put X and y values in a data.frame for plotting
df <- data.frame(A, z)
library(plotly)
z_label <- list( title = "z=f(x,y)" )
myPlotly <- plot_ly(x=~x, y=~y, z=~matrix(df$z, grid_length,grid_length),
                    type="surface", colors = colorRamp(rainbow(8)),
                    opacity=0.8, hoverinfo="none", showscale=FALSE ) %>%
  layout(scene = list(zaxis=z_label), showlegend = FALSE)
myPlotly
```

13.10.5 Nonlinear Constraint Optimization Problem

Maximize this objective function (a mixture of polynomial and exponential components)

$$f(x, y, z) = x^3 + 5y - 2^z$$

subject to

$$D = \begin{cases} x - \dfrac{y}{2} + z^2 \leq 50 \\ \mathrm{mod}\,(x,\ 4) + \dfrac{y}{2} \leq 1.5 \end{cases}.$$

Alternatively, *minimize $f^*(x, y, z) = -(x^3 + 5y - 2^z)$*. It's difficult to plot a 4D surface in 2D or 3D space, but we can try animating or cross-sectioning the $w = f(x, y, z)$ surface. The code below can be used, or modified, to generate a dynamic surface or a volume rendering of the objective function, $f^*(x, y, z)$. This code is not executed here (eval−F) to reduce the size of the output HTML output file.

It's difficult to visualize this complicated objective function; however, we can use time as the 4th dimension to show the dynamic nature of the singularities of the function. Below are two alternative displays of the surface and the point-cloud representation of the 4D object. Note that these time-animated plots are difficult to render and may display degenerate surface representations (due to singularities). Hence, we only show a point-cloud representation of the objective function as a 4D object with temporal dynamics (slider) (Fig. 13.14).

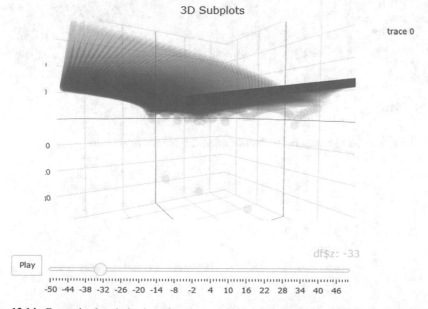

Fig. 13.14 Constrained optimization of a mixture of polynomial and exponential functions

```
library(plotly)
grid_length <- 101
BO_function <- function(A) {
  A <- matrix(A, ncol=3)
  x <- A[ , 1];    y <- A[ , 2];    z <- A[ , 3]
  w_xyz <- -(x^3 + 5*y -2^z)
  return(w_xyz)
}
x <- seq(-50, 50, length = grid_length)
y <- seq(-50, 50, length = grid_length)
z <- seq(-50, 50, length = grid_length)
A <- as.matrix(expand.grid(x, y, z))
colnames(A) <- c("x", "y", "z")
# evaluate function
w <- log(abs(BO_function(A)))   # apply log(abs()) to tamper large w
values
# put x, y and z values in a data.frame for plotting
df <- data.frame(A, w); str(df)
## 'data.frame':    1030301 obs. of  4 variables:
z_label <- list(title = "w=f(x,y_o,z)")
myPlotly <- plot_ly(df, x=~x, y=~y, z=~matrix(df$w,
                    grid_length,grid_length,grid_length),
                    frame=~df$z, type="surface",
colors=colorRamp(rainbow(8)),
                    opacity=0.8, hoverinfo="none", showscale=T ) %>%
  layout(scene = list(zaxis=z_label), showlegend = FALSE)  %>%
  animation_opts(500, easing = "elastic", redraw = F) %>%
  animation_slider(active = 50,
                    currentvalue=list(prefix="Z ",
font=list(color="red")))
myPlotly
fig <- df %>% plot_ly(x = ~x, y = ~y, z = ~w, frame=~df$z,
type="scatter3d",
                    mode = "markers", opacity=0.1, scene="scene")
%>%
  layout(title = "3D Subplots", scene = list(domain=list(x=c(-
50,50),
        y=c(-50,50)),aspectmode='cube',zaxis=list(title="f",range=c(-
40,40)))))
fig
```

Next, we can use solnp() to optimize the objective function.

```
fun3 <- function (x) {  -(x[1]^3 + 5*x[2] - 2^x[3]) }
ineq3 <- function(x) {
  z1 = x[1] - (x[2]/2) + (x[3]^2)
  z2 = (x[1] %% 4) + (x[2]/2)
  z3 = x[3]
  return(c(z1, z2, z3))
}
lb = c(-1000,-1000,-1000)
ub = c(1000,1000,100)
lh <- c(-Inf, -Inf, -Inf)
uh <- c(50, 1.5, Inf)
x0 <- c(1,0,1) # setup: Try alternative starting-parameter vector (pars)
sol3 <- solnp(x0, fun=fun3, ineqfun=ineq3, ineqLB=lh, ineqUB=uh)
## Iter: 1 fn: -11.2821  Pars:  0.000002152 2.817591348 1.488463477
## Iter: 2 fn: -11.2821  Pars:  0.000002152 2.817591348 1.488463477
## solnp--> Completed in 2 iterations
cat("Min is attained at: (", sol3$pars[1], ", ", sol3$pars[2], ", ",
    sol3$pars[1], ")\n")
## Min is attained at: ( 2.152334e-06 ,  2.817591 ,  2.152334e-06 )
cat("Min_f = ", sol3$values[length(sol3$values)])
## Min_f =  -11.28206
```

Finally, we can also try the optim() method using *simulated annealing*, a slower stochastic global optimizer that works well with difficult functions, e.g., nondifferentiable or nonconvex functions. We will use two different initialization points $(0.01, 2, -2)$ and $(0, 2, -3)$.

```
# Define the constraints with conditions returning NA to restrict SANN stochastic
walk
fun3_constraints <- function(x) {
  if (x[1] - (x[2]/2)+x[3]^2 > 50) {NA}       # constraint 1
  else if ((x[1] %% 4) + (x[2]/2) > 1.5) {NA} # constraint 2
  else { fun3(x) }                            # the objective function,
}
# Case 1: Initial conditions, chosen analytically
x0 <- c(0.01, 2, -2)
# Initialize optimization using dummy variables
x_optimal_value <- Inf
x_optimal_point <- c(NA, NA)
# Run 50 iterations of SANN and choose the optimal result
for (i in 1:50) { x_optimal <- optim(x0, fun3_constraints)
    if (x_optimal$value < x_optimal_value) {
        x_optimal_value <- x_optimal$value
        x_optimal_point <- x_optimal$par
    }
}
cat("Init: x_o = (0.01, 2, -2); fun3 minimum estimate is=", x_optimal_value,
    " which is attained at (", x_optimal_point[1], ", ", x_optimal_point[2],
    ", ", x_optimal_point[3], ")!\n")
## Init: x_o = (0.01, 2, -2); fun3 minimum estimate is= -14.76122   which is
attained at ( 7.225925e-09 ,  3 ,  -2.066219 )!
# Case 2: Initial conditions, chosen analytically
x0 <- c(0, 2, -3)
# Initialize optimization using dummy variables
x_optimal_value <- Inf
```

```r
x_optimal_point <- c(NA, NA)
# Run 50 iterations of SANN and choose the optimal result
for (i in 1:50) {
  x_optimal <- optim(x0, fun3_constraints, method="SANN")
  if (x_optimal$value < x_optimal_value) {
    x_optimal_value <- x_optimal$value
    x_optimal_point <- x_optimal$par
  }
}
cat("Init: x_o = (0, 2, -3); fun3 minimum estimate is=", x_optimal_value,
    " which is attained at (", x_optimal_point[1], ", ", x_optimal_point[2],
    ", ", x_optimal_point[3], ")!\n")
## Init: x_o = (0, 2, -3); fun3 minimum estimate is= -108827.8  which is attained
at ( 47.74684 ,  -4.505561 ,  0.01073434 )!
```

We can also check the solution $\min_{D} f(x, y, z) = f(x=0, y=3, z=-3.6) = -15$ using alternative methods. This R paper[23] on convex optimization provides a number of additional objective functions and interesting optimization problems.

13.11   Examples of Explicit Optimization Use in AI/ML

Most advanced DSPA techniques rely on some form of optimization strategies to tune parameters, estimate likelihoods, approximate unknown values, derive unobserved characteristics, or obtain solutions to various problems.

Examples of explicit optimization methods used in artificial intelligence and machine learning include:

- LASSO regularized linear modeling (Chap. 11), the regularization penalty term is not differentiable, which requires an optimization-based solution for estimating the effects and the penalty-weight.
- Training neural networks (Chap. 6) with backpropagation requires minimizing the total aggregate error to estimate the weights of the specific NN nodes.
- Boosting (Chap. 9) requires minimization of an objective function of the weighted average of weaker classifiers.
- The SVM search for the maximum margin hyperplane (MMH) (Chap. 6) requires optimization of an objective function whose extremes lead to optimal separation of the samples.
- RandomForest relies on optimization to obtain an optimal `mtry` parameter (representing the number of variables randomly sampled as candidates at each tree-node split) that minimizes the Out-of-Bag error estimate of the classifier, see `randomForest::tuneRF()`.

---

[23] https://doi.org/10.18637/jss.v060.i05

13.12   Practice Problems

Try different optimization methods to solve the following problems. For each problem, you can report your solutions including min values and the optimal location, execution-time, performance under alternative initialization points, dependence on initial conditions, and so on.

- $\min_{x=(x_1,\,x_2)} f(x_1, x_2) = \min_{x=(x_1,\,x_2)} \left\{ (x_1 - 3)^2 + (x_2 + 4)^2 + x_1 x_2 \right\}.$
- Find the extrema of the Booth's function $f(x, y) = (x + 2y - 7)^2 + (2x + y - 5)^2$ constrained to $S = \{(x, y) \in \mathbb{R}^2 | -10 \leq x, y \leq 10\}$. To start. use *plot_ly* to render the objective function as a 3D surface over the domain, S, f(x) = (x[1]+2*x [2]-7)^2 + (2*x[1]+x[2]-5)^2. Try library(quadprog) and/or library(Rsolnp). Compare your solution to the Wolfram Alpha Optimizer.
- The quantile function of a probability distribution is the inverse function of the cumulative distribution function. Review the optimization example we discussed in this chapter using the Normal distribution and try the Probability Distributome Navigator. For Cauchy and Poisson distributions, use first principles and optimization theory to compute (estimate) the inverse CDF (quantile function) for each distribution. Plot your estimates against the corresponding exact quantile functions (qpois and qcauchy). Generate creative and informative R plots. Note that in general, (1) the Cauchy distribution has two parameters that are defaulted to *location* $= 0$ and *scale* $= 1$, and (2) the Poisson distribution has one parameter, non-negative mean, e.g., $\lambda = 5$. You can either take the default parameters or specify other appropriate alternatives.
- *Google Trends*: To tie data science with optimization, gather data, model the temporal patterns, and try to predict various trends based on other factors. For instance, we will use *Google Trends* to select some relevant (interesting?) 5–10 themes, phrases, or keywords and investigate the corresponding temporal dynamics of the Google searches of these themes for the past 10–15 years. Use Chap. 12 examples as a starting point. Retrieve the trends data, plot the data, and write a few sentences summarizing the visual analytics (what is your inference in the context of the themes you chose?) Run some quantitative longitudinal data analytics to showcase some statistical inference, forecasting, or specific models of these trends or the differences between these trajectories of search popularity. Try to predict one theme trend using information about the others.

Chapter 14
Deep Learning, Neural Networks

Deep learning is a special branch of machine learning using a collage of algorithms to model high-level motifs in data. Deep learning resembles the biological communications between brain neurons in the central nervous system (CNS), where synthetic graphs represent the CNS network as nodes/states and connections/edges between them. For instance, in a simple synthetic network consisting of a pair of connected nodes, an output sent by one node is received by the other as an input signal. When more nodes are present in the network, they may be arranged in multiple levels (like a multiscale object) where the ith layer output serves as the input of the next $(i + 1)^{st}$ layer. The signal is manipulated at each layer and sent as a layer output downstream and interpreted as an input to the next, $(i + 1)^{st}$ layer, and so forth. Deep learning relies on multiple layers of nodes and many edges linking the nodes forming input/output (I/O) layered grids representing a multiscale processing network. At each layer, linear and nonlinear transformations are converting inputs into outputs.

In this chapter, we explore the R-based deep neural network learning and demonstrate state-of-the-art deep learning models utilizing CPU and GPU for fast training (learning) and testing (validation). Other powerful deep learning frameworks include *TensorFlow, Theano, Caffe, Torch, CNTK*, and *Keras*.

Neural Networks Versus Deep Learning Deep learning is a machine learning strategy that learns a deep, multilevel hierarchical representation of the affinities and motifs in the dataset. Machine learning Neural Nets tend to use shallower network models. Although there are no formal restrictions on the depth of the layers in a Neural Net, few layers are commonly utilized. Recent methodological, algorithmic, computational, infrastructure, and service advances have overcome previous limitations. In addition, the rise of *big data* accelerated the evolution of *classical Neural Nets* to *Deep Neural Nets*, which can now handle lots of layers and many hidden nodes per layer. The former is a precursor to the latter; however, there are also *non-neural* deep learning techniques. For example, *syntactic pattern recognition methods* and *grammar induction discover hierarchies*.

© The Author(s), under exclusive license to Springer Nature Switzerland AG 2023   773
I. D. Dinov, *Data Science and Predictive Analytics*, The Springer Series in Applied
Machine Learning, https://doi.org/10.1007/978-3-031-17483-4_14

Some readers may find it useful to review the previous discussions included in Chap. 6 (Black Box Machine-Learning Methods), where we presented the foundations of Neural Networks, Support Vector Machines, ensemble methods, bagging, boosting, and Random Forests.

14.1 Perceptrons

A *perceptron* is an artificial analog of a neuronal brain cell that calculates a *weighted sum of the input values* and *outputs a thresholded version of that result*. For a bivariate perceptron, P, let's denote the weights of the two inputs, (X, Y) by A and B, respectively. Then, the weighted sum could be represented as

$$W = AX + BY.$$

At each layer l, the weight matrix, $W^{(l)}$, has the following properties:

- The number of rows of $W^{(l)}$ equals the number of nodes/units in the previous $(l-1)^{\text{st}}$ layer.
- The number of columns of $W^{(l)}$ equals the number of units in the next $(l+1)^{\text{st}}$ layer.

Neuronal cells fire depending on the presynaptic inputs to the cell which cause constant fluctuations of the neuronal membrane—depolarizing or hyperpolarizing, i.e., making the cell membrane potential rise or fall. Similarly, perceptrons rely on the thresholding of the weight-averaged input signal, which for biological cells corresponds to voltage increases passing a critical threshold. Perceptrons output nonzero values only when the weighted sum exceeds a certain threshold C. In terms of its input vector (X, Y), we can describe the output of each perceptron (P) by

$$\text{Output } (P) = \begin{cases} 1, & \text{if } AX + BY > C \\ 0, & \text{if } AX + BY \le C \end{cases}.$$

Feed-forward networks are constructed as layers of perceptrons where the first layer ingests the inputs, and the last layer generates the network outputs. The intermediate (internal) layers are not directly connected to the external world and are called hidden layers. In *fully connected networks*, each perceptron in one layer is connected to every perceptron on the next layer enabling information "fed forward" from one layer to the next. There are no connections between perceptrons in the same layer.

Multilayer perceptrons (fully connected feed-forward neural networks) consist of several fully connected layers representing an input `matrix` $X_{n,m}$ and a generated `output matrix` $Y_{n,k}$. The input $X_{n,m}$ is a matrix encoding the n cases and m features per case. The weight matrix $W_{m,k}^{(l)}$ for layer l has rows (i)

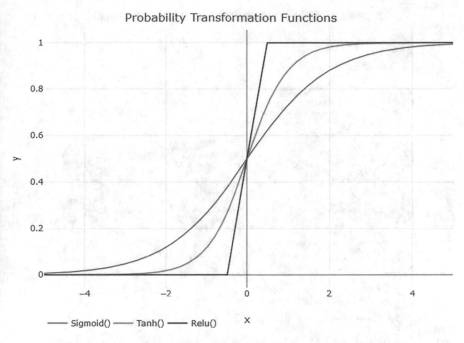

Fig. 14.1 Examples of activation functions transforming observations into likelihoods

corresponding to the weights leading from all the units i in the previous layer to all the units j in the current layer.

The hidden size parameter k, the weight matrix $W_{m,k}$, and the bias vector b_k are used to compute the outputs at each layer

$$Y_{n,k}^{(l)} = f_k^{(l)}(X_{n,m}^{(l)} W_{m,k}^{(l)} + b_k^{(l)}).$$

The role of the bias parameter is similar to the intercept term in linear regression and helps improve the prediction accuracy by shifting the decision boundary along the Y axis. The outputs are fully connected layers that feed into an `activation layer` to perform element-wise operations. Examples of *activation functions* that transform real numbers to probability-like values include the following:

- The sigmoid function, a special case of the logistic function, which converts real numbers to probabilities.
- The rectifier (`relu`, Rectified Linear Unit) function, which outputs the max(0, input).
- The tanh (hyperbolic tangent function) (Fig. 14.1).[1]

---

[1] https://doi.org/10.1109/IECBES.2018.8626714

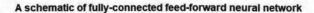

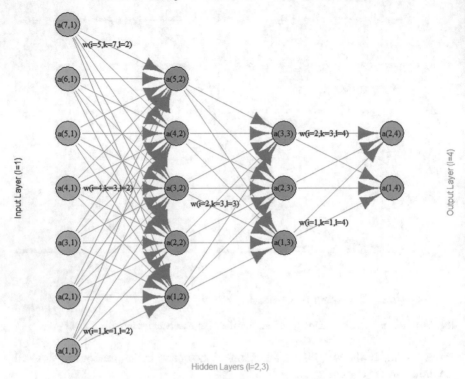

Fig. 14.2 Synthetic fully connected neural network example

The final fully connected layer may be hidden of a size equal to the number of classes in the dataset, and may be followed by a `softmax` layer mapping the input into a probability score. For example, if a size $n \times m$ input is denoted by $X_{n \times m}$, then the probability scores may be obtained by the `softmax` transformation function, which maps real valued vectors to vectors of probabilities

$$\left(\frac{e^{x_{i,1}}}{\sum\limits_{j=1}^{m} e^{x_{i,j}}}, \cdots, \frac{e^{x_{i,m}}}{\sum\limits_{j=1}^{m} e^{x_{i,j}}} \right).$$

Figure 14.2 shows a schematic of a fully connected feed-forward neural network of nodes.

$$\left\{ a_{j=\text{node index},l=\text{layer index}} \right\}_{j=1,l=1}^{n_j,4}.$$

The plot above illustrates the key elements in the action potential, or activation function, calculations and the corresponding training parameters

$$a_{\text{node}=k,\text{layer}=l} = f\left(\sum_i w^{(l)}_{k,i} \times a^{(l-1)}_i + b^{(l)}_k\right),$$

where:

- f is the *activation function*, e.g., logistic function $f(x) = \frac{1}{1+e^{-x}}$. It converts the aggregate weights at each node to probability values.
- $w^l_{k,i}$ is the weight carried from the ith element of the $(l-1)^{\text{th}}$ layer to the kth element of the current l^{th} layer.
- b^l_k is the (residual) bias present in the kth element in the lth layer. Effectively, the residual bias is the information not explained by the training model.

These parameters may be estimated using different techniques (e.g., using least squares, or stochastically using steepest descent methods) based on the training data.

14.2   Biological Relevance

There are parallels between biology (neuronal cells) and the mathematical models (perceptrons) for neural network representation. The human brain contains about 10^{11} neuronal cells connected by approximately 10^{15} synapses forming the basis of our functional phenotypes. The schematic below illustrates some of the parallels between brain biology and mathematical representation using synthetic neural networks. Every neuronal cell receives multichannel (afferent) input from its dendrites, generates output signals and disseminates the results via its (efferent) axonal and synaptic connections to dendrites of other neurons.

The perceptron is a mathematical model of a neuronal cell that allows us to explicitly determine algorithmic and computational protocols for transforming input signals into output actions. For instance, a signal arriving through an axon x_0 is modulated by some prior weight, e.g., synaptic strength, $w_0 \times x_0$. Internally, within the neuronal cell, this input is aggregated (summed, or weight-averaged) with inputs from all other axons. Brain plasticity suggests that synaptic strengths (weight coefficients w) are enhanced by training and prior experience. This learning process controls the direction and influence of neurons on other neurons. Either excitatory ($w > 0$) or inhibitory ($w \le 0$) influences are possible. Dendrites and axons carry signals to and from neurons, where the aggregate responses are computed and transmitted downstream. Neuronal cells only fire if action potentials exceed a certain threshold. In this situation, a signal is transmitted downstream through its axons. The neuron remains silent when the summed signal is below the critical threshold.

Timing of events is important in biological networks. In the computational perceptron model, a first-order approximation may ignore the timing of neuronal firing (spike events) and only focus on the frequency of the firing. The firing rate of a neuron with an activation function f represents the frequency of the spikes along the

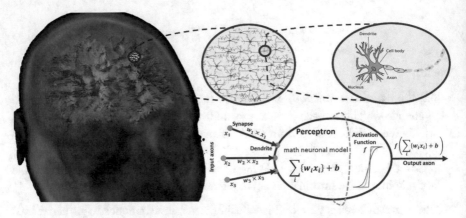

Fig. 14.3 Parallels between biological and artificial neural networks

axon. We saw some examples of activation functions earlier. This diagram illustrates the parallels between the brain network-synaptic organization and an artificial synthetic neural network (Fig. 14.3).

14.3 Simple Neural Net Examples

Before we look at examples of deep learning algorithms applied to model observed natural phenomena, we will develop a couple of simple networks for computing fundamental Boolean operations.

14.3.1 Exclusive OR (XOR) Operator

The exclusive OR (XOR) operator works as a bivariate binary-outcome function, mapping pairs of false (0) and true (1) values to dichotomous false (0) and true (1) outcomes.

We can design a simple two-layer neural network that calculates XOR, Fig. 14.4. The *values within each neuron represent its explicit threshold*, which can be normalized so that all neurons utilize the same threshold, typically 1. The *value labels associated with network connections (edges) represent the weights of the inputs*. When the threshold is not reached, the output is 0, whereas when the threshold is reached, the corresponding output is 1.

Fig. 14.4 An example
artificial neural network
representing the exclusive
OR operator

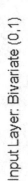

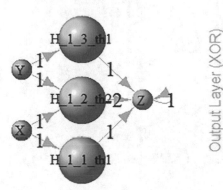

Let's work out manually the four possible outputs.

Input X	Input Y	XOR Output (Z)
0	0	0
0	1	1
1	0	1
1	1	0

We can validate that this network indeed represents an XOR operator by plugging in all four possible input combinations and confirming the expected results at the end (Fig. 14.5).

14.3.2   NAND Operator

Another binary operator is NAND (negative AND, Sheffer stroke) that produces a false (0) output if and only if both of its operands are true (1), and generates true (1), otherwise. Below is the NAND input–output table.

Input X	Input Y	NAND Output (Z)
0	0	1
0	1	1
1	0	1
1	1	0

Similar to the XOR operator, we can also design a one-layer neural network that calculates NAND, Fig. 14.6. The values within each neurons represent its explicit

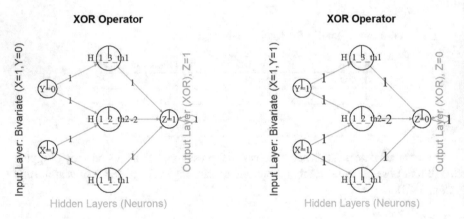

Fig. 14.5 Explicating the XOR operator input–output relation encoded via an artificial neural network

threshold, which can be normalized so that all neurons utilize the same threshold, typically 1. The value labels associated with network connections (edges) represent the weights of the inputs. When the threshold is not reached, the output is trivial (0) and when the threshold is reached, the output is correspondingly 1. Here is a shorthand analytic expression for the NAND calculation

$$\text{NAND}(X, Y) = 1.3 - (1 \times X + 1 \times Y).$$

Check that $\text{NAND}(X, Y) = 0$ if and only if $X = 1$ and $Y = 1$, otherwise it equals 1.

NAND Operator

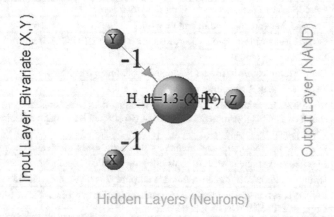

Fig. 14.6 An example artificial neural network representing the exclusive OR operator

14.3.3   Complex Networks Designed Using Simple Building Blocks

Observe that stringing some of these primitive networks together, or/and increasing the number of hidden layers, allows us to model problems with exponentially increasing complexity. For instance, constructing a 4-input NAND function would simply require repeating several of our 2-input NAND operators. This will increase the space of possible outcomes from 2^2 to 2^4. Of course, introducing more depth in the *hidden layers* further expands the complexity of the problems that can be modeled using neural nets. The interactive Google TensorFlow Deep Neural Network Webapp[2] allows dynamic manipulation to gain additional intuition and experience with the various components of deep learning networks. This ConvNetJS demo provides another hands-on example using 2D classification with a two-layer neural network.[3]

---

[2] https://playground.tensorflow.org/

[3] https://cs.stanford.edu/people/karpathy/convnetjs/demo/classify2d.html

Table 14.1   Commonly used deep neural network platforms

Package	Description
nnet	Feed-forward neural networks using 1 hidden layer
neuralnet	Training backpropagation neural networks
tensorflow	Google TensorFlow used in TensorBoard (see SOCR UKBB Demo[a])
deepnet	Deep learning toolkit
darch	Deep Architectures based on Restricted Boltzmann Machines
rnn	Recurrent Neural Networks (RRNs)
rcppDL	Multilayer machine learning methods including dA (Denoising Autoencoder), SdA (Stacked Denoising Autoencoder), RBM (Restricted Boltzmann machine), and DBN (Deep Belief Nets)
deepr	DL training, fine-tuning and predicting processes using darch and deepnet
MXNetR	Flexible and efficient ML/DL tools utilizing CPU/GPU computing
kerasR	RStudio's keras DL implementation wrapping C++/Python executable libraries
Keras	Python based neural networks API, connecting Google TensorFlow, Microsoft Cognitive Toolkit (CNTK), and Theano

[a]https://socr.umich.edu/HTML5/SOCR_TensorBoard_UKBB/

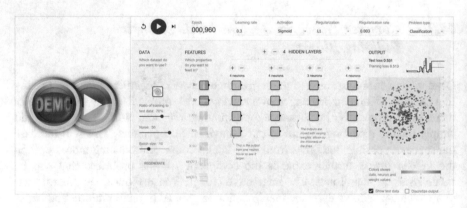

https://playground.tensorflow.org

14.4   Neural Network Modeling Using `Keras`

There are many different neural-net and deep-learning frameworks. Table 14.1 summarizes some of the main deep learning *R* packages.

14.4.1   Iterations—Samples, Batches, and Epochs

Table 14.2 shows the meanings of three complementary machine learning references to iterations. Concept definitions—sample, batch, and epoch

Iteration	Description
Sample	A singleton from the dataset, i.e., one element such as a patient, case, image, and file
Batch	An n-tuple, a set of n samples. All samples in a batch are typically processed independently, e.g., in parallel. AI training on a batch yields a single model (or model update). Dataset batches should accurately represent the underlying input data distribution, whereas a single sample represents one input. Larger batch sizes correspond to better model fits, however, they require significantly more computing processing power (cf. algorithmic complexity).
Epoch	A user-specified iterator that controls the number of passes over the entire dataset. Epochs separate training into independent model estimators and provide mechanisms for performance tracking and algorithmic evaluation.

Most DL/ML R packages provide interfaces (APIs) to libraries that are built using foundational languages like C/C++ and Java. Most of the Python libraries also act as APIs to lower-level executables compiled for specific platforms (Mac, Linux, PC).

The keras package uses the magrittr package pipe operator (%>%) to join multiple functions or operators, which streamlines the readability of the script protocol. Also, the library zeallot supplies the reverse piping function "%<-%", used in multiple assignment operators, see the brain_dataset() function later.

The kerasR package contains functions analogous to the ones in keras and utilizes the $ operator to create models. There are parallels between the core Python methods and their keras counterparts: compile() and keras_compile(), fit() and keras_fit(), predict() and keras_predict().

Below we will demonstrate using the Keras package for deep neural network analytics. This will require installation of keras and TensorFlow via R devtools::install_github("rstudio/keras"). For additional details, see the keras installation reference, user guide, and FAQs.[4]

```
# devtools::install_github("rstudio/keras")
library("keras")
# install_keras() #install.packages("tensorflow")
library(tensorflow)
```

The Keras package includes built-in datasets with load() functions, e.g., mnist.load_data() and imdb.load_data().

```
mnist <- dataset_mnist()
imdb <- dataset_imdb()
```

---

[4] https://tensorflow.rstudio.com/guide/keras/faq/

14.4.2   Use-Case: Predicting Titanic Passenger Survival

Instead of using the default data provided in the `keras` package, we will utilize one of the datasets on the DSPA Case Studies website, which can be loaded much like we previously did in Chap. 2. We start with performing some preprocessing steps on the Titanic Passengers Dataset.

```r
library(reshape)
library(caret)
dat <-
    read.csv("https://umich.instructure.com/files/9372716/download?download_frd=1")
# Inspect for missing values (empty or NA):
dat.miss <- melt(apply(dat[, -2], 2, function(x) sum(is.na(x) | x=="")))
cbind(row.names(dat.miss)[dat.miss$value>0], dat.miss[dat.miss$value>0,])
# We can exclude the "Cabin" feature which includes 80% missing values.
# Impute the few missing Embarked values using the most common value (S)
table(dat$embarked)
##       C   Q   S
##   2 270 123 914
dat$embarked[which(is.na(dat$embarked) | dat$embarked=="")] <- "S"
# Some "fare"" values may represent total cost of group purchases
# We can derive a new variable "price" representing fare per person
# Replace missing fare values with 0
dat$fare[which(is.na(dat$fare))] <- 0
# calculate ticket Price (Fare per person)
ticket.count <- aggregate(dat$ticket, by=list(dat$ticket),
                            function(x) sum( !is.na(x) ))
dat$price <- apply(dat, 1, function(x) as.numeric(x["fare"]) /
            ticket.count[which(ticket.count[, 1] == x["ticket"]), 2])
# Impute missing prices (price=0) using the median price per passenger class
pclass.price <- aggregate(dat$price, by = list(dat$pclass),
                FUN = function(x) median(x, na.rm = T))
dat[which(dat$price==0), "price"] <-
  apply(dat[which(dat$price==0), ] , 1, function(x)
    pclass.price[pclass.price[, 1]==x["pclass"], 2])
# Define "ticketcount" coding the number of passengers with same ticket number
dat$ticketcount <- apply(dat, 1,
    function(x) ticket.count[which(ticket.count[, 1] == x["ticket"]), 2])
# Capture the passenger title
dat$title <- regmatches(as.character(dat$name),
            regexpr("\\,[A-z ]{1,20}\\.", as.character(dat$name)))
dat$title <- unlist(lapply(dat$title,FUN=function(x) substr(x,3,nchar(x)-1)))
table(dat$title)
# Bin the 17 alternative title groups into 4 common 4 titles (factors)
dat$title[which(dat$title %in% c("Mme", "Mlle"))] <- "Miss"
dat$title[which(dat$title %in%
                c("Lady", "Ms", "the Countess", "Dona"))] <- "Mrs"
dat$title[which(dat$title=="Dr" & dat$sex=="female")] <- "Mrs"
dat$title[which(dat$title=="Dr" & dat$sex=="male")] <- "Mr"
dat$title[which(dat$title %in% c("Capt", "Col", "Don",
                    "Jonkheer", "Major", "Rev", "Sir"))] <- "Mr"
dat$title <- as.factor(dat$title)
table(dat$title)
## Master   Miss    Mr   Mrs
##     61    263   782   203
# Impute missing ages using median age for each title group
title.age <- aggregate(dat$age, by = list(dat$title),
                FUN = function(x) median(x, na.rm = T))
dat[is.na(dat$age), "age"] <- apply(dat[is.na(dat$age), ] , 1,
            function(x) title.age[title.age[, 1]==x["title"], 2])
```

14.4.3   EDA/Visualization

We can start by creating simple EDA plots, reporting numerical summaries, examining pairwise correlations, and showing the distributions of some features in this dataset (Figs. 14.7, 14.8 and 14.9).

```
library(ggplot2)
summary(dat)
plot_ly(dat, type="scatter", mode="markers")  %>%
    add_trace(x = ~ticketcount, y=~fare, mode = 'markers',
            color = ~as.character(survived), colors=~survived) %>%
    layout(legend = list(title=list(text='<b> Survival </b>'),
        orientation='h'),
        title="Titanic Passenger Data (TicketCount vs. Fare) Color Coded by
            Survival")
```

```
fig <- dat %>% plot_ly(type = 'violin')
fig <- fig %>% add_trace(x = ~survived[dat$survived == '1'],
    y = ~fare[dat$survived == '1'],
    legendgroup = 'survived',   scalegroup = 'survived',  name = 'survived',
    box=list(visible=T),  meanline = list(visible = T ),  color = I("green"))
fig <- fig %>% add_trace(x = ~survived[dat$survived == '0'],
    y = ~fare[dat$survived == '0'],
    legendgroup = 'died',   scalegroup = 'died',  name = 'died',
    box=list(visible = T),  meanline = list(visible = T ),  color = I("red"))
fig <- fig %>% layout(xaxis=list(title="Survival"),yaxis=list(title="Fare"),
    title='<b> Titanic Passenger Survival vs. Fare </b>', orientation='h')
fig
```

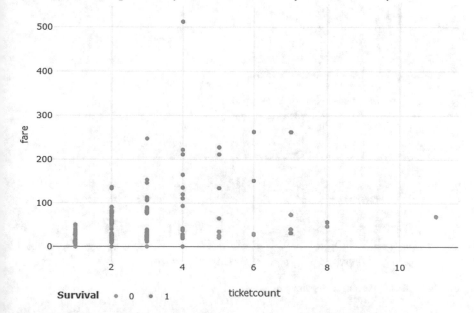

Titanic Passenger Data (TicketCount vs. Fare) Color Coded by Survival

Fig. 14.7 Titanic passengers—scatterplot of fare, ticket-count, survival indicator

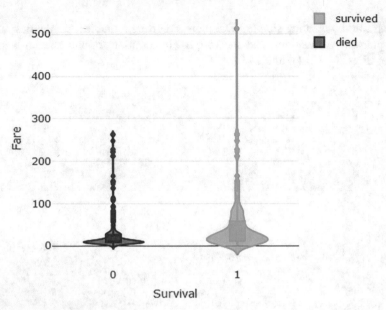

Fig. 14.8 Titanic passengers—violin plots of fare and survival

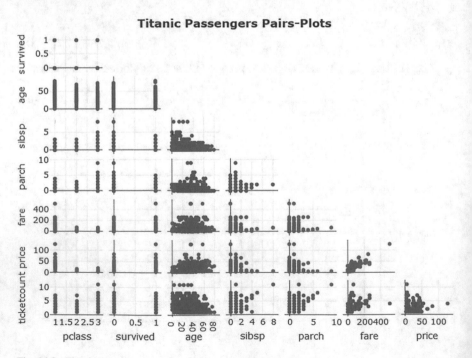

Fig. 14.9 Titanic passengers—pairs plot

```
dims <- dplyr::select_if(dat, is.numeric)
dims <- purrr::map2(dims, names(dims), ~list(values=.x, label=.y))
plot_ly(type = "splom", dimensions = setNames(dims, NULL),
         showupperhalf = FALSE, diagonal = list(visible = FALSE) ) %>%
  layout( title='<b> Titanic Passengers Pairs-Plots </b>')
```

14.4.4   Data Preprocessing

Before we go into modeling the data, we need to preprocess it, e.g., normalize the numerical values and split it into training and testing sets.

```
dat1 <- dat[ , c("pclass", "age", "sibsp", "parch", "fare",
                 "price", "ticketcount", "survived")]
dat1$pclass <- as.factor(dat1$pclass)
dat1$age <- as.numeric(dat1$age)
dat1$sibsp <- as.factor(dat1$sibsp)
dat1$parch <- as.factor(dat1$parch)
dat1$fare <- as.numeric(dat1$fare)
dat1$price <- as.numeric(dat1$price)
dat1$ticketcount <- as.numeric(dat1$ticketcount)
dat1$survived <- as.factor(dat1$survived)
dim(dat1) ## [1] 1309    8
```

Use keras::normalize() to normalize the numerical data.

```
library("keras")
summary(dat1[ , c(2,5,6,7)])
dat2 <- dat1[ , c(2,5,6,7)]
dat2 <- as.matrix(dat2)
dimnames(dat2) <- NULL
# May be best to avoid normalizing the ordinal variable "ticketcount"
dat2.norm <- keras::normalize(dat2) # Normalize the data
summary(dat2.norm)
colnames(dat2.norm) <- c("age", "fare", "price", "ticketcount")
```

Next, we'll partition the raw data into *training* (80%) and *testing* (20%) sets that will be utilized to build the forecasting model (to predict Titanic passenger survival) and assess the model performance, respectively.

```
train_set_ind <- sample(nrow(dat2.norm), floor(nrow(dat2.norm)*0.8))
# 80:20 plot training:testing
train_dat2.X <- dat2.norm[train_set_ind, ]
train_dat2.Y <- dat1[train_set_ind , 8]  # Outcome "survived" column:8
test_dat2.X <- dat2.norm[-train_set_ind, ]
test_dat2.Y <- dat1[-train_set_ind , 8]  # Outcome "survived" column:8
# check the shapes of the training and testing data (predictors & responses)
dim(train_dat2.X); length(train_dat2.Y); dim(test_dat2.X); length(test_dat2.Y)
```

14.4.5   Keras Modeling

For *multiclass classification problems* via NN modeling, the `keras::to_categorical()` function allows us to transform the outcome attribute from a vector of class labels to a matrix of Boolean features, one for each class label. In this case, we have a bivariate passenger survival indicator (binary classification). Keras modeling starts with first initializing a sequential model using the `keras::keras_model_sequential()` function.

We will try to predict the passenger survival using a fully connected multilayer perceptron NN. We will need to choose an activation function, e.g., `relu`, `sigmoid`. A rectifier activation function (relu) may be used in a hidden layer and a `softmax` activation function may be used in the final output layer so that the outputs represent (posterior) probabilities between 0 and 1, corresponding to the odds of survival. In the first layer, we can specify 8 hidden nodes (`units`), an `input_shape` of 4, to reflect the four features in the training data (*age, fare, price*, and *ticketcount*). At the end, we can specify the output layer with two output values, one for each of the survival categories.

We can also inspect the structure of the NN model using:

- `summary()`: print a summary representation of your model
- `get_config()`: return a list that contains the configuration of the model
- `get_layer()`: return the layer configuration
- `$layers`: NN model attribute retrieves a flattened list of the model's layers
- `$inputs`: NN model attribute listing the input tensors
- `$outputs`: NN model attribute retrieves the output tensors

```
model.1 <- keras_model_sequential()
model.1 %>%      # Add layers to the model
    layer_dense(units = 8, activation = 'relu', input_shape = c(4)) %>%
    layer_dense(units = 2, activation = 'softmax')
summary(model.1) # NN model summary
## Model: "sequential"
## Layer (type)                         Output Shape                      Param ##
## ========================================================================
## dense_1 (Dense)                      (None, 8)                             40
## dense (Dense)                        (None, 2)                             18
## Total params: 58
## Trainable params: 58
## Non-trainable params: 0
get_config(model.1)                 # Report model configuration
get_layer(model.1, index = 1)       # Report layer configuration
model.1$layers                      # Report model layers
model.1$inputs                      # List the input tensors
model.1$outputs                     # List the output tensors
```

Once the model architecture is specified, we need to estimate (fit) the NN model using the `training` data. The adaptive momentum (`ADAM`) optimizer along with the `categorical_crossentropy` objective function may be used to *compile* the NN model. Specifying `accuracy` as a metrics argument allows us to inspect the quality of the NN model fit during the training phase (training data validation). The *optimizer* and the *objective* (loss) functions are the pair of required arguments for model compilation.

In addition to *ADAM*, alternative optimization algorithms include Stochastic Gradient Descent (*SGD*) and Root Mean Square proportion (*RMSprop*). ADAM is essentially RMSprop with momentum whereas NADAM is ADAM RMSprop with Nesterov momentum.[5] Following the selection of the optimization algorithm, we need to tune the model parameters, e.g., learning rate or momentum. Choosing an appropriate objective function depends on the classification or regression forecasting task. For instance, for continuous outcomes, regression prediction usually utilizes Mean Squared Error (*MSE*), whereas multiclass classification problems use the *categorical_crossentropy* loss and binary classification problems commonly use the *binary_crossentropy* loss function.

```
# "Compile"" the model
model.1 %>% compile(
    loss = 'binary_crossentropy', optimizer = 'adam', metrics = 'accuracy')
```

14.4.6 NN Model Fitting

The next step fits the NN model (`model.1`) to the training data using 200 epochs, or iterations. In this case, the model-fitting process uses all the samples in `train_dat2.X` (predictors) and `train_dat2.Y` (outcomes), in batches of 10 samples. This process trains the model on a specified number of epochs (iterations or exposures) on the training data. One epoch is a single pass through the whole training set followed by comparing the model prediction results against the verification labels. The batch size defines the number of samples being propagated through the network at once (as a batch).

```
# convert the labels to categorical values
train_dat2.Y <- to_categorical(train_dat2.Y)
test_dat2.Y <- to_categorical(test_dat2.Y)
# Fit the model & Store the fitting history
track.model.1 <- model.1 %>% fit(
 train_dat2.X, train_dat2.Y, epochs=200, batch_size=10, validation_split=0.2)
```

---

[5] https://doi.org/10.1109/CVPR.2019.01138

14.4.7   Convolutional Neural Networks (CNNs)

Convolutional neural networks represent a specific type of deep learning algorithm that incorporates the topological, geometric, spatial, and temporal structure of the input data (generally images) and assigns importance by learning the weights and biases of the (image) intensities associated with the objects or affinities present in the data. These important features are then utilized to differentiate between datasets (images) or components within the data (structure and objects in images). CNNs require less preprocessing compared to other DL classification algorithms, which may depend on manually-specified filters. CNNs tend to learn these filters by iteratively extrapolating multiresolution characteristics in the data objects by convolution methods. See the DSPA Appendix for the mathematical *convolution* operation and its applications in image processing.[6]

Recall that one may attempt to learn the features of an image (or a higher dimensional tensor) by flattening the image array (matrix/tensor) into a 1D vector. This vectorization works well if there are no spatiotemporal dependencies in the data. Most of the time, there are image intensity correlations that can't be ignored. The CNN architecture facilitates a mechanism to better model the intrinsic image affinities, reduce the number of DNN parameters, and produce more reliable predictions. Many images are represented as tensors whose modes (dimensions) encode spatial, temporal, color-channel, and other information about the observed image intensity. For instance, an RGB image of size $1000 \times 1000 = 10^6$ pixels, may require 3 MB of memory/storage. A CNN learns to encode the image into a higher-dimensional multispectral hierarchical tensor encoding the intrinsic image characteristics that can lead to easy classification of similar images or generation of synthetic images. For instance, ignoring the color-channels and using a stride $= 10$, convolving the original image of dimension with a kernel of size 10×10 would yield another (smoother) lower-resolution image of size 100×100, encoding the convolved features.

The convolution process aims to extract the high-level features such as edges, borders, and contrasts from the input image. CNNs involve both convolutional and dense layers. Much like the Fourier transform, the first convolutional layer captures low-level features such as edges, color, and gradient orientation. Subsequent layers progressively add higher-level details, and the entire CNN holistically encodes the understanding of the input image structure.

Convolution, de-convolution (the reverse process) and padding reduce or increase the image dimensionality. Most CNNs mix *convolutional layers* with *pooling layers*. The latter are responsible for reducing the spatial size of the convolved features, which decreases the computational data processing demand. Pooling may be implemented as *Max Pooling* or *Average Pooling*. Max-pooling takes an image patch defined by the kernel and returns the maximum intensity value. It performs noise-suppression as it decimates noisy pixel intensities, denoises the image, and reduces the image dimensions. Average-pooling returns the average of all intensity values covered by the image-kernel and reduces the image dimension.

---

[6] https://socr.umich.edu/DSPA2/DSPA2_notes/DSPA_Appendix_6_ImageFilteringSpectralProcessing.html

Jointly, the convolutional and pooling processes form the CNN i-th layer and the number of layers may reflect the ANN complexity. Fully connected layers are typically added to the ANN architecture to enhance the classification, prediction, or regression performance of DL models. Fully connected layers provide a mechanism to learn nonlinear associations and nonaffine characteristics of high-level features captured as outputs of the convolutional layers.

14.4.8 Model Exploration

We can visualize the model fitting process using `keras::plot()` jointly depicting the loss of the objective function and the accuracy of the model, across epochs. Alternatively, we can split the pair of plots—one for the *model loss* and the other for the *model accuracy*. The $ operator is used to access the tensor data and plot it step-by-step. A sign of overfitting may be an accuracy (on training data) that keeps improving while the accuracy (on the validation data) worsens. This may be an indication that the NN model started to *learn* noise in the data instead of learning real patterns or affinities in the data. While the accuracy trends of both datasets are rising toward the final epochs, this may indicate that the model is still in the process of learning on the training dataset (and we can increase the number of epochs) (Fig. 14.10).

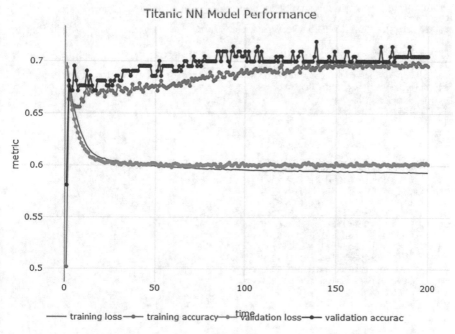

Fig. 14.10 Titanic passengers neural network model performance (loss and accuracy on training and validation data) against the iteration index

```
epochs <- 200
time <- 1:epochs
hist_df <- data.frame(time=time, loss=track.model.1$metrics$loss,
    acc=track.model.1$metrics$acc, valid_loss=track.model.1$metrics$val_loss,
    valid_acc=track.model.1$metrics$val_acc)
plot_ly(hist_df, x = ~time)  %>%
  add_trace(y = ~loss, name='training loss', mode='lines') %>%
  add_trace(y = ~acc, name='training accuracy', mode='lines+markers') %>%
  add_trace(y= ~valid_loss, name='validation loss', mode='lines+markers') %>%
  add_trace(y=~valid_acc,name='validation accuracy',mode='lines+markers') %>%
  layout(title="Titanic NN Model Performance",
         legend = list(orientation = 'h'), yaxis=list(title="metric"))
```

14.4.9 Passenger Survival Forecasting Using New Data

Once the model is fit, we can use it to predict the survival of passengers using the testing data, test_dat2.X. As we have seen before, predict() provides this functionality. Finally, we can evaluate the performance of the NN model by comparing the predicted class labels and test_dat2.Y using table() or confusionMatrix().

```
# Predict the classes for the test data
predict.survival <- model.1 %>%
        predict(test_dat2.X, batch_size = 30) %>% k_argmax()
# Confusion matrix
test_dat2.Y <- dat1[-train_set_ind , 8]
table(test_dat2.Y, predict.survival$numpy())
## test_dat2.Y   0    1
##           0 136   27
##           1  56   43
caret::confusionMatrix(test_dat2.Y, as.factor(predict.survival$numpy()))
## Confusion Matrix and Statistics
##           Reference
## Prediction   0    1
##          0 136   27
##          1  56   43
##                  Accuracy : 0.6832
##                    95% CI : (0.6231, 0.7391)
##       No Information Rate : 0.7328
##       P-Value [Acc > NIR] : 0.968572
##                     Kappa : 0.2851
##    Mcnemar's Test P-Value : 0.002116
##               Sensitivity : 0.7083
##               Specificity : 0.6143
##            Pos Pred Value : 0.8344
##            Neg Pred Value : 0.4343
##                Prevalence : 0.7328
##            Detection Rate : 0.5191
##      Detection Prevalence : 0.6221
##         Balanced Accuracy : 0.6613
##          'Positive' Class : 0
```

We can also utilize the `evaluate()` function to assess the model quality using testing data.

```
# Evaluate on test data and labels
test_dat2.Y <- to_categorical(test_dat2.Y)
model1.qual <- model.1 %>% evaluate(test_dat2.X, test_dat2.Y, batch_size=30)
print(model1.qual)
##        loss  accuracy
## 0.6059126 0.6832061
```

14.4.10 Fine-Tuning the NN Model

The main NN model parameters we can adjust to improve the model quality include the following:

- The *number of layers*
- The *number of nodes* within layers (*hidden units*)
- The *number of epochs*
- The *batch size*

Models can be improved by adding additional layers, increasing the number of hidden units, and by tuning the optimization parameters in `compile()`. Let's first try to add another layer to the N model (Fig. 14.11).

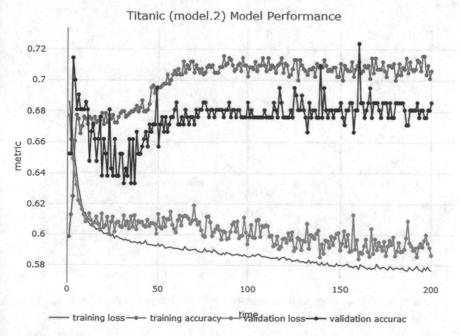

Fig. 14.11 Titanic passengers model2 performance (loss and accuracy on training and validation data) against the iteration index

```r
model.2 <- keras_model_sequential()    # Initialize the sequential model
model.2 %>%                            # Add layers to model
    layer_dense(units = 8, activation = 'relu', input_shape = c(4)) %>%
    layer_dense(units = 6, activation = 'relu') %>%
    layer_dense(units = 2, activation = 'softmax')
# Compile the model
model.2 %>% compile(
    loss = 'binary_crossentropy', optimizer = 'adam', metrics = 'accuracy')
# Fit NN model to training data & Save the training history
track.model.2 <- model.2 %>% fit(
    train_dat2.X, train_dat2.Y, epochs=200,batch_size=10,validation_split=0.2)
# Evaluate the model
model2.qual <- model.2 %>% evaluate(test_dat2.X, test_dat2.Y, batch_size= 30)
print(model2.qual)
##      loss  accuracy
## 0.5982294 0.6679389
epochs <- 200
time <- 1:epochs
hist_df2 <- data.frame(time=time, loss=track.model.2$metrics$loss,
    acc=track.model.2$metrics$acc, valid_loss=track.model.2$metrics$val_loss,
    valid_acc=track.model.2$metrics$val_acc)
plot_ly(hist_df2, x = ~time)  %>%
  add_trace(y = ~loss, name = 'training loss', mode = 'lines') %>%
  add_trace(y = ~acc, name = 'training accuracy', mode = 'lines+markers') %>%
  add_trace(y = ~valid_loss, name='validation loss',mode='lines+markers') %>%
  add_trace(y=~valid_acc,name='validation accuracy',mode='lines+markers') %>%
  layout(title="Titanic (model.2) Model Performance",
          legend = list(orientation = 'h'), yaxis=list(title="metric"))
```

Next, we can examine the effects of adding more *hidden units* to the NN model.

```r
model.3 <- keras_model_sequential()
model.3 %>%
    layer_dense(units = 30, activation = 'relu', input_shape = c(4)) %>%
    layer_dense(units = 15, activation = 'relu') %>%
    layer_dense(units = 2, activation = 'softmax')
model.3 %>% compile(
    loss = 'binary_crossentropy', optimizer = 'adam', metrics = 'accuracy')
track.model.3 <- model.3 %>% fit(
    train_dat2.X,train_dat2.Y,epochs=200,batch_size=10,validation_split=0.2)
# Evaluate the model
model3.qual <- model.3 %>% evaluate(test_dat2.X, test_dat2.Y, batch_size=30)
print(model3.qual)
##      loss  accuracy
## 0.5922436 0.6793893
epochs <- 200
time <- 1:epochs
hist_df3 <- data.frame(time=time, loss=track.model.3$metrics$loss,
    acc=track.model.3$metrics$acc, valid_loss=track.model.3$metrics$val_loss,
    valid_acc=track.model.3$metrics$val_acc)
plot_ly(hist_df3, x = ~time)  %>%
  add_trace(y = ~loss, name = 'training loss', mode = 'lines') %>%
  add_trace(y = ~acc, name = 'training accuracy', mode = 'lines+markers') %>%
  add_trace(y = ~valid_loss, name='validation loss',mode='lines+markers') %>%
  add_trace(y=~valid_acc,name='validation accuracy',mode='lines+markers') %>%
  layout(title="Titanic (model.3) NN Model Performance",
          legend = list(orientation = 'h'), yaxis=list(title="metric"))
```

Finally, we can attempt to fine-tune the optimization parameters provided to the compile() function. For instance, we can experiment with alternative optimization algorithms, like the Stochastic Gradient Descent (SGD), `optimizer_sgd()`, and adjust the *learning rate*, `lr`. In addition, we can specify alternative learning rate to train the NN, typically by 10-fold increase or decrease, which trades algorithmic accuracy, speed of convergence, and avoidance of local minima.

```
model.4 <- keras_model_sequential()
model.4 %>%        # Add layers and Node-Units to model
    layer_dense(units = 30, activation = 'relu', input_shape = c(4)) %>%
    layer_dense(units = 15, activation = 'relu') %>%
    layer_dense(units = 2, activation = 'softmax')
# Define an optimizer
SGD <- optimizer_sgd(lr = 0.001)
# Compile the model
model.4 %>% compile(optimizer=SGD, loss = 'binary_crossentropy',
                    metrics = 'accuracy')
# Fit NN model to training data & Save the training history
set.seed(1234)
track.model.4 <- model.4 %>% fit(
  train_dat2.X,train_dat2.Y, epochs=200, batch_size=10, validation_split=0.1)
# Evaluate the model
model4.qual <- model.4 %>% evaluate(test_dat2.X, test_dat2.Y, batch_size=30)
print(model4.qual)
##       loss   accuracy
## 0.6221561 0.6793893
epochs <- 200
time <- 1:epochs
hist_df4 <- data.frame(time=time, loss=track.model.4$metrics$loss,
    acc=track.model.4$metrics$acc, valid_loss=track.model.4$metrics$val_loss,
    valid_acc=track.model.4$metrics$val_acc)
plot_ly(hist_df3, x = ~time)  %>%
  add_trace(y = ~loss, name = 'training loss', mode = 'lines') %>%
  add_trace(y = ~acc, name = 'training accuracy', mode = 'lines+markers') %>%
  add_trace(y = ~valid_loss, name='validation loss',mode='lines+markers') %>%
  add_trace(y=~valid_acc,name='validation accuracy',mode='lines+markers') %>%
  layout(title="Titanic (model.4) NN Model Performance",
         legend = list(orientation = 'h'), yaxis=list(title="metric"))
```

14.4.11   Model Export and Import

Intermediate and final NN models may be saved, (re)loaded, and exported as PyTorch (.pt) or Keras Hierarchical Data Format (HDF5, .h5) files. For example, we can use `save_model_hdf5()` and `load_model_hdf5()` based on the HDF5 file format (h5).[7] We can operate on *complete models* on just on the *model weights*. the models can also be exported in JavaScript Object Notation (JSON) or YAML (Yet Another Multicolumn Layout) formats using `model_to_json()` and `model_to_yaml()`, and their load counterparts `model_from_json()` and `model_from yaml()`.

---

[7] https://support.hdfgroup.org/HDF5/whatishdf5.html

```
save_model_hdf5(model.4, "model.4.h5")
model.new <- load_model_hdf5("model.4.h5")
save_model_weights_hdf5("model_weights.h5")
model.old %>% load_model_weights_hdf5("model_weights.h5")
json_string <- model_to_json(model.old)
model.new <- model_from_json(json_string)
yaml_string <- model_to_yaml(model.old)
model.new <- model_from_yaml(yaml_string)
```

Let's demonstrate loading several pretrained models, resnet50, VGG16, VGG19,[8] and using them for simple out-of-the-box image classification and automated labeling of an image of New Zealand's Lake Mapourika, Fig. 14.12. This image recognition example will be expanded later. For now, we will simply illustrate the quick and efficient utilization of an existing pretrained neural network to qualitatively describe an image in a narrative form.

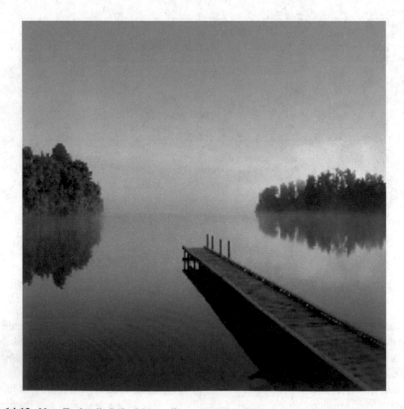

Fig. 14.12   New Zealand's Lake Mapourika

---

[8]https://keras.io/api/applications/

```r
library(keras)
# report info about local version of Python installation
reticulate::py_config()
# The first time you run this install Pillow!
# tensorflow::install_tensorflow(extra_packages='pillow')
# Load the image
download.file(
   "https://upload.wikimedia.org/wikipedia/commons/2/23/Lake_mapourika_NZ.jpeg",
        paste(getwd(),"results/image.png", sep="/"), mode = 'wb')
img <- image_load(paste(getwd(),"results/image.png", sep="/"),
        target_size = c(224,224))
# Preprocess input image
x <- image_to_array(img)
# ensure we have a 4d tensor with single element in the batch dimension,
# the preprocess the input for prediction using resnet50
x <- array_reshape(x, c(1, dim(x)))
x <- imagenet_preprocess_input(x)
# Specify and compare Predictions based on different Pre-trained Models
# Model 1: resnet50
model_resnet50 <- application_resnet50(weights = 'imagenet')
# make predictions then decode and print them
preds_resnet50 <- model_resnet50 %>% predict(x)
imagenet_decode_predictions(preds_resnet50, top = 10)
## [[1]]
##    class_name class_description       score
## 1   n09332890         lakeside 0.6543883085
## 2   n02859443        boathouse 0.1122922450
...
## 10  n03028079           church 0.0003251492
# Model2: VGG19
model_vgg19 <- application_vgg19(weights = 'imagenet')
preds_vgg19 <- model_vgg19 %>% predict(x)
imagenet_decode_predictions(preds_vgg19, top = 10)[[1]]
##    class_name class_description       score
## 1   n09332890         lakeside 0.7257616520
## 2   n02894605       breakwater 0.2156531066
...
## 10  n03873416           paddle 0.0004235525
# Model 3: VGG16
model_vgg16 <- application_vgg16(weights = 'imagenet')
preds_vgg16 <- model_vgg16 %>% predict(x)
imagenet_decode_predictions(preds_vgg16, top = 10)[[1]]
##    class_name class_description       score
## 1   n09332890         lakeside 0.656819046
## 2   n02894605       breakwater 0.201264054
...
## 10  n09421951          sandbar 0.001799420
```

14.5   Case Studies

Let's demonstrate deep neural network regression-modeling and classification-prediction using several biomedical case studies.

14.5.1   Classification Example Using Sonar Data

In this section, we will illustrate a number of AI data classification examples.
Let's load the mlbench packages which include a Sonar data mlbench::
Sonar containing information about sonar signals bouncing off a metal cylinder
or a roughly cylindrical rock. Each of the 208 observations includes a set of
60 numbers (features) in the range 0.0–1.0, and a label *M* (metal) or *R* (rock).
Each feature represents the energy within a particular frequency band, integrated
over a certain period of time. The M and R labels associated with each observation classify the record as rock or mine (metal) cylinder. The numbers in the
labels are in increasing order of aspect angle, but they do not encode the angle
directly.

```
library(mlbench)
data(Sonar, package="mlbench")
table(Sonar[,61])
##   M   R
## 111  97
Sonar[,61] = as.numeric(Sonar[,61])-1 # R = "1", "M" = "0"
set.seed(123)
train.ind = sample(1:nrow(Sonar),0.7*nrow(Sonar))
train.x = data.matrix(Sonar[train.ind, 1:60])
train.y = Sonar[train.ind, 61]
test.x = data.matrix(Sonar[-train.ind, 1:60])
test.y = Sonar[-train.ind, 61]
```

Let's start by using a *multilayer perceptron* as a classifier using a general
multilayer neural network that can be utilized to do classification or regression
modeling. It relies on the following parameters:

- Training data and labels
- Number of hidden nodes in each hidden layer
- Number of nodes in the output layer
- Type of activation
- Type of output loss

Here is one example using the *training* and *testing* data we defined above
(Fig. 14.13).

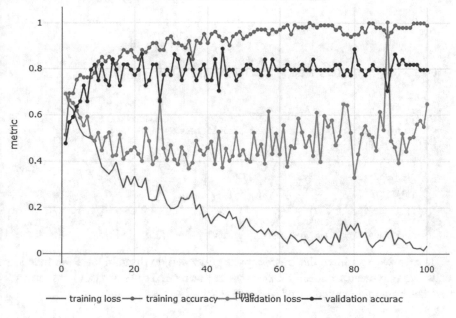

Fig. 14.13 Sonar data model performance (loss and accuracy on training and validation data) against the iteration index

```
library(plotly)
dim(train.x)  # [1] 145  60
## [1] 145  60
dim(test.x)   # [1] 63 60
## [1] 63 60
model <- keras_model_sequential()
model %>%
  layer_dense(units = 256, activation='relu', input_shape=ncol(train.x)) %>%
  layer_dropout(rate = 0.4) %>%
  layer_dense(units = 128, activation = 'relu') %>%
  layer_dropout(rate = 0.3) %>%
  layer_dense(units = 2, activation = 'sigmoid')
model %>% compile(
  loss = 'binary_crossentropy', optimizer = 'adam', metrics = c('accuracy'))
one_hot_labels <- to_categorical(train.y, num_classes = 2)
# Train the model, iterating on the data in batches of 25 samples
history <- model %>% fit(
  train.x, one_hot_labels, epochs = 100, batch_size=5, validation_split=0.3)
# Evaluate model
metrics <- model %>% evaluate(test.x, to_categorical(test.y, num_classes=2))
metrics
##       loss   accuracy
## 1.0744098 0.7301587
epochs <- 100
time <- 1:epochs
hist_df <- data.frame(time=time, loss=history$metrics$loss,
        acc=history$metrics$accuracy, valid_loss=history$metrics$val_loss,
        valid_acc=history$metrics$val_accuracy)
plot_ly(hist_df, x = ~time)  %>%
  add_trace(y=~loss, name='training loss', type="scatter", mode='lines') %>%
  add_trace(y=~acc, name='training accuracy',type="scatter",mode='lines') %>%
  add_trace(y=~valid_loss,name='valid loss',type="scatter",mode='lines') %>%
  add_trace(y=~valid_acc,name='validation accuracy',
            type="scatter",mode='lines') %>%
  layout(title="Sonar Data NN Model Performance",
         legend = list(orientation = 'h'), yaxis=list(title="metric"))
```

```
# Finally prediction of binary class labels and Confusion Matrix
predictions <- model %>% predict(test.x) %>% k_argmax()
table(factor(predictions$numpy()),factor(test.y))
##     0  1
##   0 29 10
##   1  7 17
# inspect the corresponding probabilities of the binary classification labels
prediction_probabilities <- model %>% predict(test.x)
prediction_probabilities
##               [,1]          [,2]
##   [1,] 1.130471e-01 8.933094e-01
##   [2,] 9.955512e-01 5.039215e-03
##   [3,] 9.285519e-01 7.906529e-02
...
##  [61,] 1.000000e+00 1.716803e-07
##  [62,] 9.991487e-01 9.450018e-04
##  [63,] 9.994618e-01 5.978942e-04
```

In case we also have the `caret` package loaded, to disambiguate the function calls, we may need to specify `crossval::confusionMatrix()`, as caret also has a function called `confusionMatrix()`.

```
library("crossval")
diagnosticErrors(confusionMatrix(predictions$numpy(),test.y,negative=0))
##       acc      sens      spec       ppv       npv       lor
## 0.7301587 0.7083333 0.7435897 0.6296296 0.8055556 1.9520139
```

We can plot the ROC curve and calculate the AUC (Area under the curve). Specifically, we will show computing the *area under the curve (AUC)* and drawing the *receiver operating characteristic (ROC)* curve. Assuming "positive" ranks higher than "negative," the AUC quantifies the probability that a classifier will rank a randomly chosen positive instance higher than a randomly chosen negative instance. For binary classification, interpreting the AUC values, $0 \leq AUC \leq 1$, corresponds to (poor) *uninformative classifiers* when AUC = 0.5 and perfect classifiers when $AUC \rightarrow 1^-$ (Fig. 14.14).

```
# install.packages("pROC"); install.packages("plotROC");
# install.packages("reshape2")
library(pROC); library(plotROC); library(reshape2);
get_roc = function(preds) {       # compute AUC
  roc_obj <- roc(test.y, preds, quiet=TRUE)
  auc(roc_obj)
}
get_roc(predictions$numpy()) # Area under the curve: 0.7176
predictions <- predictions$numpy()
#plot roc
dt <- data.frame(test.y, predictions)
colnames(dt) <- c("class","scored.probability")
# Compute the AUC and draw the ROC curve
roc_curve <- function(df) {
```

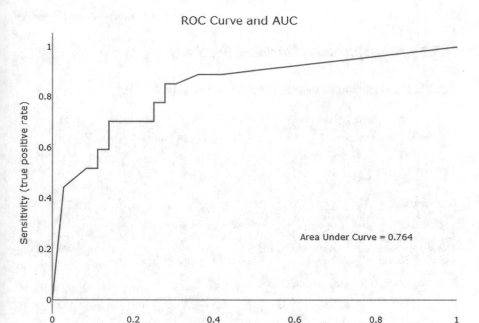

Fig. 14.14 The area under the ROC curve (AUC) quantifies the algorithmic performance

```
x <- c();   y <- c()
true_class = df[, "class"];    probabilities = df[, "scored.probability"]
thresholds = seq(0, 1, 0.01);   rx <- 0;   ry <- 0
for (threshold in thresholds) {
  predicted_class <- c()
  for (val in probabilities) {
    if (val > threshold) { predicted_class <- c(predicted_class, 1) }
    else { predicted_class <- c(predicted_class, 0)    }
  }
  df2 <- as.data.frame(cbind(true_class, predicted_class))
  TP <- nrow(filter(df2, true_class == 1 & predicted_class == 1))
  TN <- nrow(filter(df2, true_class == 0 & predicted_class == 0))
  FP <- nrow(filter(df2, true_class == 0 & predicted_class == 1))
  FN <- nrow(filter(df2, true_class == 1 & predicted_class == 0))
  specm1 <- 1 - ((TN) / (TN + FP))
  sens <- (TP) / (TP + FN)
  x <- append(x, specm1)
  y <- append(y, sens)
}
dfr <- as.data.frame(cbind(x, y))
plot_ly(dfr, x = ~ x, y = ~ y, type = 'scatter', mode = 'lines') %>%
  layout(title = paste0("ROC Curve and AUC"), annotations = list(
    text = paste0("Area Under Curve = ", round(get_roc(predictions)[[1]],3)),
    x = 0.75, y = 0.25, showarrow = FALSE),
  xaxis= list(showgrid=FALSE, title="1-Specificity (false positive rate)"),
  yaxis= list(showgrid=FALSE, title="Sensitivity (true positive rate)"),
  legend= list(orientation = 'h'))
}
roc_curve(data.frame(class=test.y,
    scored.probability=prediction_probabilities[,2]))
```

14.5.2   Schizophrenia Neuroimaging Study

The SOCR Schizophrenia dataset is available here (Fig. 14.15).[9]

```r
library("XML"); library("xml2")
library("rvest");
wiki_url <-
read_html("https://wiki.socr.umich.edu/index.php/SOCR_Data_Oct2009_ID_NI")
html_nodes(wiki_url, "#content")
SchizoData<- html_table(html_nodes(wiki_url, "table")[[1]])
# View (SchizoData): Select an outcome response "DX"(3), "FS_IQ" (5)
set.seed(1234)
test.ind = sample(1:63, 10, replace = F)
# select 10/63 cases for testing, train on remaining (63-10)/63 cases
train.x=scale(data.matrix(SchizoData[-test.ind,c(2, 4:9)])) # exclude outcome
train.y = ifelse(SchizoData[-test.ind, 3] < 2, 0, 1) # Binarize the outcome
test.x = scale(data.matrix(SchizoData[test.ind, c(2, 4:9)]))
test.y = ifelse(SchizoData[test.ind, 3] < 2, 0, 1)
model <- keras_model_sequential()
model %>%
  layer_dense(units = 256, activation='relu', input_shape=ncol(train.x)) %>%
  layer_dropout(rate = 0.4) %>%
  layer_dense(units = 128, activation = 'relu') %>%
  layer_dropout(rate = 0.3) %>%
  layer_dense(units = 64, activation = 'relu') %>%
  layer_dropout(rate = 0.1) %>%
  layer_dense(units = 32, activation = 'relu') %>%
  layer_dropout(rate = 0.1) %>%
  layer_dense(units = 2, activation = 'sigmoid')
model %>% compile(
  loss = 'binary_crossentropy', optimizer = 'adam', metrics = c('accuracy'))
one_hot_labels <- to_categorical(train.y[,1])
# Train the model, iterating on the data in batches of 25 samples
history <- model %>% fit(
  train.x, one_hot_labels, epochs=100, batch_size = 5, validation_split=0.1)
metrics <- model %>% evaluate(test.x, to_categorical(test.y[ , 1]))
metrics  # Evaluate model
##      loss accuracy
## 1.813025 0.800000
plot(history)
```

[9] http://wiki.stat.ucla.edu/socr/index.php/SOCR_Data_Oct2009_ID_NI, and https://wiki.socr.umich.edu/index.php/SOCR_Data_Oct2009_ID_NI

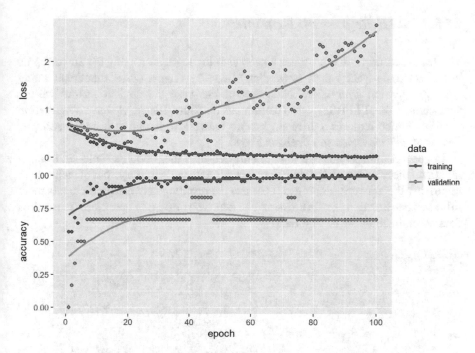

Fig. 14.15 Schizophrenia study—training and validation data algorithmic performance

```
epochs <- 100
time <- 1:epochs
hist_df <- data.frame(time=time, loss=history$metrics$loss,
    acc=history$metrics$accuracy, valid_loss=history$metrics$val_loss,
    valid_acc=history$metrics$val_accuracy)
plot_ly(hist_df, x = ~time)  %>%
  add_trace(y= ~loss, name='training loss', type="scatter", mode='lines') %>%
  add_trace(y=~acc,name='training accuracy', type="scatter",mode='lines') %>%
  add_trace(y=~valid_loss,name='validation loss',type="scatter",mode='lines') %>%
  add_trace(y=~valid_acc, name='validation accuracy', type="scatter",
            mode='lines') %>%
  layout(title="Schizophrenia Study NN Model Performance",
         legend = list(orientation = 'h'), yaxis = list(title="metric"))
# Finally prediction of binary class labels and Confusion Matrix
predictions <- model %>% predict(test.x) %>% k_argmax()
prediction_probabilities <- model %>% predict(test.x)
prediction_probabilities
##                  [,1]           [,2]
## [1,] 5.437903e-06 9.999892e-01
## [2,] 9.999998e-01 7.379477e-08
...
## [10,] 5.319853e-06 9.999871e-01
table(factor(predictions$numpy()),factor(test.y))
##      0 1
##    0 4 1
##    1 1 4
```

14.5.3 ALS Regression Example

The second example demonstrates a deep learning regression using the amyotrophic lateral sclerosis (ALS) data to predict `ALSFRS_slope` (ALS functional rating scale progression over time). Note that in this case the clinical feature we are predicting, $Y = \text{ALSFRS}_{slope}$, is a continuous outcome. Hence, we have a *regression problem*, which requires a different `keras` network formulation from the *categorical or binary classification problem* above.

In general, normalizing all data features ensures the model is scale- and range-invariant. Feature normalization may not be always necessary, but it helps with improving the network training and ensures the resulting network prediction is more robust. The function `tfdatasets::feature_spec()` provides tensorflow data normalization for tabular data.

```
library(tfdatasets)
als <-
    read.csv("https://umich.instructure.com/files/1789624/download?download_frd=1")
ALSFRS_slope <- als[,7]
als <- as.data.frame(als[,-c(1,7,94)])
colnames(als)
##  [1] "Age_mean"                          "Albumin_max"
##  [3] "Albumin_median"                    "Albumin_min"
...
## [95] "trunk_range"                       "Urine.Ph_max"
## [97] "Urine.Ph_median"                   "Urine.Ph_min"
spec <- feature_spec(als, ALSFRS_slope ~ . ) %>%
   step_numeric_column(all_numeric(), normalizer_fn=scaler_standard()) %>% fit()
spec
```

The `feature_spec` output *spec* is used together with the `keras::layer_dense_features()` method to directly perform preprocessing in the TensorFlow graph. We can take a look at the output of a dense-features layer created by the `feature_spec`, which is a matrix (2D tensor) with scaled values.

```
layer <-
    layer_dense_features(feature_columns=dense_features(spec),dtype=tf$float32)
layer(als)
## tf.Tensor(
## [[-0.3184486    0.13492961    0.24731219 ...    0.98161167   1.7149795
##    -0.9971952 ]
##  [ 0.9987701    0.8886633     0.13080972 ...    0.98161167   0.86683726
##    -0.38858187]
##  [-1.4474932   -1.9755248    -1.1507174  ...   -2.2801561   -1.2535185
##     0.39815933]
##  ...
##  [-1.071145    -0.6188041     0.01430727 ...   -0.41628885   0.44276613
##    -1.1794543 ]
##  [ 0.4342478    0.3610497     0.13080972 ...   -0.18330544  -0.40537617
##     0.794734  ]
##  [ 0.9987701    1.03941       -1.0342149  ...    1.4475784   -0.82944727
##     1.99725   ]], shape=(2223, 98), dtype=float32)
```

Next, we design the network architecture model using the `feature_spec` API by passing the `dense_features` from the new *spec* object.

```
input <- layer_input_from_dataset(als)
output <- input %>%
  layer_dense_features(dense_features(spec)) %>%
  layer_dense(units = 256, activation = "relu") %>%
  layer_dense(units = 128, activation = "relu") %>%
  layer_dense(units = 64, activation = "relu") %>%
  layer_dense(units = 16, activation = "relu") %>%
  layer_dense(units = 1)
model <- keras_model(input, output)
```

It's time to compile the deep network model and wrap it into a function `build_model()` that can be reused for different experiments. Remember that `keras::fit()` modifies the model in-place.

```
model %>% compile(loss = "mse", optimizer = optimizer_rmsprop(),
          metrics = list("mean_absolute_error"))
build_model <- function() {
  input <- layer_input_from_dataset(als)
  output <- input %>%
  layer_dense_features(dense_features(spec)) %>%
  layer_dense(units = 256, activation = "relu") %>%
  layer_dense(units = 128, activation = "relu") %>%
  layer_dense(units = 64, activation = "relu") %>%
  layer_dense(units = 16, activation = "relu") %>%
  layer_dense(units = 1)
  model <- keras_model(input, output)
  model %>% compile(loss = "mse", optimizer = optimizer_rmsprop(),
            metrics = list("mean_absolute_error"))
  model
}
```

Model training follows with 200 epochs where we record the training and validation accuracy in a *keras_training_history* object. For tracking the learning progress, we use a custom callback to replace the default training output at each epoch by a single dot (period) printed in the console.

```
# Display training progress - printing a single dot for each completed epoch
print_dot_callback <- callback_lambda(
  on_epoch_end = function(epoch, logs) {
    if (epoch %% 80 == 0) cat("\n")
    cat(".")
  }
)
model <- build_model()
history <- model %>% fit(x = als, y = ALSFRS_slope, epochs = 200,
  validation_split = 0.2, verbose=0, callbacks = list(print_dot_callback))
```

Let's visualize the model's training data performance using the metrics stored in the history object. This graph provides clues to determine training duration and confirm model performance convergence.

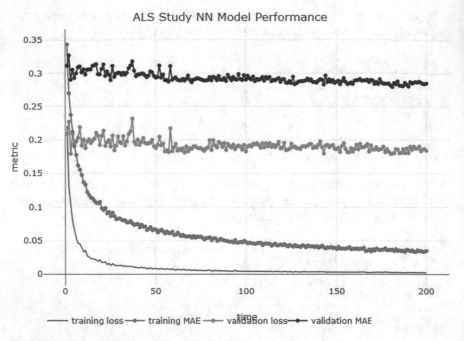

Fig. 14.16 ALS study—the training and validation data algorithmic performance

This graph shows little improvement in the model after about 200 epochs. Let's update the fit method to automatically stop training when the validation score doesn't improve. We'll use a callback that tests a training condition for every epoch. If a set number of epochs elapses without showing improvement, it automatically stops the training (Fig. 14.16).

```
epochs <- 200
time <- 1:epochs
hist_df <- data.frame(time=time, loss=history$metrics$loss,
  mae=history$metrics$mean_absolute_error,valid_loss=history$metrics$val_loss,
  valid_mae=history$metrics$val_mean_absolute_error)
plot_ly(hist_df, x = ~time) %>%
  add_trace(y=~loss, name='training loss', type="scatter", mode='lines') %>%
  add_trace(y=~mae, name='training MAE',
            type="scatter", mode='lines+markers')%>%
  add_trace(y=~valid_loss,name='validation loss',type="scatter",mode='lines') %>%
  add_trace(y=~valid_mae,name='validation MAE', type="scatter", mode='lines') %>%
  layout(title="ALS Study NN Model Performance",
         legend = list(orientation = 'h'), yaxis=list(title="metric"))
# This graph shows little improvement in the model after about 100 epochs
```

Have a look at the Google TensorFlow API.[10] It shows the importance of *learning rate* and the *number of rounds*. We can test different sets of parameters.

---

[10] https://www.tensorflow.org/versions

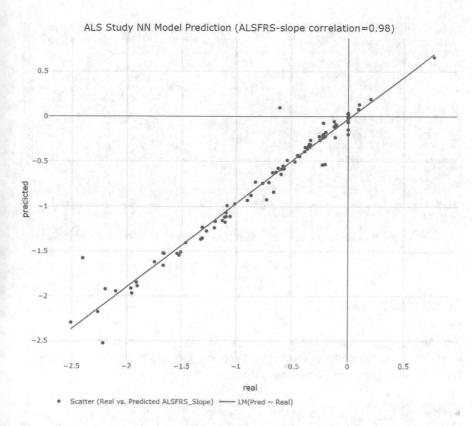

Fig. 14.17 ALS study—scatterplot of observed vs. NN-predicted outcome (ALSFRS-slope)

- Too small *learning rate* may lead to long computations.
- Too large *learning rate* may cause the algorithm to fail to converge, as large step size (learning rate) may by-pass the optimal solution and then oscillate or even diverge.

Finally, we can forecast and predict the ALSFRS_slope using data in the testing set (Fig. 14.17).

```
cases <- 100
test_sample <- sample(1:dim(als)[1], size=cases)
test_predictions <- model %>% predict(als[test_sample, ])
# test_predictions[ , 1]
print(paste0("Corr(real_ALSFRS_Slope, predicted_ALSFRS_Slope)=",
              round(cor(test_predictions, ALSFRS_slope[test_sample]), 3)))
## [1] "Corr(real_ALSFRS_Slope, predicted_ALSFRS_Slope)=0.984"
cases <- 1:cases
hist_df <- data.frame(cases=cases, real=ALSFRS_slope[test_sample],
              predicted=test_predictions)
corr1 <- round(cor(hist_df$real, hist_df$predicted), 2)
plot_ly(hist_df, x = ~real)  %>%
  add_trace(y = ~predicted, name='Scatter (Real vs. Predicted ALSFRS_Slope)',
            type="scatter", mode = 'markers') %>%
  add_lines(x = ~real, y = ~fitted(lm(predicted ~ real, hist_df)),
            name="LM(Pred ~ Real)") %>%
  layout(title= paste0("ALS Study NN Model Prediction (ALSFRS-slope
            correlation =", corr1,")"),
            legend = list(orientation = 'h'), yaxis=list(title="predicted"))
```

14.5.4   IBS Study

Let's try another example using the irritable bowel syndrome (IBS) neuroimaging study.[11] Again, we will use deep neural network learning to predict a categorical/ binary classification label (diagnosis, DX).

```
# IBS NI Data
library(xml2)
library(rvest)
# UCLA Data
wiki_url <-
  read_html("http://wiki.stat.ucla.edu/socr/index.php/SOCR_Data_April2011_NI_IBS_Pain")
IBSData <- html_table(html_nodes(wiki_url, "table")[[2]]) # table 2
set.seed(1234)
# select 50/354 of cases for testing, train on remaining (354-50)/354 cases
test.ind = sample(1:354, 50, replace = F)
html_nodes(wiki_url, "#content")
# scale/normalize all input variables
IBSData <- na.omit(IBSData)
IBSData[,4:66] <- scale(IBSData[,4:66])  # scale the entire dataset
train.x = data.matrix(IBSData[-test.ind, c(4:66)]) # exclude outcome
train.y = IBSData[-test.ind, 3]-1
test.x = data.matrix(IBSData[test.ind, c(4:66)])
test.y = IBSData[test.ind, 3]-1
train.y <- train.y$Group
test.y <- test.y$Group
model <- keras_model_sequential()
model %>%
  layer_dense(units = 256, activation='relu', input_shape=ncol(train.x)) %>%
  layer_dropout(rate = 0.4) %>%
  layer_dense(units = 128, activation = 'relu') %>%
  layer_dropout(rate = 0.3) %>%
  layer_dense(units = 64, activation = 'relu') %>%
  layer_dropout(rate = 0.1) %>%
```

---

[11] http://wiki.stat.ucla.edu/socr/index.php/SOCR_Data_April2011_NI_IBS_Pain

```
    layer_dense(units = 32, activation = 'relu') %>%
  layer_dropout(rate = 0.1) %>%
  layer_dense(units = 16, activation = 'relu') %>%
  layer_dropout(rate = 0.1) %>%
  layer_dense(units = 2, activation = 'sigmoid')
model %>% compile(
  loss = 'binary_crossentropy', optimizer = 'adam', metrics = c('accuracy'))
one_hot_labels <- to_categorical(train.y, num_classes = 2)
# Train the model, iterating on the data in batches of 25 samples
history <- model %>% fit(
  train.x, one_hot_labels, epochs = 100, batch_size=5, validation_split=0.1)
# Evaluate model
metrics <- model %>% evaluate(test.x, to_categorical(test.y, num_classes=2))
metrics
plot(history)
epochs <- 100
time <- 1:epochs
hist_df <- data.frame(time=time, loss=history$metrics$loss,
      acc=history$metrics$accuracy, valid_loss=history$metrics$val_loss,
      valid_acc=history$metrics$val_accuracy)
plot_ly(hist_df, x = ~time)  %>%
  add_trace(y=~loss, name='training loss', type="scatter", mode='lines') %>%
  add_trace(y=~acc, name='training accuracy',type="scatter",mode='lines') %>%
  add_trace(y=~valid_loss,name='validation loss',type="scatter",mode='lines') %>%
  add_trace(y=~valid_acc, name='validation accuracy', type="scatter",
            mode='lines')%>%
  layout(title="IBS Study NN Model Performance",
          legend = list(orientation = 'h'), yaxis=list(title="metric"))
# Finally prediction of binary class labels and Confusion Matrix
predictions <- model %>% predict(test.x) %>% k_argmax()
table(factor(predictions$numpy()),factor(test.y))
##      0  1
##   0 21 16
##   1  9  4
```

These results suggest that the DNN classification of IBS diagnosis is not particularly good, at least under the specific network topology and training conditions.

14.5.5   Country QoL Ranking Data

Another case study we have seen before is the country quality of life (QoL) dataset.[12] Let's try to fit a network model and use it to predict the overall QoL. This is another binary classification problem categorizing countries as either *developed* or *developing*. In this case, the results indicate that the DNN model performs exceptionally well (Fig. 14.18).

---

[12] http://wiki.stat.ucla.edu/socr/index.php/SOCR_Data_2008_World_CountriesRankings

```r
wiki_url <-
  read_html("http://wiki.stat.ucla.edu/socr/index.php/SOCR_Data_2008_World_CountriesRankings")
html_nodes(wiki_url, "#content")
CountryRankingData<- html_table(html_nodes(wiki_url, "table")[[2]])
set.seed(1234)
# select 15/100 of cases for testing, train on remaining 85/100 cases
test.ind = sample(1:100, 30, replace = F)
CountryRankingData[,c(8:12,14)] <- scale(CountryRankingData[,c(8:12,14)])
# scale/normalize all input variables
train.x=data.matrix(CountryRankingData[-test.ind,c(8:12,14)])#exclude outcome
train.y = ifelse(CountryRankingData[-test.ind, 13] < 50, 1, 0)
test.x = data.matrix(CountryRankingData[test.ind, c(8:12,14)])
test.y = ifelse(CountryRankingData[test.ind, 13] < 50, 1, 0) # developed country
(high overall rank)
model <- keras_model_sequential()
model %>%
  layer_dense(units = 16, activation = 'relu', input_shape=ncol(train.x)) %>%
  layer_dropout(rate = 0.4) %>%
  layer_dense(units = 4, activation = 'relu') %>%
  layer_dropout(rate = 0.1) %>%
  layer_dense(units = 2, activation = 'sigmoid')
model %>% compile(
  loss = 'binary_crossentropy', optimizer = 'adam', metrics = c('accuracy'))
one_hot_labels <- to_categorical(train.y, num_classes = 2)
# Train the model, iterating on the data in batches of 25 samples
history <- model %>% fit(
  train.x, one_hot_labels, epochs = 50, batch_size = 5, validation_split=0.1)
# Evaluate model
metrics <- model %>% evaluate(test.x, to_categorical(test.y, num_classes=2))
metrics
##      loss  accuracy
## 0.1235760 0.9666666
epochs <- 50
time <- 1:epochs
hist_df <- data.frame(time=time, loss=history$metrics$loss,
      acc=history$metrics$accuracy, valid_loss=history$metrics$val_loss,
      valid_acc=history$metrics$val_accuracy)
plot_ly(hist_df, x = ~time) %>%
  add_trace(y=~loss, name='training loss', type="scatter", mode='lines') %>%
  add_trace(y=~acc,name='training accuracy',type="scatter", mode='lines') %>%
  add_trace(y=~valid_loss,name='validation loss',type="scatter",mode='lines') %>%
  add_trace(y = ~valid_acc, name = 'validation accuracy', type="scatter",
            mode = 'lines+markers') %>%
  layout(title="Country QoL Ranking NN Model Performance",
         legend = list(orientation = 'h'), yaxis=list(title="metric"))


# Finally prediction of binary class labels and Confusion Matrix
predictions <- model %>% predict(test.x) %>% k_argmax()
table(factor(predictions$numpy()),factor(test.y))
##      0  1
## 0  13  1
## 1   0 16
```

Note that in this case, even a simple DNN network rapidly converges to an accurate model.

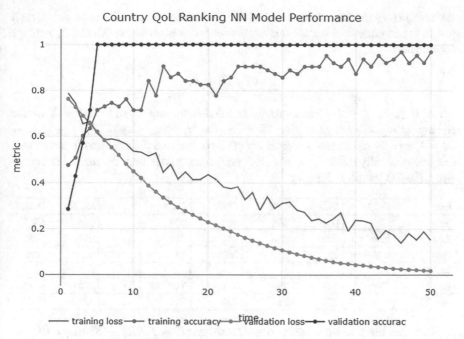

Country QoL Ranking NN Model Performance

— training loss —•— training accuracy —•— validation loss —•— validation accurac

Fig. 14.18 QoL study—the training and validation data algorithmic performance

14.5.6   *Handwritten Digits Classification*

In Chap. 6 (Black Box ML Methods), we discussed Optical Character Recognition (OCR). Specifically, we analyzed handwritten notes (unstructured text) and converted it to printed text.

The Modified National Institute of Standards and Technology (MNIST) database includes a large handwritten digits imaging dataset with human annotated labels.[13] Every digit is represented by a 28 × 28 thumbnail image. You can download the training and testing data from Kaggle.[14] The train.csv and test.csv data files contain gray-scale images of hand-drawn digits, 0, 1, 2, ..., 9. Each 2D image is 28 × 28 in size and each of the 784 pixels has a single pixel-intensity representing the lightness or darkness of that pixel (stored as a 1 byte integer [0, 255]). Higher intensities correspond to darker pixels.

The training data, train.csv, has 785 columns, where the first column, *label*, codes the actual digit drawn by the user. The remaining 784 columns contain the 28 × 28 = 784 pixel-intensities of the associated 2D image. Columns in the training

---

[13] https://yann.lecun.com/exdb/mnist/

[14] https://www.kaggle.com/c/digit-recognizer/data

set have $pixel_K$ names, where $0 \leq K \leq 783$. To reconstruct a 2D image out of each row in the training data we use this relation between pixel-index (K) and X, Y image coordinates

$$K = Y \times 28 + X,$$

where $0 \leq X, Y \leq 27$. Thus, $pixel_K$ is located on row Y and column X of the corresponding 2D Image of size 28×28. For instance, $pixel_{60 \ = \ (2 \ \times \ 28 \ + \ 4)} \leftrightarrow$ $(X = 4, Y = 2)$ represents the pixel on the 3-rd row and 5-th column in the image. Diagrammatically, omitting the "pixel" prefix, the pixels may be ordered to reconstruct the 2D image as follows

Row	Col0	Col1	Col2	Col3	Col4	...	Col26	Co27
Row0	000	001	002	003	004	...	026	027
Row1	028	029	030	031	032	...	054	055
Row2	056	057	058	059	060	...	082	083
RowK	...	...	...	...	...	...	...	...
Row26	728	729	730	731	732	...	754	755
Row27	756	757	758	759	760	...	782	783

Note that the point-to-pixelID transformation $(K = Y \times 28 + X)$ may easily be inverted as a pixelID-to-point mapping $X = K$ mod 28, where mod gives the remainder of the integer division $(K/28)$ and $Y=$ integer part of the division $K/28$. Here is one example.

```
K <- 60
X <- K %% 28 # X= K mod 28, remainder of integer division 60/28
Y <- K%/%28  # integer part of the division
# This validates that the application of both, the back and forth
transformations, leads to an identity
K; X; Y; Y * 28 + X
## [1] 60
## [1] 4
## [1] 2
## [1] 60
```

The test data (test.csv) has the same organization as the training data, except that it does not contain the first *label* column. It includes 28,000 images and we can predict image labels that can be stored as *ImageId, Label* pairs, which can be visually compared to the 2D images for validation/inspection.

```
# train.csv
pathToZip <- tempfile()
download.file("https://www.socr.umich.edu/people/dinov/2017/Spring/DSPA_HS650/data/D
igitRecognizer_TrainingData.zip", pathToZip)
train <- read.csv(unzip(pathToZip))
dim(train) ## [1] 42000    785
unlink(pathToZip)
# test.csv
pathToZip <- tempfile()
download.file("https://www.socr.umich.edu/people/dinov/2017/Spring/DSPA_HS650/data/D
igitRecognizer_TestingData.zip", pathToZip)
test <- read.csv(unzip(pathToZip))
dim(test) ## [1] 28000    784
unlink(pathToZip)
train <- data.matrix(train)
test <- data.matrix(test)
train.x <- train[,-1]
train.y <- train[,1]
# Scaling will be discussed below
train.x <- t(train.x/255)
test <- t(test/255)
# We can also load the MNIST dataset (training & testing directly from keras)
# mnist <- dataset_mnist()
```

Let's look at some examples of these handwritten-digits MNIST images
(Fig. 14.19).

```
library("imager")
# first convert the CSV data (one row per image, 28,000 rows)
array_3D <- array(test, c(28, 28, 28000))
mat_2D <- matrix(array_3D[,,1], nrow = 28, ncol = 28)
plot(as.cimg(mat_2D))
# extract all N=28,000 images
N <- 28000
img_3D <- as.cimg(array_3D[,,], 28, 28, N)
# plot the k-th image (1<=k<=N)
k <- 5
plot(img_3D, k)
image_2D <- function(img,index) {    img[,,index,,drop=FALSE] }
plot(image_2D(img_3D, 1))
# Plot a collage of the first 4 images
imappend(list(image_2D(img_3D, 1), image_2D(img_3D, 2), image_2D(img_3D, 3),
        image_2D(img_3D, 4)),"y") %>% plot
```

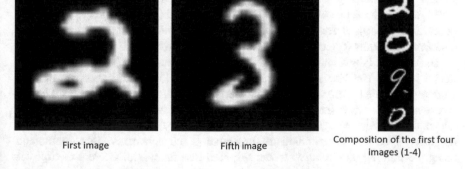

First image   Fifth image   Composition of the first four
                                                                          images (1-4)

Fig. 14.19 Instances of the MNIST handwritten digits imaging dataset

In these CSV data files, each 28×28 image is represented as a single row. Grayscale images are 1 byte, in the range $[0, 255]$, which we linearly transformed into $[0, 1]$. Note that we only scale the X input, not the output (labels). Also, we don't have manual gold-standard validation labels for the testing data, i.e., test.y is not available for the handwritten digits data. Next, we can transpose the input matrix to n (*pixels*) $\times m$ (*examples*), as the column major format required by the classifiers. The image labels are evenly distributed.

```
table(train.y); prop.table(table(train.y))
## train.y
## 0 1 2 3 4 5 6 7 8 9
## 4132 4684 4177 4351 4072 3795 4137 4401 4063 4188
## train.y
## 0 1 2 3 4 5 6 7 8 9
## 0.10 0.11 0.10 0.10 0.10 0.09 0.10 0.11 0.10 0.10
```

The majority class (1) in the training set includes 11.2% of the observations.

14.5.6.1   Configuring the Neural Network

The neural network model is trained by feeding the training data, i.e., *training images (train.x)* and *training labels (train.y)*. The network learns to associate specific images with concrete labels. Then, the network generates label predictions for (new) *testing images* that can be compared to the true labels of test-images (if these are available) or visually inspected to confirm correct auto-classification.

The magrittr package pipe operator, %>%, is commonly used for short-hand notation to allow left-and-right feed-and-assignment that can be interpreted as "do ... then feed into ... and do ...".

Nodes and layers represent the basic building-blocks of all artificial neural networks. Both are generalizations of brain neuron and network data processing that effectively transform, compress, or filter the input data. *Inputs* go in a node or a layer, and *outputs* come out. Network layers learn to extract effective representations of the inputs that are coded as meaningful outputs that can be connected by chaining together multiple layers that progressive distill the information into compressed generic knowledge (patterns) that can be used to predict, forecast, classify, or model the mechanistic relations in the process. That is, we use data as a proxy of observable processes for which we don't have explicit closed-form probability distribution models (typically complex multivariate processes).

The network below chains a pair of layers densely connected (i.e., fully connected neural layers). The keras_model_sequential() method specifies the network architecture before we start with training (i.e., estimating the weights). The *loss function* specifies how the network measures its performance on the training data to adjust the network weights (using train.x and train.y) to optimize the loss. The *optimizer* specifies the mechanism for updating the network weight coefficients using the training data relative to the specified loss function. Different metrics can be used to track the performance during the iterative training and testing process. For instance, accuracy represents the fraction of the images that were correctly classified. The second layer is a *10-way softmax layer* that returns a vector of 10 probability scalars (all positive and summing to 1) each representing the probability that the current hand-written image represents any of the 10 digits (0, 1, 2, $\cdots$, 9). The `compile()` function modifies the network in place to specify the optimization strategy, the loss function and the assessment metric that will be used in the learning process.

In this network example, we chain two dense layers to each layer and apply simple tensor operations (tensor-dot-product/matrix multiplication and tensor addition) to the input data to estimate the weight parameter tensors, i.e., attributes of the layers encoding the persistent knowledge of the network. The `categorical_crossentropy` is the specific loss function that is optimized in the training phase to provide a feedback signal for learning the weight tensors. The loss optimization relies on mini-batch stochastic gradient descent, which is defined by the `rmsprop` optimizer argument.

```
network <- keras_model_sequential() %>%
  layer_dense(units = 512, activation - "relu", input_shape = c(28 * 28)) %>%
  layer_dense(units = 10, activation = "softmax")
network %>% compile(optimizer = "rmsprop", loss = "categorical_crossentropy",
                    metrics = c("accuracy"))
```

Concatenating dense layers allows us to build a neural network whose depth is determined by the number of layers that are specified by a version of `layer_dense(units = 512, activation = "relu")`, which represents a function of the input (2D tensor) and output (a different 2D tensor) that may be fed as an input tensor to the next layer. Let $ReLu(x) = \max(x, 0)$. W and b represent two of the attributes of the layer (trainable weight parameters of the layer), i.e., the 2D kernel tensor and the bias vector. Then the layer-output O is

$$O = ReLu(W \times Input + b).$$

Deep learning network models are represented as directed, acyclic graphs of layers. Often, these networks constitute a linear stack of layers mapping a single input to a single output. Different types of network layers are appropriate for different kinds of data tensors:

- Simple vector data, stored in *2D tensors* of shape (*samples, features*), are often modeled using densely connected layers, i.e., fully connected dense layers (`keras::layer_dense function()`).
- Sequence data, stored in *3D tensors* of shape (*samples, timesteps, features*), are typically modeled by recurrent layers such as `keras::layer_lstm()`.
- Image data, stored in *4D tensors*, is usually processed by 2D convolution layers (`keras::layer_conv_2d()`).

14.5.6.2 Training

We are ready to start the network training process. At the initialization step of the learning process, the weight matrices are filled with random values (random initialization). At the start, when W and b are random, the output `relu(W*input) + b` is likely going to be meaningless. However, the subsequent iterative process optimizing the objective (loss) function will gradually adapt to these weights (training process) by repeating the following steps until certain stopping criterion is met:

- Draw a (random) batch of training samples x and their corresponding targets y.
- Forward pass: Run the network on x to obtain predictions y_{pred}.
- Estimate the loss of the network on the batch data assessing the mismatch between y and y_{pred}.
- Update all weights (W and b) of the network to reduce the overall loss on this batch.

Iterating this process eventually yields a network that has a low loss on its training data, indicating good fidelity (match between predictions y_{pred} and expected targets y). This reflects the network learning process progressed and accurately maps inputs to correct targets.

Stochastic gradient descent (SGD) is a powerful function optimization strategy for differentiable multivariate functions. Recall that a function's extrema are attained at points where the derivative (gradient, $\nabla(f)$) is trivial (0) or at the domain boundary. Hence, to minimize the loss, we need to find all points (parameter vectors/tensors) that correspond to trivial derivatives/gradients of the objective function f. Then, we can pick the parameter vectors/tensors/points leading to the smallest values of the loss. In neural network learning, this means analytically finding the combination of weight values corresponding to the smallest possible loss values.

This optimization is achieved at W_o when $\nabla(f)(W_o) = 0$. Often, this gradient equation is a polynomial equation of N parameters (variables) corresponding to the number of coefficients (W and b) in the network.

For large networks (with millions of parameters), this optimization is difficult. An approximate solution may be derived using alternative numerical solutions. This involves incrementally modifying the parameters and assuming the loss function is differentiable. We can then compute its gradient, which points the direction of the fastest growth or decay of the objective function.

- Draw a (random) batch of training samples x and their corresponding targets y.
- Forward pass: Run the network on x to obtain predictions y_{pred}.
- Estimate the loss of the network on the batch data assessing the mismatch between y and y_{pred}.
- Compute the gradient of the loss $\nabla(f)$ with regard to the network's parameters (a backward pass).

- Slightly update/adjust the parameters in the opposite direction of the gradient, e.g., $W = W - (\text{step} \times \text{gradient})$, which reduces the loss function value on the batch data.

In practice, neural network learning depends on chaining many tensor operations. For instance, a network f composed of three tensor operations a, b, and c, with weight matrices W_1, W_2, and W_3 can be expressed as $f(W_1, W_2, W_3) = a(W_1, b(W_2, c(W_3)))$. The chain-rule for differentiation yields that $f(g(x)) = f'(g(x)) \times g'(x)$ leads to a corresponding neural network optimization algorithm (*backpropagation*), which starts with the final loss value and works backward from the top layers to the bottom layers, sequentially applying the chain rule to compute the contribution of each parameter to the aggregate loss value.

```
train_images <- t(train.x)   # (42000, 28 * 28))
test_images <- t(test)        # (28000, 28 * 28))
# categorically encode the training-image labels
train_labels <- to_categorical(train.y)
```

Let's now train (fit or estimate) the neural network model using `keras`. In general, the first mode (axis) in the data tensors is typically the sample axis (sample dimension). Often, it's difficult to process all data at the same time, so breaking the data into small *batches*, e.g., batch_size=128, allows for more effective, efficient, and tractable processing (learning). The MNIST tensor consists of images, saved as 3D color arrays indexed by height, width, and depth, where gray-scale images (like the MNIST digits) have only one color channel. In general, image tensors are always 3D. Hence, a batch of 128 gray-scale images of size 256×256 is stored in a tensor of *shape* $(128, 256, 256, 1)$, whereas a batch of 128 color (RGB) images is stored as a $(128, 256, 256, 3)$ tensor.

```
network %>% fit(train_images, train_labels, epochs = 10, batch_size = 128)
```

Invoking the method `fit ()` launches the iterative network learning on the training data using mini-batches of 128 samples. Each iteration over all the training data is called an *epoch*. Here, we use epoch $= 10$ to indicate looping 10 times over. At each iteration, the network computes the gradients of the weights with regard to the loss on the batch and updates the tensor weights. After completing 10 epochs, the network learning performed 3290 gradient updates (329 per epoch), which progressively reduced the loss of the network from 10^{-2} to 10^{-4}. This low loss indicates the network learned to classify handwritten digits with high accuracy (0.99).

During the training process, two graphs are dynamically shown that illustrate the parity between the network loss function (expected to decrease) and the accuracy of the network, using the training data. Note that the accuracy approaches 0.99, but remember, this is training-data sample-accuracy, which is biased. To get a more realistic performance estimate, we can test the model on an independent set of 10,000 testing data images.

```
# Load and preprocess the testing data
mnist <- dataset_mnist()
test_images <- mnist$test$x
test_labels <- mnist$test$y
dim(test_images)    # [1] 10000    28    28
length(test_labels) # [1] 10000
test_images <- array_reshape(test_images, c(10000, 28 * 28))
test_images <- test_images / 255
test_labels <- to_categorical(test_labels)
metrics <- network %>% evaluate(test_images, test_labels)
metrics
##        loss    accuracy
## 0.03420694 0.99129999
```

The testing data accuracy is 0.9886, on par with the training data performance, which indicates no evidence of overfitting.

14.5.6.3   Forecasting

Next, we will generate forecasting using the model on testing data and evaluate the prediction performance. The `preds` matrix has 28, 000 rows and 10 columns, containing the desired classification probabilities from the `output layer` of the neural net. To extract the maximum label for each row, we can use the `max.col` (Fig. 14.20).

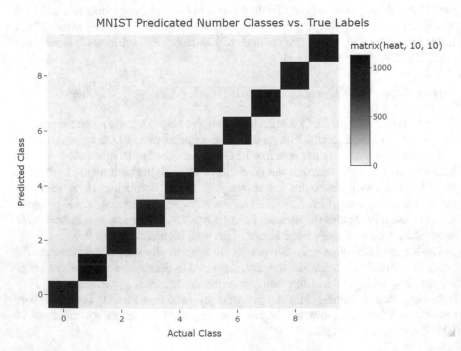

Fig. 14.20 Results show an excellent agreement between the actual and the DNN-predicted digit class labels for the MNIST handwritten digits imaging dataset

```
pred.label <- network %>% predict(test_images) %>% k_argmax()
heat <- table(factor(pred.label$numpy()),factor(mnist$test$y))
keys = c(0:9)
plot_ly(x =~keys, y =~keys, z =~matrix(heat, 10,10),
        name="NN Model Performance",
        hovertemplate=paste('<i>Matching</i>: %{z:.0f}',
                            '<br><b>True</b>: %{x}<br>','<b>Pred</b>: %{y}'),
        colors = 'Reds', type = "heatmap") %>%
  layout(title="MNIST Predicated Number Classes vs. True Labels",
        xaxis=list(title="Actual Class"), yaxis=list(title="Predicted Class"))
```

The predictions are stored in a 1D vector, 28, 000 (rows), including the predicted classification labels generated by the network output layer (Fig. 14.21).

```
# For example, the ML-classification labels assigned to the first 7 images
(from the 28,000 testing data collection) are
pred.label <- pred.label$numpy()
head(pred.label, n = 7L)
## [1] 7 2 1 0 4 1 4
library(knitr)
kable(head(pred.label, n = 7L), format = "markdown", align='c')
```

x	7	2	1	0	4	1	4

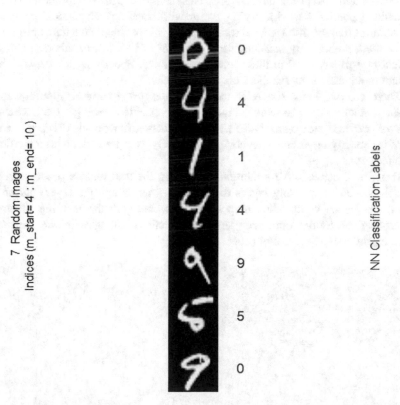

Fig. 14.21 Pairing a set of 7 images (4–10) on the left with their corresponding DNN-predicted digit class labels on the right

```
label.names <- c("0", "1", "2", "3", "4", "5", "6", "7", "8", "9")
# initialize a list of m=7 images from the N=28,000 available images
m_start <- 4
m_end <- 10
if (m_end <= m_start) { m_end = m_start+1 }  # check that m_end > m_start
label_Ypositons <- vector() # initialize array of label positions on the plot
for (i in m_start:m_end) {
  if (i==m_start) img1 <- as.cimg(test_images[m_start,], 28, 28)
  else img1 <- imappend(list(img1, as.cimg(test_images[i,], 28, 28)),"y")
  label.names[i+1-m_start] <- pred.label[i]
  label_Ypositons[i+1-m_start] <- 15 + 28*(i-m_start)
}
plot(img1, axes=FALSE)
text(40, label_Ypositons, labels=label.names[1:(m_end-m_start)],
    cex= 1.2, col="blue")
mtext(paste((m_end+1-m_start)," Random Images \n Indices (m_start=", m_start,
    " : m_end=", m_end, ")"), side=2, line=-6, col="black")
mtext("NN Classification Labels", side=4, line=-5, col="blue")
```

14.5.6.4 Examining the Network Structure

There are a variety of network topologies, e.g., two-branch networks, multihead networks, and inception blocks, that encode the *a priori* hypothesis space of predefined possibilities. Specifying the network topology constrains the space of possibilities to a specific series of tensor operations that map input data onto outputs. Then, the learning only searches for a good set of network parameter values (the weight tensors involved in these tensor operations). Specifying the network architecture in advance is as much an art as it is science.

There are two main strategies to define an *a priori* network topology model. Linear stacks of network layers are specified using the keras::keras_model_sequential() method, whereas functional APIs provide interfaces for specifying directed acyclic graph (DAG) layer networks with more flexible architectures.

Functional network APIs facilitate managing the data tensors processed by the model as well as applying layers to tensors just as though the layers are abstract functions. In the compilation step below, we configure the learning process by specifying the model optimizer and loss functions, along with the metrics for tracking the iterative learning process.

```
#  Linear stacks of network layers
network <- keras_model_sequential() %>%
  layer_dense(units = 512, activation = "relu", input_shape = c(28 * 28)) %>%
  layer_dense(units = 10, activation = "softmax")
# vs. functional API network (DAG)
input_tensor  <- layer_input(shape = c(784))
output_tensor <- input_tensor %>%
  layer_dense(units = 32, activation = "relu") %>%
  layer_dense(units = 10, activation = "softmax")
model <- keras_model(inputs = input_tensor, outputs = output_tensor)
model %>% compile(
    optimizer = optimizer_adam(), loss = "mse", metrics = c("accuracy"))
model %>% fit(train_images, train_labels, epochs = 10, batch_size = 128)
```

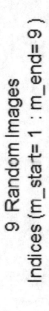

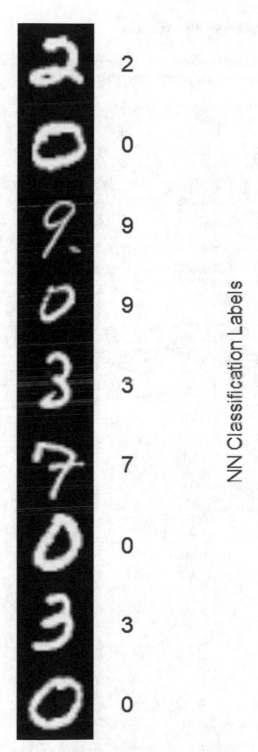

Fig. 14.22 Comparing a set of nine images (1–9) with their corresponding derived digital labels

14.5.6.5   Model Validation

We can use *accuracy* to track the performance of the NN training during the learning process on new (prospective) data (Fig. 14.22).

```r
# randomly choose 10K images
val_indices <- sample(1:dim(train_images)[1], size=10000)
x_val <- train_images[val_indices, ]
y_val <- to_categorical(train.y[val_indices])
partial_x_train <- train_images[-val_indices, ]
partial_y_train <- to_categorical(train.y[-val_indices])
# train the model for 20 iterations over all samples in the x_train and y_train
tensors (20 epochs),
# using mini-batches of 512 samples and track the loss and accuracy on the 10,000
validation samples
model %>% compile(optimizer = "rmsprop", loss = "binary_crossentropy",
      metrics = c("accuracy"))
history <- model %>% fit(partial_x_train, partial_y_train, epochs = 20,
      batch_size = 512, validation_data = list(x_val, y_val) )
tic <- proc.time()
print(paste0("Total Compute Time: ", proc.time() - tic))
library(plotly)
epochs <- 20
time <- 1:epochs
hist_df <- data.frame(time=time, loss=history$metrics$loss,
      acc=history$metrics$accuracy, valid_loss=history$metrics$val_loss,
      alid_acc=history$metrics$val_accuracy)
plot_ly(hist_df, x = ~time)  %>%
  add_trace(y = ~loss, name = 'training loss', mode = 'lines') %>%
  add_trace(y = ~acc, name = 'training accuracy', mode = 'lines+markers') %>%
  add_trace(y = ~valid_loss, name='validation loss',mode='lines+markers') %>%


  add_trace(y=~valid_acc,name='validation accuracy',mode='lines+markers') %>%
  layout(title="MNIST Digits NN Model Performance",
        legend = list(orientation = 'h'), yaxis=list(title="metric"))
# Finally prediction of MNIST testing image classification (auto-labeling):
pred.label <- model %>% predict(t(test))
for (i in 1:9) {
  print(sprintf("NN predicted Label for image %d is %s", i,
      which.max(pred.label[i,])-1))
}
## [1] "NN predicted Label for image 1 is 2"
## [1] "NN predicted Label for image 2 is 0"
…
## [1] "NN predicted Label for image 9 is 0"
array_3D <- array(t(test), c(28000, 28, 28))
plot(as.cimg(array_3D[1,,], nrow = 28, ncol = 28))
# initialize a list of m=9 testing images from the N=28,000 available images
m_start <- 1
m_end <- 9
label_Ypositons <- vector() # initialize array of label positions on the plot
for (i in m_start:m_end) {
  if (i==m_start) img1 <- as.cimg(array_3D[1,,], nrow = 28, ncol = 28)
  else img1 <-imappend(list(img1,as.cimg(array_3D[i,,],nrow=28,ncol=28)),"y")
  label.names[i] <- which.max(pred.label[i,])-1
  label_Ypositons[i+1-m_start] <- 15 + 28*(i-m_start)
}
plot(img1, axes=FALSE)
text(40, label_Ypositons, labels=label.names, cex= 1.2, col="blue")
mtext(paste((m_end+1-m_start), " Random Images \n Indices (m_start=",
      m_start, " : m_end=", m_end, ")"), side=2, line=-6, col="black")
mtext("NN Classification Labels", side=4, line=-5, col="blue")
```

Note that the `keras::predict()` method only works with *Sequential* network models. However, when using the functional API network model we need to use the `keras::predict()` method to obtain a vector of probabilities and then get the *argmax* of this vector to find the most likely class label for the image.

14.6 Classifying Real-World Images Using Pretrained *Tensorflow* and *Keras* Models

A real-world example of deep learning is the classification of 2D images (pictures) or 3D volumes (e.g., neuroimages). In this section, we will demonstrate the use of *pretrained* network models (resnet50, vgg16, and vgg19) to predict the class-labels of real-world images. Later, we will also show the process of training DNNs on images and volumes.

There are dozens of pretrained models that are made available to the entire community.[15] These advanced Deep Network models yield state-of-the-art predictions that accurately label different types of 2D images. We will use the `keras` and `tensorflow` packages to load the pretrained network models and classify the images, along with the `imager` package to load and preprocess raw images in *R*.

14.6.1 Load the Pretrained Model

You can download, unzip. and examine this pretrained model.[16] There are many different types of pretrained deep neural network models. For instance, in our experiments, we will utilize the following three pretrained deep neural network models:

- Resnet50: Deep Residual Learning for Image Recognition
- VGG16: Very Deep Convolutional Networks for Large-Scale Image Recognition, by Oxford's Visual Geometry Group
- VGG19: Very Deep Convolutional Networks for Large-Scale Image Recognition

The VGGs are deep convolutional networks, trained to classify images, with VGG19 model layers comprised of the following *ordered* list of operations: Conv3x3 (64), Conv3x3 (64), *MaxPool,* Conv3x3 (128), Conv3x3 (128), *MaxPool,* Conv3x3 (256), Conv3x3 (256), Conv3x3 (256), Conv3x3 (256), *MaxPool,* Conv3x3 (512), Conv3x3, (512), Conv3x3 (512), Conv3x3 (512), *MaxPool,* Conv3x3 (512), Conv3x3 (512), Conv3x3 (512), Conv3x3 (512), *MaxPool,* Fully Connected (4096), Fully Connected (4096), Fully Connected (1000), and finally *SoftMax.* More information about the VGG architecture is available online.[17]

---

[15] https://keras.io/api/applications/

[16] https://www.socr.umich.edu/people/dinov/2017/Spring/DSPA_HS650/data/Inception.zip

[17] https://iq.opengenus.org/vgg19-architecture/

14.6.2   Load and Preprocess a New Image

To classify a new image, start with selecting and importing the image into R. Below, we show the classifications of several different types of images.

```
library("imager")
library("EBImage")
library("keras")
# download file to local working directory, use "wb" mode to avoid problems
download.file("https://wiki.socr.umich.edu/images/6/69/DataManagementFig1.png",
              paste(getwd(),"results/image.png", sep="/"), mode = 'wb')
paste(getwd(),"results/image.png", sep="/")
img <- image_load(paste(getwd(),"results/image.png", sep="/"),
                  target_size = c(224,224))
# dim(image_to_array(img))  # [1] 1084 1875     3
img <- rgbImage(red=t(image_to_array(img)[,,1]/255),
  green=t(image_to_array(img)[,,2]/255),blue=t(image_to_array(img)[,,3]/255))
display(img)
```

Before feeding the image to the deep learning network for classification, we *may* need to do some preprocessing to make it fit the network input requirements. This image preprocessing (e.g., cropping, intensity mean-centralization, and scaling) can be done manually in R. For example, below is an instance of an image-preprocessing function. In practice, we can also use the function `keras::` `imagenet_preprocess_input()`.

```
preproc.image <- function(im) {
    # crop the image  # Reshape to format (width, height, channel, num)
    mean.img <- mean(im)
    shape <- dim(im)
    resized <- resize(im, 224, 224)
    plot(resized)
    dim(resized) <- c(224, 224, 3, 1)
    return(resized)
}
normed <- preproc.image(img)
```

Figure 14.23 shows the initial image along with the result of the preprocessing function generating a conforming (normalized) image ready for auto-classification.

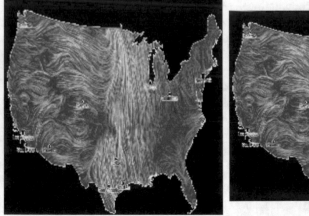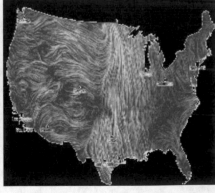

Fig. 14.23 Initial (left) and preprocessed (right) image (low resolution US weather pattern)

14.6.3   Image Classification

Next, we use the `predict()` function to get the probability estimates over all (learned) classes and classify the image type using alternative pretrained DNN models (e.g., *resnet50, VGG16, VGG19*).

```
# get info about local version of Python installation
reticulate::py_config()
# Preprocess input image
x <- image_to_array(img)
# ensure we have a 4d tensor with 1 element in the first (batch) dimension,
# then preprocess the input for prediction using resnet50
x <- array_reshape(x, c(1, dim(x)))
x <- imagenet_preprocess_input(x)
# Specify and compare Predictions based on different Pre-trained Models
# Model 1: resnet50
model_resnet50 <- application_resnet50(weights = 'imagenet')
# make predictions then decode and print them
preds_resnet50 <- model_resnet50 %>% predict(x)
imagenet_decode_predictions(preds_resnet50, top = 10)
## [[1]]
##    class_name class_description    score
## 1   n04404412        television 0.05130376
## 2   n03196217     digital_clock 0.05040657
...
## 10  n0363/318         lampshade 0.01786401
# Model2: VGG19
model_vgg19 <- application_vgg19(weights = 'imagenet')
preds_vgg19 <- model_vgg19 %>% predict(x)
imagenet_decode_predictions(preds_vgg19, top = 10)[[1]]
##    class_name class_description    score
## 1   n03729826        matchstick 0.076670796
## 2   n01930112          nematode 0.055275645
...
## 10  n03759954        microphone 0.008829281
# Model 3: VGG16
model_vgg16 <- application_vgg16(weights = 'imagenet')
preds_vgg16 <- model_vgg16 %>% predict(x)
imagenet_decode_predictions(preds_vgg16, top = 10)[[1]]
##    class_name class_description    score
## 1   n03729826        matchstick 0.077248417
## 2   n01930112          nematode 0.048016328
...
## 10  n04456115             torch 0.007933105
dim(preds_vgg16)
## [1]    1 1000
```

The `probability` prediction generates a 1000×1 array representing the (vector) of probabilities reflecting the likelihood that the input image resembles (is classified as) each of the top 1000 known image categories. We can report the indices of the top-10 closest image classes to the input image. Clearly, this US weather pattern image is not well classified by either of the three different deep networks. The optimal predictions include *television*, *digital_clock*, and *theater_curtain*. However, the confidence of these predictions is very low, Prob < 0.052. None of the other top-10 class-labels capture the type of this weather-pattern image.

14.6.4   Additional Image Classification Examples

The machine learning image classification results won't always be this poor. Let's try classifying several alternative images.

14.6.4.1   Lake Mapourika, New Zealand

Let's try the automated image classification of this lakeside panorama, New Zealand's Lake Mapourika, which we saw earlier, Fig. 14.12.

```
# load the image
download.file("https://upload.wikimedia.org/wikipedia/commons/2/23/Lake_mapourika_NZ.jpeg",
            paste(getwd(),"results/image.png", sep="/"), mode = 'wb')
img <- image_load(paste(getwd(),"results/image.png", sep="/"),
        target_size = c(224,224))
imgRGB <- rgbImage(red=t(image_to_array(img)[,,1]/255),
 green=t(image_to_array(img)[,,2]/255), blue=t(image_to_array(img)[,,3]/255))
display(imgRGB)
x <- image_to_array(img)  # Preprocess input image
# ensure we have a 4d tensor with single element in the batch dimension,
# the preprocess the input for prediction using resnet50
x <- array_reshape(x, c(1, dim(x)))
x <- imagenet_preprocess_input(x)
# Specify and compare Predictions based on different Pre-trained Models
# Model 1: resnet50
model_resnet50 <- application_resnet50(weights = 'imagenet')
# make predictions then decode and print them
preds_resnet50 <- model_resnet50 %>% predict(x)
imagenet_decode_predictions(preds_resnet50, top = 10)
## [[1]]
##     class_name class_description        score
## 1   n09332890           lakeside 0.6543883085
## 2   n02859443          boathouse 0.1122922450
...
## 10  n03028079             church 0.0003251492
# Model2: VGG19
model_vgg19 <- application_vgg19(weights = 'imagenet')
preds_vgg19 <- model_vgg19 %>% predict(x)
imagenet_decode_predictions(preds_vgg19, top = 10)[[1]]
##     class_name class_description        score
## 1   n09332890           lakeside 0.7257616520
## 2   n02894605         breakwater 0.2156531066
...
## 10  n03873416             paddle 0.0004235525
# Model 3: VGG16
model_vgg16 <- application_vgg16(weights = 'imagenet')
preds_vgg16 <- model_vgg16 %>% predict(x)
imagenet_decode_predictions(preds_vgg16, top = 10)[[1]]
##     class_name class_description       score
## 1   n09332890           lakeside 0.656819046
## 2   n02894605         breakwater 0.201264054
...
## 10  n09421951            sandbar 0.001799420
dim(preds_vgg16)
## [1]    1 1000
```

This photo does represent a lakeside, which is reflected by the top three class labels:

- Model 1 (resnet50): lakeside, boathouse, dock, breakwater.
- Model 1 (VGG19): lakeside, breakwater, boathouse, dock.
- Model 1 (VGG16): lakeside, breakwater, dock, canoe.

14.6.4.2   Beach

Another coastal boundary between water and land is represented in this beach image (Fig. 14.24).

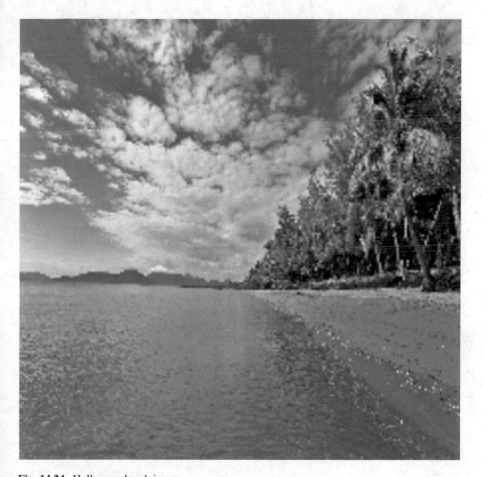

Fig. 14.24 Holloways beach image

```
download.file("https://upload.wikimedia.org/wikipedia/commons/9/90/Holloways_beach_1920x1080.jpg",
            paste(getwd(),"results/image.png", sep="/"), mode = 'wb')
img <- image_load(paste(getwd(),"results/image.png", sep="/"),
          target_size = c(224,224))
imgRGB <- rgbImage(red=t(image_to_array(img)[,,1]/255),
 green=t(image_to_array(img)[,,2]/255), blue=t(image_to_array(img)[,,3]/255))
display(imgRGB)
```

```
x <- image_to_array(img)
x <- array_reshape(x, c(1, dim(x)))
x <- imagenet_preprocess_input(x)
# Model 1: resnet50
model_resnet50 <- application_resnet50(weights = 'imagenet')
# make predictions then decode and print them
preds_resnet50 <- model_resnet50 %>% predict(x)
imagenet_decode_predictions(preds_resnet50, top = 10)
## [[1]]
##    class_name class_description       score
## 1   n09421951            sandbar 0.5721765161
## 2   n09332890           lakeside 0.2440176159
...
## 10  n04606251              wreck 0.0003732552
# Model2: VGG19
model_vgg19 <- application_vgg19(weights = 'imagenet')
preds_vgg19 <- model_vgg19 %>% predict(x)
imagenet_decode_predictions(preds_vgg19, top = 10)[[1]]
##    class_name class_description       score
## 1   n09421951            sandbar 0.359486282
## 2   n09332890           lakeside 0.292688996
...
## 10  n09288635             geyser 0.001652389
# Model 3: VGG16
model_vgg16 <- application_vgg16(weights = 'imagenet')
preds_vgg16 <- model_vgg16 %>% predict(x)
imagenet_decode_predictions(preds_vgg16, top = 10)[[1]]
##    class_name class_description       score
## 1   n09421951            sandbar 0.508114755
## 2   n09332890           lakeside 0.275204331
...
## 10  n09472597            volcano 0.001169212
```

This photo was classified appropriately and with high confidence as sandbar or lakeside.

14.6.4.3   Volcano

Here is another natural image representing the Mount St. Helens volcano (Fig. 14.25).

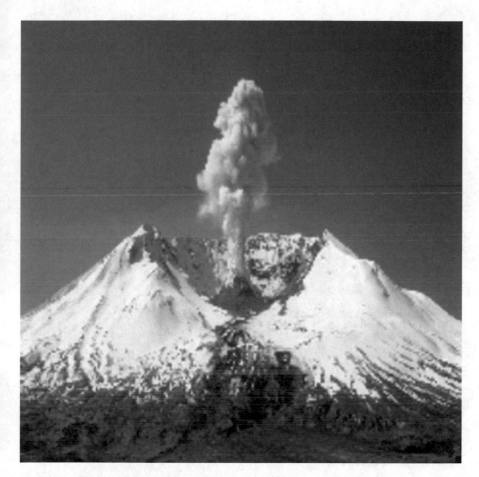

Fig. 14.25 Mount St. Helens volcano image

```
download.file("https://upload.wikimedia.org/wikipedia/commons/thumb/d/dc/MSH82_st_helens_plume_
from_harrys_ridge_05-19-82.jpg/1200px-MSH82_st_helens_plume_from_harrys_ridge_05-19-82.jpg",
              paste(getwd(),"results/image.png", sep="/"), mode = 'wb')
img <- image_load(paste(getwd(),"results/image.png", sep="/"),
        target_size = c(224,224))
imgRGB <- rgbImage(red=t(image_to_array(img)[,,1]/255),
 green=t(image_to_array(img)[,,2]/255), blue=t(image_to_array(img)[,,3]/255))
display(imgRGB)
```

```
x <- image_to_array(img)
x <- array_reshape(x, c(1, dim(x)))
x <- imagenet_preprocess_input(x)
# Model 1: resnet50
model_resnet50 <- application_resnet50(weights = 'imagenet')
preds_resnet50 <- model_resnet50 %>% predict(x)
imagenet_decode_predictions(preds_resnet50, top = 10)
## [[1]]
##    class_name class_description       score
## 1   n09472597           volcano 9.999564e-01
## 2   n09193705               alp 4.145014e-05
...
## 10  n03773504           missile 1.750468e-08
# Model2: VGG19
model_vgg19 <- application_vgg19(weights = 'imagenet')
preds_vgg19 <- model_vgg19 %>% predict(x)
imagenet_decode_predictions(preds_vgg19, top = 10)[[1]]
##    class_name class_description       score
## 1   n09472597           volcano 9.992106e-01
## 2   n09193705               alp 7.414014e-04
...
## 10  n09332890          lakeside 5.683109e-07
# Model 3: VGG16
model_vgg16 <- application_vgg16(weights = 'imagenet')
preds_vgg16 <- model_vgg16 %>% predict(x)
imagenet_decode_predictions(preds_vgg16, top = 10)[[1]]
##    class_name class_description       score
## 1   n09472597           volcano 9.998018e-01
## 2   n09193705               alp 1.845273e-04
...
## 10  n09246464             cliff 1.076844e-07
```

The predicted top-class labels for this image are perfect volcano, alps, mountain, tent, geyser.

14.6.4.4   Brain Surface

The next image represents a 2D snapshot of 3D shape reconstruction of a cortical brain surface. This image is particularly difficult to automatically classify because (1) few people have ever seen a real brain and typical ML/AI methods and not trained to recognize cortical surfaces, (2) the mathematical and computational models used to obtain the 2D manifold representing the brain surface do vary, and (3) the patterns of sulcal folds and gyral crests are quite inconsistent between people (Fig. 14.26).

```
download.file("https://wiki.socr.umich.edu/images/e/ea/BrainCortex2.png",
          paste(getwd(),"results/image.png", sep="/"), mode = 'wb')
im <- load.image(paste(getwd(),"results/image.png", sep="/"))
download.file("https://wiki.socr.umich.edu/images/e/ea/BrainCortex2.png",
          paste(getwd(),"results/image.png", sep="/"), mode = 'wb')
img <- image_load(paste(getwd(),"results/image.png", sep="/"),
          target_size = c(224,224))
imgRGB <- rgbImage(red=t(image_to_array(img)[,,1]/255),
  green=t(image_to_array(img)[,,2]/255), blue=t(image_to_array(img)[,,3]/255))
display(imgRGB)
```

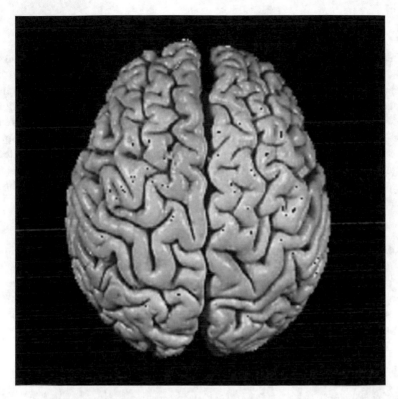

Fig. 14.26 A 2D image of a 3D reconstruction of a cortical brain surface

```
x <- image_to_array(img)
x <- array_reshape(x, c(1, dim(x)))
x <- imagenet_preprocess_input(x)
# Model 1: resnet50
model_resnet50 <- application_resnet50(weights = 'imagenet')
preds_resnet50 <- model_resnet50 %>% predict(x)
imagenet_decode_predictions(preds_resnet50, top = 10)
## [[1]]
##    class_name class_description       score
## 1  n01917289        brain_coral 0.49230418
## 2  n03724870               mask 0.05836945
…
## 10 n03598930       jigsaw_puzzle 0.01429038
# Model2: VGG19
model_vgg19 <- application_vgg19(weights = 'imagenet')
preds_vgg19 <- model_vgg19 %>% predict(x)
imagenet_decode_predictions(preds_vgg19, top = 10)[[1]]
##    class_name class_description       score
## 1  n01917289        brain_coral 0.48069310
## 2  n12267677              acorn 0.09673864
## 3  n07715103        cauliflower 0.07138743
…
## 10 n01943899              conch 0.01397455
# Model 3: VGG16
model_vgg16 <- application_vgg16(weights = 'imagenet')
preds_vgg16 <- model_vgg16 %>% predict(x)
imagenet_decode_predictions(preds_vgg16, top = 10)[[1]]
##    class_name class_description        score
## 1  n01917289        brain_coral 0.878696144
## 2  n12267677              acorn 0.029935000
….
## 10 n01910747          jellyfish 0.003211482
```

The top-class labels for the brain image are brain coral, mask, knot, cauliflower, and acorn.

Imagine if we can train a brain image classifier that labels individuals (volunteers or patients), solely based on their brain scans into different classes reflecting their development, clinical phenotypes, disease states, or aging profiles. This will require a substantial amount of expert-labeled brain scans, significant model training, and extensive validation. However, any progress in this direction may lead to effective computational clinical decision support systems that can assist physicians with diagnosis, tracking, and prognostication of brain growth and aging in health and disease.

14.6.4.5   Face Mask: Synthetic Face Image

We can also try the deep learning methods to see if they can uncover the core deterministic model or structure used to generate designed, synthetic, or simulated images. This example represents a synthetic computer-generated image of a cartoon face or a mask (Fig. 14.27).

```
download.file("https://wiki.socr.umich.edu/images/f/fb/FaceMask1.png",
              paste(getwd(),"results/image.png", sep="/"), mode = 'wb')
img <- image_load(paste(getwd(),"results/image.png", sep="/"),
                  target_size = c(224,224))
imgRGB <- rgbImage(red=t(image_to_array(img)[,,1]/255),
  green=t(image_to_array(img)[,,2]/255), blue=t(image_to_array(img)[,,3]/255))
display(imgRGB)
```

Fig. 14.27 A synthetically generated 2D face image

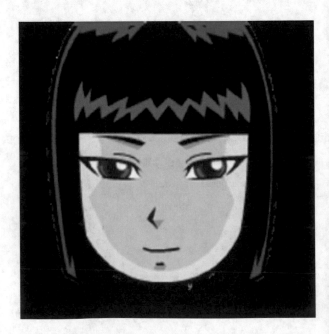

```
x <- image_to_array(img)
x <- array_reshape(x, c(1, dim(x)))
x <- imagenet_preprocess_input(x)
# Model 1: resnet50
model_resnet50 <- application_resnet50(weights = 'imagenet')
preds_resnet50 <- model_resnet50 %>% predict(x)
imagenet_decode_predictions(preds_resnet50, top = 10)
## [[1]]
##    class_name class_description       score
## 1   n06596364        comic_book 0.16772421
## 2   n02667093             abaya 0.11260374
...
## 10  n03916031           perfume 0.02765948
# Model2: VGG19
model_vgg19 <- application_vgg19(weights = 'imagenet')
preds_vgg19 <- model_vgg19 %>% predict(x)
imagenet_decode_predictions(preds_vgg19, top = 10)[[1]]
##    class_name class_description       score
## 1   n02708093       analog_clock 0.23986669
## 2   n03916031            perfume 0.10508933
...
## 10  n02865351           bolo_tie 0.01694274
# Model 3: VGG16
model_vgg16 <- application_vgg16(weights = 'imagenet')
preds_vgg16 <- model_vgg16 %>% predict(x)
imagenet_decode_predictions(preds_vgg16, top = 10)[[1]]
##    class_name class_description       score
## 1   n02667093             abaya 0.404464602
## 2   n03724870              mask 0.182569548
...
## 10  n04584207               wig 0.008511139
```

The top-class labels for the face mask are comic book, mask, analog clock, shield, abaya.

Readers can easily test these pretrained DNN image classifiers with other images and identify classes of pictures that are either well classified or poorly labeled by the deep learning-based machine learning models.

14.7   Data Generation: Simulating Synthetic Data

Next, we will present AI strategies to synthetically generate data.

14.7.1   Fractal Shapes

One way to design fractal shapes relies on using iterated function systems (IFS).[18] Each IFS is represented by finite set of contractive maps acting on complete metric spaces

---

[18] https://doi.org/10.1098/rspa.1985.0057

$$\{f_i : X \to X \mid i = 1, 2, \ldots, N\}, \ N \in \mathbb{N}.$$

A map $f : X \to X$ is *contractive*, if $\exists 0 \leq k < 1$, such that $\forall x, y \in X$ the range distance is bounded by the domain distance between the pair of points in the space

$$d(f(x), f(y)) \leq k\, d(x, y).$$

The smallest such value of the parameter k is called the *Lipschitz constant* of the map f. In the case of 2D sets and images, linear and contracting IFS's can be represented as linear operators

$$w = f(x, y) = A \begin{bmatrix} x \\ y \end{bmatrix} + \begin{bmatrix} e \\ f \end{bmatrix} = \begin{bmatrix} a & b \\ c & d \end{bmatrix} \begin{bmatrix} x \\ y \end{bmatrix} + \begin{bmatrix} e \\ f \end{bmatrix}.$$

Computationally, these linear IFS contraction maps can be expressed as $N \times 7$ matrices, where N is the number of maps and 7 is the number of parameters needed to describe an affine transformation in $\mathbb{R}^2$.

Map	$A_{1,1}$	$A_{1,2}$	$A_{2,1}$	$A_{2,2}$	B_1	B_2	Probability
w	a	b	c	d	e	f	p

For example, let's look at the Barnsley's fern, which is designed to model real lady ferns (*athyrium filix-femina*). It can be defined by a set of $N = 4$ IFS contraction maps

Map	$A_{1,1}$	$A_{1,2}$	$A_{2,1}$	$A_{2,2}$	B_1	B_2	Probability	Fern portion
f_1	0	0	0	0.16	0	0	0.01	Stem
f_2	0.85	0.02	−0.02	0.85	0	1.60	0.85	Successively smaller leaflets
f_3	0.20	−0.26	0.23	0.22	0	1.60	0.1	Largest left-hand leaflet
f_4	−0.15	0.28	0.26	0.24	0	0.44	0.05	Largest right-hand leaflet

Here is how the *Barnsley Fern* can be generated in R (Fig. 14.28).

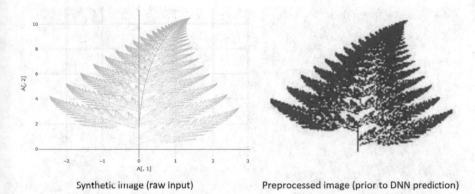

Synthetic image (raw input)   Preprocessed image (prior to DNN prediction)

Fig. 14.28 Barnsley's fern as a fixed point of an IFS (synthetically generated fractal image)

```
# Barnsley's Fern
# (1) create the 4-IFS functions of the probability and the current point
fractal_BarnsleyFern <- function(x, p){
    if (p <= 0.01) {
        A <- matrix(c(0, 0, 0, 0.16), 2, 2)
        B <- c(0, 0)
    } else if (p <= 0.86) {
        A <- matrix(c(.85, -.02, .02, .85), 2, 2)
        B <- c(0, 1.6)
    } else if (p <= 0.95) {
        A <- matrix(c(.2, .23, -.26, .22), 2, 2)
        B <- c(0, 1.6)
    } else {
        A <- matrix(c(-.15, .26, .28, .24), 2, 2)
        B <- c(0, .44)
    }
    return(A %*% x + B)
}
# Fern resolution depends on the number of iterative applications of the IFS
reps <- 100000
# create a vector with probability values, and a matrix to store coordinates
p <- runif(reps)
# initialize a point at the origin
init_coords <- c(0, 0)
# compute the list of reps fractal coordinates: (X,Y) pairs
A <- Reduce(fractal_BarnsleyFern, p, accumulate = T, init = init_coords)
A <- t(do.call(cbind, A)) # unwind list of (X,Y) pairs as (reps * 2) array
plot_ly(x=~A[,1], y=~A[,2], type="scatter", mode="markers",
    name="Barnsley's Fern", marker=list(color='rgb(157, 255, 157)', size=1))
# export Fern as JPG image
jpeg(paste(getwd(), sep="/", "results/FernPlot.jpg"))
plot(A, type = "p", cex = 0.1, col="darkgreen", xlim=c(-3, 3), ylim=c(0, 15),
    xlab = NA, ylab = NA, axes = FALSE)
dev.off()
# load the image back in and test the DNN classification
img <- image_load(paste(getwd(),"results/FernPlot.jpg", sep="/"),
                target_size = c(224,224))
# Preprocess the Fern image and predict its class (label)
imgRGB <- rgbImage(red=t(image_to_array(img)[,,1]/255),
 green=t(image_to_array(img)[,,2]/255), blue=t(image_to_array(img)[,,3]/255))
display(imgRGB)
```

Next, we can feed this synthetic image into the DNN predictor and report the
corresponding qualitative image descriptions.

```
x <- image_to_array(img)
x <- array_reshape(x, c(1, dim(x)))
x <- imagenet_preprocess_input(x)
# Model 1: resnet50
model_resnet50 <- application_resnet50(weights = 'imagenet')
preds_resnet50 <- model_resnet50 %>% predict(x)
imagenet_decode_predictions(preds_resnet50, top = 10)
## [[1]]
##    class_name class_description        score
## 1   n03485794       handkerchief 0.18395340
## 2   n04208210             shovel 0.11467008
...
## 10  n03991062                pot 0.02632549
# Model2: VGG19
model_vgg19 <- application_vgg19(weights = 'imagenet')
preds_vgg19 <- model_vgg19 %>% predict(x)
imagenet_decode_predictions(preds_vgg19, top = 10)[[1]]
##    class_name class_description        score
## 1   n03476684         hair_slide 0.17450647
## 2   n01943899              conch 0.05162914
## 3   n04153751              screw 0.04990320
...
## 10  n03658185     letter_opener 0.01346772
# Model 3: VGG16
model_vgg16 <- application_vgg16(weights = 'imagenet')
preds_vgg16 <- model_vgg16 %>% predict(x)
imagenet_decode_predictions(preds_vgg16, top = 10)[[1]]
##    class_name class_description        score
## 1   n03476684         hair_slide 0.08098602
## 2   n03595614             jersey 0.03968396
...
## 10  n03804744               nail 0.01775864
```

The prediction results are not optimal and correspond to low probability estimates.

14.7.2   Fake Images

You can also try to use TensorFlow and Keras to generate some "fake" *synthetic images* that can be then classified. This can be accomplished by using a Generative Adversarial network (GAN) to synthetically sample from a collection of images like the MNIST image sets, e.g., keras::dataset_fashion_mnist and keras::cifar10, and keras::dataset_mnist. In this initial demonstration, we will use the 10-class Canadian Institute For Advanced Research (CIFAR10) image archive, which will be described in greater detail below (Fig. 14.29).

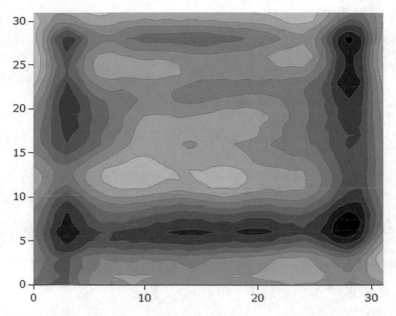

Fig. 14.29 Simple example of synthetically generated images using a Generative Adversarial Network (GAN) using the CIFAR-10 dataset (from the Canadian Institute For Advanced Research)

```
library(keras)
latent_dim <- 32
height <- 32
width <- 32
channels <- 3
generator_input <- layer_input(shape = c(latent_dim))
generator_output <- generator_input %>%
  layer_dense(units = 128 * 16 * 16) %>%
  layer_activation_leaky_relu() %>%
  layer_reshape(target_shape = c(16, 16, 128)) %>%
  layer_conv_2d(filters = 256, kernel_size = 5, padding = "same") %>%
  layer_activation_leaky_relu() %>%
  layer_conv_2d_transpose(filters = 256, kernel_size = 4,
                          strides = 2, padding = "same") %>%
  layer_activation_leaky_relu() %>%
  layer_conv_2d(filters = 256, kernel_size = 5, padding = "same") %>%
  layer_activation_leaky_relu() %>%
  layer_conv_2d(filters = 256, kernel_size = 5, padding = "same") %>%
  layer_activation_leaky_relu() %>%
  layer_conv_2d(filters = channels, kernel_size = 7,
                activation = "tanh", padding = "same")
generator <- keras_model(generator_input, generator_output)
discriminator_input <- layer_input(shape = c(height, width, channels))
discriminator_output <- discriminator_input %>%
  layer_conv_2d(filters = 128, kernel_size = 3) %>%
  layer_activation_leaky_relu() %>%
  layer_conv_2d(filters = 128, kernel_size = 4, strides = 2) %>%
  layer_activation_leaky_relu() %>%
  layer_conv_2d(filters = 128, kernel_size = 4, strides = 2) %>%
  layer_activation_leaky_relu() %>%
  layer_conv_2d(filters = 128, kernel_size = 4, strides = 2) %>%
  layer_activation_leaky_relu() %>%
```

```r
  layer_flatten() %>%
  layer_dropout(rate = 0.4) %>%
  layer_dense(units = 1, activation = "sigmoid")
discriminator <- keras_model(discriminator_input, discriminator_output)
discriminator_optimizer <- optimizer_rmsprop(
                                lr = 0.0008, clipvalue = 1.0,   decay = 1e-8)
discriminator %>% compile(
  optimizer = discriminator_optimizer, loss = "binary_crossentropy")
# freeze_weights(discriminator)                                  1
gan_input <- layer_input(shape = c(latent_dim))
gan_output <- discriminator(generator(gan_input))
gan <- keras_model(gan_input, gan_output)
gan_optimizer <- optimizer_rmsprop(
  lr = 0.0004, clipvalue = 1.0, decay = 1e-8)
gan %>% compile(
  optimizer = gan_optimizer, loss = "binary_crossentropy")
cifar10 <- dataset_cifar10()  # shape (num_samples, 3, 32, 32)
c(c(x_train, y_train), c(x_test, y_test)) %<-% cifar10
x_train <- x_train[as.integer(y_train) == 6,,,]
x_train <- x_train / 255
iterations <- 100
batch_size <- 20
save_dir <- getwd()
start <- 1
for (step in 1:iterations) {


  random_latent_vectors <- matrix(rnorm(batch_size * latent_dim),
                                  nrow = batch_size, ncol = latent_dim)
  generated_images <- generator %>% predict(random_latent_vectors)
  stop <- start + batch_size - 1
  real_images <- x_train[start:stop,,,]
  rows <- nrow(real_images)
  combined_images <- array(0, dim = c(rows * 2, dim(real_images)[-1]))
  combined_images[1:rows,,,] <- generated_images
  combined_images[(rows+1):(rows*2),,,] <- real_images
  labels <- rbind(matrix(1, nrow = batch_size, ncol = 1),
                  matrix(0, nrow = batch_size, ncol = 1))
  labels <- labels + (0.5 * array(runif(prod(dim(labels))),
                                  dim = dim(labels)))
  d_loss <- discriminator %>% train_on_batch(combined_images, labels)
  random_latent_vectors <- matrix(rnorm(batch_size * latent_dim),
                                  nrow = batch_size, ncol = latent_dim)
  misleading_targets <- array(0, dim = c(batch_size, 1))
  a_loss <- gan %>% train_on_batch(
    random_latent_vectors,  misleading_targets)
  start <- start + batch_size
  if (start > (nrow(x_train) - batch_size)) start <- 1
  if (step %% 10 == 0) {
    # save_model_weights_hdf5(gan, "gan.h5")  # Status Reporting
    cat("Completion Status: ", round((100*step)/iterations,0), "% \n")
    cat("\t discriminator loss:", d_loss, "\n")
    cat("\t adversarial loss:", a_loss, "\n")
    # Optionally save the real/generated images
```

```
    # image_array_save(generated_images[1,,,]*255, path="/path/*.png")
  }
}
## Completion Status:  10 %
##   discriminator loss: 0.6526977 ##   adversarial loss: 0.8566464
...
## Completion Status:  100 %
##   discriminator loss: 0.6212658 ##   adversarial loss: 1.679258
# Generated images: generated_images[batch_size=20, x=32, y=32, channels=3]
# Upscale the last generated image 32*32 -> 128*128*
normed <- EBImage::resize(generated_images[10,,,2]*255, w = 224, h = 224)
plot_ly(z = ~generated_images[15,,,1], type="contour", showscale=F)
```

Clearly, we don't expect to get particularly useful narrative prediction on this
synthetically generated pseudo image using one of the pretrained DNN models.

```
normed4D <- rbind (normed, normed, normed)
dim(normed4D) <- c(224, 224, 3, 1)
x <- image_to_array(img)
x <- array_reshape(x, c(1, dim(x)))
x <- imagenet_preprocess_input(x)
# Model 1: resnet50
model_resnet50 <- application_resnet50(weights = 'imagenet')
preds_resnet50 <- model_resnet50 %>% predict(x)
imagenet_decode_predictions(preds_resnet50, top = 10)
## [[1]]
##    class_name class_description       score
## 1   n03485794     handkerchief 0.18395340
## 2   n04208210           shovel 0.11467008
...
## 10  n03991062              pot 0.02632549
```

In this very simple image, the DNN classification is not very informative. The
results reported above will vary with the draw of the randomly generated synthetic
image from the GAN generator.

14.7.3   Generative Adversarial Networks (GANs)

The articles "Generating Sequences with Recurrent Neural Networks"[19] by Alex
Graves, and "Generative Adversarial Nets"[20] by Goodfellow and colleagues, introduced a novel strategy to use recurrent neural networks to generate realistic signals,
including audio generation (music, speech, dialogue), image generation, text-
synthesis, and molecule design. GANs represent an alternative strategy to variational
auto-encoders (VAE) to generate synthetic data.

  GAN frameworks estimate generative models using an adversarial process that
simultaneously trains a pair of network models—a *generative model G* that captures
the data distribution, and a separate *discriminative model D* that estimates the

---

[19] https://arxiv.org/abs/1308.0850

[20] https://proceedings.neurips.cc/paper/2014/file/5ca3e9b122f61f8f06494c97b1afccf3-Paper.pdf

probability that a previously generated (synthetic) sample was real, i.e., came from the training data, rather than a synthetic G output.

For a binary classification, the G training maximizes the probability of D making a mistake (adversity), which corresponds to a *mini-max* optimization of a two-player game. The *state-space* of all potential G and D permits a unique solution where G recovers the training data distribution and $D = \frac{1}{2}$ is a constant, which corresponds to 50–50 change (largest entropy). Often, the G and D networks are defined as multilayer perceptrons (MLP) that can be jointly fit using backpropagation.

GAN learning requires iterative estimation of the generator's distribution p_g using the training data x, subject to some prior on noisy input latent variables $Z \sim p_Z(z)$. Denote a generator mapping to the data space as $G(z; \theta_g)$, where G is a differentiable function representing a multilayer perceptron network with parameters θ_g. Also denote by $D(x; \theta_g)$ the second multilayer perceptron network, which represents the output scalar probability that the input x came from the training data, rather than from generator's distribution p_g.

The iterative NN modeling fitting (learning) involves the following:

- D maximization of the probability of assigning the correct labels (true=real or false=synthetic) to both types of inputs x, either from training examples of synthetic samples from G.
- Simultaneously training G to minimize $\log(1 - D(G(z)))$.

This dual optimization process for D and G corresponds to a two-player *mini-max* game with an objective value function $V(G, D)$

$$\min_G \max_D V(D, G) = \mathbb{E}_{x \sim p_{\text{data}}(x)}[\log D(x)] + \mathbb{E}_{x \sim p_Z(z)}[\log(1 - D(G(z)))].$$

This training approach enables recovering the *data generating distribution* using iterative numerical approaches. Note that for finite datasets, a perfect optimization of D in the inner loop of training is computationally impractical and, in general, may result in overfitting. Therefore, the algorithm alternates the estimation process by performing k steps of optimizing D followed by 1 step of optimizing G. When G updates change slowly, repeating this process yields a D estimation near its optimal solution. In practice, direct gradient optimization of the objective value function $V(G, D)$ may be insufficient to learn/estimate G. Therefore, early in the learning process when G may be poorly estimated, D can reject samples with higher confidence because these early generations are expected to be obviously simple and fake, i.e., different from the training data and unrealistic, as for the early initial iterations, $\log(1 - D(G(z)))$ may saturate. Hence, in the early training process, rather than training G to minimize $\log(1 - D(G(z)))$, the G training may focus on maximizing $\log D(G(z))$. Eventually, we transition to minimizing the correct cost $\log(1 - D(G(z)))$ and the final result of this dynamic optimization still has the same fixed point for G and D, but provides stronger gradients during the early learning iterations.

14.7.3.1 CIFAR10 Archive

We will demonstrate GAN training using the 10-classes Canadian Institute For Advanced Research (CIFAR10) image archive containing 50,000 32 × 32 RGB images, representing 10 classes (5K images per class). Let's focus on `birds` (label = 2). All (low-resolution) images are of dimension $(\underbrace{32,32}_{\text{pixels}}, \underbrace{3}_{\text{RGB colors}})$. Note the 3-channel RGB intensities. Below is a 10 × 10 collage of the first 100 bird images in the CIFAR10 archive (Fig. 14.30).

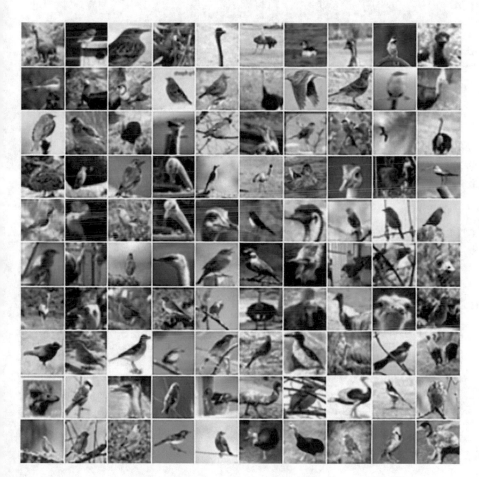

Fig. 14.30 A collage of 100 CIRAF-10 bird images (class # 2)

```
library(plotly)
library(keras)
library(tensorflow)
# CIFAR10 original labels: https://www.cs.toronto.edu/~kriz/cifar.html
# The label data is just a list of 10,000 numbers ranging from 0 to 9, which
corresponds to each of the 10 classes in CIFAR-10.
#      airplane : 0  |  automobile : 1    |     bird : 2  | …    truck : 9
# Focus on CIFAR10 BIRD images(label 2)!
# Loads CIFAR10 data
cifar10 <- dataset_cifar10()
c(c(x_train, y_train), c(x_test, y_test)) %<-% cifar10
# Selects bird images (class 2)
x_train <- x_train[as.integer(y_train) == 2,,,]
# Normalizes image intensities (bytes [0,255] --> [0,1])
x_train <- x_train / 255
bird_images <- x_train[1:(10*10),,,]
plt_list <- list()
N=100
for (i in 1:10) {
  for (j in 1:10) {
    plt_list[[i+(j-1)*10]] <-
      plot_ly(z=255*bird_images[i+(j-1)*10,,,],type="image",showscale=FALSE)
  }
}  # plot a single image plt_list[[2]]
plt_list %>%     # plot image collage
  subplot(nrows = 10, margin = 0.0001, which_layout=1) %>%
  layout(title="CIFAR-10 - a collage of random birds")
```

14.7.3.2   Generator (*G*)

Recall that the GAN represents a forger (adversarial) network *G* and an expert network *D* duking it out for superiority. Let's first examine *G* and experiment with a generator network which takes a random vector input (a stochastic point in the latent space) and outputs a decoded synthetic image that is sent to the expert (discriminator) for auto-labeling.

We will demonstrate a keras implementation of GAN modeling using deep convolutional GAN (DCGAN). Both the generator *G* and discriminator *D* will be deep convolutional networks, `convnets`.

The method `layer_conv_2d_transpose()` is used for image upsampling in the generator. GAN model includes the following:

- A generator network *G* mapping vectors of shape (*latent_dim*) to (fake) RGB images of dimension (32,32, $\underbrace{3}_{\text{RGB colors}}$).

  $\underbrace{}_{\text{pixels}}$

- A discriminator network *D* mapping images of the same dimension to a binary score estimating the probability that the image is real.
- A GAN network concatenating the generator and the discriminator together: `gan(x) <- discriminator(generator(x))` to map latent space

vectors *x* to the discriminator decoding real/fake and an assessment of the realism of generator output images.

- *D* is trained using examples of *real* and *synthetic* *G*-output images along with their corresponding "real" or "synth" labels.
- *G* training uses the gradients of the generator's weights, which reflects the loss of the GAN objective function. At each iteration, these *G* weights are updated to optimize the cost function in a direction improving the performance of *D* to correctly identify "real" and "synthetic" images supplied by the generator, *G*.
- To avoid getting the generator stuck with generating purely noisy images, we use dropout on both the discriminator and the generator.

14.7.3.3 Discriminator

The expert (Discriminator) network takes an input image and outputs a label (or probability prediction) about the chance that the image came from the real training set or was synthetically created by the generator network (*G*). Note that *G* is trained to confuse the discriminator network *D* and evolve toward generating increasingly more realistic output images. As the number of training epochs increases, the artificially created images become similar to the real training data images. Thus, *D* continuously adapts its neural network to increase the probability of catching fake images. However, this process also gradually improves the *G* capability to generate highly realistic output images. As the dual optimization process stabilizes and the training terminates, the generator is producing realistic images from random points in the state space, and the discriminator improves with detection of fakes.

Below is an implementation of a discriminator model taking a real or synthetic candidate image as input and outputting a classification label "generated (synth) image" or "real image from the training set."

14.7.3.4 Training the DCGAN

Just like most other deep learning processes, the DCGAN *design*, *training*, and *tuning* involve significant scientific rigorous and artistry. The theoretical foundations are intertwined with heuristic approaches, translating intuition and human-intelligence into computational modeling. Some of the exemplary heuristics involved in DCGAN modeling and the implementation of the GAN *generator* and *discriminator* include the following:

- Using the tanh() function in the last activation of the generator, as opposed to the more standard `sigmoid` function commonly employed in other types of DL models.
- Random sampling points from the latent space rely on *Gaussian (normal)* distribution, rather than a high-entropy *uniform* distribution. This randomness

and stochasticity during training yields more reliability and robustness in the final models.

- DCGAN training aims to achieve a dynamic equilibrium (tug-of-war between G and D nets). To ensure the GAN models avoid local minima (suboptimal solutions), randomness is embedded in the training process. Stochasticity is introduced by using dropout in the discriminator (omitting or dropping out the feedback of each discriminator in the framework with some probability at the end of each batch) and by adding random noise to the labels for the discriminator.

- Sparse gradients can negatively impact the GAN training process. Sparsity is often a desirable property in DL, as it makes many theoretically intractable computational problems solvable in practice. Gradient sparsity in DCGANs is the result of (1) *max-pooling* operations for calculating the largest value in each patch of each feature map, i.e., down sampling or pooled feature maps to highlight the most salient feature in the patch (instead of averaging the signal as is the case of average pooling); or (2) *ReLU activations* (rectified linear activation function, ReLU, is a piecewise linear function that will output the input directly if it is positive, otherwise, it will output zero). Max-pooling can be swapped with strided convolutions for downsampling. ReLU activation can be replaced by layer_activation_leaky_relu, which is similar to ReLU, but it relaxes sparsity constraints by allowing small negative activation values.

- The G generated output images may exhibit checkerboard artifacts caused by unequal coverage of the pixel space in the generator. This problem may be addressed by employing a kernel of size divisible by the image stride size whenever we use a strided layer_conv_2d_transpose or layer_conv_2d in both the generator and the discriminator. The stride, or pitch, is the number of bytes from one row of pixels in memory to the next row of pixels in memory; the presence of padding bytes widens the stride relative to the width of the image.

Recall that stochastic gradient descent optimization facilitates iterative learning using a training dataset to update the learned model at each iteration:

- The *batch size* is a hyperparameter of gradient descent that controls the number of training samples to work through before the model's internal parameters are updated.
- The *number of epochs* is a hyperparameter of gradient descent that controls the number of complete passes through the training dataset.

Let's demonstrate the synthetic image generation using the CIFAR10 imaging data archive of 10K images labeled in ten different categories (e.g., airplanes, horses). The example below just does 2 epochs. Increasing the *iterations* parameter ($k \times 100$) would generate more, and increasingly accurate synthetic images (in this case we are focusing on birds, label 2).

14.7.3.5 Elements of the DCGAN Training

The DCGAN training involves looping (iterating over each epoch) the following steps:

- Randomly traverse the latent space (introduce random noise by random sampling).
- Use *G* to generate images based on the random noise in the previous step.
- Mix the synth-generated images with real real-images (from training data).
- Train *D* to discriminate (label) these mixed images, outputting "real" or "fake" class labels.
- Again, randomly traverse the latent space drawing new random points (in the latent space).
- Train the DCGAN model using these random vectors, with a fixed target label="real" for all images. This process updates only the network weights of the generator! The discriminator is static inside the GAN. Hence, these updates force the discriminator to predict "real images" for synthetically generated images. This is the adversarial phase, as it trains the generator to fool the (frozen) discriminator.
- In the experiment below, we use a low number of iterations <- 200. To generate more realistic results, this number needs to be much higher (e.g., 10, 000).

GPU computing Note: these DCGAN models are very computationally intensive. The performance is enhanced by installing CUDA Toolkit and NVIDIA cuDNN, which facilitates running the calculations on the GPU, instead of the default CPU chipset (Fig. 14.31).

```
## Step= 100 ; discriminator loss= 0.6647896
## Step= 100 ; adversarial loss= 1.161157
## Step= 200 ; discriminator loss= 0.5714389
## Step= 200 ; adversarial loss= 4.558217
```

The *generator* transforms *random latent vectors* into *images*. The *discriminator* attempts to correctly identify the real and synthetically generated images. The generator is trained to fool the discriminator.

Iterative Protocol
- *Inputs*: Random vector from the latent space (random_latent_vectors <- matrix(rnorm(batch_size * latent_dim), nrow = batch_size, ncol = latent_dim)) and Real Images (real_images [1,,,] * 255).
- Generator (decoder) receives *Inputs* and *training feedback* from Discriminator including real and synth images and their discriminated labels (real or synthetic).

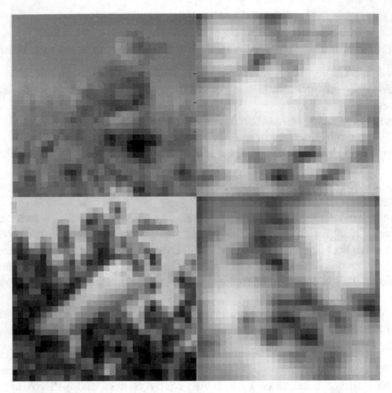

Fig. 14.31 Examples of real bird images (left column) and simple GAN-generated synthetic images (right column)

- Generator outputs new synth (decoded) image that is sent along with another real image as input to the Discriminator for another subsequent real vs. synth labeling
- Discriminator receives a pair of (real and synth) images as inputs, and outputs labels (real or synth) to them and forwards the results to generator.
- This iterative process continues until a certain stopping criterion is reached.

The GAN (generator network) is iteratively trained and tuned to fool the discriminator network (i.e., pass synth images as real). This training cycle continues and the neural network evolves toward generating increasingly realistic images. Simulated artificial images begin to look indistinguishable from their real counterparts. The discriminator network becomes less effective in telling the two types of images apart. In this iterative process, the discriminator is constantly adapting to the gradually improving capabilities of the generator. This constant reinforcement yields realistic versions of synthetic computer-generated images. At the end of the training process, which is highly nonlinear and discontinuous, the generator churns out input latent space points into realistic-looking images.

14.8   Transfer Learning

Humans learn complex tasks by capitalizing on their prior experiences, no matter how remote these previous encounters may appear to be. By the age of five, most kids can learn how to ride a bicycle in a couple of training sessions. This riding ability is acquired after they have already mastered the arts of *running*, also known as *controlled falling*, navigating complex 3D environments, and anticipating dynamic 4D spatiotemporal events. In effect, before kids start pedaling, their many prior holistic training experiences ensure that they "know" the basics of bike balancing. Children's formative years include a very large number of trial-and-errors, parental guidance sessions, and societal cues. These events already provide the basic building blocks necessary to learn bicycle riding. And this is well in advance of the actual "bicycle training" experience, which we typically associate with bicycle riding.

This learning process is very different for machines. It's extremely difficult to train a machine (a robot) to ride a bike, because these prior experiences kids go through are missing and cannot be easily built and transferred to complete the new task of learning how to balance a bike. In a way, humans learn new tasks easily as (1) they build on a large collection of skills they have already mastered, and (2) they can *transfer*, mix, match, integrate, and harness their prior experiences to the process of learning a *new task*. *Transfer machine learning* attempts to replicate this human transfer learning process into the domain of artificial intelligence. The goals are to expedite the ML training process by capitalizing on prior knowledge, expand the realm of ML/AI applications, and enable their "last mile" training to ensure they generate "reasonable decisions and actions" without starting with blank slate *de novo* learning.

14.8.1   Text Classification Using Deep Network Transfer Learning

One of the main challenges of AI/ML interpretation of free text is the extreme heterogeneity of the information and the unstructured format of the text content. This problem can be resolved by structurizing the input text and establishing homologies between multiple text samples (e.g., clinical notes). In a nutshell, transfer learning facilitates this process and enables (1) synthetic text generation (new data) that simulates realistic textual content (nonhuman data); and (2) transformation of unstructured text to structured data elements. For instance, if an *input* = *clinical notes*, a DNN model generates *output* = *vector* representing a quantitative signature vector of the input text; think of it as a vector of principal components associated with the specific free text.

The result of this AI process is that independent of the text length or type, DNN always generates a numeric vector of a fixed size (say 128 values). This canonical representation establishes *homologies* between any given set of strings (character arrays).

Let's demonstrate *transfer machine learning* using the medical specialty text-mining of clinical notes example that we saw in Chap. 5. This data includes a binary outcome indicating whether the medical specialty unit (there are 40 such units) is a *surgical* unit or not. We'll split the 4999 cases each containing 6 data elements (including the medical-specialty unit and clinical notes) into training and testing sets.

The key will be to use keras to build and train a ML model for predicting surgical vs. nonsurgical units from the content in the corresponding medical notes by using a previously trained text-mining DNN that quantizes text of any size.

```
library(keras)
library(reticulate)
library(tfhub)
library(tfds)
library(tfdatasets)
library(utf8)
# specify r-reticulate or r-tensorflow python Anaconda environment
# use_condaenv("r-tensorflow")
use_condaenv("r-reticulate", required = TRUE)
# Check tensorflow install configuration
tensorflow::tf_config()
py_module_available("tensorflow_hub")
```

14.8.1.1   Binary Transfer Learning Label-Classification of Clinical Text

Let's now *design a full DNN binary-classification model* composed of 4 layers stacked sequentially. The first *transfer learning* layer represents the pretrained TensorFlow Hub layer (prior model), which is loaded as the a priori left-most base layer in the full DNN, and maps clinical notes (description sentences) into its embedding vector (canonical signature vector). There are a number of *pretrained text embedding models* we can choose in this transfer-learning example. For instance, we can use google/tf2-preview/gnews-swivel-20dim/1, which splits the sentences into tokens, embeds each token, and then combines the embedding yielding an output of dimensions: (num_examples, embedding_dimension). The output of this initial *transfer learning prior model layer* is a fixed-length output vector, which is fed into the next fully connected (dense) *layer-2* with 16 hidden units. Layer-2 output feeds into the next (dense) *layer-3* with 6 nodes. Finally,

Layer-3 output goes into the last *layer-4*, which also is a densely connected layer with a single output (class label). Using the `sigmoid` activation function, this output represents a probability value between 0 and 1 indicating the model predicted chance (or confidence level) that the medical note text was written in a hospital *surgical unit*.

Other examples of pretrained text mining models that can be used for transfer learning include the following:

- https://tfhub.dev/google/tf2-preview/gnews-swivel-20dim/1
- https://tfhub.dev/google/tf2-preview/nnlm-en-dim128/1
- https://tfhub.dev/google/tf2-preview/gnews-swivel-20dim-with-oov/1, which is similar to https://tfhub.dev/google/tf2-preview/gnews-swivel-20dim/1, but with 2.5% of the vocabulary converted to OOV buckets; this helps when the training and testing vocabularies are not fully overlapping
- https://tfhub.dev/google/tf2-preview/nnlm-en-dim50/1   is   a   much   larger pretrained model with vocabulary of size 1M and 50 dimensions
- https://tfhub.dev/google/tf2-preview/nnlm-en-dim128/1, another large model, vocabulary of size 1M, and 128 dimensions

We will demonstrate NN-augmentation (transfer learning) modifying the base-model using the pretrained NN English Google News 200B corpus. Specifically, we will add four extra layers at the end, which will be tuned for our specific clinical text (medical notes). Of course, similarly, any of the other pretrained models can be used as alternatives.

Download the clinical dataset and split it into training:training (80:20). Note that in this clinical-notes example, the input data consists of medical text transcriptions stored as string sentences. In the first demonstration, we will try to predict a binary integer label, 0 or 1, representing a nonsurgical or surgical clinical unit where the clinical note was transcribed. To structurize the free-text as a computable data object (a matrix), we will automatically convert sentences into embedding vectors. This can be accomplished using text2vec or keras::layer_text_vectorization() transformations, or by including a pretrained text embedding as the first layer. This takes care of the text preprocessing, facilitates transfer learning, and makes the text-to-matrix independent of the text and the size of the clinical note.

```
dataCT <-
    read.csv('https://umich.instructure.com/files/21152999/download?download_frd=1',
             header=T)
str(dataCT)
## 'data.frame':    4999 obs. of  6 variables:
##  $ Index           : int  0 1 2 3 4 5 6 7 8 9 ...
##  $ description     : chr  " A 23-year-old white female presents with
…
##  $ medical_specialty: chr  " Allergy / Immunology" " Bariatrics" " Bariatrics"
…
##  $ sample_name     : chr  " Allergic Rhinitis "
…
##  $ transcription   : chr  "SUBJECTIVE:,  …"
…
##  $ keywords        : chr  "allergy / immunology, allergic rhinitis,…"
…
# 'data.frame': 4999 obs. with  6 variables
colnames(dataCT)
## [1] "Index"            "description"        "medical_specialty"
## [4] "sample_name"      "transcription"      "keywords"
# Binarize the 40 hospital units as Surgery-type and Non-Surgery types
dataCT$surgLabel <- ifelse(grepl('Surg', dataCT$medical_specialty), 1, 0)
table(grepl('Surg', dataCT$medical_specialty))
## FALSE   TRUE
##  3869   1130
# Fix the descriptions to UTF-8 encoding
library(stringi)
# table(stri_enc_mark(dataCT$description)) # ASCII native #  4994       5
dataCT$description   <- stri_encode(dataCT$description, "", "UTF-8")
dataCT$transcription <- stri_encode(dataCT$transcription, "", "UTF-8")
dataCT$clinicalNotes <- paste(dataCT$description, dataCT$transcription)
# Clean the clinical notes
library(tm)
## Vectorize the text
train_corpus <- VCorpus(VectorSource(dataCT$clinicalNotes))
## Remove Punctuation
train_corpus <- tm_map(train_corpus, content_transformer(removePunctuation))
## Remove numbers
train_corpus <- tm_map(train_corpus, removeNumbers)
## Convert text to lower case
train_corpus <- tm_map(train_corpus, content_transformer(tolower))
## Remove stop words
train_corpus <- tm_map(train_corpus, content_transformer(removeWords),
stopwords("english"))
## Stemming
train_corpus <- tm_map(train_corpus, stemDocument)
## Remove multiple whitespaces
train_corpus <- tm_map(train_corpus, stripWhitespace)
# Extract only the simplified text from the complex train_corpus object
dataCT$clinicalNotes <- unlist(lapply(train_corpus, `[[`, 1))
# Split the data 80:20
train_set_ind <- sample(nrow(dataCT), floor(nrow(dataCT)*0.8)) # 80:20 split
train_data <- dataCT[train_set_ind , ]
test_data <- dataCT[-train_set_ind , ]
num_words <- 10000
max_length <- 300
text_vectorization <- layer_text_vectorization(max_tokens = num_words,
                                        output_sequence_length = max_length)
```

14.8.1.1.1   Define a Fresh New `model1` De Novo

Let's define a fresh new neural network model architecture.

```
# 1. Define a new fresh model1 de novo
# for raw text input as string, needs to match exp next layer
input <- layer_input(shape = c(1), dtype = "string")
output <- input %>%
  text_vectorization() %>%
  layer_embedding(input_dim = num_words + 1, output_dim = 32) %>%
  layer_global_average_pooling_1d() %>%
  layer_dense(units = 16, activation = "relu") %>%
  layer_dropout(0.5) %>%
  layer_dense(units = 1, activation = "sigmoid")
model1 <- keras_model(input, output)
model1 %>% compile(
  optimizer = 'adam', loss='binary_crossentropy', metrics=list('accuracy'))
history <- model1 %>% fit(train_data$clinicalNotes,
            as.numeric(train_data$surgLabel),
            epochs = 10, batch_size = 512, validation_split = 0.2, verbose=2)
# Evaluate the model1 performance
results <- model1 %>% evaluate(test_data$clinicalNotes,
as.numeric(test_data$surgLabel), verbose = 0)
results
##      loss  accuracy
## 0.5299311 0.7800000
```

14.8.1.2   Naïve, Out-of-the-Box, Prior-Model Assessment (Without Retraining)

In a naïve approach, we can even evaluate the performance of the *prior model* (English Google News 200B[21]), i.e., assess transfer learning without any additional add-on training using the new problem-specific data. Remember that we have a univariate (binary) outcome and if we use `dataset_batch(32)`, the output will include a vector of 32 probability estimates.

We will see next that Keras knows how to extract elements from TensorFlow Datasets automatically making it a much more memory efficient alternative than loading the entire dataset to RAM before passing to Keras. To build the DNN model, we need to specify the network topology as a stack of network layers that include (1) a schema representing the unstructured text data (clinical note descriptions), and (2) the number and complexity of each subsequent layer in the model. For simplicity, in this example we will convert the 40 different medical units into binary "surgical" unit labels; 0 or 1 factors.

The unstructured text can be converted into embedding vectors of a fixed size, which simplifies the text processing. Using the transfer learning *prior* model, which includes a pretrained text embedding and appears as the first DNN layer. This allows

---

[21] https://tfhub.dev/google/tf2-preview/nnlm-en-dim128/1

us to outsource the text preprocessing and transformation into a quantitative information tensor. This is the key step illustrating the benefits of add-on transfer-learning in fine-tuning previously pretrained models.

The result of using this transfer-learning prior is that the model is *invariant* with respect to the length of the input clinical text—the output shape of the embeddings is (num _ examples × embedding _ dimension).

```
# 2. Naive - out-of-the-box prior-model assessment (without any retraining)
# Transfer Learning based on nnlm-en-dim128 (prior model)
# Define only output layer structure
library(keras)
###### May need to first remove outputs from prior runs!!!!! ###############
model2 <- keras_model_sequential() %>%
  layer_hub(
    handle = "https://tfhub.dev/google/tf2-preview/nnlm-en-dim128/1",
    input_shape = list(), dtype = tf$string,
    trainable = FALSE   # Set to TRUE for full model retraining
  ) %>%                 # add the binary labeling output layer format
  layer_dense(units = 1, activation = "sigmoid")
summary(model2)
## Model: "sequential_8"
##
## _____
## Layer (type)                    Output Shape                  Param ##
## ======================================================================
## keras_layer (KerasLayer)        (None, 128)                124642688
##
## _____
## dense_44 (Dense)                (None, 1)                        129
## ======================================================================
## Total params: 124,642,817
## Trainable params: 129
## Non-trainable params: 124,642,688
model2 %>% compile(
  optimizer = 'adam', loss = 'binary_crossentropy', metrics=list('accuracy'))
# Just estimate the final 128+1 coefficients of the final layer
history <- model2 %>% fit(
  train_data$clinicalNotes, train_data$surgLabel,
  epochs = 5, ### increase epochs for better performance
  batch_size = 128
)
# Assess performance
score <- model2 %>% evaluate(test_data$clinicalNotes, test_data$surgLabel)
print(score)
##      loss   accuracy
## 0.4693258 0.7790000
y_pred <- ifelse((model2 %>% predict(test_data$clinicalNotes)) > 0.4, 1, 0)
table(y_pred, test_data$surgLabel)
## y_pred   0    1
##      0 721  176
##      1  59   44
```

Clearly these surgical unit predictions can't be expected to be very reliable, as the model is not yet fine-tuned to respond specifically to *clinical text*.

The next step is to *compile the transfer-learning model* by specifying a *loss function* and an *optimizer* to facilitate the transfer-learning during the iterative network model fitting (fine-tuning). In this binary classification problem, we will use the `binary_crossentropy()` loss function. The model results in generating a probability value, which is presented as the output of the final DNN layer (the right-most single-unit layer with a sigmoid activation).

Another possible loss function for binary outcome is `mean_squared_error` (). However, binary_crossentropy is often better for dealing with probabilities as it measures the "distances" between probability distributions representing the predicted outcome and the ground-truth in supervised problems. Yet, `mean_squared_error`() is also applicable in a regression model setting. We will also employ Adaptive Moment Estimation (ADAM), as it's an effective optimizer.

14.8.1.3   Simple Transfer Learning

Let's use the `nnlm-en-dim128` (prior model) to define an expanded DNN model by adding additional four layers at the end to customize the deep neural network to our specific clinical data.

```r
# 3. Transfer Learning based on the nnlm-en-dim128 (prior model)
# Define expanded DNN model structure + 4 layers
model3 <- keras_model_sequential() %>%
  layer_hub(
    handle = "https://tfhub.dev/google/tf2-preview/nnlm-en-dim128/1",
    input_shape = list(), dtype = tf$string,
    trainable = FALSE    # Set to TRUE for full model retraining
  ) %>%
  # modify default pre-trained model by adding 4 extra layers at the end
  # tuned for our clinical text (medical notes)
  layer_dense(units = 64, activation = "sigmoid") %>%
  layer_dense(units = 32, activation = "sigmoid") %>%
  #layer_dropout(rate = 0.5) %>%
  layer_dense(units = 16, activation = "sigmoid") %>%
  layer_dense(units = 1, activation = "sigmoid")
  #    layer_dense(units = 16, activation = "relu") %>%
  #    layer_dense(units = 6, activation = "relu") %>%
  #    layer_dense(units = 1, activation = "sigmoid")
summary(model3)
## Model: "sequential_9"
##
## Layer (type)                        Output Shape                      Param
## ================================================================================
## keras_layer_1 (KerasLayer)          (None, 128)                  124642688
##
## dense_48 (Dense)                    (None, 64)                        8256
##
## dense_47 (Dense)                    (None, 32)                        2080
##
## dense_46 (Dense)                    (None, 16)                         528
##
## dense_45 (Dense)                    (None, 1)                           17
## ================================================================================
## Total params: 124,653,569
## Trainable params: 10,881
## Non-trainable params: 124,642,688
model3 %>% compile(
  optimizer = 'adam', loss = 'binary_crossentropy', metrics=list('accuracy'))
```

```
history <- model3 %>% fit(
  train_data$clinicalNotes, train_data$surgLabel,
  epochs = 10, ### increase epochs for better performance
  batch_size = 128
)
# Assess performance
score <- model3 %>% evaluate(test_data$clinicalNotes, test_data$surgLabel)
print(score)
##       loss  accuracy
## 0.3993433 0.7700000
y_pred <- ifelse((model3 %>% predict(test_data$clinicalNotes)) > 0.48, 1, 0)
table(y_pred, test_data$surgLabel)
## y_pred   0   1
##      0 682 134
##      1  98  86
```

14.8.1.4   Full-Scale Transfer Learning

Next, we will use the structure/topology of the pretrained model but estimate all $124M$ network parameters, not only the final $11K$ parameters at the end, as we did earlier.

```
# 4. Full-scale Transfer learning using the skeleton of the pre-trained model,
# but estimating all parameters
model4 <- keras_model_sequential() %>%
  layer_hub(
    handle = "https://tfhub.dev/google/tf2-preview/nnlm-en-dim128/1",
    input_shape = list(), dtype = tf$string,
    trainable = TRUE    # Set to FALSE for simple TL-model retraining
  ) %>%
  # modify default pre-trained model by adding 4 extra layers at the end
  # tuned for our clinical text (medical notes)
  layer_dense(units = 64, activation = "sigmoid") %>%
  layer_dense(units = 32, activation = "sigmoid") %>%
  layer_dense(units = 16, activation = "sigmoid") %>%
  layer_dense(units = 1, activation = "sigmoid")
summary(model4)
## Model: "sequential_10"
##
## _____
## Layer (type)                    Output Shape                   Param ##
## ========================================================================
## keras_layer_2 (KerasLayer)      (None, 128)                124642688
##
## dense_52 (Dense)                (None, 64)                      8256
##
## dense_51 (Dense)                (None, 32)                      2080
##
## dense_50 (Dense)                (None, 16)                       528
##
## dense_49 (Dense)                (None, 1)                         17
## ========================================================================
## Total params: 124,653,569
## Trainable params: 124,653,569
## Non-trainable params: 0
model4 %>% compile(
```

```
  optimizer = 'adam', loss = 'binary_crossentropy', metrics=list('accuracy'))
history <- model4 %>% fit(
  train_data$clinicalNotes, train_data$surgLabel,
  epochs = 10, ### increase epochs for better performance
  batch_size = 128
)
# Assess performance
score <- model4 %>% evaluate(test_data$clinicalNotes, test_data$surgLabel)
print(score)
##      loss   accuracy
## 0.4504241 0.7030000
y_pred <- ifelse((model4 %>% predict(test_data$clinicalNotes)) > 0.47, 1, 0)
table(y_pred, test_data$surgLabel)
## y_pred   0   1
##      0 563  83
##      1 217 137
```

The final pair of steps include the following:

- *Training.* *Transfer learning* involving fine-tuning the model starting with a prior pretrained model, which is re-trained on the specific medical text (training) data.
- *Validation.* The learning process involves repeated model estimation using mini-batches of 512 samples (see `dataset_batch()`) with 10 (for speed) or more (e.g., 100+, for accuracy and precision) epochs. This process involves 10 (or 100+) iterations over all samples in the dataset. During the fine-tuning training process, the transfer learner will report the initial and each subsequent model *loss-value* (optimization measure) and *accuracy* (fidelity measure) on sets of 10,000 samples from the validation set (see `dataset_shuffle()`) (Fig. 14.32).

```
# Evaluate the model. Examine the model performance.
# Inspect the trajectories of the Loss (representing the error,
# lower values are better), and accuracy (high values are better)
library(plotly)
plot_ly(x = ~c(1:history$params$epochs),  y = ~history$metrics$loss,
       type = "scatter", mode="markers+lines", name="Loss") %>%
  add_trace(x = ~c(1:history$params$epochs),  y = ~history$metrics$accuracy,
       type = "scatter", mode="markers+lines", name="Accuracy") %>%
  layout(title="DNN Training Performance", xaxis=list(title="epoch"),
       yaxis=list(title="Metric Value"), legend = list(orientation='h'),
       hovermode = "x unified")
```

This simple transfer learning approach achieves an accuracy of about 73–76%. More model customization and longer training are expected to significantly improve the performance of the fine-tuned transfer-learning DNN model.

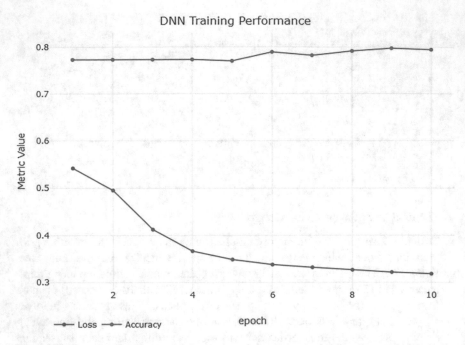

Fig. 14.32 Transfer learning model fine-tuning performance (estimating the parameters in the newly added layers at the end of the pretrained DNN model)

14.8.2   *Multinomial Transfer Learning Classification of Clinical Text*

Load all the appropriate R/Python packages and set up the RStudio environment. The same clinical data can be used for multinomial classification, where the *outcome* is the clinical specialty unit (there are 40 hospital units in this case study) and the *input* is the given clinical text. Start by defining the special labels (clinical units). The prediction of the 40-class labels will depend on the input x consisting of the string `clinicalNotes`, representing the concatenated *transcriptions* and *descriptions*.

In this transfer learning example of multiclass text classification, we will utilize the gnews-swivel-20dim model with text embedding trained on the English Google News 130 GB corpus (Fig. 14.33).[22]

---

[22] https://tfhub.dev/google/tf2-preview/gnews-swivel-20dim/1

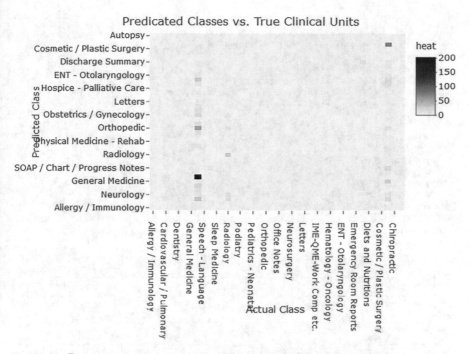

Fig. 14.33 Congruence between the 40 actual clinical units and their DNN-predicted counterparts

```
library(stringi)
dataCT <- read.csv('https://umich.instructure.com/files/21152999/download?download_frd=1',
        header=T)
dataCT$description <- stri_encode(dataCT$description, "", "UTF-8")
dataCT$transcription <- stri_encode(dataCT$transcription, "", "UTF-8")
# Concatenate Transcriptions and Descriptions into 1 string: clinicalNotes
dataCT$clinicalNotes <- paste(dataCT$description, dataCT$transcription)
convert_specialty <- list()
keys <- unique(dataCT$medical_specialty)
medical_specialtyNames <- dataCT$medical_specialty
values <- 1:length(keys)
for(i in 1:length(keys)) { convert_specialty[keys[i]] <- values[i] }
specialty <- c()
for (i in 1:length(dataCT$medical_specialty)){
  specialty[i] <- as.numeric(convert_specialty[dataCT$medical_specialty[i]])
}
dataCT$medical_specialty <- specialty
dataCT$medical_specialty <- matrix(dataCT$medical_specialty,
                        nrow=length(dataCT$medical_specialty), ncol=1)
# Convert labels to categorical one-hot encoding
one_hot_SpecialtyLabels <- to_categorical(dataCT$medical_specialty,
              num_classes = length(unique(dataCT$medical_specialty))+1)
one_hot_SpecialtyLabels<-one_hot_SpecialtyLabels[,-1] # remove empty column 1
# sum(one_hot_SpecialtyLabels)  [1] 4999
num_words  <- 10000
max_length <- 300
text_vectorization <- layer_text_vectorization(max_tokens = num_words,
```

```
                                                    output_sequence_length = max_length)
# 80:20 plot training:testing
train_set_ind <- sample(nrow(dataCT), floor(nrow(dataCT)*0.8))
train_data <- dataCT[train_set_ind, ]
test_data <- dataCT[-train_set_ind, ]
one_hot_SpecialtyLabels_trainY <- one_hot_SpecialtyLabels[train_set_ind, ]
one_hot_SpecialtyLabels_testY  <- one_hot_SpecialtyLabels[-train_set_ind, ]
model3 <- keras_model_sequential() %>%
  layer_hub(
    handle = "https://tfhub.dev/google/tf2-preview/gnews-swivel-20dim/1",
    input_shape = list(), dtype = tf$string, trainable = TRUE) %>%
  layer_dense(units = 256, activation = "relu") %>%
  layer_dropout(0.25) %>%
  layer_dense(units = 128, activation = "relu") %>%
  layer_dropout(0.25) %>%
  layer_dense(units = 64, activation = "relu") %>%
  layer_dense(units = length(keys), activation = 'softmax')
summary(model3)
```

```
## Model: "sequential_11"
## _____
## Layer (type)                      Output Shape                     Param
## ========================================================================
## keras_layer_3 (KerasLayer)        (None, 20)                      400020
##
## _____
## dense_56 (Dense)                  (None, 256)                       5376
##
## _____
## dropout_17 (Dropout)              (None, 256)                          0
##
## _____
## dense_55 (Dense)                  (None, 128)                      32896
##
## _____
## dropout_16 (Dropout)              (None, 128)                          0
##
## _____
## dense_54 (Dense)                  (None, 64)                        8256
##
## _____
## dense_53 (Dense)                  (None, 40)                        2600
## ========================================================================
## Total params: 449,148
## Trainable params: 449,148
## Non-trainable params: 0
model3 %>% compile(
  loss = 'categorical_crossentropy', metrics = list('accuracy'),
  optimizer = optimizer_sgd(learning_rate = 0.01, decay = 1e-6,
                      momentum = 0.9, nesterov = TRUE))
history3 <- model3 %>% fit(train_data$clinicalNotes,
          one_hot_SpecialtyLabels_trainY,
          epochs = 100, batch_size = 512, validation_split = 0.2, verbose=2)
results3 <- model3 %>% evaluate(test_data$clinicalNotes,
                      one_hot_SpecialtyLabels_testY, verbose = 2)
print(paste0("Mind that the testing-case performance metrics (Loss=",
  round(results3["loss"], 3)," and Accuracy=",round(results3["accuracy"],3),
      ") of the DNN text classification reflect results of ", length(keys),
      " medical specialties (classes), not a binary classification!"))
## [1] "Mind that the testing-case performance metrics (Loss=2.186 and
```

```
Accuracy=0.356) of the DNN text classification reflect results of 40 medical
specialties (classes), not a binary classification!"
score <- model3 %>%
        evaluate(test_data$clinicalNotes, one_hot_SpecialtyLabels_testY)
print(score)
##      loss accuracy
## 2.185851 0.356000        # pretty good performance, relative to 40 classes
y_pred <- model3 %>% predict(test_data$clinicalNotes)
head(apply(y_pred, 1, which.max))  # table(apply(y_pred, 1, which.max))
## [1]  3 10  8 13  8  8
y_pred_class <- apply(y_pred, 1, which.max)  # hist(y_pred[,8])
table(y_pred_class, test_data$medical_specialty[,1])
heat <- matrix(0, 40, 40)
for ( i in 1:length(test_data$clinicalNotes)) {
  heat[test_data$medical_specialty[i, 1], y_pred_class[i]] =
    heat[test_data$medical_specialty[i, 1], y_pred_class[i]] + 1
}
plot_ly(x =~keys, y = ~keys, z = ~heat, name="Model Performance",
        hovertemplate = paste('<i>Matching</i>: %{z:.0f}',
                              '<br><b>True</b>: %{x}<br>', '<b>Pred</b>: %{y}'),
        colors = 'Reds', type = "heatmap") %>%
  layout(title="Predicated Classes vs. True Clinical Units",
         xaxis=list(title="Actual Class"),yaxis=list(title="Predicted Class"))
```

14.8.3 Binary Classification of Film Reviews

All readers are encouraged to try text-based transfer learning using alternative datasets,
e.g., the 50,000 movie reviews dataset. The code skeleton below illustrates the basic
pipeline workflow for the movie review's binary classifications (Fig. 14.34).

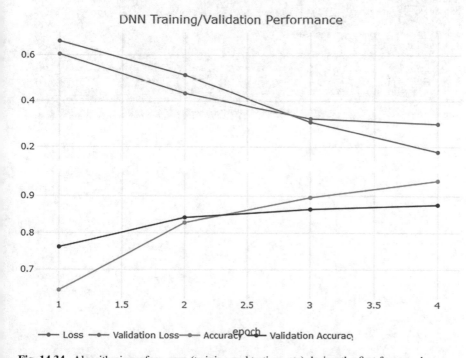

Fig. 14.34 Algorithmic performance (training and testing sets) during the first few epochs

```r
# Load Movie Reviews (50K)
# split the entire dataset into a List of 3 objects:
# imdb[[1]]=training_set, imdb[[2]]=testing_set, imdb[[3]]=validation_set
imdb <-
    tfds::tfds_load (
    "imdb_reviews:1.0.0",split = list("train[:60%]", "train[-40%:]", "test"),
    as_supervised = TRUE
)
# summary(imdb)
# tfds_Load returns a TensorFlow Dataset, an abstraction representing a List
# of elements, in which each element consists of one or more components.
# To access individual elements of a Dataset:
firstBatch <- imdb[[1]] %>%
  dataset_batch(1) %>% # Used to get only the first example
  reticulate::as_iterator() %>%
  reticulate::iter_next()
str(firstBatch)
## List of 2
##  $ :tf.Tensor([b"This was an absolutely terrible movie. Don't be lured in by
Christopher Walken or Michael Ironside. Both are great actors, but this must
simply be their worst role in history. Even their great acting could not redeem
this movie's ridiculous storyline. This movie is an early nineties US propaganda
piece. The most pathetic scenes were those when the Columbian rebels were making
their cases for revolutions. Maria Conchita Alonso appeared phony, and her
pseudo-love affair with Walken was nothing but a pathetic emotional plug in a
movie that was devoid of any real meaning. I am disappointed that there are
movies like this, ruining actor's like Christopher Walken's good name. I could
barely sit through it."], shape=(1,), dtype=string)
##  $ :tf.Tensor([0], shape=(1,), dtype=int64)
review1 <- as_utf8(as.character(firstBatch[1][[1]]$numpy()[1][[1]])) # get text-
review (string)
label1 <- as.numeric(firstBatch[2][[1]]$numpy())     # get binary class (0/1)
embedding_layer <- layer_hub(
  handle ="https://tfhub.dev/google/tf2-preview/nnlm-en-dim128/1")
embedding_layer(firstBatch[[1]])
# build the complete model
model <- keras_model_sequential() %>%
  layer_hub(
    handle = "https://tfhub.dev/google/tf2-preview/nnlm-en-dim128/1",
    input_shape = list(), dtype = tf$string, trainable = TRUE) %>%
  layer_dense(units = 16, activation = "relu") %>%
  layer_dense(units = 8, activation = "relu") %>%
  layer_dense(units = 1, activation = "sigmoid")
summary(model)
```

```
## Model: "sequential_12"
##
## _____
## Layer (type)                        Output Shape                    Param
## ========================================================================
## keras_layer_5 (KerasLayer)          (None, 128)                 124642688
##
## _____
## dense_59 (Dense)                    (None, 16)                       2064
##
## _____
## dense_58 (Dense)                    (None, 8)                         136
##
## _____
## dense_57 (Dense)                    (None, 1)                           9
## ========================================================================
## Total params: 124,644,897
## Trainable params: 124,644,897
## Non-trainable params: 0
# compile model
model %>%
  compile(optimizer="adam", loss="binary_crossentropy", metrics="accuracy")
# model training
history <- model %>%
  fit(imdb[[1]] %>% dataset_shuffle(10000) %>% dataset_batch(512),
    epochs = 4,  # for convergence, use larger number of epochs (e.g., 20+)
    validation_data = imdb[[2]] %>% dataset_batch(512), verbose = 2)
# plot performance
pl_loss <- plot_ly(x = ~c(1:history$params$epochs), y=~history$metrics$loss,
          type = "scatter", mode="markers+lines", name="Loss") %>%
  add_trace(x = ~c(1:history$params$epochs),  y = ~history$metrics$val_loss,
          type = "scatter", mode="markers+lines", name="Validation Loss") %>%
  layout(title="DNN Training/Validation Performance",
          hovermode = "x unified",  xaxis=list(title="epoch"),
          yaxis=list(title="Metric Value"), legend=list(orientation='h'))
pl_acc <- plot_ly(x = ~c(1:history$params$epochs),
          y=~history$metrics$accuracy,
          type = "scatter", mode="markers+lines", name="Accuracy") %>%
  add_trace(x = ~c(1:history$params$epochs), y=~history$metrics$val_accuracy,
          type="scatter", mode="markers+lines", name="Validation Accuracy") %>%
  layout(title="DNN Training/Validation Performance",
          hovermode = "x unified",  xaxis=list(title="epoch"),
          yaxis=list(title="Metric Value"), legend = list(orientation='h'))
subplot(pl_loss, pl_acc, nrows=2, shareX = TRUE, titleX = TRUE)
```

```
# model evaluation on testing data
model %>% evaluate(imdb[[3]] %>% dataset_batch(512), verbose = 0)
##      loss  accuracy
## 0.3138316 0.8658000
```

14.9 Image Classification

Similar to the unstructured text-mining (film review case) we illustrated above, we can use DNN transfer learning for *image classification*. However, to quantify the algorithmic performance, we may need to consider some alternative distance and similarity measures. The latter will allow us to track the iterative improvements and drive the algorithm in direction of performance enhancement.

14.9.1   Performance Metrics

Binary Cross-Entropy Measure The *cross-entropy* measure of dissimilarity between two discrete probability distributions p (true state) and q (predicted state) with identical support X is defined as

$$H(p, q) = - \sum_{x_i \in X} p(x_i) \log q(x_i)$$

For binary outcomes, logistic regression transforms the log-loss over all training observations, i.e., it optimizes the average cross-entropy in the sample.

For a sample indexed by $n = 1, \cdots, N$, the expected (average) loss function is

$$J(w) = \frac{1}{N} \sum_{n=1}^{N} H(p_n, q_n) = - \frac{1}{N} \sum_{n=1}^{N} [y_n \log \widehat{y}_n + (1 - y_n) \log (1 - \widehat{y}_n)],$$

where $\widehat{y}_n \equiv g(w \cdot x_n) = \frac{1}{1 + e^{-w \cdot x_n}}$ and $g(z)$ is the logistic function. The logistic loss is the *cross-entropy loss* or *log-loss*, and binary refers to the situation of binary outcome labels $\{-1, +1\}$.

Hence, the *binary cross-entropy (BCE)* is simply

$$H(p, q) = - \sum_{x_i \in X} p(x_i) \log q(x_i) = - y \log \widehat{y} - (1 - y) \log (1 - \widehat{y}),$$

where $p \in \{y, 1 - y\}$ and $q \in \{\widehat{y}, 1 - \widehat{y}\}$ represent the probability of the *true* and *predicted* binary outcomes, respectively.

High or low BCE values indicate "bad" or "good" model performance, respectively, with a perfect model having a $BSE \approx 0$.

Dice Coefficient The Sørensen–Dice coefficient (*Dice Coefficient*) is another measure to assess the similarity between two sets, samples, or distributions. In our case we are applying the dice coefficient to track the overlap between the true brain-tumor masks, and the DCNN-derived mask-estimate (prediction) of the tumor based on the raw brain image.

Discrete sets X and Y	(Boolean) Binary Data	Probabilities (e.g., quantiles)
$D = \frac{2\|X \cap Y\|}{\|X\| + \|Y\|}$, $\|\cdot\|$ is set cardinality	TP=true positive, FP=false positive, FN=false negative, $D = \frac{2TP}{2TP + FP + FN}$	$D = \frac{2\|\mathbf{p} \cdot \mathbf{q}\|}{\|\mathbf{p}\|^2 + \|\mathbf{q}\|^2}$

Next, we will demonstrate two different deep neural network frameworks *torch* and *tensorflow*.

14.9.2   *Torch Deep Convolutional Neural Network (CNN)*

The Convolutional Networks for Biomedical Image Segmentation (Unet),[23] shown on this figure, is an example of a DCNN (Fig. 14.35).

The U-shaped DCNN (Unet) represents successive convolutional layers with max-pooling. During the auto-encoding (left-down-hill branch) the Unet reduces image resolution (downsampling), whereas the subsequent decoding phase (right-uphill branch) upsamples the images to arrive at an output of the same size as the original input. The information analysis (encoding) and synthesis (decoding) facilitate the labeling of each output image pixel by feeding information in each decoding layer from the corresponding encoding layer with matching resolution in the downsizing encoding layer.

Each upsampling (decoding) step concatenates the output from the previous layer with that from its counterpart in the compression (encoding) step. The final decoding output is a mask of the same size as the original image, derived by a 1×1-convolution, which does not require a dense layer at the end as the output convolutional layer represents a single filter. Below we show how to load, train, and use a Unet for transfer learning in 2D image segmentation. Note that this model has over $3M$ trainable parameters. You can see an R example of a Unet model for

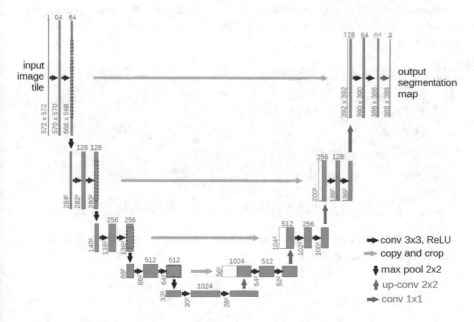

Fig. 14.35 A Unet schematic as an example of a deep convolutional neural network

---

[23] https://doi.org/10.1007/978-3-319-24574-4_28

input–output tensors of shape=c(128,128),[24] see lines 73–183 in the *unet.R* source code.

```
# when necessary, download the U-Net package, before you load it into R
# remotes::install_github("r-tensorflow/unet")
library(unet)
library(tibble)
model <- unet(input_shape = c(256, 256, 3))
# To print the model as text output, run: model
# Results: # Trainable params: 31,031,745
```

14.9.2.1   Data Import

Let's first download and load the Brain Tumor Imaging dataset. These data come from a 2019 study on association of genomic subtypes of lower-grade gliomas with shape features automatically extracted by a deep learning algorithm.[25] The 2D brain MR images are paired with 2D tumor masks, which are trivial for controls and nontrivial for patients, using The Cancer Imaging Archive (TCIA).[26] The data represent 110 patients with lower-grade glioma and include fluid-attenuated inversion recovery (FLAIR) MRI scans.[27] There are three channels of the MRI data: *precontrast, FLAIR*, and *postcontrast*. The corresponding tumor masks were obtained ,by manual-delineations on the FLAIR images by board-certified radiologists.

```
# To start a clean fresh run, remove all old files first! Be careful!
##### First check > list.files("/data/")
##### do.call(file.remove, list(list.files("/data", full.names = TRUE)))
##### unlink("/data/*", recursive=TRUE, force=TRUE)
pathToZip <- tempfile()
download.file("https://umich.instructure.com/files/21813670/download?download_frd=1",
              pathToZip, mode = "wb")
zip::unzip(pathToZip, files=NULL, exdir = "/data")
library(tibble)
library(rsample)
train_dir <- "/data/data"
valid_dir <- "/data/mri_valid"
library(magick)    # Needed for TIFF-->PNG image conversion & other processing
```

Create the necessary directories to store the training and validation imaging data (brain MRIs and tumor masks).

---

[24] https://github.com/rstudio/keras/blob/master/vignettes/examples/unet.R

[25] https://doi.org/10.1016/j.compbiomed.2019.05.002

[26] https://wiki.cancerimagingarchive.net/display/Public/TCGA-LGG

[27] https://doi.org/10.1109/JTEHM.2022.3176737

```
# check if ReadMe file is accessible
file.rename("/data/ReadMe_TCGA_MRI_Segmentation_Data_Phenotypes.txt", train_dir)
# Import the meta-data
meta_data <- read.csv("/data/TCGA_MRI_Segmentation_Data_Phenotypes.csv")
# note that these are relative file/directory names
# Create a validation folder
dir.create(valid_dir)
# Check all n=110 patients are accessible
patients <- list.dirs(train_dir, recursive = FALSE)
length(patients)
# Randomly select 20 Patients for validation, remaining 90 are for training
valid_indices <- sample(1:length(patients), 20); valid_indices
patients[valid_indices] # prints the actual folders with validation data
# Extract & Relocate the Validation cases (separate them from training data)
for (i in valid_indices) {
  dir.create(file.path(valid_dir, basename(patients[i])))
  for (f in list.files(patients[i])) {
    file.rename(file.path(train_dir, basename(patients[i]), f),
      file.path(valid_dir, basename(patients[i]), f))
  }
  unlink(file.path(train_dir, basename(patients[i])), recursive=TRUE) # clean
}
# Confirm that only 80 patients are left in the standard data folder
# list all training data imaging files: list.dirs(train_dir, recursive=FALSE)
length(list.dirs(train_dir, recursive = FALSE))
# and 30-60 validation cases are in the validation folder
length(list.dirs(valid_dir, recursive = FALSE))
# and check validation data
length(list.files(valid_dir, recursive = T)) # [1] 1268
```

Define data-frames containing the filenames for all training and validation data.

```
# Identify TRAINING / VALIDATION data (raw images + tumor masks) as filenames
data_train <- tibble(
  img = grep(list.files(train_dir, full.names = TRUE,
        pattern = "tif", recursive = TRUE),
        pattern = 'mask', invert = TRUE, value = TRUE),
  mask = grep(list.files(train_dir, full.names = TRUE, pattern = "tif",
        recursive = TRUE), pattern = 'mask', value = TRUE)
)
data_valid <- tibble(
  img = grep(list.files(valid_dir, full.names = TRUE, pattern = "tif",
        recursive = TRUE), pattern = 'mask', invert = TRUE, value = TRUE),
  mask = grep(list.files(valid_dir, full.names = TRUE, pattern = "tif",
        recursive = TRUE), pattern = 'mask', value = TRUE)
)
```

(Optionally) convert all 2D TIFF images to PNG RGB format; this may be necessary to ensure the input images are three channels and are correctly interpreted as tensorflow objects.

```
# If all training + testing data are in one folder, split them by:
#   data <- initial_split(data_train, prop = 0.8)
# convert all Training Data: TIFF images and masks to PNG format (for easier TF
processing downstream)
files_img_tif <- data_train$img[grepl("\\.tif$", data_train$img), drop=TRUE]
data_train_img_png <- lapply(files_img_tif,
    function(x) {
        # image_write(image_read(x), path=gsub(".tif$",".png",x), format="png")
        a = image_convert(image_read(x), format = ".png")
        image_write(a, path = gsub(".tif$", ".png", x), format = "png")
    }
)
files_mask_tif <- data_train$mask[grepl("\\.tif$",data_train$mask),drop=TRUE]
data_train_mask_png <- lapply(files_mask_tif,
    function(x) {
        a = image_convert(image_read(x), format = ".png")
        image_write(a, path = gsub(".tif$", ".png", x), format = "png")
    }
)
# Similarly convert all Validation Data
# convert all TIFF images and masks to PNG format (for easier TF processing)
files_valid_img_tif <-
        data_valid$img[grepl("\\.tif$", data_valid$img), drop = TRUE]
data_valid_img_png <- lapply(files_valid_img_tif,
        function(x) {
        a = image_convert(image_read(x), format = ".png")
        image_write(a, path = gsub(".tif$", ".png", x), format = "png")
    }
)
files_valid_mask_tif <-
        data_valid$mask[grepl("\\.tif$", data_valid$mask), drop = TRUE]
data_valid_mask_png <- lapply(files_valid_mask_tif,
        function(x) {
        a = image_convert(image_read(x), format = ".png")
        image_write(a, path = gsub(".tif$", ".png", x), format = "png")
    }
)
# Check that the TIF --> PNG conversion worked, inspect one case
head(list.files("/data/data/TCGA_HT_A61A_20000127"))
```

Derive a binary class label: cancer (for nontrivial tumor masks) or control (for empty tumor masks).

```
# Compute a new binary outcome variable 1=Brain Tumor
# (mask has at least 1 white pixel), 0=Normal Brain, no white pixels in mask
pos_neg_diagnosis <- sapply(data_train$mask,
    function(x) {  value = max(imager::magick2cimg(image_read(x)))
        ifelse (value > 0, 1, 0)  }
)
table(pos_neg_diagnosis)   #; head(data_train)
## pos_neg_diagnosis
##    0    1
## 2113 1127
# Add the normal vs. cancer label to training and testing datasets
data_train$label <- pos_neg_diagnosis
pos_neg_diagnosis_valid <- sapply(data_valid$mask,
    function(x) {   value = max(imager::magick2cimg(image_read(x)))
        ifelse (value > 0, 1, 0)  }
)
table(pos_neg_diagnosis_valid)
## pos_neg_diagnosis_valid
##    0    1
## 443 246
data_valid$label <- pos_neg_diagnosis_valid
```

14.9.2.2   Torch-Based Transfer Learning

Next, we will ingest the *three-channel (RGB) imaging data* and the corresponding *tumor masks* (binary images) for each participant. The method `torch::dataset()` allows specifying `initialize()` and `.getitem()` methods for complex computable data objects. The first method `initialize()` creates the archive of *imaging* and *mask* file names that can be utilized by the second method `.getitem()` for iterating over all cases. The method `.getitem()` returns ordered input–output pairs, and performs weighted sampling with prevalence to large lesion images, which is useful for accounting for DNN training with imbalanced classes.

The training sets can be enhanced by *data augmentation*—a process expanding the set of training images and masks via operations such as *flipping, resizing, and rotating* based on certain specifications.

Below we use PyTorch to define a `brain_dataset()` method providing a larger *augmented training* dataset, new size `length(train_ds)` ~ 2K, and a larger *validation* set, new size `length(valid_ds)` ~1K. In practice, we can use any alternative transfer-learning strategy including `pytorch`, `tensorflow`, and `theano`.

Note that `unet` training takes significant computational time; training 20-epochs took a total of 600 compute hours, which translates into a couple of days of computing on a 20-core server. We have provided several precomputed/pretrained *.pt models on Canvas.[28]

Next, we define a function `brain_dataset()` required for iterative retrieval of pytorch datasets. All such datasets need to have a method called `initialize()` instantiating the inventory of *imaging* and *mask* file names that will be used by the second method, `.getitem()`, to ingest the imaging data from these files, return input-image plus mask-target pairs, and perform data-augmentation. The parameter `random_sampling=TRUE`, `.getitem()` controls the weighted sample loading of image-mask pairs with larger size tumors. This option is used with the training set to counter any class-label imbalances.

The training sets, but not the validation sets, use of *data augmentation* to ensure DCNN-invariance to specific spatiotemporal and intensity transformations. During imaging-data augmentation, the training images/masks may be *flipped, resized*, and *rotated* with specifiable probabilities for each type of augmentation transformation.

---

[28] https://umich.instructure.com/courses/38100/files/folder/Case_Studies/36_TCGA_MRI_Seg mentation_Data_Phenotypes

```r
library(torch)
library(torchvision)
library(tidyverse) # data wrangling
library(zeallot)    # needed for piping function "%<-%" in "brain_dataset()"
library(magick)     # image processing and visualization
library(pins)
library(zip)
torch_manual_seed(1234)
set.seed(1234)
brain_dataset <- dataset(
  name = "brain_dataset",
  # 1. Initialize
  initialize = function(img_dir, augmentation_params = NULL,
         random_sampling = FALSE) {
    self$images <- tibble(img = grep(list.files(img_dir, full.names = TRUE,
                pattern = "png", recursive = TRUE),
                pattern = 'mask', invert = TRUE, value = TRUE),
                mask = grep(list.files(img_dir, full.names = TRUE,
                pattern = "png", recursive = TRUE),
                    pattern = 'mask',value = TRUE)
                )
    self$slice_weights <- self$calc_slice_weights(self$images$mask)
    self$augmentation_params <- augmentation_params
    self$random_sampling <- random_sampling
  },
  # 2. Load and transform images from files into TF object elements (tensors)
  .getitem = function(i) {
        index <- if (self$random_sampling == TRUE) sample(1:self$.length(),
                        1, prob = self$slice_weights)
                else i
    img <- self$images$img[index] %>% image_read() %>% transform_to_tensor()
    mask <- self$images$mask[index] %>% image_read() %>%
            transform_to_tensor() %>% transform_rgb_to_grayscale() %>%
            torch_unsqueeze(1)
    img <- self$min_max_scale(img)
    if (!is.null(self$augmentation_params)) {
      scale_param <- self$augmentation_params[1]
      c(img, mask) %<-% self$resize(img, mask, scale_param)
      rot_param <- self$augmentation_params[2]
      c(img, mask) %<-% self$rotate(img, mask, rot_param)
      flip_param <- self$augmentation_params[3]
      c(img, mask) %<-% self$flip(img, mask, flip_param)
    }
    list(img = img, mask = mask)
  },
  # 3. Save the total number of imaging files
  .length = function() { nrow(self$images)  },
  # 4. Estimate 2D image weights: Bigger tumor-masks correspond to higher weights
  calc_slice_weights = function(masks) {
    weights <- map_dbl(masks, function(m) {
      img <- as.integer(magick::image_data(image_read(m), channels = "gray"))
      sum(img / 255)
    })
    sum_weights <- sum(weights)
    num_weights <- length(weights)
    weights <- weights %>% map_dbl(function(w) {
      w <- (w + sum_weights * 0.1 / num_weights) / (sum_weights * 1.1)
    })
    weights
  },
```

```
  # 5. Estimate the image intensity range (min, max)
  min_max_scale = function(x) {
    min = x$min()$item()
    max = x$max()$item()
    x$clamp_(min = min, max = max)
    x$add_(-min)$div_(max - min + 1e-5)
    x
  },
  # 6. Image tensor shape resizing (when necessary)
  resize = function(img, mask, scale_param) {
    img_size <- dim(img)[2]
    rnd_scale <- runif(1, 1 - scale_param, 1 + scale_param)
    img <- transform_resize(img, size = rnd_scale * img_size)
    mask <- transform_resize(mask, size = rnd_scale * img_size)
    diff <- dim(img)[2] - img_size
    if (diff > 0) {
      top <- ceiling(diff / 2)
      left <- ceiling(diff / 2)
      img <- transform_crop(img, top, left, img_size, img_size)
      mask <- transform_crop(mask, top, left, img_size, img_size)
    } else {
      img <- transform_pad(img,
        padding =
            -c(ceiling(diff/2),floor(diff/2),ceiling(diff/2),floor(diff/2)))
      mask <- transform_pad(mask,
        padding =
            -c(ceiling(diff/2), floor(diff/2),ceiling(diff/2),floor(diff/2)))
    }
    list(img, mask)
  },
  # 7. Rotation (if/when augmentation is requested)
  rotate = function(img, mask, rot_param) {
    rnd_rot <- runif(1, 1 - rot_param, 1 + rot_param)
    img <- transform_rotate(img, angle = rnd_rot)
    mask <- transform_rotate(mask, angle = rnd_rot)
    list(img, mask)
  },
  # 8. Flipping (if/when augmentation is requested)
  flip = function(img, mask, flip_param) {
    rnd_flip <- runif(1)
    if (rnd_flip > flip_param) {
      img <- transform_hflip(img)
      mask <- transform_hflip(mask)
    }
    list(img, mask)
  }
)
```

Next, using the `brain_dataset()` method, we actually generate the (training and validation) imaging datasets as computable objects using the raw filenames in the training and validation data-frames defined above.

```
train_ds <- brain_dataset(
  train_dir,
  augmentation_params = c(0.05, 15, 0.5),
  random_sampling = TRUE
)
length(train_ds)  ## [1] 3240 # ~3K
valid_ds <- brain_dataset(
  valid_dir, augmentation_params = NULL, random_sampling = FALSE)
length(valid_ds)  ## [1] 689 # ~700
```

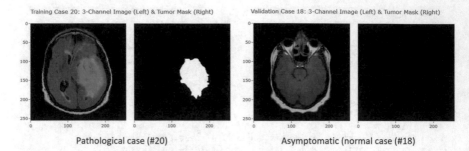

Fig. 14.36 A pair of training datasets, including a RGB brain image (left) and a manual (expert-derived) tumor mask (right). Note that different executions of the protocol will randomly sample different cases from the (training and validation) archives; at each runtime, the algorithm will plot different images (brains and their corresponding masks)

Let's visualize one testing and one validation image-mask pairs using `plot_ly()`. Notice that due to random sampling, each time we draw cases from the training and validation cohorts, we can get either patients (with nontrivial tumor masks) or asymptomatic controls (with empty tumor masks) (Fig. 14.36).

```
library (plotly)
rasterPlotly <- function (image, name="", hovermode = NULL) {
  myPlot <- plot_ly(type="image", z=image, name=name, hoverlabel=name,
              text=name, hovertext=name, hoverinfo="name+x+y") %>%
            layout(hovermode = hovermode, xaxis = list(hoverformat = '.1f'),
                yaxis = list(hoverformat = '.1f'))
  return(myPlot)
}
# Training Case #20
img_and_mask <- train_ds[20]
img <- img_and_mask[[1]]  # 3-channel image
img <- img_and_mask[[1]]$permute(c(2, 3, 1)) %>% as.array() # 3-channel image
mask <- img_and_mask[[2]]$squeeze() %>% as.array() # tumor mask
mask <- EBImage::rgbImage(255*mask, 255*mask, 255*mask)
# manually generate a gray scale mask image
p1 <- rasterPlotly(image=255*img, name = "RGB Image", hovermode="y unified")
p2 <- rasterPlotly(mask, name = "Tumor Mask", hovermode = "y unified")
subplot(p1,p2, shareY = TRUE) %>% layout(title="Training Case 20: 3-Channel
                                Image (Left) & Tumor Mask (Right)")

# Validation Case 18
img_and_mask <- valid_ds[18]
img <- img_and_mask[[1]]
mask <- img_and_mask[[2]]
img <- img_and_mask[[1]]$permute(c(2, 3, 1)) %>% as.array()  # 3-channel image
mask <- img_and_mask[[2]]$squeeze() %>% as.array() # tumor mask
mask <- EBImage::rgbImage(255*mask, 255*mask, 255*mask)  # manually generate a
gray scale mask image

p1 <- rasterPlotly(image=255*img, name = "RGB Image", hovermode = "y unified")
p2 <- rasterPlotly(mask, name = "Tumor Mask", hovermode = "y unified")
subplot(p1,p2, shareY = TRUE) %>% layout(title="Validation Case 18: 3-Channel
Image (Left) & Tumor Mask (Right)")
```

It is also important to demonstrate the process of training-data image-augmentation by using one image to generate seven rows of four augmented images. In this

Validation Case 77: Random Rotation/Flop/Scale Image Augmentation

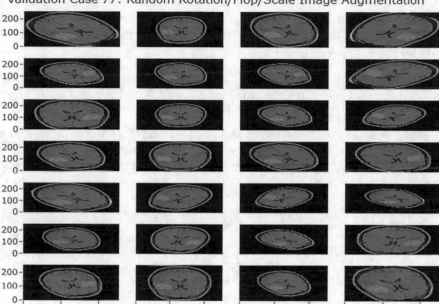

Fig. 14.37 Visual depiction of imaging data augmentation, a process of enriching a data archive of limited size by perturbing the observed data. In this case, these perturbations involve applying random affine transformations to the pairs of brain images and tumor masks

experiment, image augmentation represents *affine transformations* (Chap. 3) expressed as concatenations of three operations, image resizing, flipping, and rotation (Fig. 14.37).

```
N <- 7*4
img_and_mask <- valid_ds[77]
img <- img_and_mask[[1]]
mask <- img and_mask[[2]]
imgs <- map (1:N, function(i) {
  # spatial-scale factor
  c(img, mask) %<-% train_ds$resize(img, mask, 0.25)
  c(img, mask) %<-% train_ds$flip(img, mask, 0.3)
  c(img, mask) %<-% train_ds$rotate(img, mask, 45)
  img %>%
    transform_rgb_to_grayscale() %>%
    as.array() %>%
    plot_ly(z=.,type="heatmap",showscale=FALSE,name=paste0("AugmImg=",i)) %>%
    layout(showlegend=FALSE,  hovermode = "y unified")
})
imgs %>%
  subplot(nrows = 7, shareX = TRUE, shareY = TRUE, which_layout=1) %>%
  layout(title="Validation Case 77: Random Rotation/Flop/Scale Image
         Augmentation")
```

Completing the data augmentation allows us to instantiate both the training and the validation data loaders using `torch::dataloader()`. These processes combine a data-set and a sampler-iterator into a single, or multiple, process iterator over the entire dataset.

```
batch_size <- 25
train_dl <- dataloader(train_ds, batch_size)
valid_dl <- dataloader(valid_ds, batch_size)
```

Next, we specify the Unet model indicating the number of "down" or encoding (analysis) depth for shrinking the input images and incrementing the number of filters, as well as specify how do we go "up" again during the decoding (synthesis) phase.

```
unet <- nn_module(name="unet",
  initialize = function(channels_in=3, n_classes=1, depth=5, n_filters=6) {
    self$down_path <- nn_module_list()
    prev_channels <- channels_in
    for (i in 1:depth) {
      self$down_path$append(down_block(prev_channels, 2^(n_filters+i-1)))
      prev_channels <- 2^(n_filters+i-1)
    }
    self$up_path <- nn_module_list()
    for (i in ((depth - 1):1)) {
      self$up_path$append(up_block(prev_channels, 2^(n_filters+i-1)))
      prev_channels <- 2^(n_filters+i-1)
    }
    self$last = nn_conv2d(prev_channels, n_classes, kernel_size = 1)
  },
# forward(), keeps track of layer outputs going "down" added back when going "up"
  forward = function(x) {
    blocks <- list()
    for (i in 1:length(self$down_path)) {
      x <- self$down_path[[i]](x)
      if (i != length(self$down_path)) {
        blocks <- c(blocks, x)
        x <- nnf_max_pool2d(x, 2)
      }
    }
    for (i in 1:length(self$up_path)) {
     x <- self$up_path[[i]](x,blocks[[length(blocks)-i+1]]$to(device=device))
    }
    torch_sigmoid(self$last(x))
  }
)
# unet utilizes `down_block` and `up_block`
# down_block delegates to its conv_block() method, up_block bridges the Unet
down_block <- nn_module(
  classname="down_block",
  initialize = function(in_size, out_size) {
    self$conv_block <- conv_block(in_size, out_size)
  },
  forward = function(x) { self$conv_block(x)  }
)
up_block <- nn_module(
  classname="up_block",
  initialize = function(in_size, out_size) {
    self$up = nn_conv_transpose2d(in_size, out_size, kernel_size=2, stride=2)
    self$conv_block = conv_block(in_size, out_size)
  },
  forward = function(x, bridge) {
```

```
    up <- self$up(x)
    torch_cat(list(up, bridge), 2) %>% self$conv_block()
  }
)
conv_block <- nn_module(
  classname="conv_block",
  initialize = function(in_size, out_size) {
    self$conv_block <- nn_sequential(
      nn_conv2d(in_size, out_size, kernel_size = 3, padding = 1),
      nn_relu(),
      nn_dropout(0.6),
      nn_conv2d(out_size, out_size, kernel_size = 3, padding = 1),
      nn_relu()
    )
  },
  forward = function(x){
    self$conv_block(x)
  }
)
```

Before we start the unet model training, we need to specify the CPU/GPU device and optimization scheme.

```
# Initialize the model with appropriate CPU/GPU
device <- torch_device(if(cuda_is_available()) "cuda" else "cpu")
model <- unet(depth = 5)$to(device = device)
# OPTIMIZATION
# DCNN model training using cross entropy and dice_loss
calc_dice_loss <- function(y_pred, y_true) {
  smooth <- 1
  y_pred <- y_pred$view(-1)
  y_true <- y_true$view(-1)
  intersection <- (y_pred * y_true)$sum()
  1 - ((2*intersection+smooth)/(y_pred$sum()+y_true$sum()+smooth))
}
dice_weight <- 0.3
optimizer <- optim_sgd(model$parameters, lr = 0.1, momentum = 0.9)
```

On a multicore machine, each epoch of training the UNET model will require a couple of hours of compute time. This step can be skipped if you load in a previously pretrained model (model) that is saved (torch_save(model, "/path/model.pt")) and available for import via (torch_load("/path/model.ptt")). Several *.pt models are available here.[29]

---

[29] https://umich.instructure.com/courses/38100/files/folder/Case_Studies/36_TCGA_MRI_Segmentation_Data_Phenotypes

```
num_epochs <- 1  # for knitting demo, otherwise increase to 5+
scheduler <- lr_one_cycle(optimizer, max_lr = 0.1,
                    steps_per_epoch = length(train_dl), epochs = num_epochs)
# TRAINING
train_batch <- function(b) {
  optimizer$zero_grad()
  output <- model(b[[1]]$to(device = device))
  target <- b[[2]]$to(device = device)
  bce_loss <- nnf_binary_cross_entropy(output, target)
  dice_loss <- calc_dice_loss(output, target)
  loss <-  dice_weight*dice_loss + (1-dice_weight)*bce_loss
  loss$backward()
  optimizer$step()
  scheduler$step()
  list(bce_loss$item(), dice_loss$item(), loss$item())
}
valid_batch <- function(b) {
  output <- model(b[[1]]$to(device = device))
  target <- b[[2]]$to(device = device)
  bce_loss <- nnf_binary_cross_entropy(output, target)
  dice_loss <- calc_dice_loss(output, target)
  loss <-  dice_weight * dice_loss + (1-dice_weight)*bce_loss
  list(bce_loss$item(), dice_loss$item(), loss$item())
}
```

Start the Unet training process; this is a very computationally intensive step that
should be suspended for live demos or for real-time knitting of the Rmd source as an
HTML, PDF, or DOCX output.

```
for (epoch in 1:num_epochs) {
  model$train()
  train_bce <- c()
  train_dice <- c()
  train_loss <- c()
  coro::loop(for (b in train_dl) {
    c(bce_loss, dice_loss, loss) %<-% train_batch(b)
    train_bce <- c(train_bce, bce_loss)
    train_dice <- c(train_dice, dice_loss)
    train_loss <- c(train_loss, loss)
  })
  torch_save(model, paste0("model_", epoch, ".pt"))
  cat(sprintf("\nEpoch %d, training: loss:%3f, bce: %3f, dice: %3f\n",
              epoch, mean(train_loss), mean(train_bce), mean(train_dice)))
  model$eval()
  valid_bce <- c()
  valid_dice <- c()
  valid_loss <- c()
  i <- 0
  coro::loop(for (b in valid_dl) {
    i <<- i + 1
    c(bce_loss, dice_loss, loss) %<-% valid_batch(b)
    valid_bce <- c(valid_bce, bce_loss)
    valid_dice <- c(valid_dice, dice_loss)
    valid_loss <- c(valid_loss, loss)
  })
  cat(sprintf("\n Epoch %d, validation: loss: %3f, bce: %3f, dice: %3f\n",
              epoch, mean(valid_loss), mean(valid_bce), mean(valid_dice)))
}
# note that DCNN model mask prediction will be based on the model complexity!
# Epoch 1, training: loss:0.495716, bce: 0.307674, dice: 0.934480
# Epoch 1, validation: loss: 0.336556, bce: 0.070743, dice: 0.956785
...
# Epoch 20, training: loss:0.161496, bce: 0.079807, dice: 0.352102
# Epoch 20, validation: loss: 0.221487, bce: 0.051793, dice: 0.617438
# > proc.time()  # In Seconds! About 2,154,523 sec ~ 598 hours
#      user     system   elapsed
# 2154523.7  776791.3  141279.2
```

Evaluate the trained DCNN model using `model_6.pt` and a batch of $n = 10$ validation datasets; in this case, the validation data represent 2D brain imaging scans (Fig. 14.38).

```r
# EVALUATION
# without random sampling, we'd mainly see lesion-free patches
N <- 10 # number of cases to predict the masks for
eval_ds <-
        brain_dataset(valid_dir,augmentation_params=NULL,random_sampling=TRUE)
eval_dl <- dataloader(eval_ds, batch_size = N)
batch <- eval_dl %>% dataloader_make_iter() %>% dataloader_next()
# Load a previously saved torch model, e.g., epoch = 1
# torch_load(model, paste0("model_", epoch, ".pt"))
##### Requirements for loading a pre-trained model .....
# load torch packages above
model <- torch_load("/path/model_6.pt")
# train_dir <- "/data/data"
# valid_dir <- "/data/mri_valid"
imgsTruePred <- map (1:N, function(i) {
  # Get the 3 images
  img <- batch[[1]][i, .., drop=FALSE]  # Image to predict the tumor mask for
  inferred_mask <- model(img$to(device = device))        # Predicted MASK
  # True manual mask delineation
  true_mask <- batch[[2]][i, .., drop = FALSE]$to(device = device)
  # compute/report the BCE/Dice performance metrics
  bce<-nnf_binary_cross_entropy(inferred_mask,true_mask)$to(device="cpu") %>%
        as.numeric()
  dc <- calc_dice_loss(inferred_mask, true_mask)$to(device = "cpu") %>%
        as.numeric()
  cat(sprintf("\nSample %d, bce: %3f, dice: %3f\n", i, bce, dc))
  # extract inferred predicted mask as a 2D image/array of probability values
  inferred_mask <- inferred_mask$to(device="cpu") %>% as.array() %>% .[1,1,,]
  # Binarize the probability tumor prediction to binary mask
  inferred_mask <- ifelse(inferred_mask > 0.48, 1, 0)
  # In a real run, use "inferred_mask > 0.5, 1, 0"
  imgs <- img[1, 1, ,] %>% as.array() %>% as.array() %>%
    plot_ly(z=., type="heatmap", showscale = FALSE, name="Image")  %>%
        layout(showlegend=FALSE,  yaxis=list(scaleanchor="x", scaleratio = 1))
  masks <-true_mask$to(device="cpu")[1,1,,] %>% as.array() %>% as.array() %>%
  plot_ly(z=., type="heatmap", showscale = FALSE, name="True Mask") %>%
        layout(showlegend=FALSE,  yaxis = list(scaleanchor="x", scaleratio=1))
  predMasks <- inferred_mask %>% as.array() %>%
  plot_ly(z=., type="heatmap", showscale=FALSE, name="Unet-Derived Mask") %>%
     layout(showlegend=FALSE, yaxis = list(scaleanchor = "x", scaleratio=1))
  rowSubPlots <- subplot(imgs, masks, predMasks, nrows = 1, shareY=TRUE) %>%
             layout(hovermode = "y unified")
})
## Sample 1, bce: 0.086216, dice: 0.533167
...
## Sample 10, bce: 0.047822, dice: 0.299237
```

Finally, we can assess the `unet model` performance on the independent validation images, and report the DCNN-derived tumor masks (as images) and some quantitative measures (e.g., Binary Cross-Entropy, Dice coefficient). The figure displays the results—raw brain image, true tumor mask, and the corresponding DCNN-estimated mask.

Fig. 14.38 DCNN model
validation using 10 cases.
The columns illustrate the
original brain images (left),
the true tumor mask
(middle) and the Unet-
derived predicted mask
(right)

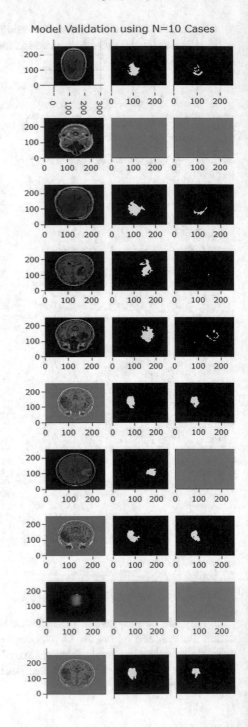

```
imgsTruePred %>% subplot(nrows = N) %>%
                 layout(title="Model Validation using N=10 Cases")
```

Next, we will demonstrate the same DCNN modeling and prediction protocol using Unet DCNN for the brain tumor data archive via the *tensorflow* framework.

14.9.3 Tensorflow Image Preprocessing Pipeline

The image prepossessing steps above use `torch` syntax. There are similarities and differences between the `torch/pytorch/libtorch` and the `tensorflow/keras` approaches.

Next, we will use `tensorflow` to illustrate some of these synergies, starting with the independent import of the images using `tf$image` functions, e.g., `decode_png()`. Assuming the data is already loaded, see the previous section (*Torch Data Import*), we will first preload all the necessary `tensorflow` libraries.

```
# clean environment, gc(), garbage collection
rm(list = ls()); gc()
# Load TensorFlow libraries
library(tensorflow)
library(tfdatasets)
library(rsample)   # for training() method
library(reticulate)
library(purrr)
library(keras)
library(unet)
library(tibble)
library(plotly)
```

Remember that we already have the ZIP data (*training=data* and *validation=mri_valid*) downloaded and expanded in a local partition `/data/`. Again, we will split the data into training:testing 80 : 20 and read the imaging/masking data from the PNG files into the tensorflow data objects `training_dataset` and `testing_dataset` (this is the separate *validation set*).

```r
train_dir <- "/data/data"
valid_dir <- "/data/mri_valid"
# Load PNG images
data_train <- tibble(
  img = grep(list.files(train_dir, full.names = TRUE,
  pattern="\\.png$",recursive=TRUE), pattern='mask', invert=TRUE,value=TRUE),
  mask = grep(list.files(train_dir, full.names = TRUE,
  pattern = "\\.png$", recursive = TRUE), pattern = 'mask', value = TRUE)
)
length(data_train$mask)    ## [1] 3240
data_train$img[[1]] # [1] "/data/data/TCGA_CS_4941_19960909/TCGA_CS_4941_19960909_1.tif"
data_train_valid <- initial_split(data_train, prop = 0.8)
training_dataset <- training(data_train_valid) %>%
  tensor_slices_dataset() %>%
  dataset_map(~.x %>% list_modify(
    # decode_jpeg yields a 3d tensor of shape (256, 256, 3)
    # Check tensor shapes!
    img = tf$image$decode_png(tf$io$read_file(.x$img), channels = 3),
    mask = tf$image$decode_png(tf$io$read_file(.x$mask))
  ))
testing_dataset <- testing(data_train_valid) %>%
  tensor_slices_dataset() %>%
  dataset_map(~.x %>% list_modify(
    img = tf$image$decode_png(tf$io$read_file(.x$img), channels = 3),
    mask = tf$image$decode_png(tf$io$read_file(.x$mask))
  ))
# Check the size of the entire (training & testing) TF datasets
tf$data$experimental$cardinality(training_dataset)$numpy() ## [1] 2592
tf$data$experimental$cardinality(testing_dataset)$numpy()  ## [1] 648
example <- training_dataset %>% reticulate::as_iterator() %>%
reticulate::iter_next(); example
# Confirm all images (tensors) use the same RGB 3-channel shape (256, 256, 3)
ind2 <- list(); i <- 1
iter <- make_iterator_one_shot(training_dataset)
until_out_of_range({
    case <- iterator_get_next(iter)
    ind2[[i]] <- ifelse (as.character(case[[1]]$shape)=="(256, 256, 1)",
                           "Incorrect", "Correct")
    if (ind2[[i]] =="Incorrect") print(".")
    i <- i+1
})
print("Check if any brain-images (tensors) are NOT of the correct RGB 3-channel
shape (256, 256, 3)")
## Correct
##    2592
```

In practice, the *uint8* data type of the RGB values in PNG/TIFF files is human-interpretable, and the Unet expects floating point tensor elements. Thus, we will convert the three-channel input images to real numbers and scale them to values in the interval $[0, 1]$.

For improving computational efficiency, sometimes it may be necessary to reduce the computational burden by downsizing the images, e.g., to 128×128 or even 32×32. In principle, we want to protect the native aspect ratio in the images, keep the pixels isotropic, and avoid distortion. In this case we won't reduce the image size, but it may be useful sometimes.

The tensorflow protocol also includes augmentation of the imaging data. Earlier, we used `torch` augmentation, now we use `tensorflow`. Of course, we will apply

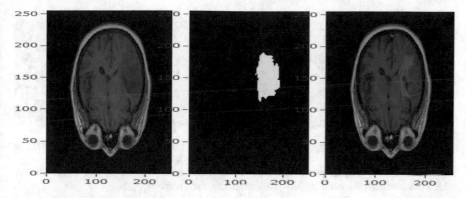

Fig. 14.39 Brightness, saturation, and contrast hue image intensity augmentation. The three images show the original brain (left), the corresponding mask (middle), and the intensity-augmented image (right column)

the same augmentation-transformations (scale, rotate, flip) to the tumor-mask as well as the brain images; see these three methods resize(), flip(), and rotate() in the create_dataset() function above. In addition, we can augment the data by intensity-transformations that preserve the spatial image structure but alter the contrast, brightness, and image saturation; see this random_bsh() method (Figs. 14.39 and 14.40).

```r
# For data augmentation - contrast, brightness & saturation perturbations
random_bsh <- function(img) {
  img %>%
    tf$image$random_brightness(max_delta = 0.2) %>%
    tf$image$random_contrast(lower = 0.3, upper = 0.6) %>%
    tf$image$random_saturation(lower = 0.5, upper = 0.6) %>%
    tf$clip_by_value(0, 1)
}
# Test Brightness-Saturation-Contrast Hue intensity augmentation
myIterator <- training_dataset %>% reticulate::as_iterator()
example <- myIterator$get_next(); example <- myIterator$get_next()
example <- myIterator$get_next() # example
bshExample <-
    random_bsh(tf$image$convert_image_dtype(example$img, dtype = tf$float32))
arr1 <- array(as.numeric(unlist(example$img)), dim=c(256, 256, 3))
p1   <- plot_ly(type="heatmap", z=~arr1[,,1], name="Image")
arr2 <- array(as.numeric(unlist(example$mask)), dim=c(256, 256, 1))
p2   <- plot_ly(type="heatmap", z=~arr2[,,1], name="Mask")
arr3 <- 255*array(as.numeric(unlist(bshExample)), dim=c(256, 256, 3))
p3   <- plot_ly(type="heatmap", z=~arr3[,,1], name="BSC-Image")
subplot(p1, p2, p3, nrows=1) %>%
layout(title="Brightness-Saturation-Contrast Hue Image Intensity Augmentation") %>%
hide_colorbar()
```

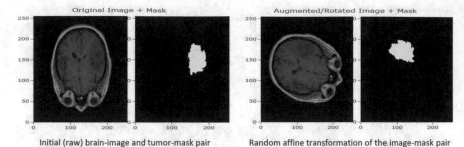

Initial (raw) brain-image and tumor-mask pair   Random affine transformation of the image-mask pair

Fig. 14.40 Spatial data augmentation using affine transformation of the special image domain, which complements the intensity image augmentation shown above

```r
# Random Rotation -- requires TF-Addon package
# reticulate::py_install(c('tensorflow-addons'), pip = TRUE)
# tfaddons::install_tfaddons()
library(tfaddons)
## This is a work-around for the data-augmentation rotation problem related to
## the zeallot right operator `%->%` and the `magrittr` pipe operator `%>%`
rot_param <- 15 # max degrees of rotation
rnd_rot <- runif(1000, -rot_param, rot_param)
randomRotationPaired <- c(rbind(rnd_rot, rnd_rot)) #double the random rotations
currentRotationIndex <- 1
random_rotate = function(img, mask) {
    img  <- img_rotate(img, angle=randomRotationPaired[currentRotationIndex])
    mask <- img_rotate(mask, angle=randomRotationPaired[currentRotationIndex])
    currentRotationIndex <- (currentRotationIndex + 1) %% 1000
    return (list(img=img, mask=mask))
}
# Test rotator
myIterator <- training_dataset %>% reticulate::as_iterator()
example <- myIterator$get_next()
example <- myIterator$get_next(); example <- myIterator$get_next() # example
arr1 <- array(as.numeric(unlist(example$img)), dim=c(256, 256, 3))
p1 <- plot_ly(type="heatmap", z=~arr1[,,1], name="Raw Img")
arr2 <- array(as.numeric(unlist(example$mask)), dim=c(256, 1, 256))
p2 <- plot_ly(type="heatmap", z=~arr2[,1,], name="Raw Mask")
subplot(p1, p2, nrows=1) %>% layout(title="Original Image + Mask") %>%
hide_colorbar()
rotExample <- random_rotate(example$img, example$mask)
rotExample$img$shape; rotExample$mask$shape
## TensorShape([256, 256, 3])
## TensorShape([256, 256, 1])
arr1 <- array(as.numeric(unlist(rotExample$img)), dim=c(256, 256, 3))
p1 <- plot_ly(type="heatmap", z=~arr1[,, 1], name="Rotated Img")
arr2 <- array(as.numeric(unlist(rotExample$mask)), dim=c(256, 256, 1))
p2 <- plot_ly(type="heatmap", z=~arr2[,, 1], name="Rotated Mask")
subplot(p1, p2, nrows=1) %>% layout(title="Augmented/Rotated Image + Mask") %>%
hide_colorbar()
currentRotationIndex <- 1 # reset the currentRotationIndex
```

The core functions we built above can be integrated into a new function, create_dataset(), which represents the complete end-to-end image preprocessing pipeline. The *input* to this pipeline is a data-frame of filenames containing the brain-images and tumor-masks, and the corresponding output contains the training_dataset and the validation_dataset as tensorflow dataset-objects that will be used in the model-fitting phase (Fig. 14.41).

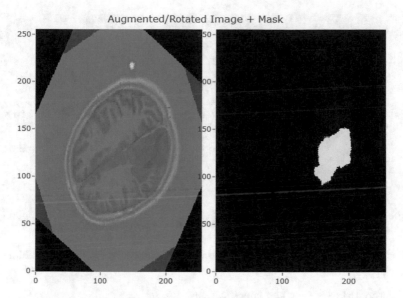

Fig. 14.41 Testing the generic image preprocessing method `create_dataset()`, which will be invoked during the DCNN training

```
library(zeallot)    # for the reverse-piping assignment operator %<-%
create_dataset <- function(data, train, batch_size = 32L) {
  dataset <- data %>%    # Load all PNG files as images
    tensor_slices_dataset() %>%
    dataset_map(~.x %>% list_modify(
      img = tf$image$decode_png(tf$io$read_file(.x$img), channels = 3),
      mask = tf$image$decode_png(tf$io$read_file(.x$mask))
    )) %>%      # convert image intensities from int8 to 32-bit float
    dataset_map(~.x %>% list_modify(
      img = tf$image$convert_image_dtype(.x$img, dtype = tf$float32),
      mask = tf$image$convert_image_dtype(.x$mask, dtype = tf$float32)
    )) %>%  # reshape all tensor-shapes to (256*256) for spatial-index homology
    dataset_map(~.x %>% list_modify(
      img = tf$image$resize(.x$img, size = shape(256, 256)),
      mask = tf$image$resize(.x$mask, size = shape(256, 256))
    ))
  # data augmentation performed on training set only
  if (train) {
    dataset <- dataset %>%
      dataset_map(~.x %>% list_modify(
          img = random_rotate(img=.x$img, mask=.x$mask)$img,
          mask= random_rotate(img=.x$img, mask=.x$mask)$mask)) %>%
      dataset_map(~.x %>% list_modify(
        img = random_bsh(.x$img)
      ))
  }
  # shuffling on training set only
  if (train) {
    dataset <- dataset %>%
      dataset_shuffle(buffer_size = batch_size*4)
  }
```

```
  # train in batches; adapt batch size to fit available RAM
  dataset <- dataset %>% dataset_batch(batch_size)
  dataset %>% # output needs to be unnamed as required by Keras
    dataset_map(unname) # makes example$img -> example[[1]]
}
# Generate the Training and Testing data as iterated TF-Data objects
training_dataset   <- create_dataset(training(data_train_valid), train=TRUE)
validation_dataset <- create_dataset(testing(data_train_valid), train=FALSE)
myIterator <- training_dataset %>% reticulate::as_iterator()
example    <- myIterator$get_next()
c(img,mask) %<-% random_rotate(img=example[[1]][1,,,1],
                               mask=example[[2]][1,,,1])
img$shape; mask$shape  ## TensorShape([256, 256])  ## TensorShape([256, 256])
arr1 <- array(as.numeric(img), dim=c(256, 256))
p1   <- plot_ly(type="heatmap", z=~arr1, name="Rotated Img")
arr2 <- array(as.numeric(mask), dim=c(256, 256))
p2   <- plot_ly(type="heatmap", z=~arr2, name="Rotated Mask")
subplot(p1, p2, nrows=1) %>%
layout(title="Augmented/Rotated Image + Mask") %>% hide_colorbar()
```

The reported Unet DCNN model summary, summary(model), includes the
following columns.

- Column 1: Layer type and specifications.
- Column 2: "output shape" contains the expected network U-shape parameters.
  Note that during the encoding phase, the image *Width* and *Height* sizes decrease
  initially (until the middle of the "U," reaching a minimum resolution of 8×8).
  Then, they start increasing again during the decoding phase, until reaching the
  sizes of the original image resolution. Similarly, the number of filters increases
  during encoding and then decreases during the decoding phase, terminating with
  an output layer having a single filter. Finally, the model architecture includes
  concatenation layers in the decoding phase that aggregate information from
  "below" with information that comes "laterally" from the parallel nodes in the
  encoding phase.
- Column 3: shows the number of parameters used in each layer of the DCNN.
- Column 4: for each layer (row), column 4 shows the parent (previous) layer in the
  network.

In this *image-segmentation problem*, the loss function needs to account for the
result of labeling ALL pixel intensities in the brain images. Hence, every pixel
location contributes equally to the total loss measure. As Binary classification yields
a 1 (tumor) or 0 (normal brain tissue), the binary_crossentropy() method is
one appropriate choice of a loss function. During the iterative transfer learning
process, we can track the classification accuracy, dice coefficient or other evaluation
metrics that capture the proportion of correctly classified pixels.

Next, we will define, compile, and test the base (pretraining default) model, prior
to model fitting. This is a naïve prediction without model tuning or transfer learning
(Fig. 14.42).

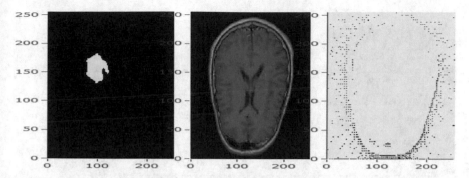

Fig. 14.42 A naïve (oversimplified) approach to DCNN tumor-mask prediction. The three columns show the original true tumor mask (left), the corresponding brain image input into the Unet (middle) and the predicted mask (right). The quality of the derived mask is not important here, recall that we used a pretrained Unet model out-of-the-box, without any finetuning. However, the end-to-end pipeline protocol is important, as subsequent improvements will slightly modify this workflow and generate significantly better tumor predictions

```
# Model Training - Starting with a pre-trained U-net model and
# then expanding it using Transfer-Learning
library(unet)
model <- unet::unet(input_shape = c(256, 256, 3))  # for RGB use 3-channels:
input_shape = c(256, 256, 3)
summary(model)
## Model: "model_11"
##
## Layer (type)             Output Shape      Param #  Connected to
## ===============================================================
## input_35 (InputLayer)    [(None, 256, 256, 0
##
## conv2d_35 (Conv2D)       (None, 256, 256,  1792     input_35[0][0]
##
## conv2d_36 (Conv2D)       (None, 256, 256,  36928    conv2d_35[0][0]
##
## max_pooling2d_4 (MaxPooli (None, 128, 128,  0        conv2d_36[0][0]
##
## conv2d_37 (Conv2D)       (None, 128, 128,  73856    max_pooling2d_4[0][0]
##
## conv2d_38 (Conv2D)       (None, 128, 128,  147584   conv2d_37[0][0]
##
## max_pooling2d_5 (MaxPooli (None, 64, 64, 12 0        conv2d_38[0][0]
##
## conv2d_39 (Conv2D)       (None, 64, 64, 25 295168   max_pooling2d_5[0][0]
##
## conv2d_40 (Conv2D)       (None, 64, 64, 25 590080   conv2d_39[0][0]
##
## max_pooling2d_6 (MaxPooli (None, 32, 32, 25 0        conv2d_40[0][0]
##
## conv2d_41 (Conv2D)       (None, 32, 32, 51 1180160  max_pooling2d_6[0][0]
##
## conv2d_42 (Conv2D)       (None, 32, 32, 51 2359808  conv2d_41[0][0]
##
## max_pooling2d_7 (MaxPooli (None, 16, 16, 51 0        conv2d_42[0][0]
##
```

```
## dropout_19 (Dropout)         (None, 16, 16, 51 0       max_pooling2d_7[0][0]
##
## conv2d_43 (Conv2D)           (None, 16, 16, 10 4719616 dropout_19[0][0]
##
## conv2d_44 (Conv2D)           (None, 16, 16, 10 9438208 conv2d_43[0][0]
##
## conv2d_transpose_6 (Conv2     (None, 32, 32, 51 2097664 conv2d_44[0][0]
##
## concatenate_4 (Concatenat    (None, 32, 32, 10 0       conv2d_42[0][0]
##                                                        conv2d_transpose_6[0][0]
##
## conv2d_45 (Conv2D)           (None, 32, 32, 51 4719104 concatenate_4[0][0]
##
## conv2d_46 (Conv2D)           (None, 32, 32, 51 2359808 conv2d_45[0][0]
##
## conv2d_transpose_7 (Conv2     (None, 64, 64, 25 524544  conv2d_46[0][0]
##
## concatenate_5 (Concatenat    (None, 64, 64, 51 0       conv2d_40[0][0]
##                                                        conv2d_transpose_7[0][0]
##
## conv2d_47 (Conv2D)           (None, 64, 64, 25 1179904 concatenate_5[0][0]
##
## conv2d_48 (Conv2D)           (None, 64, 64, 25 590080  conv2d_47[0][0]
##
## conv2d_transpose_8 (Conv2     (None, 128, 128,  131200  conv2d_48[0][0]


##
## concatenate_6 (Concatenat    (None, 128, 128,  0       conv2d_38[0][0]
##                                                        conv2d_transpose_8[0][0]
##
## conv2d_49 (Conv2D)           (None, 128, 128,  295040  concatenate_6[0][0]
##
## conv2d_50 (Conv2D)           (None, 128, 128,  147584  conv2d_49[0][0]
##
## conv2d_transpose_9 (Conv2     (None, 256, 256,  32832   conv2d_50[0][0]
##
## concatenate_7 (Concatenat    (None, 256, 256,  0       conv2d_36[0][0]
##                                                        conv2d_transpose_9[0][0]
##
## conv2d_51 (Conv2D)           (None, 256, 256,  73792   concatenate_7[0][0]
##
## conv2d_52 (Conv2D)           (None, 256, 256,  36928   conv2d_51[0][0]
##
## conv2d_53 (Conv2D)           (None, 256, 256,  65      conv2d_52[0][0]
## ================================================================================
## Total params: 31,031,745
## Trainable params: 31,031,745
## Non-trainable params: 0
##
# define a custom loss function (dice coefficient)
dice <- custom_metric("dice", function(y_true, y_pred, smooth = 1.0) {
  y_true_f <- k_flatten(y_true)
  y_pred_f <- k_flatten(y_pred)
  intersection <- k_sum(y_true_f * y_pred_f)
```

```
   (2 * intersection + smooth) / (k_sum(y_true_f) + k_sum(y_pred_f) + smooth)
})
# Compile DCNN model, package the optimizer, loss and performance metrics
model %>% compile(
  optimizer = optimizer_rmsprop(learning_rate = 1e-5),
  loss = "binary_crossentropy",
  metrics = list(dice, metric_binary_accuracy)
)
# Naïve Prediction using the default model (prior to Re-Training or Transfer
Learning)
batch <- validation_dataset %>% reticulate::as_iterator() %>%
reticulate::iter_next()
predictions <- predict(model, batch[[1]])
images <- tibble(
  image = batch[[1]] %>% array_branch(1),
  predicted_mask = predictions[,,,1] %>% array_branch(1),
  mask = batch[[2]][,,,1]  %>% array_branch(1)
)
# Check performance of the default base model on one case (# 22)
i=22
z1 <- ifelse(as.matrix(as.data.frame(images$predicted_mask[i])) > 0.5, 1, 0)
pl1 <- plot_ly(z = ~ 255*as.matrix(as.data.frame(images$mask[i])[,1:256]),
type="heatmap", name=paste0("Tumor Mask ", i))
pl2 <- plot_ly(z = ~ 255*as.matrix(as.data.frame(images$image[i])[,1:256]),
type="heatmap", name=paste0("Brain Image ", i))
pl3 <- plot_ly(z = ~ z1, type="heatmap", name=paste0("Pred Mask ", i))
subplot(pl1, pl2, pl3, nrows=1) %>% hide_colorbar()
```

The part below shows the UNct/DCNN model fitting for a single epoch. When running interactive demos, or for translating the Rmd source to output reports, this block of code should not be run (set eval=FALSE) as it takes hours to complete. Below, we show the results from offline DCNN trainings with different settings.

```
# MODEL FITTING
epochs = 1
history <- model %>% fit(training_dataset, epochs = epochs,
                        validation_data = validation_dataset)
# ASSESSMENT - Actual Model Evaluation (after Transfer-Learning retraining)
# Naive Prediction
batch <- validation_dataset %>% reticulate::as_iterator() %>%
reticulate::iter_next()
predictions <- predict(model, batch[[1]])
images <- tibble(
  image = batch[[1]] %>% array_branch(1),
  predicted_mask = predictions[,,,1] %>% array_branch(1),
  mask = batch[[2]][,,,1]  %>% array_branch(1)
)
i=22
pl1 <- plot_ly(z = ~ 255*as.matrix(as.data.frame(images$mask[i])[,1:256]),
            type="heatmap", name=paste0("Tumor Mask ", i))
pl2 <- plot_ly(z = ~ 255*as.matrix(as.data.frame(images$image[i])[,1:256]),
            type="heatmap", name=paste0("Brain Image ", i))
```

```r
pl3 <- plot_ly(
      z = ~ 255*as.matrix(as.data.frame(images$predicted_mask[i])[,1:256]),
      type="heatmap", name=paste0("Pred Mask ", i))
subplot(pl1, pl2, pl3, nrows=1)
library(keras)
dice <- custom_metric("dice", function(y_true, y_pred, smooth = 1.0) {
  y_true_f <- k_flatten(y_true)
  y_pred_f <- k_flatten(y_pred)
  intersection <- k_sum(y_true_f * y_pred_f)
  (2 * intersection + smooth) / (k_sum(y_true_f) + k_sum(y_pred_f) + smooth)
})
model %>% compile(
  optimizer = optimizer_rmsprop(learning_rate = 1e-5),
  loss = "binary_crossentropy",
  metrics = list(dice, metric_binary_accuracy)
)
```

When training the DCNN model, keep in mind that this step is very computationally intensive (each epoch can take hours to complete). Running a small number of epochs may be feasible in an interactive RStudio session, but in practice, dozens of epochs are necessary to train the network to perform well (e.g., yield high Dice coefficient values).

```r
# MODEL FITTING
history <- model %>%
            fit(training_dataset, epochs = 1,
                validation_data = validation_dataset, verbose = 2)
# 81/81 [==============================] - 3313s 41s/step -
# loss: 0.3121 - dice: 0.0106 - binary_accuracy: 0.9604 - val_loss: 0.1762 -
val_dice: 1.7162e-04 - val_binary_accuracy: 0.9900
# EVALUATION
pl_loss <- plot_ly(x = ~c(1:history$params$epochs), y = ~history$metrics$loss,
          type = "scatter", mode="markers+lines", name="Loss") %>%
  add_trace(x = ~c(1:history$params$epochs), y = ~history$metrics$val_loss,
          type = "scatter", mode="markers+lines", name="Validation Loss") %>%
  layout(title="DNN Training/Validation Performance",
          xaxis=list(title="epoch"),
          yaxis=list(title="Metric Value"), legend = list(orientation='h'))
pl_acc <- plot_ly(x = ~c(1:history$params$epochs), y =
~history$metrics$binary_accuracy,
          type = "scatter", mode="markers+lines", name="Accuracy") %>%
  add_trace(x=~c(1:history$params$epochs),y=~history$metrics$binary_accuracy,
          type = "scatter", mode="markers+lines",
          name="Validation Binary Accuracy") %>%
  layout(title="DNN Training/Validation Performance",
          xaxis=list(title="epoch"),
          yaxis=list(title="Metric Value"), legend = list(orientation='h'))
subplot(pl_loss, pl_acc, nrows=2, shareX = TRUE, titleX = TRUE)
model %>% evaluate(validation_dataset, verbose = 0)
#          loss          dice       binary_accuracy
#    0.1762175262    0.0001716204      0.9899647236
# Save/Load the pretrained model in HDF5 format
save_model_hdf5(model, "/path/model_TF_Brain_epoch_1.h5",
                overwrite = TRUE, include_optimizer = TRUE)
# Mind that loading a model with custom layers/functions, e.g., dice()
# method, requires special import using a list,
# https://github.com/rstudio/keras/issues/1240
```

Once we have pretrained (`history <- model %>% fit()`) and saved (`save_model_hdf5()`) the model, we can load it back as `mod1` the interactive session and use it for prediction. Several pretrained models (e.g., 50 and 100 epochs)

Tensorflow Transfer-Learning Performance (Brain Imaging), Epochs=100

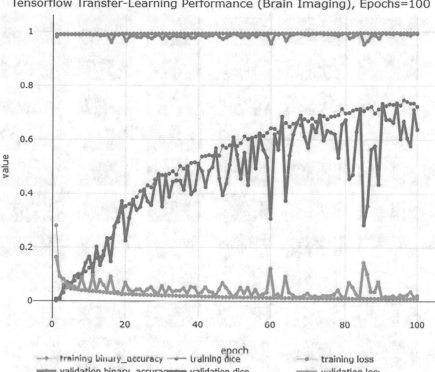

Fig. 14.43 DCNN algorithm training convergence

are available on the Canvas site. Below, we are using one of the pretrained Unet models (model_TF_Brain_epoch_100.h5, 250MB) to illustrate the prediction performance, i.e., automated brain-tumor segmentation using 2D neuroimaging data. Notice the steady model improvement (accuracy, binary tumor-labeling, and dice-coefficient) with respect to the epoch index (Figs. 14.43 and 14.44).

```
# This HDF5 model is available on Canvas:
#https://umich.instructure.com/courses/38100/files/folder/Case_Studies/36_TCGA_MRI_Segmentation_Data_Phenotypes
# REPORT Training and Validation Performance: Load the performance metrics
(history_df) over 100 epochs
load(url("https://umich.instructure.com/files/22647027/download?download_frd=1"))
lineWidth <- ifelse(history_df$data=='training', 1, 4)
lineNames <- paste0(history_df$data, " ", history_df$metric)
plot_ly(history_df, x = ~epoch, y=~value, color=~metric, type="scatter",
        mode="lines+markers", name=~lineNames,
        line = list(color = ~metric, width = lineWidth))  %>%
  layout(legend = list(orientation = 'h'),
title="Tensorflow Transfer-Learning Performance (Brain Imaging), Epochs=100")
```

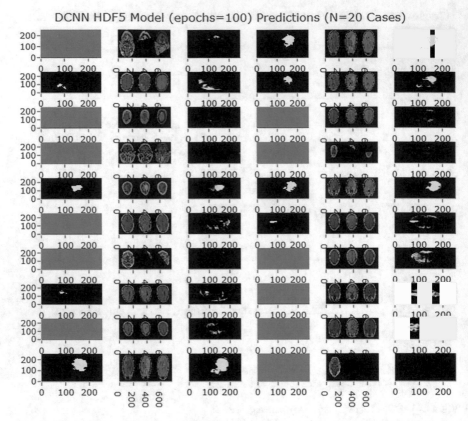

Fig. 14.44 Unet algorithm performance on 20 cases. The 20 random cases are displayed in 10 rows and 2 columns. Each element of this 10×2 matrix contains three images—the true tumor-mask (left), the corresponding three-channel brain imaging data (middle), and the Unet-predicted tumor mask (right)

```
# PREDICTION
dice <- custom_metric("dice", function(y_true, y_pred, smooth = 1.0) {
  y_true_f <- k_flatten(y_true)
  y_pred_f <- k_flatten(y_pred)
  intersection <- k_sum(y_true_f * y_pred_f)
  (2 * intersection + smooth) / (k_sum(y_true_f) + k_sum(y_pred_f) + smooth)
})
# Download pre-trained models, e.g., model_TF_Brain_epoch_100.h5 from Canvas
# The pre-computed model_TF_Brain_epoch_100.h5 model file is available in Canvas:
#
https://umich.instructure.com/courses/38100/files/folder/Case_Studies/36_TCGA_MRI
_Segmentation_Data_Phenotypes
mod1 <- load_model_hdf5("model_TF_Brain_epoch_100.h5", compile = FALSE)
# Recompile the model with our  custom dice() loss function
mod1 %>% compile(
  optimizer = optimizer_rmsprop(learning_rate = 1e-5),
  loss = "binary_crossentropy", metrics = list(dice, metric_binary_accuracy)
)
# Check re-loaded mod1 and evaluate performance metrics on validation dataset
```

```
mod1 %>% evaluate(validation_dataset)
##              loss            dice binary_accuracy
##       0.01682611      0.64169705      0.99429780
# Finally display some of the results -
# ASSESSMENT -- Actual Model Evaluation (after Transfer-Learning retraining)
batch <- validation_dataset %>% reticulate::as_iterator() %>%
reticulate::iter_next()
predictions <- predict(mod1, batch[[1]])
images <- tibble(
  image = batch[[1]] %>% array_branch(1),
  predicted_mask = predictions[,,,1] %>% array_branch(1),
  mask = batch[[2]][,,,1]  %>% array_branch(1)
)
pl_list <- list()
n = 10
for (i in 1:n) {    # to limit to only 1-channel, restrict the column range to
1:256: images$mask[i])[,1:256]
  pl1 <- plot_ly(z = ~ 255*as.matrix(as.data.frame(images$mask[i])),
          type="heatmap", name=paste0("Tumor Mask ", i)) %>%
     layout(hovermode = "y unified", xaxis = list(hoverformat = '.1f'),
          yaxis = list(hoverformat = '.1f'))
  pl2 <- plot_ly(z = ~ 255*as.matrix(as.data.frame(images$image[i])),
          type="heatmap", name=paste0("Brain Image ", i)) %>%
     layout(hovermode = "y unified", xaxis = list(hoverformat = '.1f'),
          yaxis = list(hoverformat = '.1f'))
  pl3 <- plot_ly(z = ~ 255*as.matrix(as.data.frame(images$predicted_mask[i])),
          type="heatmap", name=paste0("Pred Mask ", i)) %>%
     layout(hovermode = "y unified", xaxis = list(hoverformat = '.1f'),
          yaxis = list(hoverformat = '.1f'))
  pl4 <- plot_ly(z = ~ 255*as.matrix(as.data.frame(images$mask[1+n])),
          type="heatmap", name=paste0("Tumor Mask ", i+n)) %>%
     layout(hovermode = "y unified", xaxis = list(hoverformat = '.1f'),
          yaxis = list(hoverformat = '.1f'))
  pl5 <- plot_ly(z = ~ 255*as.matrix(as.data.frame(images$image[i+n])),
          type="heatmap", name=paste0("Brain Image ", i+n)) %>%
     layout(hovermode = "y unified", xaxis = list(hoverformat = '.1f'),
          yaxis = list(hoverformat = '.1f'))
  pl6 <- plot_ly(z=~255*as.matrix(as.data.frame(images$predicted_mask[i+n])),
          type="heatmap", name=paste0("Pred Mask ", i+n)) %>%
     layout(hovermode = "y unified", xaxis = list(hoverformat = '.1f'),
          yaxis = list(hoverformat = '.1f'))
pl_list[[i]] <- subplot(pl1,pl2,pl3, pl4, pl5, pl6, nrows=1, shareY=TRUE) %>%
  layout(title=paste0("DCNN HDF5 Model (epochs=100) Validation on Case ", i)) %>%
  hide_colorbar()
}
pl_list %>% subplot(nrows = length(pl_list)) %>%
     layout(title=paste0("DCNN HDF5 Model (epochs=100) Predictions (N=",
          2*n, " Cases)"))
```

```
PredictedMasks <- list(predictions=predictions, images=images)
save(PredictedMasks, file="/path/predictionsModel_TF_Brain_Epochs100.Rda")
# Then load it with: load("/path/predictionsModel_TF_Brain_Epochs100.Rda")
```

Finally, we can explicate some of the *Transfer Learning* process by modifying the pretrained model mod2 and obtaining a new model, modTransferLearning, which demonstrates synthetic image generation. This new modified modTransferLearning DCNN will output three-channel brain-images, not tumor masks (predicted by mod2). Note that 31M parameters part of the original pretrained mod2 are fixed and we are only estimating the remaining 16,931 parameters in this transfer-learning tuning process (Fig. 14.45).

Training Case: 3-Channel Input Image (Left) & Output Image (Right)

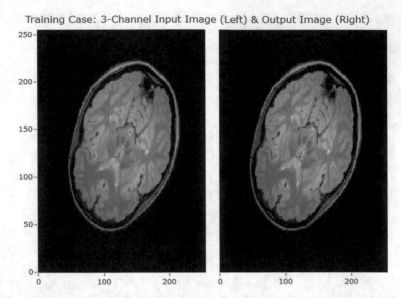

Fig. 14.45 Retraining a Unet with identical inputs and outputs representing the raw brain images. Such trained DCNN may then be used for synthetic generation of realistic brain images

```
# This HDF5 model (model_TF_Brain_epoch_100.h5) is available on Canvas:
mod2 <-   load_model_hdf5("/path/model_TF_Brain_epoch_100.h5", compile=FALSE)
# Freeze the first 32 layers
# Inspect the number of trainable and non-trainable (frozen DCNN parameters)
for (layer in mod2$layers) layer$trainable <- FALSE
input <- mod2$input                       # Pretrained UNet input layer
base <- (mod2 %>% get_layer(index=32))$output
# Get the prior-to-last output layer of "mod2", total #layers =33
target <- base %>%       # Replace the output layer by a new conv2D layer
                         # outputting a 3-channel 2D brain image, not a mask
  layer_conv_2d(filters = 64, kernel_size = c(1,1), activation = "relu") %>%
  layer_max_pooling_2d(pool_size = c(2,2)) %>%
  layer_conv_2d(filters = 64, kernel_size = c(1,1), activation = "relu") %>%
  layer_max_pooling_2d(pool_size = c(2,2)) %>%
  layer_conv_2d_transpose(filters = 32, kernel_size = c(2,2), strides = 2,
       padding = "same", activation = "relu") %>%  # deconvolution layers
  layer_conv_2d_transpose(filters = 3, kernel_size = c(2,2), strides = 2,
       padding = "same", activation = "relu")
modTransferLearning <- keras_model(input, target)
          # Update mod2 for transfer learning
summary(modTransferLearning); length(modTransferLearning$layers)
## Model: "model_12"
##
## _____
## Layer (type)            Output Shape        Param #   Connected to
## ========================================================================
## input_1 (InputLayer)    [(None, 256, 256, 0
##
## _____
## conv2d (Conv2D)         (None, 256, 256,    1792      input_1[0][0]
##
## _____
```

```
…
## max_pooling2d_8 (MaxPooli (None, 64, 64, 64 0          conv2d_54[0][0]
##  _____
## conv2d_transpose_11 (Conv (None, 128, 128,  8224     max_pooling2d_8[0][0]
##  _____
## conv2d_transpose_10 (Conv (None, 256, 256,  387      conv2d_transpose_11[0][0]
##  ==================================================================
## Total params: 31,048,611
## Trainable params: 16,931
## Non-trainable params: 31,031,680
##  _____
# 31M parameters are fixed and we are only estimating 16K parameters in the
Transfer-Learning tuning.
## MODEL RE-TRAINING (for Transfer Learning)
# Compile the DCNN model, packaging an optimizer, loss and performance metrics
modTransferLearning %>% compile(
  optimizer = optimizer_rmsprop(learning_rate = 1e-5),
  # loss = 'loss_kullback_leibler_divergence',
  loss = 'mse',
  # as we are looking at minimizing ||OrigImage - SynthImage||, i.e., RMSE
  metrics = list(metric_mean_absolute_error, metric_poisson)
)
currentRotationIndex <- 1 # reset
### PREP New Data (replace masks by the native brain images)
create_TL_dataset <- function(data, train, batch_size = 32L) {
  dataset <- data %>%   # load all PNG files as images
    tensor_slices_dataset() %>%
    dataset_map(~.x %>% list_modify(
      img =tf$image$decode_png(tf$io$read_file(.x$img), channels=3),#IMG
      mask=tf$image$decode_png(tf$io$read_file(.x$img), channels=3) #MASK--IMG
    )) %>%    # convert image intensities from int8 to 32-bit float
    dataset_map(~.x %>% list_modify(


      img = tf$image$convert_image_dtype(.x$img, dtype = tf$float32),
      mask= tf$image$convert_image_dtype(.x$mask, dtype = tf$float32)
    )) %>% #reshape all tensor-shapes to (256*256) for spatial-index homology
    dataset_map(~.x %>% list_modify(
      img = tf$image$resize(.x$img, size = shape(256, 256)),
      mask= tf$image$resize(.x$mask, size = shape(256, 256))
    ))
  # data augmentation performed on training set only
  if (train) {
    dataset <- dataset %>%
      dataset_map(~.x %>% list_modify(
        img  = random_bsh(.x$img) # ,
        # mask = img
      )) %>%
      dataset_map(~.x %>% list_modify(  # see discussion in create_dataset()
        img = random_rotate(img=.x$img, mask=.x$mask)$img,
        mask= random_rotate(img=.x$img, mask=.x$mask)$mask
      ))
  }
  # shuffling on training set only
  if (train) {
    dataset <- dataset %>%
      dataset_shuffle(buffer_size = batch_size*4)
  }
  # train in batches; batch size might need to be adapted depending on
  # available memory
  dataset <- dataset %>%
    dataset_batch(batch_size)
  dataset %>%
    # output needs to be unnamed
    dataset_map(unname)
```

```
}
# Generate the Transfer Learning (TL) Training and
# Testing data at iterated TF-Data objects
training_TL_dataset  <- create_TL_dataset(training(data_train_valid),
                                           train=TRUE)
validation_TL_dataset<- create_TL_dataset(testing(data_train_valid),
                                           train=FALSE)
example_TL <- training_TL_dataset %>% reticulate::as_iterator() %>%
reticulate::iter_next()
# example_TL
rasterPlotly <- function (image, name="", hovermode = NULL) {
  myPlot <- plot_ly(type="image", z=image, name=name, hoverlabel=name,
             text=name, hovertext=name, hoverinfo="name+x+y") %>%
    layout(hovermode = hovermode, xaxis = list(hoverformat = '.1f'),
           yaxis = list(hoverformat = '.1f'))
  return(myPlot)
}
# Training Case   # shape=(batch=32, 256, 256, channel=3)
img_and_mask <- training_TL_dataset %>%
     reticulate::as_iterator() %>% reticulate::iter_next()
img <- img_and_mask[[1]][1,,,1]  %>% as.array()    # 3-channel Input image
target<- img_and_mask[[2]][1,,,1]  %>% as.array()  # 3-channel Output image
p1 <- plot_ly(z=~255*img, type="heatmap", name = "Input Image") %>%
      hide_colorbar()
p2 <- plot_ly(z=~255*target, type="heatmap", name = "Output Image") %>%
      hide_colorbar()
subplot(p1,p2, shareY = TRUE) %>%
layout(title="Training Case: 3-Channel Input Image (Left) & Output Image
(Right)")
```

Once we have trained (history <- model %>% fit(()) and saved (save_model_hdf5()) the model (model), we can load it back as mod1 in the interactive session and use it for prediction (Figs. 14.46 and 14.47).

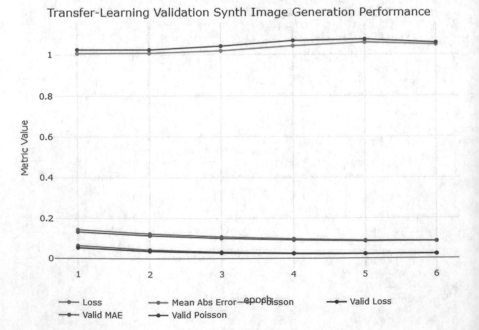

Fig. 14.46 Performance tracking metrics of DCNN transfer learning

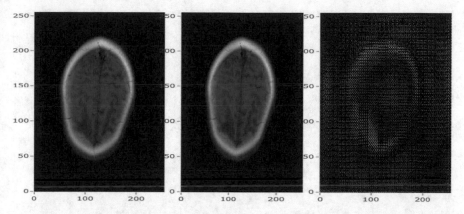

Fig. 14.47 Synthetic image generation using a pretrained DCNN model with transfer learning retraining. The identical left and middle images show the UNet input and output, and the right-most images show instances of synthetic DCNN-generated brain images. Again, this result is not particularly good, since the pretrained model is trained to predict a tumor mask, not a brain image, and the add-on transfer-learning model we designed has few simple layers, which is insufficient to capture more complex brain structure. Fine-tuning this protocol, enhancing the transfer-learning training architecture, and utilizing more computational resources (e.g., memory, compute cycles) will significantly improve the results of this DCNN synthetic image generation

```
// mod3_TL <- modTransferLearning
mod3_TL <- load_model_hdf5("/path/model_TF_TL_SynthBrainImages_epoch_6.h5",
                           compile = FALSE)
# Recompile the model with our  custom dice() loss function
mod3_TL %>% compile(
  optimizer = optimizer_rmsprop(learning_rate = 1e-5),
  # loss = 'loss_kullback_leibler_divergence',
  loss = 'mse',
  # as we are looking at minimizing ||OrigImage - SynthImage||, i.e., RMSE
  metrics = list(metric_mean_absolute_error, metric_poisson)
)
# Load the performance metrics of pre-computed 6-epoch
# model(modTransferLearning_History_6Epochs_DF.csv)
modTransferLearning_History_6Epochs_DF <-
    read.csv("https://umich.instructure.com/files/22825191/download?download_frd=1",
        header = T)
head(modTransferLearning_History_6Epochs_DF)
# EVALUATION
plot_ly(data=modTransferLearning_History_6Epochs_DF, x = ~epoch,
        y = ~loss, type = "scatter", mode="markers+lines", name="Loss") %>%
  add_trace(x = ~epoch, y = ~mean_absolute_error, type = "scatter",
            mode="markers+lines", name="Mean Abs Error") %>%
  add_trace(x = ~epoch, y = ~poisson, type = "scatter",
            mode="markers+lines", name="Poisson") %>%
  add_trace(x = ~epoch, y = ~val_loss, type = "scatter",
            mode="markers+lines", name="Valid Loss") %>%
  add_trace(x = ~epoch, y = ~val_mean_absolute_error,
            type = "scatter", mode="markers+lines", name="Valid MAE") %>%
  add_trace(x = ~epoch, y = ~val_poisson, type = "scatter",
            mode="markers+lines", name="Valid Poisson") %>%
  layout(
    title="Transfer-Learning Validation Synth Image Generation Performance",
    xaxis=list(title="epoch"), yaxis=list(title="Metric Value"),
    legend = list(orientation='h'))
```

```
# mod3_TL %>% evaluate(training_TL_dataset %>% dataset_batch(25), verbose=0)
mod3_TL %>% evaluate(validation_TL_dataset, verbose = 0)
##               loss mean_absolute_error              poisson
##         0.02072175          0.08333734           1.03864968
# TL Model Prediction using the default (prior to Transfer Learning) model
batch <- validation_TL_dataset %>% reticulate::as_iterator() %>%
reticulate::iter_next()
predictions <- predict(mod3_TL, batch[[1]])
images <- tibble(
  image     = batch[[1]][,,,1]    %>% array_branch(1),
  synth_img = predictions[,,,1]   %>% array_branch(1),
  target    = batch[[2]][,,,1]    %>% array_branch(1)
)
# Check performance of the Transfer-Learning model on one case (# 22)
i=22
pl1 <- plot_ly(z = ~ 255*as.matrix(as.data.frame(images$image[i])[,1:256]),
               type="heatmap", name=paste0("Input Image ", i))
pl2 <- plot_ly(z = ~ 255*as.matrix(as.data.frame(images$target[i])[,1:256]),
               type="heatmap", name=paste0("Target ", i))
pl3 <- plot_ly(
               z = ~ 255*as.matrix(as.data.frame(images$synth_img[i])[,1:256]),
               type="heatmap", name=paste0("Synth Image ", i))
subplot(pl1, pl2, pl3, nrows=1) %>% hide_colorbar()
```

```
pl_list <- list()
for (i in 1:10) {
  image = as.matrix(as.data.frame(images$image[i])[,1:256])
  synth_img = as.matrix(as.data.frame(images$synth_img[i])[,1:256])
  target = as.matrix(as.data.frame(images$target[i])[,1:256])
  p1 <- plot_ly(z=~255*image, type="heatmap", name=paste0("Image ", i))
  p2 <- plot_ly(z=~255*target,type="heatmap",name=paste0("Target=Image ", i))
  p3 <- plot_ly(z=~255*synth_img,type="heatmap",name=paste0("Synth Img ", i))
  pl_list[[i]] <- subplot(p1, p2, p3, nrows=1) %>% hide_colorbar() # %>%
}
pl_list %>%
  subplot(nrows = length(pl_list)) %>%
    layout(title="Input Brain Images, Targets, and Synth Reconstructions for N=10 Cases")
```

Figures 14.47 and 14.48 show examples of input brain images (left column), targets (middle), and DCNN synthetic reconstructions (right) for ten cases. The results are not particularly good since, the computational complexity of the problem prevents real-time execution. The outcomes can be significantly improved by running the script offline.

14.9.3.1   Notes About the Tensorflow Pipeline Protocol

The preprocessing pipeline allows inspecting intermediate results using `reticulate::as_iterator()` on the dataset.

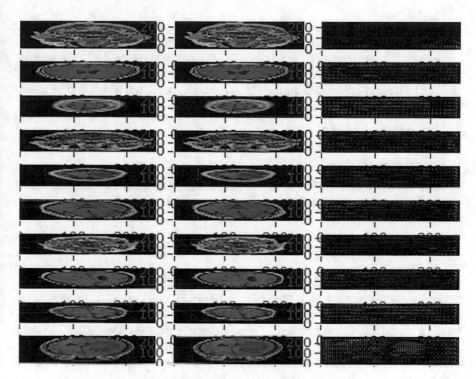

Fig. 14.48 A set of 10 synthetically generated brain images. The left and middle columns represent the inputs and outputs DCNN, and the right column shows instances of network-simulated brain scans. These results can be significantly improved by better transfer learning DCNN designs, a higher number of training epochs, a larger number of training datasets, and alternative add-on layer configurations augmenting the pretrained Unet core network

```
library(reticulate)
# display one brain image
batch <- training_dataset %>% reticulate::as_iterator()
pl_list <- list()
for (i in 1:10) {
  record <- reticulate::iter_next(batch)
  image = record[[1]] %>% as.array()
  mask = record[[2]] %>% as.array()
  p1 <- plot_ly(z=~image[i,,,3], type="heatmap", name=paste0("Image ", i))
  p2 <- plot_ly(z=~mask[i,,,1], type="heatmap", name=paste0("Mask ", i))
  pl_list[[i]] <- subplot(p1,p2, nrows=1) %>% hide_colorbar() # %>%
}
pl_list %>% # show brain Images & corresponding Masks for N=10 random cases
  subplot(nrows = length(pl_list)) %>%
    layout(title="Brain Images and Masks for N=10 Cases")
```

For the subsequent transfer-learning, we need to add additional layers to the base-model (mod1). The output of every Conv2D and MaxPooling2D layer is a 3D tensor of shape (height, width, channels). In our-case, the final mask-output is a single-channel image. The *width* and *height* dimensions typically shrink with network layer depth. The number of output channels for each Conv2D layer is controlled by the `filters` parameter (e.g., 32 or 64). As the width and height shrink, we can add more output channels in each `Conv2D` layer in the NN.

Note that the new transfer-learning model (`TL_model`) has only $17K$ parameters to estimate, as the $31M$ parameters of the base model (`mod`) are now frozen, i.e., they will not be tuned or estimated during the `TL_model` re-fitting, which will be much faster than the estimation of the original model.

- Total params: 31,048,611
- Trainable params: 16,931
- Nontrainable params: 31,031,680

After we design the DCNN model (Unet), we need to again compile and fit the model, i.e., estimate the remaining *trainable parameters*.

14.9.3.2   Network Layers

Convolutional Layers   In the late 1990s, LeCun introduced one of the most popular strategies for generating signature (feature) vectors corresponding to single- or multichannel 2D images. Previously, alternative methods, such as wavelet or spectral decomposition, could be used to map images as features. Then more classical AI/ML techniques, such as support vector machine, knn, logistic regression, among others, may be employed to model, analyze, predict, and classify images.

Transforming 2D or higher-dimensional images as feature-vectors disregard some of the spatial interaction between pixels, voxels, and tensors. *Convolution layers* tend to capture and protect some of the spatial information from neighboring spatial locations. This is accomplished by down-sampling the image into features by convolving the images with *kernels* (*filters*) and then using the resampled convolution images to predict specific outcomes (images, values, classes, etc.) The use of multiple convolution kernels to "filter" the image involves computing a product to extract different features from the images.

For a discrete image $f(m, n)$ and a kernel $g(k, l)$ defined over an integer grid $\{m, n, k, l \in \mathbb{Z}\}$, the discrete convolution of f and g is

$$\underbrace{(f * g)}_{\text{convolution}} [m, n] = \sum_{m = -\infty}^{\infty} \sum_{n = -\infty}^{\infty} (f[k, \ l] \times g[m - k, \ n - l]),$$

where typically, the support of f and g is compact, e.g., $0 \leq m, k \leq M - 1$ and $0 \leq n, l \leq N - 1$.

The convolution of two finite sequences is defined by extending the sequences to finitely supported functions on the set of integers. When the sequences are the coefficients of two polynomials, then the coefficients of the ordinary product of the two polynomials are the convolution of the original two sequences. This is known as the Cauchy product of the coefficients of the sequences.

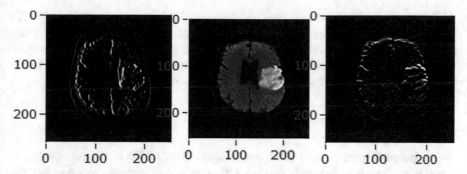

Fig. 14.49 Image convolution with Sobel Kernel Filters (Left=f*SobelX, Middle=f, Right=f*SobelY)

For instance, edge detection in an image can be done using a Sobel kernel matrix for vertical (y) and horizontal (x) edges (Fig. 14.49)

$$
g_x = \begin{bmatrix} +1 & 0 & -1 \\ +2 & 0 & -2 \\ +1 & 0 & -1 \end{bmatrix} \quad \text{and} \quad g_y = \begin{bmatrix} +1 & +2 & +1 \\ 0 & 0 & 0 \\ -1 & -2 & -1 \end{bmatrix}.
$$

```
sobelX = matrix(c(1,2,1, 0,0,0, -1,-2,-1), nrow = 3, ncol = 3); sobelX
##      [,1] [,2] [,3]
## [1,]    1    0    1
## [2,]    2    0   -2
## [3,]    1    0   -1
sobelY=t(sobelX); sobelY
##      [,1] [,2] [,3]
## [1,]    1    2    1
## [2,]    0    0    0
## [3,]   -1   -2   -1
library(jpeg)
img_url <- "https://umich.instructure.com/files/1627149/download?download_frd=1"
f <- image_read(img_url)
plot(f)
# To apply the convolution process manually, we use a convolve() function of the
'magick' package.
library(magick)
imgX <- image_convolve(f, sobelX)
imgY <- image_convolve(f, sobelY)
# Rotate 90 degrees
F <- imager::mirror(imager::imrotate(imager::magick2cimg(f), 90), "x")
ImgX <- imager::mirror(imager::imrotate(imager::magick2cimg(imgX), 90), "x")
ImgY <- imager::mirror(imager::imrotate(imager::magick2cimg(imgY), 90), "x")
p1 <- plot_ly(z=~255*(ImgX)[,,1,], type="image", name="(f*SobelX)")
p2 <- plot_ly(z=~255*(F)[,,1,], type="image", name="f")
p3 <- plot_ly(z=~255*(ImgY)[,,1,], type="image", name="(f*SobelY)")
subplot(p1, p2, p3, nrows=1) %>%
  layout(title="Image convolution with Sobel Kernel Filters (Left=f*SobelX,
                Middle=f, Right=f*SobelY)")
```

During the DCNN training process, the encoding phase typically includes 2D convolutional layers (`layer_conv_2d()`) paired with pooling layers. The latter reduce the size of the tensor shape and transform images by sliding the kernel filter across pixel grid, by a stride (e.g., 1, 2, 3), to the right and down. The relation between the resulting feature-vector size and the kernel size is represented by

$$\text{Feature size} = \frac{\text{Image size} - \text{Kernel size}}{\text{Stride}} + 1.$$

For instance, given a 10×10 square image, a filter of size 4×4, and a stride of 2 pixels, the Feature size $= \frac{10-4}{2} + 1 = 3$. Similarly, during the decoding phase, we include deconvolutional layers (`layer_conv_2d_transpose()`) that reverse the process by increasing the grid-size (tensor shape sizes) until we reach the desired output layer shape, usually the same as the input images, but they could also be different. More information about `tensorflow/keras` layers, loss functions and DCNN model performance metrics is available on the RStudio Tensorflow/Keras website.[30]

Max Pooling Layer Max pooling layers shrink the spatial extent of the convolved features and reduce overfitting by providing an abstracted feature representation. Instead of convolving (i.e., dot-product multiplying the image and the kernel) between the input and the kernel, Max-Pooling layers take the maximum value of image intensity over the region covered by the kernel filter. There are many alternatives to max-pooling, e.g., average-pooling, which computes the mean (arithmetic-average) of all image intensities covered by the kernel filter.

Fully Connected layers Input nodes (from the left) in fully connected layers are connected to every node in the subsequent layer to the right. One or several fully connected layers may be common toward the end of a DCNN to provide support for learning nonlinear affinities between high-level features generated as outputs of the prior convolutional layer. Good network designs typically include *dropout layers* between two consecutive fully connected layers (to reduce overfitting) and specify *activation functions* to capture nonlinearity.

The final fully connected layer allows us to control the output tensor shape size which reflects the expected type of classification, prediction, or forecasting. For instance, if the output is expected to have 6 class labels, the final layer will output a vector of size 6, i.e., one node for each possible class label. A *softmax* of this 6-feature vector would yield a 6D vector containing probabilities ($0 \leq p_i \leq 1$, $\forall 1 \leq i \leq 6$), one for each class label. Dropout layers provide a mechanism for regularizing the model and reducing overfitting of the DCNN. Dropout layers may follow fully connected layers or appear after other max-pooling layers to generate image noise augmentation. Dropout layers randomly annihilate (set to zero) some of

---

[30] https://tensorflow.rstudio.com/reference/keras

the connections of the input tensor, according to a Bernoulli distribution; hence some inputs are triaged with probability p.

14.9.3.3   Model Tracking and Network Visualization

One can use `tensorboard` to dynamically track the progression of an ongoing training process as well as to visualize a neural network structure as a graph. The basic mechanism for this involves the following steps.

- Install `tensorboard` (in a terminal/shell outside R/RStudio): This can be done in different ways and is system/OS dependent. Some examples include the following:
  - `python -m pip install --user --upgrade pip`
  - `conda install -c conda-forge tensorboard`
  - `conda activate tensorflow`
- Launch the `tensorboard` UI (from terminal shell): `> tensorboard --logdir logs/run_a`. Alternatively, you can launch tensorboard from RStudio directly via *Rstudio -> Tools -> Shell* and entering this command in the shell `tensorboard --logdir logs/run_a`.
- Open a local browser and point to this URL address: `http://localhost:6006/`
- The code has to use a callback mechanism for tracking, `print_dot_callback()`.
- Start the NN training process in the Rmd/R/RStudio environment and observe the tracking metrics dynamically updating in the browser. Note that your python/conda/anaconda shell needs to be open/live for this (*localhost*) process to work, and to keep the browser portal active and listening to python updates during the fitting/training process.

14.10   Additional References

- Ghatak A. (2019) Deep learning with R, Springer[31].
- Boehmke B, Greenwell B. (2019) Hands-on machine learning with R, Chapman and Hall/CRC[32].
- Lantz B. (2019) Machine learning with R: expert techniques for predictive modeling, Packt publishing ltd.

---

[31] https://doi.org/10.1007/978-981-13-5850-0
[32] https://doi.org/10.1201/9780367816377

- Chollet, F and Allaire, JJ. (2018) Deep Learning with R textbook (ISBN 9781617295546)[33] and the corresponding code notebook supporting site
- Google's TensorFlow API[34].
- Ronneberger, O, Fischer, P, Brox, T. (2015) U-Net: Convolutional Networks for Biomedical Image Segmentation,[35] Medical Image Computing and Computer-Assisted Intervention (MICCAI), Springer, LNCS, Vol.9351: 234–241, 2015, arXiv:1505.04597.

14.11   Practice Problems

14.11.1   Deep Learning Classification

- Download the SOCR Alzheimer's disease data[36].
- Preprocess the data and pool the MCI and AD cohorts (patients).
- Build a multilayer perceptron as a classifier (patients vs. controls) and select proper parameters.
- Classify AD and NC and report detailed evaluations, including cross table, accuracy, sensitivity, specificity, LOR, AUC.
- Provide some model visualizations, e.g., histograms, line plots, and model structure graphs.
- Then, try to perform a multiclasses modeling (i.e., AD, NC and MCI) and report the classification results.

14.11.2   Deep Learning Regression

- Download the Allometric relationship data from the SOCR data archive[37].
- Preprocess the data and set density as outcome response feature.
- Create a MXNet feed-forward neural net model and properly specify the parameters.
- Train and predict the density using this model and report RMSE on the test data, evaluate the result and justify your evaluation.
- Output the model structure.

---

[33] https://www.manning.com/books/deep-learning-with-r

[34] https://playground.tensorflow.org/

[35] https://doi.org/10.48550/arXiv.1505.04597

[36] https://wiki.socr.umich.edu/index.php/SOCR_Data_July2009_ID_NI

[37] https://wiki.socr.umich.edu/index.php/SOCR_Data_Dinov_032708_AllometricPlanRels

14.11.3 Image Classification

Apply the deep learning neural network techniques to classify some images with pretrained model we saw in this Chapter to some data from the following archives.

- Google images[38]
- SOCR neuroimaging data[39]
- Using your own images

14.11.4 (Challenging Problem) Deep Convolutional Networks for 3D Volume Segmentation

Use these 3D Brain Tumor Segmentation (BraTS) volumes[40] for DCNN training and testing. The brain MR dataset contains 257 training images with corresponding labels and the dimensions of these MR images are 240 × 240 with 155 and 4 different imaging modalities including T1 (T1-weighted), T1C (contrast enhanced T1-weighted), T2 (T2-weighted), and FLAIR (Fluid Attenuation Inversion Recovery).

- See this recent publication[41].
- Design a clever 3D affine transformation mapping for volume augmentation (can use ITK affine transformation).
- For pilot testing, subsample the data by 5 in each dimension, try to fit 3D volume in the existing TF/Keras/PyTorch tensor framework.
- Configure and train the network, test with augmented volumes you generate.

---

[38] https://www.google.com/search?safe=active&biw=1152&bih=728&tbm=isch&q=image

[39] https://wiki.socr.umich.edu/index.php/SOCR_Data#Neuroimaging_Data

[40] https://www.med.upenn.edu/cbica/brats2020/data.html

[41] https://doi.org/10.1016/j.bspc.2021.102458

Summary

The amount, complexity, and speed of aggregation of biomedical and healthcare data will rapidly increase over the next decade. It's likely to double every 1–2 years. This is fueled by enormous strides in digital and communication technologies, proliferation of IoT devices, and efficiencies of Cloud services, as well as rapid algorithmic, computational, and hardware advances. The substantial public demand for (near) real-time detection, precise interpretation, and reliable prognostication of human conditions in health and disease also accelerates that trend.

The future does look promising despite the law of diminishing returns, which dictates that sustaining the steady trajectory of clinical gains and the speed of breakthrough developments derived from this increased volume of information, paired with our ability to interpret it, will demand increasingly more resources. Even incremental advances, partial solutions, or lower rates of progress will likely lead to substantive improvements in many human experiences and enhanced medical treatments. The graphic on Fig. 1 illustrates a common predictive analytics protocol for interrogating big and complex biomedical and health datasets. The process starts by identifying a challenge, followed by determining the sources of data and meta-data, cleaning, harmonizing, and wrangling the data components, preprocessing the aggregated archive, model-based and model-free scientific inference, and ends with prediction, validation, and dissemination of data, software, protocols, and research findings (Fig. 1).

Our long-term success will require major headways on multiple fronts of data science and predictive analytics. There are urgent demands to develop new algorithms and optimize existing ones, introduce novel computational infrastructure, and enhance the abilities of the workforce by overhauling education and training activities. Data science and predictive analytics represent a new and transdisciplinary field, where engagement of heterogeneous experts, multitalented team-work, and open-science collaborations will be of paramount importance.

This DSPA textbook attempts to lay the foundation for some of the techniques, strategies, and approaches driving contemporary analytics involving big data (large

I. D. Dinov, *Data Science and Predictive Analytics*, The Springer Series in Applied Machine Learning, https://doi.org/10.1007/978-3-031-17483-4

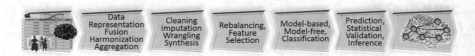

Fig. 1 Major steps in a general predictive data analytics protocol

size, complex formats, incomplete observations, incongruent features, multiple sources, multiple scales, and time-varying). It includes some of the mathematical formalisms, computational algorithms, machine learning procedures, and demonstrations for big data visualization, simulation, mining, pattern identification, forecasting, and interpretation.

This textbook (1) contains a transdisciplinary treatise of predictive health analytics; (2) provides a complete and self-contained treatment of the theory, experimental modeling, system development, and validation of predictive health analytics; (3) includes unique case studies, advanced scientific concepts, lightweight tools, web demos, and end-to-end workflow protocols that can be used to learn, practice, and apply to new challenges; and (4) includes unique interactive content supported by the active community of over 100,000 *R*-developers. These techniques can be translated to many other disciplines (e.g., social network and sentiment analysis, environmental applications, operations research, and manufacturing engineering).

The following two examples may contextually explain the need for inventive data-driven science, computational abilities, interdisciplinary expertise, and modern technologies necessary to achieve desired outcomes like improving human health and optimizing future returns on investment. These aims can only be accomplished by experienced teams of researchers who can develop robust decision support systems using modern techniques and protocols, like the ones described in this textbook.

- A *geriatric neurologist* is examining a patient complaining of gait imbalance and posture instability. To determine if the patient may have Parkinson's disease, the physician acquires clinical, cognitive, phenotypic, imaging, and genetics data (Big Healthcare Data). Most clinics and healthcare centers are not equipped with skilled data analytics that can wrangle, harmonize, and interpret such complex datasets, nor do they have access to normative population-wide summaries. *A reader that completes theDSPAcourse of study will have the basic competency and ability to manage the data, generate a protocol for deriving biomarkers, and provide an actionable decision support system*. This protocol will help the physician holistically understand the patient's health and make a comprehensive evidence-based clinical diagnosis or data-driven prognosis.
- To improve the return on investment for their shareholders, a *healthcare manufacturer* needs to forecast the demand for their new product based on observed environmental, demographic, economic, and bio-social sentiment data, another example of Big Biosocial Data. The organization's data-analytics team is tasked with building a workflow that identifies, aggregates, harmonizes, models, and

analyzes these heterogeneous data elements to generate a trend forecast. This system needs to provide an automated, adaptive, scalable, and reliable prediction of the optimal investment and R&D allocation that maximizes the company's bottom line. *Readers that complete the materials in theDSPAtextbook will be able to ingest the observed structured and unstructured data, mathematically represent the data as a unified computable object, apply appropriatemodel-basedandmodel-freeprediction techniques to forecast the expected relation between the company's investment, estimate product manufacturing costs, and project the general healthcare demand for this product by patients and healthcare service providers.* Applying this protocol to pilot data collected by the company may result in valuable predictions quantifying the interrelations between costs and benefits, supply and demand, as well as consumer sentiment and health outcomes.

The DSPA materials (chapters, code and scripts, datasets, case studies, electronic materials, and web demos) may be used as a reference, retraining or refresher guide for formal education and informal training, as well as, for health informatics, biomedical data analytics, biosocial computation courses or MOOCs. Although the textbook is intended to be utilized for one, or two, semester graduate-level courses, readers, trainees, and instructors should review the early sections of the textbook for utilization strategies and suggested completion pathways.

As acknowledged in the front matter, this textbook relies on the enormous contributions and efforts by a broad community including researchers, developers, students, clinicians, bioinformaticians, data scientists, *open-science* investigators, and funding organizations. The author strongly encourages all DSPA readers, educators, and practitioners to actively *contribute* to data science and predictive analytics, share data, algorithms, code, protocols, services, successes, failures, pipeline workflows, research findings, and learning modules. Corrections, suggestions for improvements, enhancements, and expansions of the DSPA materials are always welcome and may be incorporated in electronic updates, errata, and revised editions.

Electronic Appendix (Table 1)

Table 1 Summary of supplementary DSPA2 chapters included in a separate electronic appendix[a]

Appendix chapters	Descriptions
Bayesian simulation, modeling and inference	Includes material on applied Bayesian modeling, simulation and inference using Markov Chain Monte Carlo (MCMC) methods, as well as ergodic theorem conditions for function time averaging.
Information-theoretic foundation of statistical learning	Presents the foundations of information theory and statistical learning, summary of divergence measures based on Renyi entropy, and discussion of the relation between information theoretic learning and kernel methods.
Surface, shape, and manifold representation and visualization	An overview of the topology, visualization, and geometric primitives of orientable and nonorientable surfaces with and without boundaries.

(continued)

I. D. Dinov, *Data Science and Predictive Analytics*, The Springer Series in Applied Machine Learning, https://doi.org/10.1007/978-3-031-17483-4

Table 1 (continued)

Appendix chapters	Descriptions
Power analysis in experimental design	Includes the fundamentals of statistical power analysis in experimental design. Demonstrates R-based power analyses, Cohen's protocol for categorizing effect sizes, and many statistical power calculation examples withbivariate power-sample size plots.
Database SQL/ NoSQL Queries & Google BigQuery	Illustrates the pragmatics of SQL database connections, basic RODBC functions, SQL queries, and connecting to Google BigQuery, data joins and intersects, database management and querying automation.
Image convolution, filtering, and the Fourier transform	Protocols for representation, reading, displaying, manipulating, and writing 2D images. Spatial transformations and frequency-based image processing, image filters, morphological operations, and adaptive thresholding, high- and low-pass filtering, image segmentation and tessellation of 2D images and 3D volumes.
Causality, transfer entropy, and mechanistic effects	Review of the foundations of causal inference, prediction and probabilistic causality, and transfer entropy. Includes examples of macroeconomic market forecasting and simulated synthetic relationships.
Agent-based reinforcement learning	Outlines the mathematical foundations of reinforcement learning, decision policy, total return, and multiple agent simulations. Basics of developing computational reinforcement learning algorithms and other analytical applications.

[a]https://www.socr.umich.edu/DSPA2/

Glossary (Table 2)

Table 2 Glossary of terms and abbreviations use in the textbook

Notation	Description
ADNI	Alzheimer's Disease Neuroimaging Initiative
AD	Alzheimer's Disease patients
Allometricrelationship	Relationship of body size to shape, anatomy, physiology and behavior
ALS	Amyotrophic lateral sclerosis
API	Application program interface
Apriori	Apriori Association Rules Learning (Machine Learning) Algorithm
ARIMA	Time-series autoregressive integrated moving average model
array	Arrays are R data objects used to represent data in more than two dimensions
BD	big data
cor	correlation
CV	Cross Validation (an internal statistical validation of a prediction, classification or forecasting method)
DL	Deep Learning
DSPA	Data Science and Predictive Analytics
Eigen	Referring to the general Eigen-spectra, eigen-value, eigen-vector, eigen-function
FA	Factor analysis
GPUorCPU	Graphics or Central Processing Unit (computer chipset)
GUI	Graphical user interface
HHMI	Howard Hughes Medical Institute
I/O	Input/Output
IDF	inverse document frequency
IoT	Internet of Things
JSON	JavaScript Object Notation

(continued)

I. D. Dinov, *Data Science and Predictive Analytics*, The Springer Series in Applied Machine Learning, https://doi.org/10.1007/978-3-031-17483-4

Table 2   (continued)

Notation	Description
k-MC	k-Means Clustering
lm()	Linear model
lowess	Locally weighted scatterplot smoothing
LP or QP	Linear or quadratic programming
MCI	Mildly cognitively impaired patients
MIDAS	Michigan Institute for Data Science
ML	Machine-Learning
MOOC	Massive open online course
MXNet	Deep Learning technique using Rpackage MXNet
NAND	Negative-*AND* logical operator
NCorHC	Normal (or Healthy) control subjects
NGS	Next Generation Sequence (Analysis)
NLP	Natural Language Processing
OCR	Optical character recognition
PCA	Principal Component Analysis
PD	Parkinson's Disease patients
PPMI	Parkinson's Progression Markers Initiative
(R)AWS	(Risk for) Alcohol Withdrawal Syndrome
RMSE	Root mean square error
SEM	structural equation modeling
SOCR	Statistics Online Computational Resource
SQL	Structured Query Language (for database queries)
SVD	Singular value decomposition
SVM	Support Vector Machines
TM	Text Mining
TS	Time-series
w.r.t.	With Respect To, e.g., *"Take the derivative of this expression w.r.t. a_1 and set the derivative to 0, which yields $(S - \lambda I_N)a_1 = 0$."*
XLSX	Microsoft Excel Open XML Format Spreadsheet file
XML	eXtensible Markup Language
XOR	Exclusive *OR* logical operator

Index

Printed in the United States
by Baker & Taylor Publisher Services